NUTRITION and PERFORMANCE in MASTERS ATHLETES

NUTRITION and PERFORMANCE in MASTERS ATHLETES

Edited by
Peter R.J. Reaburn

CRC Press
Taylor & Francis Group
Boca Raton London New York

CRC Press is an imprint of the
Taylor & Francis Group, an **informa** business

CRC Press
Taylor & Francis Group
6000 Broken Sound Parkway NW, Suite 300
Boca Raton, FL 33487-2742

Printed on acid-free paper
Version Date: 20140818

International Standard Book Number-13: 978-1-4398-7187-4 (Hardback)

Library of Congress Cataloging-in-Publication Data

Nutrition and performance in masters athletes / edited by Peter R.J. Reaburn.
pages cm
Includes bibliographical references and index.
ISBN 978-1-4398-7187-4 (hardback)
1. Athletes--Nutrition. 2. Sports for older people--Physiological aspects. I. Reaburn, Peter.

RC1235.N85 2015
617.1'027--dc23 2014022398

Visit the Taylor & Francis Web site at
http://www.taylorandfrancis.com

and the CRC Press Web site at
http://www.crcpress.com

I would like to dedicate this book to Ronald (Ronnie) Cox. As a competitive young surf lifesaver and keen surfer on the Gold Coast in the late 1970s and 1980s, I had a very well-spent youth. As I matured I developed an interest in endurance sport and in particular the new sport of triathlon. As a novice to the endurance sports of distance running, open water swimming, road cycling and in particular triathlon, there were a group of 'old' athletes in their 30s and 40s leading the way. I followed.

One of these inspiring masters athletes was Ronnie Cox. A man of infinite wisdom, grace and experience who shared what he'd learnt with 'puppies' of my generation in their early 20s. Ronnie and his mates (Freddy Knudsen, Peter Forrester, Alan Davidson and Greg Reddan) inspired so many of us in those early days of triathlon in Australia. Many years later in 2005 he cheered me on with wizened words and advice as I achieved my goal of winning a national Ironman triathlon championship to then compete and complete the Hawaii Ironman that same year, a dream I'd had since I saw it on television in 1982.

Ronnie had a genuine and infectious love of fitness and the outdoor lifestyle that only multi-sport athletes enjoy and understand. More importantly now that I am older, and hopefully wiser, Ronnie always cherished family and friends. He knew the importance of balance in life! He has passed that virtue on to his son Greg, a world-champion Olympic Distance Triathlon age-group champion, well-respected sports dietician, highly applied researcher with the Australian Institute of Sport and invited contributor to this book.

Sadly, Ronnie lost his battle with advanced prostate cancer in 2011. As he did in life and sport, Ronnie handled that emotional journey with dignity and grace with close friends and family around him to the end. A few days before he passed away I spoke with him on the telephone. He was as determined as ever to live on and to inspire others as they too enjoy their journey in life.

Ronnie, this book is for you!

Contents

Preface

Just because we grow older as athletes does not mean we are not aspiring to train and compete hard. Whether it be for fun, fitness, friendships, personal bests or gold medals, people of all ages can enjoy participating in systematic training and competing in events organized for older athletes.

In 1994 I completed my PhD at the University of Queensland. The thesis focused on lifetime athletes over the age of 60 years and what factors explain the age-related declines in endurance, speed and strength performance in those athletes, despite a lifetime of physical training. In that era, few researchers were focused on older athletes. At the time the exercise physiology research was dominated by studies on young elite athletes – their aerobic capacities, their anaerobic thresholds, muscle fibre composition, blood markers and changes in these parameters with acute exercise and chronic training. Older athletes were for the most part not seen as a cohort of interest in research.

Through my PhD studies I became aware of an academic book titled *Sports Medicine for the Mature Athlete*. It was edited by a hero of mine, Professor John Sutton, a man who practiced what he preached as both a researcher and masters athlete. John had a gift for bringing people together to share research outcomes and to lead research teams focusing on applied sports science research. His book was the first book I had seen that brought the then-limited research related to older athletes together in one source.

This book you are now reading is my dream – to bring the increasing body of knowledge pertaining to masters athletes together in one coherent and highly applied book. My aim was to do what John's book did for me: To encourage young sports scientists to pursue research related to masters athletes. After many years on the bureaucracy treadmill within academia, I am now able to pursue that aim.

For this book, I have carefully invited a cast of contributors knowing that they too can bridge the gap between theory and practice. I have asked each of the contributors to focus on the topic of their chapter and to discuss the limited available research related to that topic that has specifically focused on masters athletes. Their biggest challenge related to their chapter topic was to interpolate from the many studies undertaken in younger athletes and the relatively smaller number of studies in healthy older non-athletes. They have met this challenge with style.

Critically, from an applied perspective, the primary goal of this book, I have asked the contributors to include three major headings at the end of each chapter. These are

1. Implications for Sports Medicine Professionals and Clinicians
2. Implications for Masters Athletes and Coaches
3. Future Research Directions

The aims of these sections are to both bridge the gap between theory and practice as well as stimulate young researchers to undertake research focused on masters athletes to provide them with research ideas, and to encourage them to undertake applied research with a cohort of highly-motivated athletes with a lot of experience to offer and share with young and old sports scientists alike.

I sincerely hope this book contributes to the growing field of masters athlete sports. Importantly, I hope it also contributes, as John Sutton's book did for me, to the field of applied sports science. I also hope this book assists readers from all walks of life in achieving their goals whether it be as an athlete, coach, sports administrator, sports medicine professional or sports scientist. Train and exercise for life I say, knowing that exercise is indeed medicine!

Finally, let me thank each of the 38 contributors who individually or in teams brought their chapters together. I know how much work these things take! Thanks also to my endnote referencing guru, Libbie Blanchard, for her experience in helping bring the referencing lists together at the click of a few buttons! Also thanks to Randy Brehm and Kari Budyk at Taylor & Francis and Amor Nanas at MTC. I thank you all for your patience over the journey. To all 42 of you who helped me bring this dream to a reality, I hope you are as proud of the end product as I am.

Peter R.J. Reaburn, PhD
Central Queensland University

Editor

Peter R.J. Reaburn, PhD, is an Associate Professor of Exercise and Sports Science at Central Queensland University in Australia. Peter received his Bachelor of Human Movement Studies (Education) at the University of Queensland in 1981 and spent 7 years teaching health and physical education throughout Queensland, Australia. In 1988 he returned to his alma mater to complete a first class Honours degree and then a PhD, both of which were focussed on masters athlete research. While completing his PhD, he was offered a lecturing position in exercise physiology at the University of Queensland and concurrently managed a commercial athlete testing and consulting service within the university. In 1997 he was offered and accepted a position as a Senior Lecturer at Central Queensland University in Rockhampton, Queensland. In 2000 he became Head (Dean) of the School of Health and Human Performance and served in that role for 8 years. During this time he was elected and served as Vice-President (Sports Science) for Exercise and Sports Science Australia, elected and served on the University's Academic Board for 6 years, and supervised 14 post-graduates to completion. In 2009 he was seconded as the only academic into the Central Queensland University five-person quality audit team that won the 2010 Vice-Chancellor's Award for Excellence for Professional Staff.

Since returning to his first love of teaching and bridging the gap between sports science and sports in 2011, Peter won the 2012 Vice-Chancellor's Award for Teaching Excellence and a National Office of Learning and Teaching Citation for his innovative use of research projects in second- and third-year undergraduate exercise physiology courses. In 2013 he was nominated by his current cohort of nine post-graduates and won the 2013 Vice-Chancellor's Award for Excellence in Research Higher Degree Supervision. Six of his current post-graduates are undertaking applied research projects focused on masters athlete recovery and training methodologies.

Peter has authored, edited or co-edited five books including *Training for Speed and Endurance, Guiding the Young Athlete, Practical Skills in Sports and Exercise Science, Masters Sport: Training for Enhanced Performance*, and *The Masters Athlete*. He has published 12 book chapters and over 50 peer-reviewed research articles. He writes monthly 'theory to practice' articles for *Cycling Australia* and quarterly 'bridging the gap' articles for *AUSSI Masters Swimming Australia*. He regularly gives presentations to both professional and community groups at the local, state and national levels. Peter is also the webmaster and blogger for www.mastersathlete.com.au, a website that aims to bring the latest health and sports science research to masters athletes in layman's terms.

Peter is a practicing masters athlete. In his younger years he won state and national surf lifesaving titles, state and national masters swimming and open-water championships, and in 2005 won the national Ironman Triathlon championship of Australia that qualified him to complete the Hawaii Ironman that same year. He still trains regularly and races in open-water swimming, road cycling and running events. If his aging knees hold up, he hopes to return again to the Hawaii Ironman after placing in the top 10 in his age group in 2005.

Peter has been happily married to Claire for 25 years, has two daughters, Rebecca and Megan, who are undertaking undergraduate studies in business and communications, respectively. He loves watching elite sports on television (except cricket, horse racing and motor sport), reading Gerald Seymour, John Grisham and Stephen Leather novels as well as Peter FitzSimons history yarns, and taking surfing holidays overseas with his brothers and/or friends.

Contributors

Kate Bolam
School of Human Movement Studies
University of Queensland
Brisbane, Queensland, Australia

Jeanick Brisswalter
Education, Sport and Health
University of Nice Sophia Antipolis
Nice, France

Thomas W. Buford
Department of Aging and Geriatric Research
University of Florida
Gainesville, Florida

Nuala M. Byrne
Bond Institute of Health and Sport
Faculty of Health Science and Medicine
Bond University
Gold Coast, Queensland, Australia

Ian D. Caterson
Boden Institute for Obesity Nutrition Exercise and Eating Disorders
University of Sydney
Sydney, New South Wales, Australia

Aaron J. Coutts
Faculty of Health
University of Technology, Sydney
Sydney, New South Wales, Australia

Gregory R. Cox
Sports Nutrition
Australian Institute of Sport
Canberra, Queensland, Australia

Vincent J. Dalbo
School of Medical and Applied Sciences
Central Queensland University
Rockhampton, Queensland, Australia

Benjamin J. Dascombe
Applied Sports Science and Exercise Testing Laboratory
Faculty of Science and Information Technology
University of Newcastle
New South Wales, Australia

Hans Degens
Institute for Biomedical Research into Human Movement and Health
Manchester Metropolitan University
Manchester, England

Ben Desbrow
School of Allied Health Sciences and Griffith Health Institute
Griffith University
Gold Coast, Queensland, Australia

Rob Duffield
Faculty of Health
University of Technology, Sydney
Sydney, New South Wales, Australia

Nathan Elsworthy
Applied Sports Science and Exercise Testing Laboratory
Faculty of Science and Information Technology
University of Newcastle
New South Wales, Australia

Janelle A. Gifford
Faculty of Health Sciences
University of Sydney
New South Wales, Australia

Marko Haverinen
Varala Sports Institute
Tampere, Finland

Andrew P. Hills
Mater Research Institute
University of Queensland
and
Griffith Health Institute
Griffith University
Brisbane, Queensland, Australia

Erica Hirsch
Department of Nutrition Sciences
Drexel University
Philadelphia, Pennsylvania

Alexandra L. Honey
Rheumatology Department
Royal Prince Alfred Hospital
New South Wales, Australia

Kathryn Jackson
Department of Nutrition and Dietetics
Flinders University
Adelaide, South Australia, Australia

David Jenkins
School of Human Movement Studies
University of Queensland
Brisbane, Queensland, Australia

Nathan A. Johnson
Faculty of Health Sciences
University of Sydney
New South Wales, Australia

Kathleen M. Knights
Department of Clinical Pharmacology
Flinders University
Adelaide, South Australia, Australia

Marko T. Korhonen
Gerontology Research Centre
Department of Health Sciences
University of Jyväskylä
Jyväskylä, Finland

Paul B. Laursen
Sports Performance Research Institute New Zealand
Auckland University of Technology
Auckland, New Zealand

Michael Leveritt
School of Human Movement Studies
University of Queensland
Brisbane, Queensland, Australia

Arduino A. Mangoni
Department of Clinical Pharmacology
Flinders University
Adelaide, South Australia, Australia

Amy E. Mendham
School of Human Movement Studies
Charles Sturt University
Bathurst, New South Wales, Australia

Helen T. O'Connor
Faculty of Health Sciences
University of Sydney
New South Wales, Australia

Peter R.J. Reaburn
School of Medical and Applied Sciences
Central Queensland University
Rockhampton, Queensland, Australia

Michael D. Roberts
School of Kinesiology
Auburn University
Auburn, Alabama

Aaron T. Scanlan
School of Medical and Applied Sciences
Central Queensland University
Rockhampton, Queensland, Australia

Brendan Scott
Applied Sports Science and Exercise Testing Laboratory
Faculty of Science and Information Technology
University of Newcastle
New South Wales, Australia

Dean V. Sculley
School of Biomedical Sciences and Pharmacy
University of Newcastle
New South Wales, Australia

Mrinalini Sharma
Department of Chemical and Biological Engineering
Drexel University
Philadelphia, Pennsylvania

Greg Shaw
Sports Nutrition
Australian Institute of Sport
Canberra, Queensland, Australia

Tina Skinner
School of Human Movement Studies
University of Queensland
Brisbane, Queensland, Australia

Gary Slater
School of Health and Sport Sciences
University of the Sunshine Coast
Sippy Downs, Queensland, Australia

Stephen R. Stannard
School of Sport and Exercise
Massey University
Palmerston North, New Zealand

Mark A. Tarnopolsky
Department of Pediatrics and Medicine
McMaster University
Hamilton, Ontario, Canada

Stella Lucia Volpe
Department of Nutrition Sciences
Drexel University
Philadelphia, Pennsylvania

Juliet Wiseman
School of Allied Health Sciences
Griffith University
Gold Coast, Queensland, Australia

1 Physiological Changes Affecting the Nutritional Needs of Masters Athletes

David Jenkins, Tina Skinner and Kate Bolam

CONTENTS

1.1 INTRODUCTION

Ageing is associated with major changes in almost all physiological systems. These age-related changes influence both the health and exercise capacity of the masters athlete. On one level, many of these age-related changes affect appetite, food intake and nutrient absorption and thus the potential to affect substrate availability at the exercising muscle. On another level, age-related changes to the cardiovascular and musculoskeletal systems affect the energy systems used during exercise in addition to the force-generating capacity of the muscles. This chapter reviews a number of age-related changes that occur to several physiological systems and the affect these changes may have on the nutritional needs of masters athletes. Furthermore, the chapter will examine the extent to which regular physical activity across the lifespan is likely to impact on these changes.

1.2 CHANGES IN BODY COMPOSITION AND ENERGY NEEDS

1.2.1 Sarcopenia

Sarcopenia is a syndrome which can be characterised by progressive and generalised loss of muscle mass and strength with a risk of adverse outcomes such as physical disability poor quality of life and death. In normal ageing, the rate of muscle mass decline after 40 years of age has been shown to be approximately 0.5%–1% per year which is heightened in the sixth decade of life [1]. Both men and women between the ages of 40 and 80 years lose 30%–50% of their skeletal muscle mass [2]. For most older adults, the decrease in muscle mass is accompanied by a 1%–1.5% per year reduction in strength [3] and power [4], independent of body mass [5].

Sarcopenia occurs in response to endocrine, inflammatory and nutritional changes; genetic and reduced levels of physical activity are also strong influences [6]. A change in the mass of a given muscle is due primarily to a change in the cross sectional area of individual fibres and/or a loss in the number of fibres. Age-related changes in the nervous system contribute to sarcopenia via a reduction in the number of functioning motor units [7]. The loss of motor units is marked by a gradual reduction during the first seven decades of life followed by a sharp decline into very old age [8].

The loss of motor units with ageing appears to involve almost exclusively the type II muscle fibres [9] and reductions in both the size and number of type II fibres is believed to explain most of the age-related loss of skeletal muscle mass, strength and power [3]. Although the loss in the number of fibres within muscles appears inevitable, the magnitude of loss may be ameliorated to some degree by adequate dietary protein intake and resistance training [10]. The protein needs of the masters athlete will be addressed in Chapter 6. Below we provide a brief summary of the benefits of resistance training.

1.2.2 Resistance Training

Although the influence of chronic resistance exercise on muscle mass and muscle function has been extensively studied in older populations, the specific effects of ageing on muscular performance or efficiency has been difficult to assess because of the confounding effects of a reduction in physical activity levels, changes in body composition and development of clinical diseases. Elite masters weightlifters appear to lose lean lower limb volume at a slower rate than age-matched untrained control subjects; however, they lose normalised (relative to body weight) isometric (static hold) strength and power in specific muscle groups at a slightly higher rate [11]. Interestingly, women appear to experience greater age-related declines in muscular strength and power than men, particularly in the upper extremities [12]. However, resistance-trained masters athletes have significantly greater muscle mass, higher strength per muscle thickness ratio and muscle performance characteristics than their age-matched sedentary peers, supporting the suggestion that chronic resistance exercise has the potential to delay and diminish alterations in skeletal muscle mass and function with ageing [13]. In addition, older strength-trained individuals have been reported to have greater muscle quality as a function of power per muscle volume [14]. This is likely due to less fat intrusion and maintenance of muscle architecture.

1.2.3 Endurance Training

The influence of chronic endurance training on age-related changes in muscle mass and function has also been extensively researched. Both total body mass and fat-free mass appear to be maintained in ageing endurance-trained adults, whereas sedentary adults demonstrate a significant increase in fat and total body mass with age [15]. Skeletal muscle in endurance-trained masters athletes adapts structurally and metabolically to chronic endurance training [16] with evidence suggesting that chronic intense exercise preserves muscle mass and prevents fat infiltration of muscle in masters athletes [15].

Endurance-trained masters athletes have significantly greater values of maximal oxygen uptake (VO_{2max}) compared with age-matched sedentary individuals. However, endurance-trained men and women appear to have greater absolute rates of decline in VO_{2max} with advancing age compared with healthy sedentary adults. Yet, when expressed as a percent reduction, the approximate 10% decline in VO_{2max} per decade from 25 years of age is similar between endurance-trained masters athletes and sedentary adults [17]. Both Katzel and others [18] and Eskurza and others [17] suggest that high-intensity endurance training may delay age-associated decrements in VO_{2max}; however, training load reductions which appear to be inevitable with ageing, lead to accelerated losses in VO_{2max}. Differences in the absolute rate of decline in VO_{2max} observed between these groups may be attributed to declines in maximal stroke volume (and therefore maximal cardiac output) and/or skeletal muscle oxidative capacity. Decreases in VO_{2max} appear to be greater than the age-related decline in endurance performance; the lactate threshold did not appear to change with age when expressed as a percentage of VO_{2max} [19].

Despite an age-related reduction in VO_{2max}, masters athletes retain a high capacity to store glycogen in liver and muscle, to use glycogen as a source of energy-producing substrate during submaximal endurance exercise and to restore muscle glycogen levels post-exercise [20]. Slight reductions in glycogen concentration have been reported in older sedentary adults, possibly due to lower resting levels of insulin-regulated glucose transporter (GLUT4) and relatively reduced muscle activity [21]. However, short-duration exercise training can increase GLUT4 levels in older previously sedentary adults similar to the response seen in younger adults [22]. As well, compared to younger athletes, masters athletes may consume less than optimal amounts of carbohydrate (i.e. 6 g/kg/d) due to changes in taste and smell. This may potentially reduce muscle glycogen concentrations and potentially limit performance.

In summary, masters athletes who engage in regular exercise that involves the recruitment of type II (and particularly the type IIb) fibres are likely to slow the age-related loss in muscle mass and strength. In addition, the timely intake of high-quality protein may assist not only in the short-term recovery of muscle following exercise but benefit the longer-term maintenance of muscle mass. Although endurance training results in higher VO_{2max} values compared to inactive age-matched controls, there appears an inevitable decline in maximal aerobic capacity with age.

1.3 CHANGES IN TASTE AND SMELL

1.3.1 Taste and Smell Perception

The gradual loss of taste and smell that occurs with advancing age has been extensively investigated [23]. Taste changes are broadly classified into three categories: total loss of taste (ageusia), reduced ability to taste (hypogeusia) or distortion of taste (dysgeusia). While total loss of taste is rare at any age, taste perception generally changes with age. Individuals with a reduced ability to taste have a diminished capacity to detect or recognise taste stimuli. Moreover, the intensity of taste thresholds (detection thresholds and recognition thresholds) is elevated. A taste detection threshold is the concentration for the absolute threshold of taste sensation while a taste recognition threshold is the lowest concentration at which a taste source is correctly identified. The significance of this is that taste distortions may contribute to less than optimal food choices, which potentially may result in failure to meet the nutritional needs that accompany advancing age. This has clear implications for older masters athletes who require an adequate intake of carbohydrate and fluid (pre-, during and post-exercise) in order to delay fatigue during exercise and facilitate recovery following training and competition.

Sensations of food in the mouth are presumed to be related to taste, but are in fact partially produced by aroma or smell. When food is placed in the oral cavity, the odorous molecules move up the back of the throat, and the smell is perceived retro-nasally. Odours sensed at a meal are predominantly perceived retro-nasally. With ageing, anatomical and physiological changes result in olfactory deficits and taste and smell signals cannot serve as cues for the metabolic consequences of food ingestion. Again, an awareness of these changes by masters athletes can help individuals compensate for potential changes in food choices that could compromise an adequate intake essential nutrients.

1.3.2 Taste Sensitivity

The decline in taste sensitivity with age appears to be greater in men than in women. Cohen and Gitman found that men had a higher incidence of taste errors than women when they had to recognise the basic tastes of sour, sweet, salty and bitter [24]. Glanville and others showed a gradual increase in sensitivity up to the age of 16–20 years, followed by an exponential decline in both men and women [25]. Weiffenbach and others [26] found that within each age group the thresholds for citric acid of men were higher than those of women, whilst other investigators did not find gender differences [27,28]. A few researchers have reported gender differences in sensitivity to just one or two substances. For example, Fikentscher and others [29] found that women were more sensitive than men to salt (NaCl), cane sugar, citric acid and quinine; this difference became significant in individuals older than 50 years of age. However, others reported the perception of salt was more affected by age in men compared to women, and was more pronounced for sucrose, citric acid, caffeine and quinine [23]. Therefore, older endurance-trained athletes, especially males, need to be aware of this potential reduction in perception of salt intake with age, particularly when exercising in hot/humid conditions where sports drinks and salt tablets may be consumed.

Older adults often have a lower salivary response to food intake [30], and dissatisfaction with the ability to taste food is associated with dry mouth during chewing [31]. With 50% of older adults experiencing saliva deficiency and dryness of the mouth [32], this dry mouth has clear implications for the masters athlete with regard to food and fluid intake, hydration and electrolyte balance during endurance training and competition. Given that there are currently no effective treatments for persistent impairment of the sense of taste, older athletes need to be aware of potential taste alterations and the impact these may have on their nutritional needs during training and competition.

Schiffman and others have suggested that taste impairment with age may be partially due to an increase in medication use [33]. The degree of loss in taste sensitivity may depend on the chemical structure of the compounds tested as well as the medical condition and pharmacological regimen of the individual [34]. It is important to be aware of individual differences observed for most compounds because individuals age physiologically at different rates and therefore the loss of taste and smell may occur earlier for some than for others [35].

In summary, loss of appetite may be experienced by many masters athletes following demanding exercise and when age-related changes in tastes and smell are considered. The masters athlete needs to consume foods with richer tastes and relatively strong but appetising smells in order for them to meet the nutritional requirements that support high-quality training and competition.

1.4 CHANGES IN THE GASTROINTESTINAL TRACT

1.4.1 Motility

Many older adults experience minor yet significant deterioration in gastrointestinal motility and function [36,37]. For masters athletes this may increase the risks of malnutrition and negatively impact on their capacity to train and compete. Age-related changes in gastrointestinal motility include impaired oesophageal peristalsis, delayed gastric emptying, an increase in colon transit times and eventual weight loss and nutritional deficiencies [37]. For older athletes the challenge is to ensure that these changes do not compromise energy and fluid intake. Awareness of such changes allow for the possibility to compensate so that both training and competition performances are maintained.

1.4.2 Absorption

Reduced absorption of certain nutrients is a common cause of malnutrition in older adults with the primary cause being a reduced production of gastric acid (atrophic gastritis) which leads to bacterial overgrowth and a reduction in the formation of gastric intrinsic factor [32]. Sufficient stomach acid and intrinsic factor are required for the absorption of a variety of micronutrients, including iron, folate, calcium, vitamin K and vitamin B12. In addition to a reduced uptake of a number of essential nutrients, atrophic gastritis can result in anaemia, abdominal discomfort, nausea, diarrhoea and weight loss [32]. Moreover, a higher bacterial content in the intestines increases the fermentation of carbohydrate which can cause flatulence, diarrhoea, obstipation (severe or chronic constipation) and abdominal cramps. This may influence the ability or willingness of the older athlete to exercise [32].

In addition to an age-related decrease in the synthesis of vitamin D in the skin, there is decreased absorption of vitamin D in the gastrointestinal tract with age due to decline in the number of vitamin D receptors in the intestinal epithelium [37]. Irrespective of whether the older individual is physically active, there will be a reduced capacity for them to synthesise Vitamin D which in turn will reduce their capacity to absorb dietary calcium and increase their risk of bone fractures. Supplementation with vitamin D and calcium may therefore be needed for older masters athletes [38].

The heterogeneity of the older population with regard to biological age, disease and medication intake makes evaluations of normal/abnormal function of the gastrointestinal tract complex. An individualised approach is therefore required to determine specific nutritional requirements of the older masters athlete or older exerciser, particularly in those individuals who have gastrointestinal issues. These individuals should consult with a dietitian to optimise their diet.

1.5 CHANGES IN WATER BALANCE

1.5.1 Water Loss

Water balance is critical for both health and maintenance of exercise capacity. Indeed, a meta-analyses has found body water reductions in excess of 4% of body mass impairs endurance time trial performance [39]. Ingestion of both fluids and food provides the major route of water intake, though there is additional water liberated in muscle as a result of glycogen metabolism during exercise [40]. Water is lost from the body through urine, faeces, sweat, evaporation from the respiratory tract and diffusion through the skin [41]. Normal ageing is associated with a tendency toward negative water balance, suggesting that masters athletes may be more susceptible to dehydration.

Total body water decreases with age. While approximately 80% of a child's body mass is water, the average total body water of adults aged 61–74 years is 43% for women and 51% for men [42]. This decrease is observed even when taking into account body mass and energy intake [43]. Thus, even small decreases in fluid intake may cause proportionately greater dehydration in a masters athlete than in a younger athlete. Unchecked dehydration can cause changes in body chemistry, kidney failure, kidney stones, urinary tract infections, bowel cancer and death [44]. Therefore, educating and promoting adequate fluid intake in masters athletes may be the most important modifiable health behaviour for ensuring fluid homeostasis.

Masters athletes may be at increased risk of dehydration due to age-related changes in total body water, thirst perception, fluid intake, kidney function and insensible water loss. Although thirst and volume of fluid ingested are separate entities, some researchers suggest they seem to be affected in parallel by age [45]. However, other researchers report dissociated thirst ratings from fluid intake where older adults have increased thirst but consume the same volume of water [46]. Other factors that make masters athletes at higher risk to dehydration include a greater use of medications including diuretics but also sedatives and non-steroidal anti-inflammatory drugs (NSAIDs) [47].

1.5.2 Water Intake

A key factor contributing to an increased risk of dehydration in older athletes is inadequate water intake due to decreased thirst perception. Thirst manifests as a combination of sensations that increase with dehydration and decrease with rehydration (restoration of fluid balance), including a dry, scratchy mouth and throat, chapped and dry lips, light-headedness, dizziness, tiredness, irritability, headache, loss of appetite and feeling of an empty stomach. Thirst results from a complex interaction of behavioural influences such as beverage availability, taste, temperature and palatability, knowledge of the importance of adequate hydration, drinking in association with meals, social and societal norms and habits and even the presence of others who are consuming a beverage [48]. However, increasing the availability or palatability of fluids does not seem to significantly increase fluid intake in older men and women [49]. Of additional concern is that many older adults deliberately avoid drinking beverages, especially in the evening, due to fear of incontinence [50].

1.5.3 Thirst

Physiological thirst is stimulated by increases in cellular tonicity (cellular dehydration) and decreases in extracellular fluid volume (extracellular dehydration) [48]. The former senses the level of dehydration by central, and possibly peripheral osmoreceptors which feed back to the hypothalamus to maintain homeostasis. The latter involves monitoring decreases in blood volume from baroreceptors in large vessels and renal mechanisms which elicit the renin-angiotensin-aldosterone system in response to decreased renal perfusion and other stimuli. A third mechanism which helps regulate the volume of fluid ingested, the act of swallowing, also deserves mention as it provides an integrated signal proportional to the cumulative ingested volume (termed oropharyngeal metering).

Exercise, exogenous heat stress and/or fluid deprivation will decrease blood volume and increase tonicity. Fluid deprivation and exercise both create a hypovolemic (decreased volume of blood plasma), hyperosmotic (increased concentration of penetrating and non-penetrating solute within plasma) condition, the most common environment associated with dehydration. Older individuals appear to be sensitive to increased tonicity but not to fluid volume changes. When the sole stimulus for thirst and drinking is osmotic, there appears to be little difference in thirst sensation in older adults compared to younger individuals [51].

A deficit in the sensitivity of volume receptors appears to be a more important mechanism accounting for reduced thirst with ageing. Available evidence suggests that older men and women have a higher osmotic operating point for thirst sensation under normal daily conditions [45] and diminished sensitivity to thirst and satiety reflexes arising from unloading (hypovolemia) and loading (hypervolemia) of baroreceptors, respectively. Fluid restoration in older adults is eventually effective, but restoration of fluid balance is slower. In the longer term (i.e. days to weeks), fluid intake in response to repeated dehydrating stimuli also appears to be reduced, which may contribute to a relative inability to expand plasma volume [48]. This has strong implications for fluid replacement following intense exercise in masters athletes and older exercisers. These individuals need to be diligent with their recovery practices to achieve effective restoration and maintenance of euhydration.

1.5.4 Fluid Regulation

Body fluid regulation is influenced by acclimation status. For example, in young adults, repeated bouts of exercise in hot environments have been shown to result in plasma volume expansion primarily due to increased voluntary fluid intake [52]. Following 4 days of low-intensity intermittent exercise, young men (24 years) expanded their plasma volume by 10%, whereas no change was observed in the older (67 years) active male group. During the 2-hour recovery period, participants consumed a carbohydrate-electrolyte drink. The young men replaced 80% of lost fluid on average compared to only 34% in older men. This greater involuntary dehydration was accompanied by reduced thirst ratings, plasma vasopressin, aldosterone concentrations and renin activity in the older active group [52]. Zappe and others [52] speculated that the older men may have had lower baroreflex sensitivity and the acclimation program was ineffective in attenuating this sensitivity, and thus fluid intake was not altered. The researchers concluded that the risk of dehydration is increased in elderly subjects regardless of whether they were sedentary or physically active [52].

Studies of the age-related disturbance of water balance have mostly focused on urinary concentrating ability. As people age the concentrating ability of the kidneys decline [53]. Thus, when older adults are deprived of water, urine output is not significantly reduced, increasing the likelihood of dehydration in older populations. Research suggests that ageing is also associated with kidney atrophy, decreased cortical blood flow and glomerular filtration rate and diminished maximal urinary concentrating capacity [53]. These changes can lead to electrolyte imbalances and enhanced water diuresis in older individuals [54]. The age-related reduction of urine concentrating ability may be attributed to decreased sensitivity to the anti-diuretic hormone, vasopressin (AVP) observed in rats [55]. Despite numerous studies of the effect of ageing on plasma AVP in humans, it is still not clear how ageing affects the level of AVP, especially in masters athletes. While some studies report increased basal plasma AVP with ageing, others do not, and some even report a decrease [56]. However, under normal daily living conditions, increased thirst and fluid intake defend against any threats to fluid homeostasis that may result from altered free-water clearance by the kidneys. Therefore, although an inadequate renal response to mild water deprivation may play a role in fluid volume depletion in masters athletes as a result of moderate to intense exercise, reduced thirst is likely more important.

Insensible water loss is a major component of water balance, comparable to daily urine volume. The average water loss through the respiratory tract is approximately 300–400 mL/d, similar to water loss via diffusion through the skin. This combined total of 600–800 mL/d represents 30%–50% of all water loss, depending on the level of water intake [41]. The effects of ageing on insensible water loss have not been extensively studied. Normal aged lungs have dilated alveoli, enlarged airspaces, decreased exchange surface area and loss of supporting tissue in the peripheral airways [57]. Dmitrieva and Burg [40] examined mice of different ages to investigate the factors that contribute to the disturbance of water balance with ageing, and found increased insensible water loss with age. When water was restricted, older mice compensated for increased insensible water loss by increasing AVP excretion and urine concentration and decreasing water content of their faeces. The higher AVP that maintains hydration in older mice could contribute to age-related pathology [58]. While it is acknowledged this research was related to animals, insensible water loss may be an important component of water balance in masters athletes, especially when water intake is low.

In summary, the reduced perceptions of thirst, insensible water loss, decreased urinary concentrating ability and slower restoration of fluid balance with advancing age suggests masters athletes may require greater-than-normal fluid intake to achieve and maintain adequate hydration pre-, during and post-exercise.

1.6 FAT, PROTEIN AND CARBOHYDRATE METABOLISM

1.6.1 Peripheral Oxidative Capacity

Ageing is associated with a general decrease in maximal aerobic capacity that has been attributed to both a reduced delivery of oxygen to muscles via the cardiovascular system and a reduced capacity to use oxygen to resynthesise adenosine triphosphate (ATP) within the active muscle [59]. Peripherally, sarcopenia is accompanied by a reduction in mitochondrial density and a concomitant decrease in the activity of the oxidative enzymes that regulate the use of fat and derivatives of glucose as fuel. A reduced capacity to use fat as a substrate during exercise places a greater reliance on muscle glycogen for ATP resynthesis and theoretically increases the onset of fatigue for the endurance athlete. Indeed, sedentary ageing individuals who undertake submaximal exercise have relatively high circulating lactate concentrations (reflecting a significant contribution of anaerobic metabolism to the exercise demand) and comparatively high respiratory quotients (reflecting a greater reliance on carbohydrate for energy). However, regardless of age, endurance training elicits adaptations to both the cardiovascular system and the trained skeletal muscle that favour an increased contribution of aerobic metabolism (and greater use of fat) to the energy yield [60]. While masters athletes may not have the same absolute capacity to deliver oxygen as younger athletes, there is strong evidence to suggest that peripherally, the skeletal muscle of the older athlete responds to endurance training to a similar extent as that of younger athletes [61].

1.6.2 Fat Utilisation

In considering age-related changes in the peripheral capacity to use fat as a substrate, researchers have examined whether exercise-mediated release of fat from adipose tissue changes with age. Mobilisation of fat during exercise is strongly influenced by sympathoadrenal activity and a number of researchers have reported that older sedentary individuals have a blunted catecholamine response to exercise compared to younger individuals [62,63]. This has been attributed to a smaller muscle mass being activated during exercise. However, exercise training results in an improved sympathoadrenal response to exercise in previously sedentary older people [64]. Thus, it might be suggested that the availability of fat as a substrate is not limited by the catecholamine response to submaximal exercise in masters athletes.

Taken together, the masters athlete, when compared to age-matched sedentary individuals, may have a greater capacity to mobilise fat during exercise [65] that may be characterised by a higher mitochondrial density. With oxygen delivery to the muscles also higher, the endurance-trained masters athlete can better spare muscle glycogen during exercise and delay the onset of fatigue.

1.6.3 Muscle Protein Synthesis

Sarcopenia and the known decreases in skeletal muscle protein turnover that occur with age have been attributed, at least in part, to insulin resistance, reduced cellular signalling and/or reduced availability of essential amino acids [66]. Indeed, sedentary ageing individuals have been described as being 'anabolic resistant' [67]. However, regular physical activity (and particularly resistance training) has been consistently shown to improve muscle protein synthesis and increase muscle mass in older individuals [66,68] and there is strong evidence that this can be further enhanced when resistance training is combined with the timely intake of high-quality protein [69].

Masters athletes who regularly engage in resistance-type exercise can expect to significantly reduce the age-related loss in muscle mass that occurs with sedentary living. Maintenance of muscle mass across the lifespan will not only improve athletic performance, but also reduce the risk of type II diabetes and cardiovascular disease [70]. Compared to inactive age-matched individuals, masters athletes have higher energy expenditures and greater uptake of blood glucose by skeletal muscle resulting in a lower risk of type II diabetes and the many complications associated with the disease.

When the available evidence is collectively considered, the endurance-trained masters athlete is characterised by a higher capacity to use fat during exercise. The primary advantage of this will be that glycogen during exercise will be spared and fatigue potentially delayed. For those masters athletes who engage in regular resistance-type exercise, muscle mass will also be better maintained compared to those who are inactive. In addition, the higher energy expenditure that results from regular exercise, coupled with greater clearance of glucose from the blood, reduces the risks of type II diabetes and cardiovascular disease. Compared to their sedentary peers, masters athletes can expect to enjoy better health in addition to improvements in their performance and exercise capacity.

1.7 CALCIUM AND BONE HEALTH

1.7.1 Osteoporosis

Over the lifespan, the skeletal system undergoes a dynamic process of renewal, involving cyclic coupling of the bone formation cells (osteoblasts) and bone resorption cells (osteoclasts). Following the attainment of peak bone mass at approximately 23 years of age, bone resorption increases and bone formation declines; the amount of bone formed during each remodelling cycle thus decreases [71]. Bone health is influenced by both endogenous (genetic, hormonal) and exogenous (nutritional, physical activity) factors. Nutritionally, insufficient levels of calcium and vitamin D can lead to a decline in bone mineral density (BMD) and increase the risk of osteoporosis. Osteoporosis is a disease in which the density and quality of bone are reduced, leading to weakness of the skeleton and increased risk for a fragility fracture [72].

1.7.2 Calcium

Physiologically, calcium provides rigidity to the skeleton but bone calcium also acts as a reserve to maintain blood calcium concentrations. Calcium absorption from the gastrointestinal tract is strongly dependent on vitamin D status [73] highlighting that vitamin D deficiency can therefore lead to poor bone health. Independent to nutritional factors, activities that place strain on the skeletal system also help to maintain and improve bone mass since skeletal cells adapt to suit the increased load placed upon them [74].

With regard to dietary calcium intake, Australia's National Health and Medical Research Council (NHMRC) recommends that for men aged 19–70 years and women aged 19–50 years, 1000 mg/d of calcium needs to be consumed. This increases to 1300 mg/d for men 70 years and over and women older than 50 years [75]. However, it is difficult for many older adults to achieve an intake of 1300 mg/d through their diet, as many tend to eat relatively small quantities of food and their energy intake is generally low. This has been highlighted in a recent Australian National Nutrition Survey (NNS) that found the median dietary intake of calcium was 827 mg/d and 633 mg/d for men and women, respectively. In addition to poor dietary calcium intake, both men and women experience a decline in intestinal calcium absorption and an increase in urinary calcium excretion with age [76]. Calcium bioavailability is also affected by atrophic gastritis which is common in older adults as a consequence of decreased stomach acid decreasing the dissociation of calcium from food [77]. Moreover, reduced production and absorption of vitamin D will further reduce calcium uptake in the diet. To help ensure that they gain sufficient calcium in their diets, older exercisers and master athletes need to consume calcium-rich foods and beverages perhaps, under the advice of their physician and/or dietitian, take a calcium supplement.

1.7.3 Vitamin D

Vitamin D influences calcium transport, renal calcium reabsorption and mobilisation of calcium from bone [76]. Due to both reduced production and decreased absorption of vitamin D in the diet, older individuals are at an increased risk of vitamin D deficiency (defined as 25(OH)D below 50 nmol/L) [75] and thus osteoporosis [78–80]. Given that exposure to sunlight will potentially increase vitamin D production, those masters athletes who train and compete in sunlight are likely to be at a lower risk of being vitamin D deficient compared to those who are not regularly exposed to sunlight. For masters athletes who generally train either indoors and/or do not gain regular exposure to sunlight, there may be value in gaining more sunlight exposure. In addition, and after consulting with their physician and/or dietitian, either vitamin D supplementation and/or an increased dietary intake of vitamin D-rich foods should be considered.

1.7.4 Exercise

Although exercise has long been regarded as an effective non-pharmacological way to improve bone density and reduce the risk of osteoporosis, it needs to be recognised that not all types of exercise will benefit bone health [74,81]. High-impact loading activities such as jumping, hopping, skipping, bounding and high-intensity resistance training appear to be most beneficial to bone because of the high strains these types of activities place on the bones involved [74]. In contrast, swimming and walking have a negligible effect on bone density [82]. Nichols and colleagues have compared the bone density of male master cyclists with that of age-matched controls [83,84]. They found that despite the high level of training in masters cyclists, their low bone density was no different to that of the age-matched peers. This confirms that without significant load bearing, bone density is unlikely to change with exercise training. In an earlier cross-sectional study that compared bone density between masters swimmers and masters runners, it was found that the moderate impact exercise undertaken by the runners resulted in significantly greater whole body BMD than that measured in the swimmers [85].

In summary, the age-related decline in bone density, coupled with the associated increased risk of osteoporosis, may be attenuated or reversed in older exercisers and masters athletes who regularly participate in activities that involve a degree of impact on bone. Conversely, those who engage in non-weight-bearing activities such as swimming and cycling are unlikely to gain skeletal benefits and will therefore be at a similar risk of osteoporosis as those who are inactive.

1.8 CHANGES IN THE IMMUNE SYSTEM

With ageing, the immune system deteriorates leading to increased susceptibility to infections, autoimmune diseases, malignancies [86,87] and vascular disease [88,89]. However, regular moderate-intensity exercise appears to offset the dysregulation and chronic inflammation that accompanies ageing [90]. While research is yet to compare the immune status of ageing individuals who have always maintained a commitment to regular exercise with those who take up exercise later in life, it is reasonable to assume that previously sedentary ageing individuals who take up regular activity will have a stronger resistance to infection [91]. To extend this further, it is equally likely that masters athletes who regularly participate in moderate-intensity exercise will have stronger immune systems than sedentary individuals of a similar age. This will not only contribute to their overall health and well-being, but also support higher-quality training and therefore improved exercise performance.

1.9 OXIDATIVE STRESS

1.9.1 Reactive Oxygen Species

Exercise in both younger and older individuals increases the production of reactive oxygen species (ROS) [92]. Energy produced aerobically through the mitochondria will inevitably result in leakage of electrons as a result of the chemical reactions that occur. Furthermore, higher volumes of endurance exercise are believed to result in a higher production of ROS. Theoretically, if the production of ROS surpasses the body's inherent antioxidant defences, oxidative stress can occur and damage to cellular structures may result [93]. Exercise aside, the age-related increased risks of cardiovascular disease, arterial stiffness and impaired vascular endothelial function [94] have been attributed, in part, to oxidative stress [95]. It remains speculative whether regular activity across the lifespan is likely to increase the risks of these diseases given that exercise results in an increase in the production of ROS.

1.9.2 Endogenous and Exogenous Antioxidants

As a means of countering an increased production (and the potential harmful effects) of ROS, the body increases the production of its own (endogenous) antioxidants [92]. Habitually active individuals, though they experience a higher production of ROS and oxidative stress through their training and competition, are characterised by higher antioxidant defences [96].

It should be noted that some oxidative stress is believed to be beneficial to health [97]. ROS act in cell signalling and are involved in a number of important adaptations to exercise. The prevailing view is that there is a fine and well-maintained balance between oxidative stress which is needed for normal physiological functioning and antioxidant production. This perhaps explains why the weight of evidence shows that antioxidant supplementation does not appear to reduce oxidative stress nor provide health benefits. Moreover, some studies have shown the practice to be harmful [98]. Daily intake of fruit and vegetables is the recommended means to gain an adequate source of exogenous antioxidants [92].

In summary, while masters athletes, particularly endurance athletes who maintain relatively high volumes of training, are likely to have an increased production of ROS, the body counters this by increasing its own antioxidant defences. Some degree of oxidative stress appears to be needed by the body to maintain normal function of various physiological systems and there is no evidence that antioxidant supplementation benefits either health or exercise performance. Finally, there is growing evidence to suggest that antioxidant supplementation may not only impair adaptations to training but could be harmful.

1.10 CONCLUSION

Ageing is associated with reduced functional capacity of many physiological systems and as a result, exercise capacity decreases over the lifespan. Awareness of age-related changes that occur in taste, smell and nutrient absorption can allow the masters athlete to make adjustments to compensate for the increased risks of nutrient deficiency and dehydration that will not only influence their health but also affect their exercise capacity and performance.

1.11 IMPLICATIONS FOR SPORTS MEDICINE PROFESSIONALS AND CLINICIANS

- Age-related changes in taste, smell and gastrointestinal function may affect food selection and thus nutrient availability. Choosing foods with strong tastes and appetising smells will potentially help ensure that an adequate volume and broad range of nutritious foods are consumed which will help support high-quality training and strong exercise performance.
- Due to a reduced perception of thirst, fluid intake tends to decrease with age. Fluid losses can also increase with age. Masters athletes need to voluntarily increase their fluid intake to compensate for these changes.
- Skeletal muscle mass decreases with age, as does the capacity for muscles to use fat as a fuel during exercise. This places a greater dependence on muscle glycogen to meet exercise

demands. However, endurance training results in central and peripheral adaptations that increase the capacity for fat utilisation and this spares muscle glycogen and improves exercise capacity.
- Mechanical loading of the skeleton (i.e. high-impact weight-bearing activities or strength/resistance training) and adequate intakes of calcium and vitamin D are recommended to reduce the risks of osteoporosis in masters athletes. For those masters athletes who swim or cycle, there is value in cross-training and including some weight-bearing activities such as running or resistance training.
- Ageing has been associated with oxidative stress. Some degree of oxidative stress is beneficial in eliciting adaptation at the cellular level but too much may lead to damage. Endogenous antioxidants increase in response to training and exogenous antioxidants are best acquired through consumption of fruit and vegetables. There is no consistent evidence that antioxidant supplementation is beneficial.

1.12 IMPLICATIONS FOR MASTERS ATHLETES AND COACHES

- Taste and smell deteriorate with age and food selection is likely to change. For the older athlete, the challenge is to consume a healthy, balanced diet that provides sufficient energy for exercise and adequately replenishes energy stores during recovery. In particular, carbohydrate intake (both in terms of the total amount and also the timing of intake) is critical for supporting quality training and performance. Choose foods that have strong and appealing tastes and appetising smells. This may help ensure that an adequate volume and wide range of nutritious foods are consumed.
- Masters athletes are believed to be at a greater risk of dehydration than younger athletes. In practical terms, this means that masters athletes need to make a greater effort to drink adequate volumes of fluid before, during and post-exercise. Given that thirst is not a reliable indicator of hydration, more objective measures such as changes in body mass may provide a better sense of whether sufficient fluid is being consumed.
- The risk of developing osteoporosis can be reduced through activities that involve high-impact forces or strains on bone coupled with adequate dietary intake of calcium and vitamin D. Masters athletes who only swim or cycle should consider some cross-training that involves running and/or resistance training. These activities will strengthen the bones.
- Although oxidative stress has been implicated in the ageing process, some oxidative stress is considered necessary for adaptations to occur in the body (for example the positive changes that occur in muscle following training). Intake of fruit and vegetables is recognised as the most effective means of providing protection to high levels of oxidative stress. There is no evidence that antioxidant supplementation is beneficial and some studies have shown the practice to be harmful.

1.13 FUTURE RESEARCH DIRECTIONS

- Although much is known about the adaptations to training in the older athlete through cross-sectional research, longitudinal investigations that monitor activity levels and track lifetime athletes over several decades will help us better understand the interaction between ageing, activity and relative disuse.
- Much is known about the time-course of adaptations to exercise in response to training across the lifespan. However, relative loss of exercise capacity with detraining (e.g. with injury) and then recovery of that exercise capacity with retraining is yet to be examined in the older athlete.
- The interactions between common medications and nutrient absorption specifically with older athletes warrants investigation.

REFERENCES

1. Paddon-Jones, D. and Rasmussen, B.B., Dietary protein recommendations and the prevention of sarcopenia, *Curr. Opin. Clin. Nutr. Metab. Care.* 12, 86–90, 2009.
2. Akima, H., Kano, W., Enomoto, Y. et al., Muscle function in 164 men and women aged 20–84 yr, *Med. Sci. Sports Exerc.* 33, 220–26, 2001.
3. Goodpaster, B.H., Park, S.W., Harris, T.B. et al., The loss of skeletal muscle strength, mass, and quality in older adults: The health, aging and body composition study, *J. Gerentol. A Biol. Sci. Med. Sci.* 61, 1059–64, 2006.
4. Bassey, E.J., Fiatarone, M.A., O'Neill, E.F., Kelly, M., Evans, W.J. and Lipsitz, L.A., Leg extensor power and functional performance in very old men and women, *Clin. Sci.* 82(3), 321–7, 1992.
5. Hughes, V.A., Frontera, W.R., Wood, M. et al., Longitudinal muscle strength changes in older adults: Influence of muscle mass, physical activity, and health, *J. Gerentol. A Biol. Sci. Med. Sci.* 56, B209–17, 2001.
6. Doherty, T.J., Aging and sarcopenia, *J. Appl. Physiol.* 95, 1717–27, 2003.
7. Tomlinson, B.E. and Irving, D., Numbers of limb motor neurons in human lumbosacral cord throughout life, *J. Neurol. Sci.* 34, 213–9, 1977.
8. Candow, D.G. and Chilibeck, P.D., Differences in size, strength, and power of upper and lower body muscle groups in young and older men, *J. Gerentol. A Biol. Sci. Med. Sci.* 60, 148–56, 2005.
9. Kadhiresan, V.A., Hassett, C.A. and Faulkner, J.A., Properties of single motor units in medial gastrocnemius muscles of adult and old rats, *J. Physiol.* 493, 543–52, 1996.
10. Trappe, S., Williamson, D., Godard, M. et al., Effect of resistance training on single muscle fiber contractile function in older men, *J. Appl. Physiol.* 89, 143–52, 2000.
11. Pearson, S.J., Young, A., Macaluso, A. et al., Muscle function in elite master weightlifters, *Med. Sci. Sports Exerc.* 34, 1199–206, 2002.
12. Phillips, S.K., Rook, K.M., Siddle, N.C. et al., Muscle weakness in women occurs at an earlier age than in men, but strength is preserved by hormone replacement therapy, *Clin. Sci.* 84, 95–8, 1993.
13. Hawkins, S.A. and Wiswell, R.A., Rate and mechanism of maximal oxygen consumption decline with aging: Implications for exercise training, *Sports Med.* 33, 877–88, 2003.
14. Slade, J.M., Miszko, T.A., Laity, J.H. et al., Anaerobic power and physical function in strength-trained and non-strength-trained older adults, *J. Gerentol. A Biol. Sci. Med. Sci.* 57, M168–72, 2002.
15. Wroblewski, A.P., Amati, F., Smiley, M.A. et al., Chronic exercise preserves lean muscle mass in masters athletes, *Phys. Sportsmed.* 39, 172–8, 2011.
16. Coggan, A.R., Abduljalil, A.M., Swanson, S.C. et al., Muscle metabolism during exercise in young and older untrained and endurance-trained men, *J. Appl. Physiol.* 75, 2125–33, 1993.
17. Eskurza, I., Donato, A.J., Moreau, K.L. et al., Changes in maximal aerobic capacity with age in endurance-trained women: 7-yr follow-up, *J. Appl. Physiol.* 92, 2303–8, 2002.
18. Katzel, L.I., Sorkin, J.D. and Fleg, J.L., A comparison of longitudinal changes in aerobic fitness in older endurance athletes and sedentary men, *J. Am. Geriatr. Soc.* 49, 1657–64, 2001.
19. Evans, S.L., Davy, K.P., Stevenson, E.T. et al., Physiological determinants of 10-km performance in highly trained female runners of different ages, *J. Appl. Physiol.* 78, 1931–41, 1995.
20. Meredith, C.N., Frontera, W.R., Fisher, E.C. et al., Peripheral effects of endurance training in young and old subjects, *J. Appl. Physiol.* 66(6), 2844–9, 1989.
21. Cox, J.H., Cortright, R.N., Dohm, G.L. et al., Effect of aging on response to exercise training in humans: Skeletal muscle GLUT-4 and insulin sensitivity, *J. Appl. Physiol.* 86, 2019–25, 1999.
22. Cartee, G.D., Aging skeletal muscle: Response to exercise, *Ex. Sport Sci. Rev.* 22, 91–120, 1994.
23. Mojet, J., Christ-Hazelhof, E. and Heidema, J., Taste perception with age: Generic or specific losses in threshold sensitivity to the five basic tastes? *Chem. Senses.* 26, 845–60, 2001.
24. Cohen, T. and Gitman, L., Oral complaints and taste perception in the aged, *J. Gerentol.* 14, 294–8, 1959.
25. Glanville, E.V., Kaplan, A.R. and Fischer, R., Age sex and taste sensitivity, *J. Geretol.* 19, 474–7, 1964.
26. Weiffenbach, J.M., Baum, B.J. and Burghauser, R., Taste thresholds – Quality specific variation with human aging, *J. Gerontol.* 37, 372–7, 1982.
27. Cooper, R.M., Bilash, I. and Zubek, J.P., The effect of age on taste sensitivity, *J. Gerentol.* 14(1), 56–8, 1959.
28. Hyde, R.J. and Feller, R.P., Age and sex effects on taste of sucrose, NaCl, citric-acid and caffeine, *Neurobiol. Aging* 2, 315–8, 1981.
29. Fikentscher, R., Roseburg, B., Spinar, H. et al., Loss of taste in elderly – Sex-differences, *Clin. Otolaryngol.* 2, 183–89, 1977.

30. Donini, L.M., Savina, C. and Cannella, C., Eating habits and appetite control in the elderly: The anorexia of aging, *Int. Psychogeriatr.* 15, 73–87, 2003.
31. Yoshinaka, M., Yoshinaka, M.F., Ikebe, K. et al., Factors associated with taste dissatisfaction in the elderly, *J. Oral Rehab.* 34, 497–502, 2007.
32. Gille, D., Overview of the physiological changes and optimal diet in the golden age generation over 50, *Eur. Rev. Aging Phys. Act.* 7, 27–36, 2010.
33. Schiffman, S.S., Graham, B.G., Suggs, M.S. et al., Effect of psychotropic drugs on a range of taste responses in young and elderly persons, *Chem. Senses.* 22, 786, 1997.
34. Schiffman, S.S., Perception of taste and smell in elderly persons, *Crit. Rev. Food Sci. Nutr.* 33, 17–26, 1993.
35. Stevens, J.C., Cruz, L.A., Hoffman, J.M. et al., Taste sensitivity and aging – High-incidence of decline revealed by repeated threshold measures, *Chem. Senses.* 20, 451–9, 1995.
36. Greenwald, D.A., Aging, the gastrointestinal tract, and risk of acid-related disease, *Am. J. Med.* 117(Suppl 5A), 8S–13, 2004.
37. Bhutto, A. and Morley, J.E., The clinical significance of gastrointestinal changes with aging, *Curr. Opin. Clin. Nutr. Metab. Care.* 11(5), 651–60, 2008.
38. Tang, B.M., Eslick, G.D., Nowson, C., Smith, C. and Bensoussan, A., Use of calcium or calcium in combination with vitamin D supplementation to prevent fractures and bone loss in people aged 50 years and older: A meta-analysis, *Lancet.* 370(9588), 657–66, 2007.
39. Goulet, E.D., Effect of exercise-induced dehydration on time-trial exercise performance: A meta-analysis, *Br. J. Sports Med.* 45(14), 1149–56, 2011.
40. Dmitrieva, N.I. and Burg, M.B., Increased insensible water loss contributes to aging related dehydration, *PloS One.* 6(5), e20691, 2011.
41. Guyton, A.C. and Hall, J.E., The body fluids compartments: Extracellular and intracellular fluids; interstitial fluids and edema. In *Textbook of Medical Physiology*, A.C. Guyton and J.E. Hall, eds., W.B. Saunders Company, Philadelphia, 2000, 263–379.
42. Lavizzo-Mourey, R.J., Dehydration in the elderly: A short review, *J. Natl Med. Assoc.* 79, 1033–8, 1987.
43. Zizza, C.A., Ellison, K.J. and Wernette, C.M., Total water intakes of community-living middle-old and oldest-old adults, *J. Gerentol. A Biol. Sci. Med. Sci.* 64, 481–6, 2009.
44. Kleiner, S.M., Water: An essential but overlooked nutrient, *J. Am. Diet. Assoc.* 99, 200–6, 1999.
45. Mack, G.W., Weseman, C.A., Langhans, G.W. et al., Body-fluid balance in dehydrated healthy older men – Thirst and renal osmoregulation, *J. Appl. Physiol.* 76, 1615–23, 1994.
46. Miescher, E. and Fortney, S.M., Responses to dehydration and rehydration during heat exposure in young and older men, *Am. J. Physiol.* 257, R1050–6, 1989.
47. Sansevero, A.C., Dehydration in the elderly: Strategies for prevention and management, *Nurse Pract.* 22, 41–57, 1997.
48. Kenney, W.L. and Chiu, P., Influence of age on thirst and fluid intake, *Med. Sci. Sports Exerc.* 33, 1524–32, 2001.
49. Phillips, P.A., Johnston, C.I. and Gray, L., Thirst and fluid intake in the elderly, in *Thirst: Physiological and Psychological Aspects*, D.J. Ramsay and D.A. Booth, eds., Springer-Verlag, London, 1991, pp. 403–11.
50. De Castro, J.M., Age-related changes in natural spontaneous fluid ingestion and thirst in humans, *J. Gerentol.* 47, 321–30, 1992.
51. Stachenfeld, N.S., DiPeitro, L., Nadel, E.R. et al., Mechanism of attenuated thirst in aging: Role of central volume receptors, *Am. J. Physiol. Regul. Integr. Comp. Physiol.* 272, R148–57, 1997.
52. Zappe, D.H., Bell, G.W., Swartzentruber, H. et al., Age and regulation of fluid and electrolyte balance during repeated exercise sessions, *Am. J. Physiol. Regul. Integr. Comp. Physiol.* 270, R71–9, 1996.
53. Rowe, J.W., Shock, N.W. and Defronzo, R.A., Influence of age on renal response to water-deprivation in man, *Nephron.* 17, 270–8, 1976.
54. Ayus, J.C. and Arieff, A.I., Abnormalities of water metabolism in the elderly, *Sem. Neph.* 16, 277–88, 1996.
55. Geelen, G. and Corman, B., Relationship between vasopressin and renal concentrating ability in aging rats, *Am. J. Physiol.* 262(5), R826–33, 1992.
56. Frolkis, V.V., Kvitnitskaya-Ryzhova, T.Y. and Dubiley, T.A., Vasopressin, hypothalamo-neurohypophyseal system and aging, *Arch. Gerontol. Geriatr.* 29, 193–214, 1999.
57. Janssens, J.P., Pache, J.C. and Nicod, L.P., Physiological changes in respiratory function associated with aging, *Eur. Respir. J.* 13, 197–205, 1999.
58. Knepper, M.A. and Star, R.A., Vasopressin: Friend or foe?, *Nat. Med.* 14, 14–6, 2008.

59. Coggan, A.R., Spina, R.J., King, D.S. et al., Histochemical and enzymatic comparison of the gastrocnemius muscle of young and elderly men and women, *J. Gerontol.* 47(3), 871–6, 1992.
60. Pogliaghi, S., Terziotti, P., Cevese, A., Balestreri, F. and Schena, F., Adaptations to endurance training in the healthy elderly: Arm-cranking vs leg cycling, *Eur. J. Appl. Physiol.* 97, 723–31, 2006.
61. Holloszy, J.O., Cellular adaptations to endurance exercise: Masters athletes, *Int. J. Sports Nutr. Exerc. Metab.* 11, S186–8, 2001.
62. Kohrt, W.M., Spina, R.J., Ehsani, A.A., Cryer, P.E. and Holloszy, J.O., Effects of age, adiposity and fitness level on plasma catecholamine responses to standing and exercise, *J. Appl. Physiol.* 75(4), 1828–35, 1993.
63. Ford, G.A., Dachman, W.D., Blaschke, T.F. and Hoffman, B.B., Effect of aging on beta adrenergic receptor-stimulated flux of K^+, PO4, FFA and glycerol in human forearms, *J. Appl. Physiol.* 78(1), 172–8, 1985.
64. Galbo, H., Influence of aging and exercise on endocrine function, *Int. J. Sport Nutr. Exer. Metab.* 11, S49–57, 2001.
65. Sial, S., Coggan, A.R., Hickner, R.C. and Klein, S., Training-induced alterations in fat and carbohydrate metabolism during exercise in elderly subjects, *Am. J. Physiol.* 274, E785–90, 1998.
66. Koopman, R. and van Loon, L.J.C., Aging, exercise and muscle protein metabolism, *J. Appl. Physiol.* 106, 2040–8, 2009.
67. Rennie, M.J., Anabolic resistance: The effects of aging, sexual dimorphism and immobilisation of human muscle turnover, *Appl. Physiol. Nutr. Metab.* 34, 377–81, 2009.
68. Symons, T.B., Sheffield-Moore, M., Mamerow, M.M., Wolfe, R.R. and Paddon-Jones, D., The anabolic response to resistance exercise and a protein-rich meal is not diminished by age, *J. Nutr. Health Aging* 15(5), 376–81, 2011.
69. Walker, D.K., Dickinson, J.M., Timmerman, K.L. et al., Exercise, amino acids and aging in the control of human muscle protein synthesis, *Med. Sci. Sports Exerc.* 43(12), 2249–58, 2011.
70. Beaufrere, B. and Morio, B., Fat and protein distribution with aging: Metabolic considerations, *Eur. J. Clin. Nutr.* 54(Suppl 3), S48–53, 2000.
71. Seeman, E., Structural basis of growth-related gain and age-related loss of bone strength, *Rheumatology (Oxford).* 47(Suppl 4 iv), 2–8, 2008.
72. Johnell, O. and Kanis, J.A., An estimate of the worldwide prevalence and disability associated with osteoporotic fractures, *Osteoporos Int.* 17(12), 1726–33, 2006.
73. Lips, P., Vitamin D physiology, *Prog. Biophys. Mol. Biol.* 92(1), 4–8, 2009.
74. Guadalupe-Grau, A., Fuentes, T., Guerra, B. and Calbet, J.A., Exercise and bone mass in adults, *Sports Med.* 39(6), 439–68, 2009.
75. Ross, A.C., Manson, J.E., Abrams, S.A., Aloia, J.F., Brannon, P.M. and Clinton, S.K., The 2011 report on dietary reference intakes for calcium and vitamin D from the Institute of Medicine: What clinicians need to know, *J. Clin. Endocrinol. Metab.* 96(1), 53–8, 2011.
76. Sanders, K.M., Nowson, C.A., Kotowicz, M.A., Briffa, K., Devine, A. and Reid, I.R. Calcium and bone health: Position statement for the Australian and New Zealand Bone and Mineral Society, Osteoporosis Australia and the Endocrine Society of Australia, *Med J Aust.* 190(6), 316–20, 2009.
77. Eastell, R., Yergey, A.L., Vieira, N.E., Cedel, S.L., Kumar, R. and Riggs, B.L., Interrelationship among vitamin D metabolism, true calcium absorption, parathyroid function, and age in women: Evidence of an age-related intestinal resistance to 1,25-dihydroxyvitamin D action, *J. Bone Miner. Res.* 6(2), 125–32, 1991.
78. Sambrook, P.N., Cameron, I.D., Cumming, R.G. et al., Vitamin D deficiency is common in frail institutionalised older people in northern Sydney, *Med. J. Aust.* 176(11), 560, 2002.
79. Flicker, L., Mead, K., MacInnis, R.J. et al., Serum vitamin D and falls in older women in residential care in Australia, *J. Am. Geriatr. Soc.* 51(11), 1533–8, 2003.
80. Diamond, T., Smerdely, P., Kormas, N., Sekel, R., Vu, T. and Day, P., Hip fracture in elderly men: The importance of subclinical vitamin D deficiency and hypogonadism, *Med. J. Aust.* 169(3), 138–41, 1998.
81. Gomez-Cabello, A., Ara, I., Gonzalez-Aguero, A., Casajus, J.A. and Vicente-Rodriguez, G., Effects of training on bone mass in older adults: A systematic review, *Sports Med.* 42(4), 301–25, 2012.
82. Palombaro, K.M., Effects of walking-only interventions on bone mineral density at various skeletal sites: A meta-analysis, *J. Geriatr. Phys. Ther.* 28(3), 102–7, 2005.
83. Nichols, J.F., Palmer, J.E. and Levy, S.S., Low bone mineral density in highly trained male master cyclists, *Osteoporos Int.* 14(8), 644–9, 2003.
84. Nichols, J.F. and Rauh, M.J., Longitudinal changes in bone mineral density in male master cyclists and nonathletes, *J. Strength Cond. Res.* 25(3), 727–34, 2011.

85. Velez, N.F., Zhang, A., Stone, B., Perera, S., Miller, M. and Greenspan, S.L., The effect of moderate impact exercise on skeletal integrity in master athletes, *Osteoporos Int.* 19(10), 1457–64, 2008.
86. Pawelec, G., Immunosenescence: Impact in the young as well as the old? *Mech. Ageing Dev.* 108, 1–7, 1999.
87. Haaland, D.A., Sabljic, T.F. and Baribeau, D.A., Is regular exercise a friend or foe of the aging immune system? A systematic review, *Clin. J. Sports Med.* 18(6), 539–48, 2008.
88. Haffner, S.M., The metabolic syndrome: Inflammation, diabetes mellitus and cardiovascular disease, *Am. J. Cardiol.* 97(2A), 3A–11A, 2006.
89. Ritz, P., Physiology of aging with respect to gastrointestinal, circulatory and immune system changes and their significance for energy and protein metabolism, *Eur. J. Clin. Nutr.* 54, S21–5, 2000.
90. Gleeson, M., Immune function in sport and exercise, *J. Appl. Physiol.* 103, 693–9, 2007.
91. Simpson, R.J. and Guy, K., Coupling aging immunity with a sedentary lifestyle: Has the damage already been done? A mini review, *Gerontol.* 16, 449–58, 2010.
92. Peternelj, T. and Coombes, J.S., Antioxidant supplementation during exercise training: Beneficial or detrimental?, *Sports Med.* 41(12), 1043–71, 2011.
93. McCord, J.M., The evolution of free radicals and oxidative stress, *Am. J. Med.* 108, 652–9, 2000.
94. Seals, D.R., DeSouza, C.A., Donato, A.J. and Tanaka, H., Habitual exercise and aging, *J. Appl. Physiol.* 105, 1323–32, 2008.
95. Wallace, D.C., A mitochondrial paradigm of metabolic and degenerative diseases, aging, and cancer: A dawn for evolutionary medicine, *Ann. Rev. Genet.* 39, 359–407, 2005.
96. Niess, A.M. and Simon, P., Response and adaptation of skeletal muscle to exercise: The role of reactive oxygen species, *Front. Biosci.* 12, 4826–38, 2007.
97. Valko, M., Leibfritz, D., Moncol, J. et al., Free radicals and antioxidants in normal physiological functions and human disease, *Int. J. Biochem. Cell. Biol.* 39(1), 44–84, 2007.
98. Miller, E.R., Pastor-Barriuso, R., Dalal, D., Riemersma, R.A., Appel, L.J. and Guallar, E., Meta-analysis: High dosage vitamin E supplementation may increase all-cause mortality, *Ann. Intern. Med.* 142, 37–46, 2005.

2 Physiological Changes Affecting Performance of Masters Athletes

Benjamin J. Dascombe, Nathan Elsworthy, Brendan Scott, Dean V. Sculley and Peter R.J. Reaburn

CONTENTS

2.1 INTRODUCTION

Masters athletes are classified as older individuals who systematically train for and compete in organized forms of competitive sport. Each sport's national or international governing body determines the age at which masters competition begins, normally between 30–40 years of age. During recent decades there has been an increase in the number of active older individuals who can be classified as recreational or competitive athletes who focus on sports performance. For example, the inaugural World Masters Games held in Toronto, Canada in 1985 had 8305 participants from 61 countries competing across 22 sports, while the 2009 World Masters Games held in Sydney, Australia saw 28,676 competitors from 95 countries competing in 28 sports in the largest organized sports event ever held to date. Data from the most recent 2013 World Masters Games in Torino, Italy say approximately 20,000 competitors took part in 29 different sports [1]. However, it is well documented that performance across a range of sports declines with advancing age [2–5]. Given the popularity and size of the competitive masters sports movement, it is surprising that little research data exist that reports on the physiological mechanisms responsible for the observed declines in performance with advancing age.

The primary basis for this decrease in competitive performance relates to the unavoidable and natural deterioration of several physiological systems that occur with ageing [2–5]. Importantly, there are a number of declines in physiological function that explain the reduced level of performance in older athletes. These measures include maximal aerobic capacity $\left(VO_{2max}\right)$, anaerobic power and capacity, muscular strength, body composition, muscle fibre characteristics and metabolic efficiency [4].

Despite these age-related changes, several studies have demonstrated that the continued training and competition undertaken by masters athletes slows the natural ageing-related reductions in both athletic performance and physiological function [6–9]. It should also be highlighted that many other non-physiological age-related changes occur that contribute to the decline in masters athlete performances (e.g. social circumstances, family commitments, employment situations and musculoskeletal limitations). Regardless, it is well understood that athletic performance decreases with age across endurance, sprint and strength events after approximately 35–40 years. These highlighted losses in physiological function and performance accelerate rapidly after an individual reaches 70 years of age [4,5,10–16].

2.2 CHANGES IN ATHLETIC PERFORMANCE WITH AGE

There is limited research and few reviews that provide a holistic evaluation of the changes in physiological factors that explain the reported age-related decline in athletic performance [2–4]. More frequently, these papers have discussed the age-related changes in performances with an isolated or small number of physiological capacities. As a result, it has been difficult to comprehensively explain the magnitude with which each decline in physiological capacity contributes to the age-related reduction in athletic performance. However, the inter-relationships between physiological capacities and performance have been well documented in endurance, sprint and strength-based events in younger athletes, and as such, indirect inferences can be made to older athletic populations. This chapter will focus on the physiological adaptations that occur with ageing in competitive athletes, and in so doing, highlight those adaptations and factors that are most likely to explain the age-related decline in age-related performance using models proposed from younger populations.

While other chapters (see Chapters 14–18) in this book provide more specific detail on the decrease in performance across a range of sports, this chapter aims to briefly outline the magnitude of the reported decreases in performance with age. The majority of data has demonstrated that performance across endurance, strength and sprint domains decline with age [2–5,12]. Importantly, recent data suggest that anaerobic power and performance traits are more likely to be reduced with age than the subsequent aerobic characteristics [17]. Moreover, the age-related decrease in endurance performance has been reported to be up to three times greater in women compared to men, possibly due to either biological or sociological differences or alternatively selection bias in the available research studies [4]. Briefly, some of the historical data that quantifies the changes in performance will be provided.

2.2.1 Endurance Performance

Previously, age-related declines have been reported by masters athletes in endurance events such as marathon and road running [15,18–20], track endurance running [11,21–24], orienteering [18] and long-distance swimming [12,25–29]. Examples of the age-related decrease in the world records from marathon and 1500-m swimming events are shown in Figure 2.1. As observed, such data demonstrate that the decrease in endurance performance occurs in a curvilinear fashion with the initial decreases occurring after 35 years of age, followed by modest decreases until 50 years of age. Following this, progressive decreases in endurance performance continue until 70 years of age after which the greatest declines in performance occur. Such a curvilinear relationship has been shown to occur in long-distance running [11,18,30,31] and swimming [12,26,29]. Of particular interest,

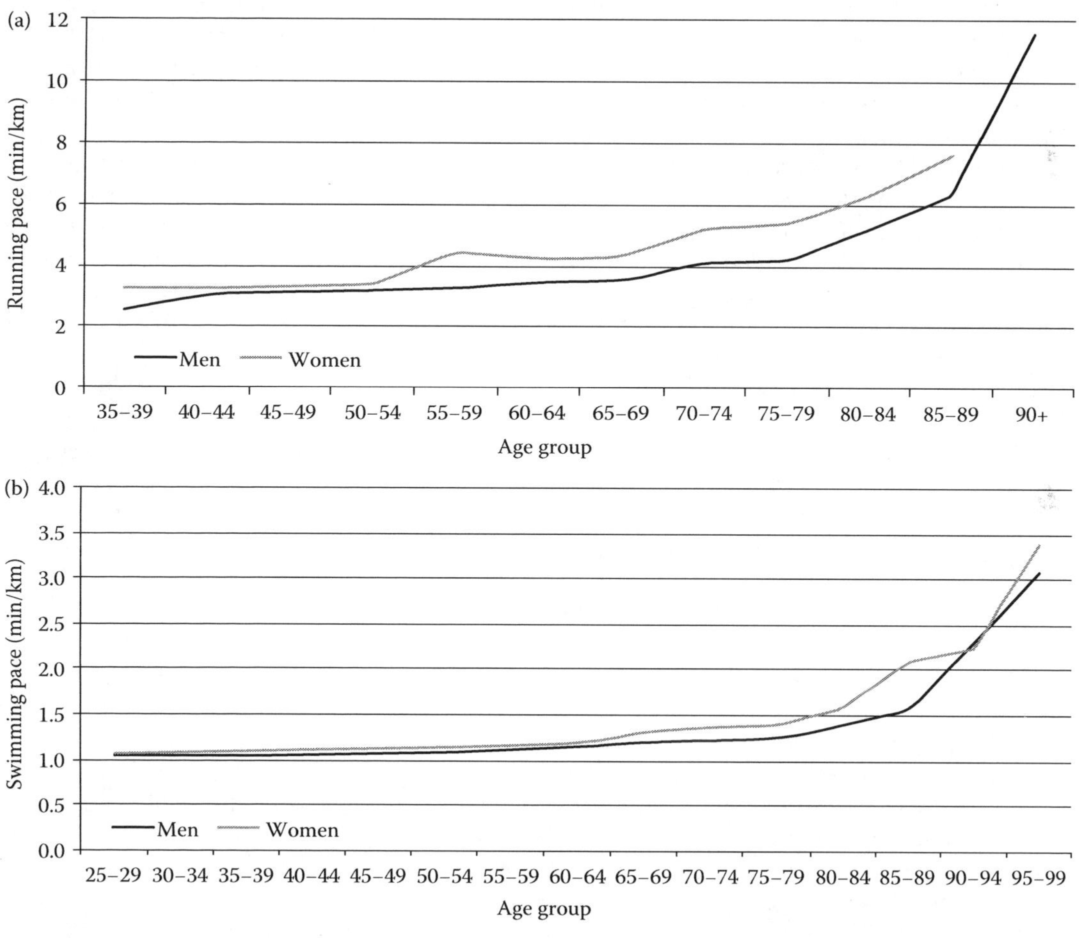

FIGURE 2.1 Respective age group world records for men and women in (a) the marathon and (b) 1500-m freestyle swimming. (From World Masters Athletics, Records. Available at http://www.world-masters-athletics.org/records/, accessed 14 January 2014; FINA, Masters World Records. Available at http://www.fina.org/H2O/index.php?option=com_wrapper&view=wrapper&Itemid=637, accessed 14 January 2014.)

endurance performance may decline earlier in running due to an increased incidence of orthopaedic injuries as a result of continued loading of joints and structures [4]. Alternatively, swimming performances appear to decrease more slowly than land-based activities which may reflect the increased importance of biomechanical techniques rather than physiological capacities and reduced load on joint structures. Hence, examination of swimming data may be more reflective of changes in physiological function that reduce competitive performance.

Previously, Tanaka and Seals observed that females exhibited a greater rate of age-related decline in swimming performance than males across all swim events from 50 to 1500 m [4]. In a follow-up longitudinal study, it was observed that the gender differences in age-related declines in swim performance were only present in the sprint events [12]. In their comment on this research, Tanaka and Seals suggested that this may be due to the greater decline in muscular strength and power of the upper extremities in females than males that may affect sprint performance [4]. On the other hand, the similar decline in long-distance swimming performance compared to males may reflect several factors, including a similar rate of decline in VO_{2max} and the reduced oxygen cost of swimming that has been shown to be particularly evident in females due to their smaller body size, lower body density, greater body fat and shorter legs than men [34].

It is also possible that other physiological factors may influence these age-related declines in endurance performance. Previously, research has suggested that swimming velocity is reduced mainly as a result of a lower stroke frequency until 65 years of age [35]. Beyond this, further decrements in performance may reflect decreases in stroke length that are dependent upon force production capacity and strongly related to swimming velocity and hydrodynamic factors. An earlier and greater decrease in stroke frequency may represent a decreased potential for anaerobic metabolism and/or a reduction in the neural pathways required for faster velocity movements [35]. This may amplify the reported anthropometrical changes that occur with ageing (i.e. ↑ fat mass, ↓ fat-free mass), given the larger surface area that must be moved through and against the water [30]. Regardless, the available research demonstrates that endurance swimming performance declines with age in competitive swimmers as a result of a combination of several physiological, biomechanical and anthropometrical changes.

2.2.2 Sprint and Strength Performance

Briefly, the decline in performance in events dominated by high force and power output suggest that there is an obvious interaction with ageing where decreases in muscular function are widely reported [10,16,36–41]. Numerous studies have conclusively shown a linear age-related decline in both anaerobic and strength sports performance between the ages of 35 and 65–70 years, followed by a quadratic decline in masters athlete performances from track and field [5,11,17,42,43], swimming [12,29,43] and weightlifting [10,16,39,40]. Figure 2.2 shows the current male and female age-group world record trends for the shot put, 400-m track run and long jump.

Continuing to focus on swimming data, Donato and others conducted a 12-year longitudinal study of high performance US Masters swimmers and observed a significant linear 3%–8%·decade^{-1} increase in 50-m swim time for both men and women until 70 years of age [12]. After this age, the reduction in performance is accelerated for both female (15%–16%·decade^{-1}) and male (13%–14%·decade^{-1}) cohorts. Similarly, Korhonen and colleagues reported that 100-m sprint running performance slowed by approximately 7%·decade^{-1} in males and 9%·decade^{-1} in females between 40–80 years of age [44]. A separate sub-sample taken from the European Veterans Athletics Championships (n = 70, age: 35–80 years) demonstrated exponential declines of 5.8%·decade^{-1} (males) and 6.9%·decade^{-1} (females) [44]. Collectively, the reported data demonstrates that the reduction in performance is magnified after 65–70 years of age.

In an earlier study examining the changes in masters athletes world records across a range of sports, Baker and Tang reported that weightlifting demonstrated the greatest decline with increasing age with respect to current elite world record performances [11]. Similarly, other strength- and

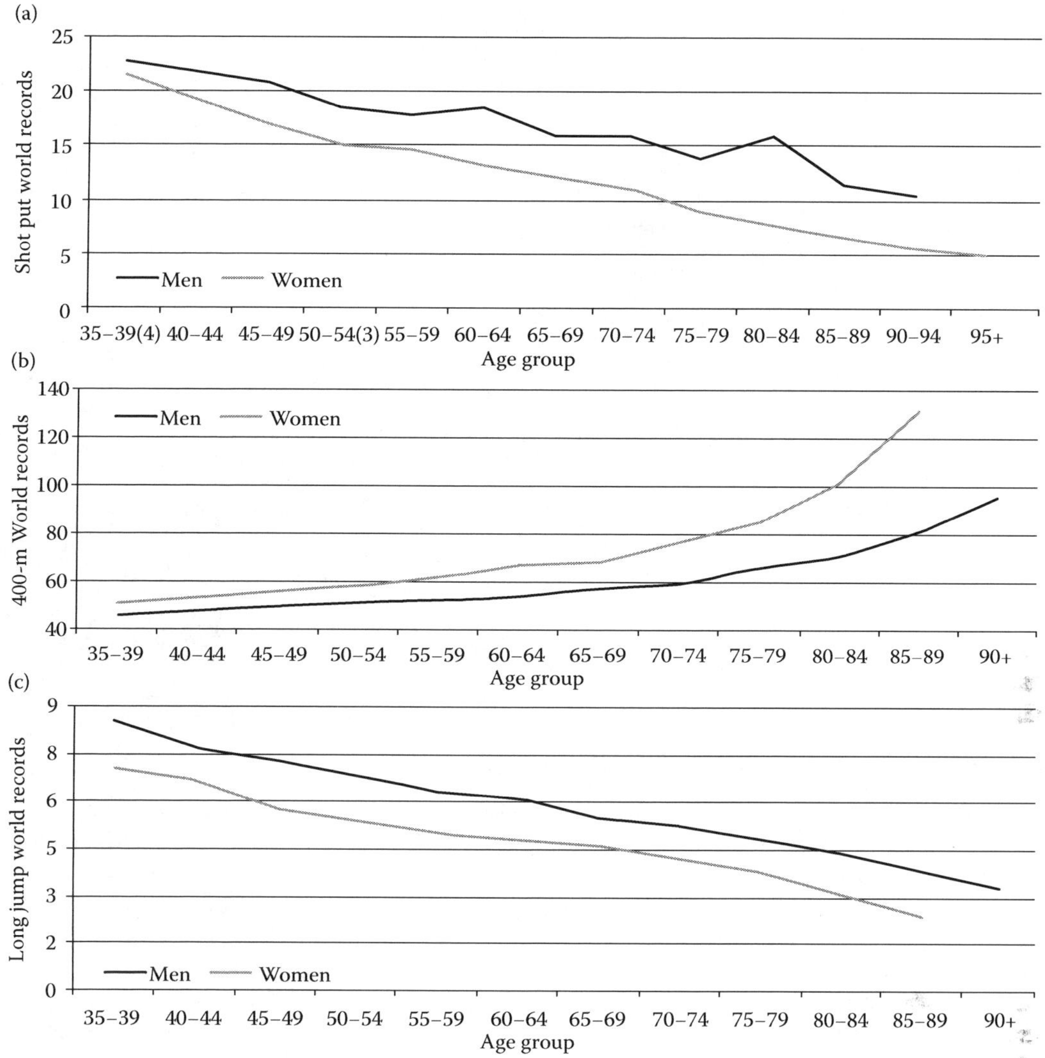

FIGURE 2.2 Respective age group world records for men and women in (a) the shot put, (b) 400-m track running and (c) long jump. (From World Masters Athletics, Records. Available at http://www.world-masters-athletics.org/records/, accessed 14 January 2014.)

power-based sports such as those based on jumping demonstrated a rapid decline in performance with age. The researchers suggested that these age-related declines in performance were reflective of major physiological changes that were occurring in the muscle with age, predominately reflected in a shift in fibre composition away from type II fibres together with a reduced fibre shortening velocity. The work of The and Ploutz-Snyder observed a similar response in the Olympic weight-lifting performance of masters athletes [16]. These researchers propose that the loss in competitive performance reflected a loss of muscle power with advancing age, most likely as a result of an interaction of changes in anthropometrical, histochemical and neuromuscular factors. Clearly, these observed reductions in performance within sprint and strength sports suggest that multiple significant physiological and morphological changes occur which limit the potential for masters athletes to complete high-intensity work and exert a high level of force production that are both needed for sprint and strength events.

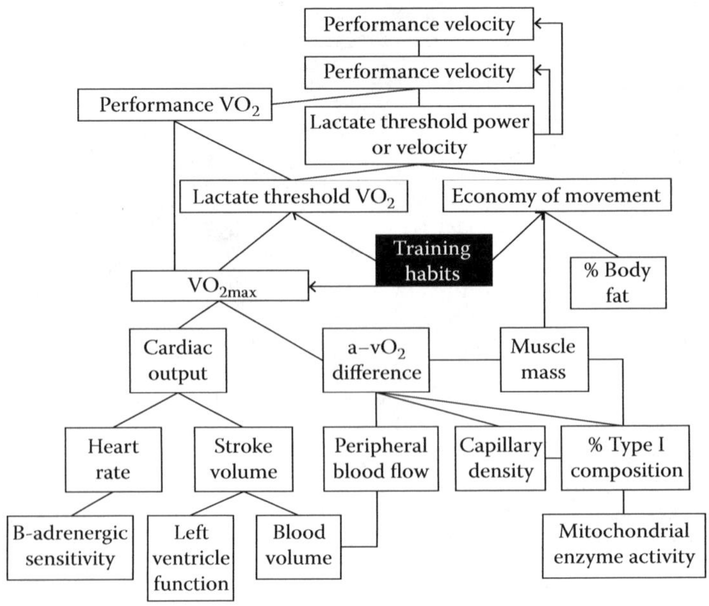

FIGURE 2.3 Physiological factors that may limit endurance performance in masters athletes. (Modified from Coyle, E.F., *Exerc. Sports Sci. Rev.* 23, 25–63, 1995.)

2.3 FACTORS AFFECTING ENDURANCE PERFORMANCE

A proposed model for physiological capacities and factors that relate to endurance performance is shown in Figure 2.3. This model allows us to examine the influence of ageing on the inter-relationships between physiological factors and performance to be examined. For example, it is well documented that VO_{2max} decreases with age after 25–30 years of age in both healthy sedentary control and competitive masters athletes at a rate of around 1%·year^{-1} [46–50]. Given the multi-factorial nature of the contributing factors that limit VO_{2max}, the basis for this observation is poorly understood, with the magnitude of the contribution of either central or peripheral factors widely debated. As demonstrated in Figure 2.3, there is a clear pathway for these functional changes to influence physiological capacities that limit endurance performance.

2.3.1 Maximum Heart Rate

An age-related decrease in an individual's maximum heart rate (HR_{max}) is commonly observed in both male and female endurance athletes, with a decrease of approximately one beat per year after the age of 20 years reported for both ageing athletes and sedentary populations [51]. Tanaka, Monahan and Seals have used both meta-analysis (351 studies, n = 18,712) and laboratory-based maximal treadmill testing (n = 514) to demonstrate that HR_{max} is strongly inversely related to age in both genders in healthy sedentary, active and endurance-trained individuals [52].

The most likely underlying physiological mechanism responsible is an age-related reduction in the sensitivity of beta-adrenergic receptors to catecholamines, although an age-related decrease in sympathetic drive may also contribute [53]. The reduction in sensitivity of the catecholamine receptors has gained support with evidence demonstrating a decrease in HR_{max} in older subjects, despite higher catecholamine concentrations being reported [54]. As such, the reduction in HR_{max} and a resultant contribution to the decline in VO_{2max} appears unavoidable with age.

2.3.2 Maximum Stroke Volume

There is conclusive evidence that maximal stroke volume is reduced with age in masters endurance athletes [55,56]. Ogawa and others observed a significant age-related decline in the maximal stroke volume of endurance-trained men during both submaximal and maximal treadmill exercise when compared to healthy young and older sedentary cohorts [55]. When compared to age-matched sedentary controls, the maximal stroke volume of both male and female masters endurance athletes has been shown to be significantly elevated [57,58]. More recently, Hagmar and others reported a significantly increased stroke volume (45 ± 10 vs. 36 ± 5 $mL \cdot m^{-2}$) in 20 post-menopausal former elite female endurance athletes compared to sedentary controls [57]. Lastly, Nottin and others assessed left ventricular relaxation characteristics and demonstrated that stroke volume was significantly higher and submaximal exercise heart rate was lower in masters athletes than aged-matched sedentary subjects [58]. They suggested that this was most likely a result of an expanded blood volume (see Section 2.3.4) allowing earlier filling of the left ventricle. Taken together, the available data suggest that masters athletes tend to maintain ventricular function as well as stroke volume with age when compared to age-matched sedentary controls.

2.3.3 Cardiac Morphology

Few studies have examined the changes in cardiac structure and function in masters athletes [59–62]. Both cross-sectional and longitudinal studies have shown that endurance training in masters athletes leads to increases in cardiac dimensions [57,61,63], posterior wall thickness and interventricular septum thickness [59,61], as well as left and right ventricular mass compared to age-matched controls [61]. Hagmar and others used echocardiography to demonstrate that both left and right ventricular dimensions were 11% and 14% larger, respectively, in a cohort of currently active former elite female endurance athletes (56 ± 3.5 years) when compared to age-matched sedentary controls [57]. However, these same researchers observed a lack of myocardial hypertrophy in the female masters athletes when compared to measures provided from ageing male exercises [61–63]. These gender differences may reflect hormonal differences, genetic factors, training status or that the blood pressure responses of women during exercise are insufficient to stimulate cardiac hypertrophy. However, such adaptations in cardiac morphology may enhance systolic and diastolic function of the left ventricle, in turn improving cardiac output and helping maintain aerobic capacity into older age.

2.3.4 Blood Volume

Typically, a decrease in blood volume is normally reported with ageing in sedentary healthy populations [60,64,65]. Previous research has reported strong correlations between VO_{2max} and blood volume in both young [66] and older male [67] and female [56] endurance athletes. Hagberg and others reported that compared to age-matched sedentary men, masters athletes possessed significantly higher peak exercise stroke volume indexes (75 vs. 57 $mL \cdot m^{-2}$), 17% larger end-diastolic volume indexes, and larger relative plasma (46 vs. 38 $mL \cdot kg^{-1}$), red cell (30 vs. 26 $mL \cdot kg^{-1}$) and total blood volumes (76 vs. 64 $mL \cdot kg^{-1}$), in addition to a significantly higher VO_{2max} [67]. These findings suggest that a continued expanded blood volume with ageing, typical of younger trained athletes, contributes to a higher peak exercise left ventricular end-diastolic volume, stroke volume and cardiac output. Taken together, the maintenance of these cardiac function assist to maintain VO_{2max} in masters endurance athletes. Further continued exercise and training undertaken by masters athletes may provide chronic volume overload and increased utilization of the Frank-Starling effect to stimulate cardiac hypertrophy and adaptation.

When comparing the central cardiac factors that influence VO_{2max}, it may be suggested that the largest influence is the age-related decrease in HR_{max} as a result of reduced sensitivity to catecholamines, rather than the smaller and more inconsistent changes in stroke volume, cardiac morphology or blood volume. However, when the age-related declines in endurance performance and VO_{2max} are compared, the loss in performance is less than that of aerobic capacity [4]. Thus, it might be suggested that peripheral factors may contribute to the age-related changes in VO_{2max} and alterations in other physiological capacities may help to explain this disproportionate relationship.

2.3.5 Fibre Composition, Morphology and Capillarization

Masters endurance athletes typically tend to maintain or increase the percentage of the oxidative type I muscle fibres [6,68–71] when compared to sedentary ageing individuals [72–75]. Several studies have demonstrated the maintenance of type I fibre composition and age-related changes in the more glycolytic type II fibres [6,69,76–79]. For example, Coggan and others reported that a group of masters (>60 years) endurance-trained runners possessed a similar gastrocnemius fibre composition (59.6 ± 13.6% type I) to a group of younger performance (60.3 ± 9.6%) and training-matched (73.2 ± 10.1%) runners [6]. Interestingly, the type I fibres of the older runners were 34% larger than the younger performance-matched cohort and 25% larger than younger competitive runners. These data highlights that a strong relationship between type I fibre composition and endurance performance is maintained with ageing, typical of younger endurance athletes. Similarly, such a change in muscle fibre composition may have a direct affect on both the nerve conduction and muscle shortening velocities of the muscle, which may directly impact performance. Furthermore, Trappe stated that prolonged endurance training with ageing is likely to cause muscle fibres to show signs of atrophy, weakness and to be less powerful despite an increased conduction velocity [80].

Further to the muscle fibre composition changes observed above, masters athletes typically demonstrate a decreased cross-sectional area (CSA) of type II fibres while maintaining or increasing the CSA of their type I fibres. This is the result of a shift towards a higher expression of the more oxidative fibres discussed above. Previously, Trappe and others have observed a 7% decrease in the type I and IIa fibre area of competitive masters endurance runners compared to age-matched sedentary controls over a 22-year period [71]. However, the longitudinal changes within the muscle most likely will reflect continued training habits of older endurance athletes [70,76,77,79–82]. Alternatively, Proctor and colleagues reported a significant ($p < 0.05$) increase in the area of type I muscle fibres between endurance-trained masters athletes (4424 ± 832 μm²) and sedentary aged-matched controls (3510 ± 813 μm²) [79]. Despite both the mean area of both type IIa and IIx fibres decreasing in the older trained individuals, no significant change was found to have occurred as a result of training. These researchers suggested that the modest hypertrophy of type I fibres observed were consistent with adaptations of chronic endurance training [79]. They also hypothesised that ageing produces natural atrophy of type IIa and type IIx fibres in the lower limbs of individuals, which is most likely caused by a reduction in the training intensity in older life. Proctor et al. suggested that prolonged endurance training may not be of sufficient training intensity to reverse the age-associated atrophy of Type II fibres, due to a failure to provide an intensity which would provide frequent recruitment of these fibres [79]. Finally, Coggan et al. reported that the masters athletes showed a significantly lower type II:I fibre CSA ratio (0.92 ± 0.15) than both the matched (1.15 ± 0.12) and competitive runners (1.23 ± 0.28) [83]. This ratio demonstrates the moderate hypertrophy of type I fibres and the selective atrophy of type II fibres CSA with ageing, even in competitive older athletes.

The age-related changes in both muscle fibre composition and CSA in masters athletes have been shown to facilitate changes within measures of capillarization and the oxidative metabolism potential within the muscle that may benefit endurance performance [83–86]. Coggan and others reported greater measures of capillarization in masters endurance runners compared against a cohort of performance-matched younger runners with capillary density (388 ± 93 vs. 367 ± 60 cap·mm^{-2}), capillary to fibre ratio (2.44 ± 0.36 vs. 1.86 ± 0.41) and CC (5.88 ± 0.86 vs. 4.79 ± 0.77 contacts/capillary), respectively [83]. Furthermore, an 18-year longitudinal study of 33 male masters endurance-trained runners (42–72 years) reported a higher degree of capillarization when compared to young and old sedentary controls [86]. Taken together, these results demonstrate that capillarization within muscles is maintained or improved in individuals that maintain training into older age [83,84], which is in contrast to the data available on the capillarization trends reported in sedentary ageing [87]. The reported maintenance and increased capillarization measures may help to compensate for the larger type I muscle fibres that have been reported in masters athletes, given that this would increase oxygen diffusion distance and slow oxygen delivery to muscle during exercise [88].

2.3.6 Oxidative Metabolism

The age-related changes in the muscle fibre properties reported above imply that the oxidative potential within the muscle is influenced by both ageing and training. Such changes in fibre composition have an obvious impact on the activities of substrate pathways and oxidative enzymes responsible for aerobic adenosine triphosphate (ATP) production within the muscle [89,90]. In sedentary ageing, it would appear that muscle oxidative capacity is somewhat maintained, with the capacity for anaerobic energy production reduced, a result that reflects an age-related loss of type II fibres [89,91,92]. However, other data suggest that ageing *per se* has a negative impact on oxidative characteristics such as aerobic enzyme activities (i.e. citrate synthase [CS], succinate dehydrogenase [SDH], 2-oxogluterate-dehydrogenase [2-OGDH], β-hydroxy-CoA dehydrogenase [β-HAD]) activity [71,79,83,93–96], mitochondrial uncoupling [97] and/or the delivery of O_2 due to capillary atrophy [84,98].

Contrasting evidence has been produced on changes in oxidative enzyme characteristics of masters endurance athletes [70,98]. Firstly, Coggan and others have reported that older (~60 years) endurance-trained masters athletes possessed significantly lower activities of CS and increased activities of SDH and β-HAD than a younger, training-matched cohort [98]. In contrast, Trappe and others reported that SDH activity was maintained across 20 years of ageing in a cohort of highly trained endurance runners [70]. Of particular interest was the finding from Trappe and colleagues that demonstrated that the activity of CS and SDH within the thigh were able to discriminate between highly trained, fitness-trained and untrained older men [70].

Taken together, the above results suggest that the oxidative potential (capacity to generate ATP using aerobic metabolism) may be maintained or slightly decreased with age [6,71,79,94–96,98]. The limited changes in the oxidative enzyme activities observed in masters endurance athletes suggest that mitochondrial function is well-maintained, which may differ from sedentary ageing where an increase in mitochondrial uncoupling and decrease in phosphate substrate kinetics has been reported [85,89,92,97]. Furthermore, the suggestion that the glycolytic capacity of muscle decreases with age may directly influence the capacity for high-intensity work and the ability of masters endurance athletes to maintain a high work capacity above lactate threshold.

2.3.7 Body Composition

Significant changes occur in body composition with advanced ageing in both sedentary and competitive individuals although the reported changes are more attenuated in active subjects. Typically these changes result in increases in the percentage of body fat and reductions in muscle mass [4,30,99–101]. Pollock et al. reported that within both moderate- and high-intensity trained cohorts of masters track runners, body mass was consistently maintained and body fat percentage increased by between 2%–2.5%·decade^{-1} across a 20-year longitudinal study [30]. Similar increases were observed in waist circumference across the latter half of the study, whereas peripheral girths (hip, thigh and bicep) remained more stable. The above data suggest that muscle mass appears to reduce with advancing age with increasing body fat percentage to allow body mass to remain relatively stable with ageing.

The age-related increase in body fat appears to be more evident on the central aspect of the trunk which most likely reflects preferred sights for adipose tissue formation. Of interest, Yataco and colleagues reported that when compared to sedentary age-matched controls, masters athletes were leaner and displayed lipoprotein profiles similar to younger individuals [102]. These researchers proposed that the more favourable lipid profile in the masters athletes was largely due to their leaner body composition. Collectively, the maintenance of an athletic body composition appears to convey significant health benefits for masters athletes. Moreover, body composition maintenance also affords a positive effect on performance through better maintenance of skeletal muscle mass, oxidative capacities and exercise economy.

A commonly reported outcome of ageing is a decrease in muscle mass [19,103–106], which appears to have a direct effect on the age-related decline in VO_{2max} and performance [107,108]. These changes in muscle mass will directly influence biomechanical factors as well as exercise intensity and economy which may increase the requirement for ATP production through oxidative metabolism in endurance athletes of any age. As such, it is likely that muscle mass also has an indirect influence on change in VO_{2max}. Previously, Fleg and Lakatta have reported a significant positive correlation between VO_{2max} and creatinine excretion (reflective of muscle mass) in both men and women [108]. The variance in the decline of VO_{2max} that was attributable to age declined from 60% to 14% in men and from 50% to 8% in women when corrected for muscle mass. Other studies have examined the relationship between decline in endurance performance and VO_{2max} and lean body mass in masters athletes [55,109]. Proctor and Joyner suggested that approximately 50% of the difference in whole-body lean body mass could be explained by reduced appendicular muscle mass between young and masters athletes [110]. As a result, ~14% of the age differences in VO_{2max} relative to appendicular muscle mass could be explained by this age-related reduction in muscle mass.

More recently, Hawkins and others examined the longitudinal changes in VO_{2max}, HR_{max}, muscle mass and training volume in 86 male (53.9 ± 1.1 years) and 49 female (49.1 ± 1.2 years) masters endurance runners over 8.5 years [51]. As expected and discussed earlier, VO_{2max} and HR_{max} declined significantly regardless of gender or age. However, one of the most interesting findings from this research was that men with the greatest loss in VO_{2max} had the greatest loss in lean body mass. This data appear to confirm that there is a relationship between declines in both muscle mass and VO_{2max} in masters athletes. It also highlights that maintenance of muscle mass may be vital for preserving physiological function and athletic performance in masters endurance athletes.

Importantly, continued strength training into older age appears to facilitate small increases in muscle mass in previously sedentary individuals [111] although this increase may be limited [112]. However, it appears that chronic endurance training into older age does not maintain overall muscle mass [77,78,113–115]. Collectively, these studies showed that masters endurance athletes maintain similar muscle masses compared to age-matched sedentary controls, though somewhat reduced relative to younger sedentary or young endurance-trained individuals. These data strongly demonstrate the need for masters athletes to continue some form of resistance training into older age to maintain their muscle mass in order to limit its affect on other physiological capacities and endurance performance. Similarly, preservation of muscle mass with ageing is also vital for the maintenance of other physiological capacities such as anaerobic capacity, strength and homeostatic metabolic function.

2.3.8 Lactate Threshold

Strictly defined, lactate threshold (LT) is defined as the exercise intensity $(\%VO_{2max})$ at which blood lactate increases significantly above baseline level and has previously been identified as a key indicator of endurance performance in younger athletes [116,117]. There are no data to suggest that this relationship changes in masters-level endurance athletes. In support of this, endurance performance has been correlated to both VO_{2max} and velocity at LT in both highly trained older male [31,118] and female runners [19,49]. When expressed as a percentage of VO_{2max}, LT does not appear to decrease significantly with age in either male [119,120] or female [19,49] distance runners. Allen and others reported that despite being matched for 10-km running performance, male masters runners (56 ± 5 years) had a significantly lower (–9%) VO_{2max} than young runners (25 ± 3 years) [119]. While running economy was not significantly different, the masters runners reached LT at a higher percentage of their VO_{2max} (92% vs. 89%), which allowed LT to occur at the same absolute running velocity and oxygen consumption in both groups. Similarly, a longitudinal study by Wiswell and others reported that LT relative to VO_{2max} $(\%VO_{2max})$ did not differ between older male and female endurance runners and increased significantly with age in both groups [120]. Taken together, these data demonstrate that LT appears to be consistently maintained with ageing and continued endurance training. This in turn may help to preserve or improve endurance performance in older individuals who continue high-intensity endurance training into older age.

Other research has examined changes in the maximal lactate steady state (MLSS), defined as the highest blood lactate concentration maintained (± 1 $mmol{\cdot}L^{-1}$) across the last 20 min of a 30-min constant-workload test. Mattern and others assessed the MLSS and VO_{2max} in three age groups: young (25.9 ± 1.0 years), middle-aged (43.2 ± 1.0 years) and older (64.6 ± 2.7 years) male competitive cyclists and triathletes matched for training intensity and duration [121]. As expected, significant differences were reported for VO_{2max} among all age groups: 67.7 ± 1.2 $mL{\cdot}kg^{-1}{\cdot}min^{-1}$, 56.0 ± 2.6 $mL{\cdot}kg^{-1}{\cdot}min^{-1}$, 47.0 ± 2.6 $mL{\cdot}kg^{-1}{\cdot}min^{-1}$ in the young, middle-aged and older endurance athletes, respectively. Similarly, a significant age-related decrease in the relative MLSS exercise intensity $(\%VO_{2max})$: 80.8 ± 0.9%, 76.1 ± 1.4%, 69.9 ± 1.5% was also reported. Thus, it would appear that the velocity at race pace and lactate steady state as well as the maximal aerobic capacity all significantly decline with age in endurance athletes.

2.3.9 Maximal Aerobic Capacity

As mentioned above, it is well known that VO_{2max} is a major contributor to endurance performance and a continued decline in VO_{2max} exists with age in highly trained male and female endurance athletes [19,50,122–126]. VO_{2max} is a function of both central (cardiac output) and peripheral (oxygen extraction and utilisation) factors that interact during exercise in order to aerobically produce ATP stores [127]. In both young adults and endurance athletes under 40 years of age, VO_{2max} appears to be a strong predictor of running speed for run distances such as 5 and 10 km [128,129]. However, it may not necessary be a strong predictor of endurance performance in older cohorts [19,31,130].

As expected, the VO_{2max} of endurance-trained athletes is significantly higher when compared to similar-aged sedentary individuals, with the rate of decline in VO_{2max} in masters athletes reported to be reduced [46,47], similar [49] or greater [123] when compared to age-matched sedentary individuals. Taken together, the available data estimates that VO_{2max} declines by approximately $10\%{\cdot}decade^{-1}$ after the age of 25 years in sedentary ageing individuals [123]. In contrast, this age-related decline is reported to be approximately $5\%{\cdot}decade^{-1}$ in endurance-trained masters athletes [67,109,131,132].

The age-related reduction in VO_{2max} has also been established across both cross-sectional and longitudinal studies of ageing male and female endurance athletes [30,46,67,109,120,122,123,125,126,133–136], suggesting that it is inevitable that VO_{2max} decreases with age, regardless of training status. In their longitudinal study, Kasch and others measured VO_{2max} in 12 physically active men aged 44–79 years of age after 10, 15, 20 and 25 years of follow-up after an initial investigation [46]. The VO_{2max} of the cohort was 60% greater than those reported for sedentary men of similar age [107,136,137]. The age-related decline in VO_{2max} was 13% ($5\%{\cdot}decade^{-1}$) over the 25-year period which equated to a rate of decline per annum of 0.24 $mL{\cdot}kg^{-1}{\cdot}min^{-1}$ for the ageing athletes. In context, this was half of the 0.45 $mL{\cdot}kg^{-1}{\cdot}min^{-1}$ previously reported for sedentary ageing men [107].

Gender differences have been reported in the rate of age-related decline in VO_{2max} in masters endurance athletes [122,138]. Brown and others reported declines of 0.65 $mL \cdot kg^{-1} \cdot min^{-1} \cdot yr^{-1}$ and 0.39 $mL \cdot kg^{-1} \cdot min^{-1} yr^{-1}$ in male (n = 36; 17–64 years) and female (n = 20; 16–54 years) in high-performance older cyclists, respectively [122]. Therefore, it would appear that ageing female athletes may maintain their VO_{2max} better than their male counterparts; however, this may be offset by the higher initial VO_{2max} values reported for young male athletes when compared to their female counterparts. Taken together, while the age-related reduction in VO_{2max} cannot be completely halted through continued physical training, it appears that the rate of the decline can be slowed [4,30,71,125,134]. The maintenance of VO_{2max} may aid in endurance exercise ability into older age.

2.3.10 Exercise Economy

Exercise economy (defined as the oxygen cost to exercise at a given exercise intensity [velocity or % VO_{2max}]) is also a major determining factor in endurance performance. Exercise economy has been shown to be a stronger predictor of endurance performance than VO_{2max} in a homogenous group of young endurance athletes [85]. However, few studies have reported on changes in exercise economy in masters endurance athletes [19,119,139]. Previously, Allen and co-workers reported similar running economies for both young (25 ± 3 years) and older (56 ± 5 years) well-trained runners [119]. Similarly, Evans and others examined whether the age-related decline in 10-km run performance in females was directly associated with decreases in VO_{2max}, lactate threshold or running economy in 31 highly trained female runners [19]. As expected, 10-km race pace declined significantly with age, though 10-km performance and age were not correlated with running economy in the highly trained and competitive female endurance runners [19]. Thus, exercise economy appears not to change with age in masters endurance athletes, suggesting that decreases in endurance performance are not related to a lower economy of exercise. This may also reflect the increased relative oxidative potential of older masters athletes due to a reduction in their glycolytic capacity, or similarly, reflect an age-related reduction in body mass that maintains exercise economy despite the inevitable declines in VO_{2max}.

Taken together, these data clearly demonstrate that a range of physiological and morphological changes occur with ageing to decrease endurance performance. There is a growing body of evidence that links these factors to changes in sports performance. In turn, these adaptations interact to influence physiological capacities such as LT and VO_{2max} that directly affect endurance exercise performance. Similarly, the ability of masters athletes to perform in sports reliant on speed and strength appears to also reduce with age due to age-related changes in a range of physiological and morphological factors.

2.4 FACTORS AFFECTING SPRINT AND STRENGTH PERFORMANCE

While the factors contributing to the age-related reduction in endurance performance in masters athletes has been examined in depth, fewer research investigations have examined the age-related decline in anaerobic performance or the physiological changes contributing to speed and strength performance in masters athletes [3].

Anaerobic energy production involves the replenishment of ATP from both the creatine kinase (CK) and adenylate kinase pathways (ATP-phosphocreatine [PCr] system), as well as the glycogenolysis and glycolysis pathways (lactic system). In order to systematically inform the current review, the influence of several influential factors towards anaerobic performance as proposed by Bouchard et al. will be discussed [140]. Typically, these factors are within the working muscle, and limit ATP production and/or neuromuscular recruitment during high-intensity exercise. A flowchart highlighting the suggested age-affected factors that may limit anaerobic performance is shown in Figure 2.4.

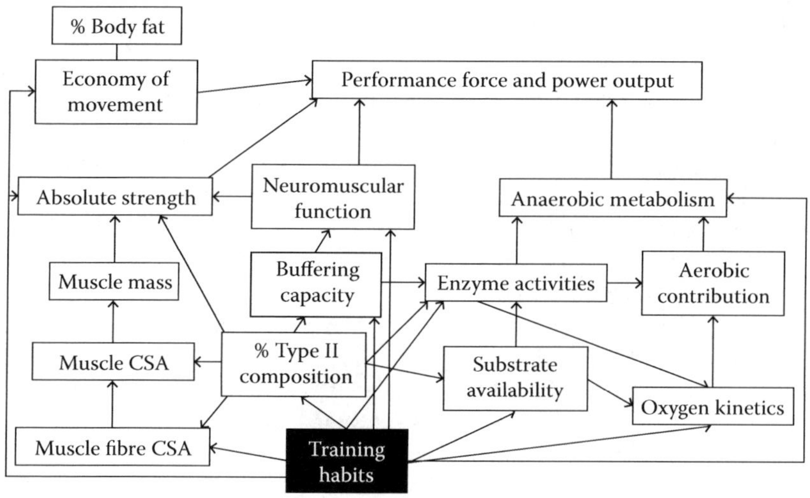

FIGURE 2.4 Physiological factors that may limit anaerobic performance in masters athletes.

2.4.1 Muscle Mass

While the role of muscle mass in endurance exercise performance of older athletes has been discussed above, it is also vital in maintaining sprint and strength performance in masters athletes. As reported above, an age-related decline in active muscle mass is a consistent finding in ageing non-athletic individuals [105,141,142] and both endurance-trained [77,78] and sprint-trained masters athletes [143]. Moreover, previous research has shown that muscle mass is highly related to anaerobic work capacity in both young men and women [140,144,145]. Furthermore, Makrides and others observed that total work performed during a maximal 30-second cycle ergometry test in 100 older sedentary males and females was strongly related (r = 0.84) to lean thigh volume, albeit estimated anthropometrically [146]. Other earlier studies have also demonstrated similar reductions in muscle mass of the quadriceps muscles using autopsy and computerized tomography with ageing [38,141]. Such data support previous data which has suggested that reductions in active muscle mass, at least in older sedentary individuals, is related to maximal short-term anaerobic performance [147].

In contrast, there exists some evidence to suggest that older strength-trained athletes may be able maintain muscle mass with age [40,78]. For example, Klitgaard et al. observed that elderly men (68 ± 0.8 years) with 12–17 years of heavy resistance training three times a week had muscle fibre sizes similar to young (28 ± 1.0 years) sedentary controls [78]. More recently, a general increase in muscle fibre areas and significant increase in type IIA fibre area has been reported in elite male and female masters sprinters (66 ± 3 years; 32 ± 7 training years) across a 20-week training program that consisted of combined sprint and strength/power training [143]. Importantly, significant increases were reported for strength, power, rate of force development, stride length, as well as 10- and 60-m sprint run performance. These findings also support previous data that have compared type I, IIA and IIX muscle fibre areas of elderly (68–78 years) endurance- and strength-trained athletes who were trained for over 50 years [76]. As expected, both muscle fibre size and mechanical muscle performance were improved in those individuals exposed to lifelong strength training.

Taken together, the above data suggest that heavy resistance training combined with high-power exercises may help prevent decreases muscle mass through protecting against type II fibre atrophy commonly observed in older individuals. In turn, the maintenance of type II fibre size may attenuate losses in explosive muscular power and strength as well as decreased sprint performance in masters athletes.

2.4.2 Muscle Fibre Composition

The reported age-related decrease in muscle mass may be in part due to either a reduction in muscle fibre number, a reduction in fibre CSA, or a combination of the two [36,141]. A common finding with ageing research is the loss of muscle fibre numbers with increasing age. Direct evidence for loss of muscle fibres with age was originally obtained by counting muscle fibres in autopsied thigh muscle in previously healthy individuals aged between 15 to 83 years [141]. Of particular interest was that these researchers reported a reduction in the total number of muscle fibres with no apparent effect for a particular fibre type. This is in contrast to the typical suggestion that in sedentary older cohorts there is a reduction in the number of type II fibres. This finding has been verified by several needle biopsy studies taken from the *vastus lateralis* in healthy, non-athletic individuals, particularly during the seventh decade of life [74,141,148–150].

In contrast, Korhonen et al. observed no age-related differences in fibre type distribution when comparing the fibre composition of young (18–33 years) and older (53–77 years) national- and international-level sprint runners [143]. These data agree with earlier findings where no significant difference in fibre composition was observed between chronically (>35 years) trained sprint- or endurance-trained masters runners and training volume and body mass-matched younger runners [151]. However, when the fibre composition data and corresponding fibre area were combined to form the relative fibre type area, there was an age-related increase in type I fibre area and a trend towards a decrease in the area of type IIB fibres with age [143]. Similarly, Reaburn observed a significant age-related decline in type II fibre area in older (>60 years) and long-term trained (>35 years) sprint runners compared to younger sprint runners [151].

Taken together, these findings suggest that highly trained masters sprint runners experience the normal age-related decrease in relative type II fibre area and a shift towards a slower myosin heavy chain (MHC) isoform profile that plays a major role in the rate of force development within muscles involved in sprint and strength performance.

2.4.3 Muscle Fibre Size

Recently, a multivariate analysis demonstrated that muscle CSA was the strongest factor that limited maximal strength performance [152]. Such decreases in muscle CSA reported in ageing studies commonly relate to the loss and atrophy of type II fibres which in turn are proposed to contribute to the age-related declines in strength and speed performance observed in older individuals. In sedentary ageing individuals, one of the most consistent findings is an age-related decrease in the size of type II muscle fibres [72,153,154]. Lexell and others observed no decrease in type I fibre size and reported a decrease in the type II muscle fibre CSA by 26% in individuals aged between 20–80 years [141]. However, data suggest that this trend may be slowed by older athletes who continue to engage in high-intensity resistance and sprint training [76,143,155]. Recent evidence from Korhonen and others suggest that while ageing sprint runners exhibit significant age-related declines in the CSA of the different type II muscle fibres, the declines were not different for type IIA (6.7%·decade^{-1}) or type IIB (11.3%·decade^{-1}) [143].

Taken together, these recent data suggest that high-intensity sprint training combined with power and strength training into older age may help reduce the decrease in type II fibre size and thus possibly slow the age-related decline in speed and strength performance commonly observed in masters athletes. Interestingly, beyond 65–70 years of age, there is a dramatic reduction in fibre size appears that is evident in all fibre types, particularly in the glycolytic type II [98,149,156–158]. Korhonen and others have observed significantly larger type I fibres than type IIB fibres in 60-plus-year-old sprint runners compared to younger runners 18–59 years of age [143]. This finding may help explain the quadratic versus linear rate of decline in performance within speed and strength sports in masters athletes [3,74,159,160].

2.4.4 Muscle Architecture

In addition to muscle CSA, a muscle's geometry (angles and lengths of the muscle's fibres or fascicles) strongly influences force production and thus anaerobic performance and strength performance [140,161,162]. Changes in muscle architecture have been proposed to partially explain the decreases in muscular strength associated with ageing [161]. The limited data available suggest that normal ageing is accompanied by both a decrease in fascicle angle and length, which appears to accompany the well-observed decrease in muscle mass in sedentary ageing individuals [161,163]. However, it appears that heavy and long-term weight training may attenuate this decline, at least in fascicle length [161].

A more recent study investigated the contribution of muscle architecture to both isometric and isokinetic torque-velocity and power-velocity relationships in older (69–82 years) and younger (19–35 years) men [163]. The age-related decrease in muscle strength and power can be partially explained through decreases in both muscle CSA and fibre fascicle length, in addition to a change towards more oxidative fibre composition. Further research needs to examine the role of neural factors in the expression of maximal strength and power. Collectively, the changes in fibre number and area as well as the alterations in muscle architecture contribute to strength declines with age and thus, anaerobic performance.

2.4.5 Neuromuscular Factors

Neural factors may also play a role in the age-related decline in both muscular strength and speed performance in masters athletes. In elite masters sprint runners, the rate of force development (RFD) has been shown to decrease significantly with age at approximately 9.7%·decade^{-1}, with the time taken to reach peak RFD almost doubling between the 18–33 years group and the >70 years group in sprint runners [143]. Crucially, there were strong correlations between the RFD and time taken to reach peak RFD to the MHC II isoform content, which decreased significantly with age while MHC I isoform content significantly increased with age. Thus, it appears that there is a slowing of muscle contractile velocity due to age-related increases in muscle cells expressing the slow MHC isoform in masters athletes, a finding commonly observed in sedentary ageing individuals [164,165]. More research is warranted into the neuromuscular changes that occur in masters athletes with age, as currently little is known in this important factor affecting muscle strength, power and speed and thus sports performance in masters athletes.

2.4.6 Availability of Substrates

Importantly, speed and strength capacities are limited by the availability of high-energy substrates such as PCr and glycogen that may limit the ATP production during maximal intensity exercise [140,143]. Intramuscular concentrations of PCr in the thigh musculature have been shown to be lower (5%) in older sedentary men and women (52–79 years) compared with younger adults (18–36 years) [166]. Furthermore, the same researchers reported similar trends in the total nucleotide pool, despite no such age-effect in resting ATP or adenosine monophosphate (AMP) concentrations. In support, using magnetic resonance spectroscopy, McCully and others reported a significant age-related decrease in the ratio of PCr to inorganic phosphate [167]. Interestingly, Moller and Brandt demonstrated that the ratios between PCr/total creatine and ATP/ADP could be increased with cycling training in a group of older, previously sedentary adults [166]. As such, these researchers concluded that age-related changes of intramuscular phosphagens in elderly subjects may be, at least in part, due to physical inactivity. While the above data suggest that age-related changes in high-energy substrates may also contribute to the decrease in anaerobic performance observed in aged sedentary population, no data have detailed the effects of age on the PCr availability in well-trained older athletes.

Similarly, limited research has examined the effects of age on glycogen concentrations within the musculature of either ageing sedentary populations or masters athletes. The available evidence has shown that resting muscle glycogen significantly declines with age in sedentary populations, with muscle glycogen levels being 61% higher in sedentary young men (~24 years) compared to sedentary older (~65 years) men [168,169]. Furthermore, glycogen content has been significantly correlated with the glycogen synthase protein content which is inversely correlated with age [170]. In summary, declines in the availability of the major substrates used in anaerobic and strength performance may contribute to age-related declines in anaerobic performance observed in masters athletes.

2.4.7 Efficiency of Metabolic Pathways

The anaerobic energy systems refer to the enzymatic breakdown of stored PCr and ATP, as well as the breakdown of glucose and glycogen to lactic acid via glycolysis without consuming oxygen [127]. It is well known that PCr metabolism is limited by CK activity across a reversible reaction that occurs in the cytosol of the cell. Previously, CK activity has been shown to be 21% lower in the *obliquus internus abdominis* muscle of older (61–74 years) men compared to middle-aged (29–54 years) men [171]. This finding supports previous data that have reported age-related decreases in CK in human skeletal muscle [172].

In contrast, other studies have observed no age-related change in CK activity within weight-bearing muscles such as *vastus lateralis*, *gastrocnemius* or *ankle dorsi flexors* [7,173,174]. Furthermore, Lanza and others reported that the rate of PCr hydrolysis and the overall and peak glycolytic rate were significantly faster in young (20–35 years) versus older (65–80 years) men during a 60-second all-out cycling sprint [174]. As such, older subjects, whether sedentary or trained, appear to be more reliant on oxidative ATP production and derive a smaller proportion of their ATP from anaerobic metabolism. Together, these data might suggest that the capacity of the ATP-PCr system is compromised in masters athletes, which may limit anaerobic performance in this cohort.

Anaerobic glycolysis is responsible for the formation of ATP within the cytosol, and is largely regulated by the enzymes phosphofructokinase (PFK) and lactate dehydrogenase (LDH). An important by-product of anaerobic metabolism is lactic acid, which, when dissociated to lactate and hydrogen ions (H^+), resulting in a decrease in muscle and blood pH. Data on age-related changes in the glycolytic pathway enzymes of ageing sedentary individuals are equivocal [6,98,156,173,175]. A cross-sectional study by Coggan and others observed no differences in LDH, PFK or phosphorylase activity in the *gastrocnemius* muscle of sedentary young (26 ± 1 years) and older (64 ± 1 years) individuals [98]. In contrast, a 5-year longitudinal study by Aniansson and others reported a significant decrease in the LDH activity of the thigh of physically active men from the age of 76 to 80 years of age [156]. However, more recent research also suggests that LDH activity is markedly decreased in older adults, at least from studies that have examined LDH activity in abdominal muscles [171,176]. Again, while Pastoris and others support this finding of a decreased LDH activity in abdominal muscles, the same research team reported no changes in LDH activity in locomotive muscles (*vastus lateralis* or *gluteus maximus*) in 76 sedentary subjects (32 males, 44 females) aged 15–91 years of age [176]. In summary, the limited available data suggest that a decline in some glycolytic enzymes may contribute to the observed age-related decline in anaerobic performance and strength that has been observed in masters athletes.

As highlighted above, continued anaerobic glycolysis results in localised metabolic acidosis due to an accumulation of H^+. This decrease in muscle pH causes an increased need for calcium for tension development, an inhibition of effective cross bridge cycling and inhibition of enzymes that regulate glycolytic flux, thus leading to a decrease in speed and strength capacities [177,178]. Though the validity of its use has been questioned, peak blood lactate concentration is sometimes used as an indirect measure of glycolytic capacity [179]. Previously, peak blood lactate concentration has been reported to be lower in sedentary men aged 60–70 years when compared to young men aged 20–30 years following a maximal 30-second cycle ergometer test [9,180]. Similarly, masters athletes have also shown an age-related decrease in peak blood lactate following both maximal sprint running [181] and swimming [182]. Studies on large numbers of high-performance masters swimmers (52 males and 56 females aged 40–79 years) [182] and track sprinters (81 males and 75 females aged 35–88 years) [181] competing in international-level competition have conclusively shown that peak blood lactate concentration following maximal anaerobic exercise decreases with age. Both studies demonstrated that the peak blood lactate values observed were much higher than values reported for aged-matched sedentary men and women.

The H^+ ions produced during anaerobic glycolysis may be partly sequestered by the body's buffering system, predominately the bicarbonate system which associates with the H^+ ion to form carbonic acid that then dissociates to carbon dioxide and water [127]. The limited data related to buffering capacity in older individuals suggest that there is a 6%–7% increase in blood acidity and 12%–16% reduction in blood bicarbonate ion concentration between 20 and 80 years of age [183]. More specifically, a previous study observed similar muscle buffering capacity within young (20–35 years) and old (65–80 years) sedentary men following a 60-second maximal voluntary isometric contraction of the ankle dorsiflexor muscles, despite a lower pH and greater glycolytic rate being observed in the younger men [174]. These data again suggest that older individuals rely more on oxidative pathways for ATP resynthesise during anaerobic performance while younger persons rely more on the PCr and glycolytic pathways, possibly as a result of common finding of a younger population possessing a greater type II muscle fibre area compared to older individuals [6,98,176], a common finding in both anaerobic [143,151] and endurance [77,151] masters athletes.

2.4.8 Contribution of Aerobic Energy System

Differences in the contribution of the aerobic energy system during high-intensity exercise may also play a significant role in the observed age-related decline in maximal short-term work performance such as speed and strength. In highly trained young athletes, the aerobic energy system contributes an increasingly greater percentage of the overall energy demand the longer the anaerobic performance duration [184–188]. An increasing number of studies have examined the aerobic contribution to anaerobic performance in older sedentary or masters athlete populations [17,146,179,180,189–194]. Early work by Makrides and others reported that the total maximal work performed in 30 seconds declined linearly for both ageing males and females by about $6\% \cdot decade^{-1}$ [146]. This finding strongly suggests that aerobic capacity is related to anaerobic performance in older individuals. This is strengthened by data that high-intensity endurance training in older sedentary individuals significantly improves 30-second maximal exercise capacity by 12.5% [195]. Therefore, in trained older individuals it appears that the ability to utilise both the aerobic and anaerobic energy systems during maximal exercise is maintained.

Importantly, the proportion of aerobic contribution to anaerobic energy metabolism is largely influenced by the initial speed of the oxygen uptake response at the onset of exercise. Previously, Babcock and colleagues reported that the increase in oxygen consumption was slowed with ageing in sedentary individuals, but later demonstrated that physical training increases that speed of the VO_2 response in older individuals [189,190]. More recently, it has been reported that sedentary older individuals (68 ± 3 years) demonstrated a slower VO_2 response to both moderate and high-intensity exercise when compared to a younger (26 ± 3 years) cohort [193,194]. However, concurrent training into older age has been shown to ameliorate the moderate-intensity VO_2 response speed in sprint and endurance-trained athletes between the ages of 45–85 years [192]. From their work, Berger and colleagues reported that sprint-trained masters athletes demonstrated a slower VO_2 response than aged-matched endurance trained cohorts between 46–55 years, 56–65 years, 66–75 years and >76 years of age [192]. Interestingly, the sprint-trained veteran athletes developed increasingly slowed VO_2 responses as age increased between 56–65 and 66–75 years, while the endurance-trained athletes showed no effect of age.

Taken together these findings suggest that ageing sprint-trained athletes are likely to possess slowed VO_2 response to exercise, which most likely reflects changes in muscle fibre characteristics and enzyme activities as discussed earlier. This slowed VO_2 response may increase the anaerobic contribution to energy production at the onset of exercise, which results in a greater disturbance in the metabolic homeostasis within the muscle, or alternatively, facilitate a decrease in the power output to match the available energy resources that is likely to decrease sprint performance. Given the importance of the aerobic contribution to anaerobic performance, it is possible that the lower VO_2 max of masters athletes [101,122] and slower oxygen uptake responses [189,190,192–194] may contribute to the age-related decreases in anaerobic performance observed in laboratory-based studies and sprint events from a range of sports. Together with reductions in muscle mass, changes in type II fibre composition and/or size and glycolytic enzyme activities, it could be suggested that the age-related reduction in sprint and strength capacities in masters athletes is reliant upon changes that appear to be an unavoidable consequence of ageing.

In summary, there is limited research that has specifically examined anaerobic capacity and strength performance in masters athletes. From the limited data available, there appears no doubt that anaerobic performance declines linearly in older athletes to around 65–70 years of age, after which the decline in anaerobic performance accelerates. While the actual mechanisms explaining these declines remain elusive, age-related changes in the many factors contributing to anaerobic performance appear to contribute. The consensus of research suggests that decreased muscle mass, type II muscle fibre atrophy and a shift towards a greater oxidative potential of muscle in older age are primarily responsible. Taken together, these changes in muscle fibre characteristics and the subsequent changes in other physiological processes (i.e. fibre contractile velocity, enzyme activity, lactate production) help to explain the majority of the reported age-related decline in speed and strength performance in masters athletes. It also appears that high-intensity sprint training, combined with hypertrophy resistance training, may potentially slow the decline in anaerobic performance of masters athletes into older age due to maintenance of muscular characteristics that allow greater anaerobic ATP production and force production.

2.5 CONCLUSIONS

As discussed above, masters athletes competition is increasing in popularity, helping to maintain physiological function and overall health in trained masters athletes. Such continued training and competition has demonstrated vast health and performance benefits when compared to sedentary ageing. However, it appears as that preventing age-related declines in sports performance is largely unavoidable, as a natural age-related decline in performance has been observed in endurance, speed and strength events. These performance declines appear to reflect changes in the limiting physiological capacities and systems that concomitantly occur as part of the ageing process.

Given the complexity of the physiological factors that limit sports performance, it remains difficult to directly explain any correlation between losses in physiological capacities and athletic performance with ageing. For example, the reductions in endurance performance appear to best reflect the age-related decrease in VO_{2max}, which is a collective measure of cardiovascular function and muscular oxidative capacity, both which appear to decline with age. However, the loss in VO_{2max} may also be affected be age-related changes in body composition, anaerobic contribution to high-intensity exercise and other physiological factors. Taken together, decreases in endurance performance appear inevitable with ageing, due to natural declines in function within several physiological systems. Continued training demonstrates that these losses in physiological capacities may be better preserved, limiting the declines observed in the endurance performance of masters athletes.

Separately, the greatest losses in physiological function and athletic performance have been reported to occur in events that rely on anaerobic metabolism or maximal muscle function. The large reductions reported in athletic performance within speed and strength events are again reflective of a decline in a range of physiological systems. In particular, performance in events that require speed and strength is most likely a result of an age-related loss of muscle mass and function. The concept of age-related loss of muscle mass is well documented in ageing sedentary populations, and is proposed to be the result of programmed losses of muscle cells. While similar events occur in masters athletes, continued training appears to be able to attenuate the losses in muscle cells and maintain their functional capacities. The preservation of muscle mass in masters athletes assists in the development of force production, anaerobic metabolism and neuromuscular traits, which collectively influence athletic performance. Taken together, masters athletes should aim to preserve lean muscle mass through both resistance training and dietary means (detailed in later chapters) to limit the age-related losses in speed and strength performance.

2.6 IMPLICATIONS FOR SPORTS MEDICINE PROFESSIONALS AND CLINICIANS

- Due to their continued training and performance within competitive sport, it is likely that masters athletes will present with superior physiological capacities than age-matched sedentary controls. Physicians and clinicians should be aware that typical age-related normative values for various physiological measures might not be specific for masters athletes.
- The age-related declines in observable physiological measures (e.g. heart rate, VO_{2max}, blood lactate) should be taken into consideration when prescribing training and monitoring exercise testing.
- Current evidence suggests that continued participation of high-intensity training and competition typical of a masters athlete helps to provide numerous health benefits and limit the decline in physiological systems that may impact on overall health. Sports medicine professionals and clinicians should advocate continued training and competition activities throughout the wider community as a means to assist in health maintenance with advancing age.

2.7 IMPLICATIONS FOR MASTERS ATHLETES AND COACHES

- It should be acknowledged that performance will decline with advancing age, and therefore relative training and performance targets should be incorporated into training plans. Consideration should be given to age, training history and the capacity of the various physiological systems that limit performance.
- The reported losses in physiological function (in particular VO_{2max}, muscle mass and type II fibre size and composition) are minimised with continued high-intensity training. Therefore, it is vital for masters athletes to continue to undertake high-intensity cardiorespiratory and resistance exercise to maintain physiological function and performance. In particular, the use of high-intensity resistance training is likely to maintain the number and size of type II fibres which could have a great impact on the performance of masters athletes.
- Masters athletes and coaches should consider the various age-related changes in physiological and physical factors such as maximum heart rate, blood volume, body composition, muscle mass and composition and the impact that they may have on capacities that affect performance.

2.8 FUTURE RESEARCH DIRECTIONS

- Researchers need to further examine how the myriads of changes in physiological systems collectively contribute to limit exercise performance in masters athletes. Attention should be directed to the impact of training on selected physiological and physical factors to determine how training may be best programmed to limit losses in performance. For example, continued attention should be provided to means of maintaining type II fibre population in masters athletes and the subsequent impact that has on performance.

- Specifically, little attention has been provided to changes in the neuromuscular responses during exercise in masters athletes. In combination with the altered muscle fibre composition and size reported for masters athletes, it is of interest as to whether superior neuromuscular responses are possessed by masters athletes. Therefore, research needs to explore whether continued training and competition with ageing helps to maintain better neuromuscular function during exercise than sedentary ageing.
- There are very few studies that have provided a holistic assessment of changes in physiological function in masters athletes compared to sedentary controls. Most studies have provided a cross-sectional assessment of a selected measure of interest, irrespective of other changes that are likely to occur. Given the complexity of the interaction between losses in physiological function and performance with age, more studies need to provide a longitudinal and holistic assessment of physiological changes that occur with ageing athletes.

REFERENCES

1. International Masters Games Association (IMGA), World Summer Masters Games, http://www.imga.ch/, accessed 14 January 2014.
2. Reaburn, P. and Dascombe, B., Endurance performance in masters athletes, *Eur. Rev. Aging Phys. Act.* 5(1), 31–42, 2008.
3. Reaburn, P. and Dascombe, B., Anaerobic performance in masters athletes, *Eur. Rev. Aging Phys. Act.* 6, 39–53, 2009.
4. Tanaka, H. and Seals, D.R., Dynamic exercise performance in masters athletes: Insight into the effect of primary human aging on physiological functional capacity, *J. Appl. Physiol.* 95, 2152–62, 2003.
5. Wright, V.J. and Perricelli, B.C., Age-related rates of decline in performance among elite senior athletes, *Am. J. Sports Med.* 36(3), 443–50, 2008.
6. Coggan, A.R., Spina, R.J. and King, D.S., Skeletal muscle adaptations to endurance training in 60- to 70-year old men and women, *J. Appl. Physiol.* 70, 1780–6, 1990.
7. Coggan, A.R., Spina, R.J., King, D.S. et al., Skeletal muscle adaptations to endurance training in 60- to 70-yr-old men and women, *J. Appl. Physiol.* 72(5), 1780–6, 1992.
8. Louis, J., Hausswirth, C., Easthope, C. and Brisswalter, J., Strength training improves cycling efficiency in master endurance athletes, *Eur. J. Appl. Physiol.* 112(2), 631–40, 2012.
9. Makrides, L., Heigenhauser, G.J. and Jones, N.L., High-intensity endurance training in 20- to 30- and 60- to 70-yr-old healthy men, *J. Appl. Physiol.* 69(5), 1792–8, 1990.
10. Anton, M.M., Spirduso, W.W. and Tanaka, H., Age-related declines in anaerobic muscular performance: Weightlifting and powerlifting, *Med. Sci. Sports Exerc.* 36(1), 143–7, 2004.
11. Baker, A.B., Tang, Y.Q. and Turner, M.J., Percentage decline in Masters superathlete track and field performance with aging, *Exp. Aging Res.* 29, 47–65, 2003.
12. Donato, A.J., Tench, K., Glueck, D.H., Seals, D.R., Eskurza, I. and Tanaka, H., Declines in physiological functional capacity with age: A longitudinal study in peak swimming performance, *J. Appl. Physiol.* 94, 764–9, 2003.
13. Medic, N., Starkes, J.L. and Young, B.W., Examining relative age effects on performance achievement and participation rates in masters athletes, *J. Sports Sci.* 25(12), 1377–84, 2007.
14. Medic, N., Young, B.W. and Medic, D., Participation-related relative age effects in Masters swimming: A 6-year retrospective longitudinal analysis, *J. Sports Sci.* 29(1), 29–36, 2011.
15. Tanaka, H. and Higuchi, M., Age, exercise, performance, and physiological functional capacities, *Adv. Exer. Sports Physiol.* 4, 51–6, 1998.
16. The, D.J. and Ploutz-Snyder, L., Age, body mass, and gender as predictors of masters Olympic weightlifting performance, *Med. Sci. Sports Exerc.* 35(7), 1216–24, 2003.
17. Gent, D.N. and Norton, K., Aging has greater impact on anaerobic versus aerobic power in trained masters athletes, *J. Sports Sci.* 31(1), 97–103, 2013.

18. Bird, S., Balmer, J., Olds, T. and Davison, R.C.R., Differences between the sexes and age-related changes in orienteering speed, *J. Sports Sci.* 19, 243–52, 2001.
19. Evans, S.L., Davy, K.P., Stevenson, E.T. and Seals, D.R., Physiological determinants of 10-km performance in highly trained female runners of different ages, *J. Appl. Physiol.* 78(5), 1931–41, 1995.
20. Jokl, P., Sethi, P.M. and Cooper, A.J., Master's performance in the New York City Marathon 1983–1999, *Br. J. Sports Med.* 38(4), 408–12, 2004.
21. Fung, L. and Ha, A., Changes in track and field performance with chronological aging, *Int. J. Aging Hum. Dev.* 38(2), 171–80, 1994.
22. Moore, D.H., A study of group track and field records to relate age and running speed, *Nature* 253(5489), 264–5, 1975.
23. Nessel, E.H., The physiology of aging as it relates to sports, *J. Am. Med. Athl. Ass.* 17, 12–7, 2004.
24. Young, B.W. and Starkes, J.L., Career-span analyses of track performance: Longitudinal data present a more optimistic view of age-related performance decline, *Exp. Aging Res.* 31, 69–90, 2005.
25. Bongard, V., McDermott, A.Y., Dallal, G.E. and Schaefer, E.J., Effect of age and gender on physical performance, *Age* 29(3), 77–85, 2007.
26. Fairbrother, J.T., Prediction of 1500-m freestyle swimming times for older masters all-American swimmers, *Exp. Aging Res.* 33(4), 461–71, 2007.
27. Hartely, A.A. and Hartely, J.T., Age differences and changes in sprint swimming performances of masters athletes, *Exp. Aging Res.* 12(2), 65–70, 1986.
28. Rahe, R.H. and Arthur, R.J., Swim performance decrement over middle life, *Med. Sci. Sports* 7(1), 53–8, 1975.
29. Tanaka, H. and Seals, D.R., Age and gender interactions in physiological functional capacity: Insight from swimming performance, *J. Appl. Physiol.* 82(3), 846–51, 1997.
30. Pollock, M.L., Mengelkoch, L.J., Graves, J.E. et al., Twenty-year follow-up of aerobic power and body composition of older track athletes, *J. Appl. Physiol.* 82(5), 1508–15, 1997.
31. Tanaka, K., Takeshima, N., Kato, T., Niihata, S. and Ueda, K., Critical determinants of endurance performance in middle-aged and elderly endurance runners with heterogeneous training habits, *Eur. J. Appl. Physiol. Occup. Physiol.* 59(6), 443–9, 1990.
32. FINA, Masters world records, http://www.fina.org/H2O/index.php?option=com_wrapper&view=wrapper&Itemid=637, accessed 14 January 2014.
33. World Masters Athletics, Records, http://www.world-masters-athletics.org/records/, accessed 14 January 2014.
34. Lavoie, J.M. and Montpetit, R.R., Applied physiology of swimming, *Sports Med.* 3(3), 165–89, 1986.
35. Gatta, G., Benelli, P. and Ditroilo, M., The decline in swimming performance with advancing age: A cross sectional study, *J. Strength Cond. Res.* 20(4), 932–8, 2006.
36. Faulkner, J.A., Davis, C.S., Mendias, C.L. and Brooks, S.V., The aging of elite male athletes: Age-related changes in performance and skeletal muscle structure and function, *Clin. J. Sport Med.* 18(6), 501–7, 2008.
37. Faulkner, J.A., Larkin, L.M., Claflin, D.R. and Brooks, S.V., Age-related changes in the structure and function of skeletal muscles, *Clin. Exp. Pharmacol. Physiol.* 34(11), 1091–6, 2007.
38. Frontera, W.R., Hughes, V.A., Fielding, R.A., Fiatarone, M.A., Evans, W.J. and Roubenoff, R., Aging of skeletal muscle: A 12-year longitudinal study, *J. Appl. Physiol.* 71(2), 644–50, 2000.
39. Meltzer, D.E., Age dependence of Olympic weightlifting ability, *Med. Sci. Sports Exerc.* 26(8), 1053–67, 1994.
40. Pearson, S.J., Young, A., Macaluso, A. et al., Muscle function in elite master weightlifters, *Med. Sci. Sports Exerc* 34(7), 1199–206, 2002.
41. Porter, M.M., Vandervoort, A.A. and Lexell, J., Aging of human muscle: Structure, function and adaptability, *Med. Sci. Sports Exerc.* 5, 129–42, 1995.
42. Medic, N., Starkes, J.L. and Young, B.W., Examining relative age effects on performance achievement and participation rates in Masters athletes, *J. Sports Sci.* 25(12), 1377–84, 2007.
43. Medic, N., Young, B.W., Starkes, J.L., Weir, P.L. and Grove, J.R., Gender, age, and sport differences in relative age effects among US Masters swimming and track and field athletes, *J. Sports Sci.* 27(14), 1535–44, 2009.
44. Korhonen, M.T., Mero, A. and Suominen, H., Age-related differences in 100-m sprint performance in male and female master runners, *Med. Sci. Sports Exerc.* 35(8), 1419–28, 2003.
45. Coyle, E.F., Integration of the physiological factors determining endurance performance ability, *Exerc. Sports Sci. Rev.* 23, 25–63, 1995.

46. Hawkins, S.A., Marcell, T.J., Victoria Jaque, S. and Wiswell, R.A., A longitudinal assessment of change in VO_2 max and maximal heart rate in masters athletes, *Med. Sci. Sports Exerc.* 33, 1744–50, 2001.
47. Kasch, F.W., Boyer, J.L., Schmidt, P.K. et al., Ageing of the cardiovascular system during 33 years of aerobic exercise, *Age Ageing* 28(6), 531–6, 1999.
48. Kasch, F.W., Boyer, J.L., Van Camp, S., Nettl, F., Verity, L.S. and Wallace, J.P., Cardiovascular changes with age and exercise. A 28-year longitudinal study, *Scand. J. Med. Sci. Sports* 5(3), 147–51, 1995.
49. Proctor, D.N., Sinning, W.E., Bredle, D.L. and Joyner, M.J., Cardiovascular and peak VO_2 responses to supine exercise: Effects of age and training status, *Med. Sci. Sports Exerc.* 28(7), 892–9, 1996.
50. Wiswell, R.A., Hawkins, S.A., Jaque, S.V. et al., Relationship between physiological loss, performance decrement, and age in Master athletes, *J. Gerontol. A-Med.* 56(10), M618–26, 2001.
51. Hawkins, S.A., Marcell, T.J., Victoria Jaque, S. and Wiswell, R.A., A longitudinal assessment of change in VO_2 max and maximal heart rate in masters athletes, *Med. Sci. Sports Exerc.* 33(10), 1744–50, 2001.
52. Tanaka, H., Monahan, K.D. and Seals, D.R., Age-predicted maximal heart rate revisited, *J. Am. Coll. Cardiol.* 37(1), 153–6, 2001.
53. Conway, J., Wheeler, R. and Sannerstedt, R., Sympathetic nervous activity during exercise in relation to age, *Cardiovasc. Res.* 5(4), 577–81, 1971.
54. Fleg, J.L., Tzankoff, S.P. and Lakatta, E.G., Age-related augmentation of plasma catecholamines during dynamic exercise in healthy males, *J. Appl. Physiol.* 59(4), 1033–9, 1985.
55. Ogawa, T., Spina, R.J., Martin, W.H. 3rd et al., Effects of aging, sex, and physical training on cardiovascular responses to exercise, *Circulation* 86(2), 494–503, 1992.
56. Wiebe, C.G., Gledhill, N., Jamnik, V.K. and Ferguson, S., Exercise cardiac function in young through elderly endurance trained women, *Med. Sci. Sports Exerc.* 31(5), 684–91, 1999.
57. Hagmar, M., Hirschberg, A.L., Lindholm, C., Schenck-Gustafsson, K. and Eriksson, M.J., Athlete's heart in postmenopausal former elite endurance female athletes, *Clin. J. Sports Med.* 15(4), 257–62, 2005.
58. Nottin, S., Nguyen, L.D., Terbah, M. and Obert, P., Long-term endurance training does not prevent the age-related decrease in left ventricular relaxation properties, *Acta Physiol. Scand.* 181(2), 209–15, 2004.
59. Bouvier, F., Saltin, B., Nejat, M. and Jensen-Urstad, M., Left ventricular function and perfusion in elderly endurance athletes, *Med. Sci. Sports Exerc.* 33(5), 735–40, 2001.
60. Davy, K.P. and Seals, D.R., Total blood volume in healthy young and older men, *J. Appl. Physiol.* 76(5), 2059–1062, 1994.
61. Giada, F., Bertaglia, E., De Piccoli, B. et al., Cardiovascular adaptations to endurance training and detraining in young and older athletes, *Int. J. Cardiol.* 149–55, 1998.
62. Hood, S. and Northcote, R.J., Cardiac assessment of veteran endurance athletes: A 12 year follow up study, *Br. J. Sports Med.* 33(4), 239–43, 1999.
63. Seals, D.R., Hagberg, J.M., Spina, R.J., Rogers, M.A., Schechtman, K.B. and Ehsani, A.A., Enhanced left ventricular performance in endurance trained older men, *Circulation* 89(1), 198–205, 1994.
64. Chien, S., Usami, S., Simmons, R.L., McAllister, F.F. and Gregersen, M.I., Blood volume and age: Repeated measurements on normal men after 17 years, *J. Appl. Physiol.* 21(2), 583–8, 1966.
65. Ito, T., Takamata, A., Yaegashi, K. et al., Role of blood volume in the age-associated decline in peak oxygen uptake in humans, *Jpn. J. Physiol.* 51(5), 607–12, 2001.
66. Convertino, V.A., Blood volume: Its adaptation to endurance training, *Med. Sci. Sports Exerc.* 23(12), 1338–48, 1991.
67. Hagberg, J.M., Allen, W.K., Seals, D.R., Hurley, B.F., Ehsani, A.A. and Holloszy, J.O., A hemodynamic comparison of young and older endurance athletes during exercise, *J. Appl. Physiol.* 58(6), 2041–6, 1985.
68. Klitgaard, H., Ausoni, S. and Damiani, E., Sarcoplasmic reticulum of human skeletal muscle: Age-related changes and effect of training, *Acta Physiol. Scand.* 137(1), 23–31, 1989.
69. Klitgaard, H., Brunet, A., Marc, R., Monod, H., Mantoni, M. and Saltin, B., The aging skeletal muscle: Effect of training on muscle force and mass, *Int. J. Sports Med.* 10, S93–4, 1989.
70. Trappe, S.W., Costill, D.L., Fink, W.J. and Pearson, D.R., Skeletal muscle characteristics among distance runners: A 20-yr follow-up study, *J. Appl. Physiol.* 78(3), 823–9, 1995.
71. Trappe, S.W., Costill, D.L., Vukovich, M.D., Jones, J. and Melham, T., Aging among elite distance runners: A 22-yr longitudinal study, *J. Appl. Physiol.* 80(1), 285–90, 1996.
72. Andersen, J.L., Muscle fibre type adaptation in the elderly human muscle, *Scand. J. Med. Sci. Sports* 13(1), 40–7, 2003.
73. Larsson, L., Physical training effects on muscle morphology in sedentary males at different ages. *Med. Sci. Sports Exerc.* 14(3), 203–6, 1982.
74. Larsson, L., Gimby, G. and Karlsson, J., Muscle strength and speed of movement in relation to age and muscle morphology, *J. Appl. Physiol.* 46(3), 451–6, 1979.

75. Larsson, L., Sjodin, B. and Karlsson, J., Histochemical and biochemical changes in human skeletal muscle with age in sedentary males, age 22–65 years, *Acta Physiol. Scand.* 103(1), 31–9, 1978.
76. Aagaard, P., Magnusson, P.S., Larsson, B., Kjaer, M. and Krustrup, P., Mechanical muscle function, morphology, and fiber type in lifelong trained elderly, *Med. Sci. Sports Exerc.* 39(11), 1989–96, 2007.
77. Harridge, S., Magnusson, G. and Saltin, B., Life-long endurance-trained elderly men have high aerobic power, but have similar muscle strength to non-active elderly men, *Aging* 9(1–2), 80–7, 1997.
78. Klitgaard, H., Mantoni, M., Schiaffino, S. et al., Function, morphology and protein expression of ageing skeletal muscle: A cross-sectional study of elderly men with different training backgrounds, *Acta Physiol. Scand.* 140(1), 41–54, 1990.
79. Proctor, D.N., Sinning, W.E., Walro, J.M., Sieck, G.C. and Lemon, P.W.R., Oxidative capacity of human muscle fibre types: Effects of age and training status, *J. Appl. Physiol.* 78(6), 2033–8, 1995.
80. Trappe, T.A., Lindquist, D.M. and Carrithers, J.A., Muscle-specific atrophy of the quadriceps femoris with aging, *J. Appl. Physiol.* 90(6), 2070–4, 2001.
81. Coggan, A.R., Spina, R.J., Rogers, M.A. et al., Histochemical and enzymatic characteristics of skeletal muscle in master athletes, *J. Appl. Physiol.* 68(5), 1896–901, 1990.
82. Houston, M.E. and Green, H.J., Skeletal muscle and physiologic characteristics of a world champion masters distance runner: A case study, *Int. J. Sports Med.* 2(1), 47–9, 1981.
83. Coggan, A.R., Spina, R.J., Rogers, M.A. et al., Histochemical and enzymatic characteristics of skeletal muscle in masters athletes, *J. Appl. Physiol.* 68(5), 1896–901, 1990.
84. Chilibeck, P.D., Paterson, D.H., Cunningham, D.A., Taylor, A.W. and Noble, E.G., Muscle capillarization O_2 diffusion distance, and VO_2 kinetics in old and young individuals, *J. Appl. Physiol.* 82(1), 63–9, 1997.
85. Conley, K.E., Esselman, P.C., Jubrias, S.A. et al., Ageing, muscle properties and maximal O_2 uptake rate in humans, *J. Physiol.* 526, 211–7, 2000.
86. Grimby, G. and Saltin, B., The ageing muscle, *Clin. Physiol.* 3(3), 209–18, 1983.
87. Parizkova, J., Eiselt, E., Sprynarova, S. and Wachtlova, M., Body composition, aerobic capacity, and density of muscle capillaries in young and old men, *J. Appl. Physiol.* 31(3), 323–5, 1971.
88. Trappe, S.W., Masters athletes, *Int. J. Sports Nutr. Exerc. Metab.* 11, S196–207, 2001.
89. Russ, D.W. and Kent-Braun, J.A., Is skeletal muscle oxidative capacity decreased in old age?, *Sports Med.* 34(3), 221–9, 2004.
90. Russell, R.M., The aging process as a modifier of metabolism, *Am. J. Clin. Nutr.* 72, S32, 2000.
91. Conley, K.E., Jubrias, S.A. and Esselman, P.C., Oxidative capacity and ageing in human muscle, *J. Physiology* 526, 203–10, 2000.
92. Taylor, A.W., Kemp, G.J., Thompson, C.H. and Radda, G.K., Ageing: Effects on oxidative function of skeletal muscle in vivo, *Mol. Cell. Biochem.* 174, 321–4, 1997.
93. Coggan, A.R., Spina, R.J., Rogers, M.A. et al., Histochemical and enzymatic comparison of the gastrocnemius muscle of young and elderly men and women, *J. Gerontol. A-Biol. Med.* 47, B71–6, 1992.
94. Houmard, J.A., Weidner, M.L., Gavigan, K.E., Tyndall, G.L., Hickey, M.S. and Alshami, A., Fibre type and citrate synthase activity in the human gastrocnemius and vastus lateralis with aging, *J. Appl. Physiol.* 85(4), 1337–41, 1998.
95. Kiessling, K.H., Pilstrom, L., Bylund, A.C., Saltin, B. and Piehl, K., Enzyme activities and morphometry in skeletal muscle of middle aged men after training, *Scand. J. Clin. Lab. Inv.* 33, 63–9, 1974.
96. Taylor, A.W., Noble, E.G., Cunningham, D.A., Paterson, D.H. and Rechnitzer, P., Ageing, skeletal muscle contractile properties and enzyme activities with exercise, *Int. Med. Sports Sci.* 37, 109–25, 1992.
97. Brierley, E.J., Johnson, M.A., James, O.F. and Turnball, D.M., Mitochondrial involvement in the ageing process. Facts and controversies, *Mol. Cell. Biochem.* 174, 325–8, 1997.
98. Coggan, A.R., Spina, R.J., King, D.S. et al., Histochemical and enzymatic comparison of the gastrocnemius muscle of young and elderly men and women, *J. Gerontol. A-Biol. Med.* 47(3), B71–6, 1992.
99. Going, S., Williams, D. and Lohman, T., Aging and body composition: Biological changes and methodological issues, *Exerc. Sport Sci. Rev.* 23, 411–53, 1995.
100. Maharam, L.G., Bauman, P.A., Kalman, D., Skolnik, H. and Perle, S.M., Masters athletes: Factors affecting performance, *Sports Med.* 28(4), 273–85, 1999.
101. Pollock, M.L., Foster, C., Knapp, D., Rod, J.L. and Schmidt, D.H., Effect of age and training on aerobic capacity and body composition of Masters athletes, *J. Appl. Physiol.* 62(2), 725–31, 1987.
102. Yataco, A.R., Busby-Whitehead, J., Drinkwater, D.T. and Katzel, L.I., Relationship of body composition and cardiovascular fitness to lipoprotein lipid profiles in masters athletes and sedentary men, *Aging* 9(1–2), 88–94, 1997.
103. Bunout, D., de la Maza, M.P., Barrera, G., Leiva, L., Gattas, V. and Hirsch, S., Assessment of sarcopenia: Longitudinal versus cross sectional body composition data, *Aging-Clin. Exp. Res.* 19(4), 295–9, 2007.

104. Hughes, V.A., Frontera, W.R., Wood, M. et al., Longitudinal muscle strength changes in older adults: Influence of muscle mass, physical activity, and health, *J. Gerontol. A-Biol. Med.* 56(5), B209–17, 2001.
105. Janssen, I., Heymsfield, S.B., Wang, Z. and Ross, R., Skeletal muscle mass and distribution in 468 men and women aged 18–88 yr, *J. Appl. Physiol.* 89(1), 81–95, 2000.
106. Tzankoff, S.P. and Norris, A.H., Effect of muscle mass decrease on age-related BMR changes, *J. Appl. Physiol.* 43(6), 1001–6, 1977.
107. Buskirk, E.R. and Hodgson, J.L., Age and aerobic power: The rate of change in men and women, *Fed. Proceed.* 46(5), 1824–9, 1987.
108. Fleg, J.L. and Lakatta, E.G., Role of muscle loss in the age-associated reduction in VO_2 max, *J. Appl. Physiol.* 65(3), 1147–51, 1988.
109. Heath, G.W., Hagberg, J.M., Ehsani, A.A. and Holloszy, J.O., A physiological comparison of younger and older endurance athletes, *J. Appl. Physiol.* 51, 634–40, 1981.
110. Proctor, D.N. and Joyner, M.J., Skeletal muscle mass and the reduction of VO_2 max in trained older subjects, *J. Appl. Physiol.* 82(5), 1411–5, 1997.
111. Miszko, T.A., Cress, M.E., Slade, J.M., Covey, C.J., Agrawal, S.K. and Doerr, C.E., Effect of strength and power training on physical function in community-dwelling older adults, *J. Gerontol. A-Biol. Med.* 58(2), 171–5, 2003.
112. Porter, M.M., The effects of strength training on sarcopenia, *Can. J. Appl. Physiol.* 26(1), 123–41, 2001.
113. Alway, S.E., Siu, P.M., Murlasits, Z. and Butler, D.C., Muscle hypertrophy models: Applications for research on aging, *Can. J. Appl. Physiol.* 30(5), 591–624, 2005.
114. Sipila, S. and Suominen, H., Ultrasound imaging of the quadriceps muscle in elderly athletes and untrained men, *Muscle Nerve* 14(6), 527–33, 1991.
115. Sipila, S. and Suominen, H., Muscle ultrasonography and computed tomography in elderly trained and untrained women, *Muscle Nerve* 16(3), 294–300, 1993.
116. Bassett, D.R., Jr. and Howley, E.T., Limiting factors for maximum oxygen uptake and determinants of endurance performance, *Med. Sci. Sports Exerc.* 32(1), 70–84, 2000.
117. Roecker, K., Schotte, O., Niess, A.M., Horstmann, T. and Dickhuth, H.H., Predicting competition performance in long-distance running by means of a treadmill test, *Med. Sci. Sports Exerc.* 30(10), 1552–7, 1998.
118. Iwaoka, K., Fuchi, T., Higuchi, M. and Kobayasji, S., Blood lactate accumulation during exercise in older endurance runners, *Int. J. Sports Med.* 9(4), 253–6, 1988.
119. Allen, W.K., Seals, D.R., Hurley, B.F., Ehsani, A.A. and Hagberg, J.M., Lactate threshold and distance-running performance in young and older endurance athletes, *J. Appl. Physiol.* 58(4), 1281–4, 1985.
120. Wiswell, R.A., Jaque, S.V., Marcell, T.J. et al., Maximal aerobic power, lactate threshold, and running performance in master athletes, *Med. Sci. Sports Exerc.* 32(6), 1165–70, 2000.
121. Mattern, C.O., Gutilla, M.J., Bright, D.L., Kirby, T.E., Hinchcliff, K.W. and Devor, S.T., Maximal lactate steady state declines during the aging process, *J. Appl. Physiol.* 95, 2576–82, 2003.
122. Brown, S.J., Ryan, H.J. and Brown, J.A., Age-associated changes in VO_2 and power output—A cross-sectional study of endurance trained New Zealand cyclists, *J. Sport Sci. Med.* 6, 477–83, 2007.
123. Fitzgerald, M.D., Tanaka, H., Tran, Z.V. and Seals, D.R., Age-related declines in maximal aerobic capacity in regularly exercising versus sedentary women: A meta-analysis, *J. Appl. Physiol.* 83(1), 160–5, 1997.
124. Joyner, M.J., Physiological limiting factors and distance running: Influence of gender and age on record performances, *Exerc. Sports Sci. Rev.* 21, 103–33, 1993.
125. Pimentel, A.E., Gentile, C.L., Tanaka, H., Seals, D.R. and Gates, P.E., Greater rate of decline in maximal aerobic capacity with age in endurance-trained than in sedentary men, *J. Appl. Physiol.* 94(6), 2406–13, 2003.
126. Wilson, T.M. and Tanaka, H., Meta-analysis of the age-associated decline in maximal aerobic capacity in men: Relation to training status, *Am. J. Physiol. Heart Circ. Physiol.* 278, H829–H34, 2000.
127. Kenney, W.L., Wilmore, J. and Costill, D., *Physiology of Sport and Exercise*, 5th Ed., Human Kinetics, Champaign, IL, 2012.
128. Morgan, D.W. and Craib, M., Physiological aspects of running economy, *Med. Sci. Sports Exerc.* 24(4), 456–61, 1992.
129. Nicholson, R.M. and Sleivert, G.G., Indices of lactate threshold and their relationship with 10-km running velocity, *Med. Sci. Sports Exerc.* 33(2), 339–42, 2001.
130. Sjodin, B. and Svedenhag, J., Applied physiology of marathon running, *Sports Med.* 2(2), 83–99, 1985.
131. Dehn, M.M. and Bruce, R.A., Longitudinal variations in maximal oxygen intake with age and activity, *J. Appl. Physiol.* 33(6), 805–7, 1972.
132. Kasch, F.W., Boyer, J.L., Van Camp, S.P., Verity, L.S. and Wallace, J.P., Effect of exercise on cardiovascular ageing, *Age Ageing* 22(1), 5–10, 1993.

133. Hagerman, F.C., Fielding, R.A., Fiatarone, M.A. et al., A 20-yr longitudinal study of Olympic oarsmen, *Med. Sci. Sports Exerc.* 28(9), 1150–6, 1996.
134. Katzel, L.I., Sorkin, J.D. and Fleg, J.L., A comparison of longitudinal changes in aerobic fitness in older endurance athletes and sedentary men, *J. Am. Geriatr. Soc.* 49(12), 1657, 2001.
135. Kavanagh, T. and Shephard, R.J., Can regular sports participation slow the aging process? Data on Masters athletes, *Physician Sportsmed.* 18, 94–104, 1990.
136. Rogers, M.A., Hagber, J.M., Martin, W.H.I., Ehsani, A.A. and Holloszy, J.O., Decline in VO_2 max with aging in Masters athletes and sedentary men, *J. Appl. Physiol.* 68(5), 1833–7, 1990.
137. Åstrand, I., Aerobic work capacity in men and women with special reference to age, *Acta Physiol. Scand.* S49(169), 1–92, 1960.
138. Weiss, E.P., Spina, R.J., Holloszy, J.O. and Ehsani, A.A., Gender differences in the decline in aerobic capacity and its physiological determinants during the later decades of life, *J. Appl. Physiol.* 101(3), 938–44, 2006.
139. Wells, C.L., Boorman, M.A. and Riggs, D.M., Effect of age and menopausal status on cardiorespiratory fitness in masters women runners, *Med. Sci. Sports Exer.* 24(10), 1147–54, 1992.
140. Bouchard, C., Taylor, A.W., Simoneau, J.A. and Dulac, S., Testing anaerobic power and capacity. In *Physiological Testing of the High Performance Athlete,* J.D. Macdougall, H.A. Wenger, and H.J. Green, eds., Human Kinetics, Champaign, IL, 1991, pp. 175–221.
141. Lexell, J., Human aging, muscle mass, and fiber type composition, *J. Gerontol. A-Biol. Med.* 2(3), 253–65, 1995.
142. Orlander, J., Kiessling, K.H., Larsson, L., Karlsson, J. and Aniansson, A., Skeletal muscle metabolism and ultrastructure in relation to age in sedentary men, *Acta Physiol. Scand.* 104, 249–61, 1978.
143. Korhonen, M.T., Cristea, A., Alenn, M. et al. Aging, muscle fiber type, and contractile function in sprint-trained athletes, *J. Appl. Physiol.* 101(3), 906–17, 2006.
144. Bouchard, C., Dionne, F.T., Simoneau, J.A. and Boulay, M.R., Genetics of aerobic and anaerobic performances, *Exer. Sport Sci. Rev.* 20, 27–58, 1992.
145. Perez-Gomez, J., Rodriguez, G.V., Ara, I. et al., Role of muscle mass on sprint performance: Gender differences?, *Eur. J. Appl. Physiol.* 102(6), 685–94, 2008.
146. Makrides, L., Heigenhauser, G.J., McCartney, N. and Jones, N.L., Maximal short term exercise capacity in healthy subjects aged 15–70 years, *Clin. Sci.* 69(2), 197–205, 1985.
147. Feretti, G., Narici, M.V., Binzoni, T. et al., Determinants of peak muscle power: Effects of age and physical conditioning, *Eur. J. Appl. Physiol. Occup. Physiol.* 68(2), 111–5, 1994.
148. Aniansson, A., Grimby, G., Rundgren, A., Svanborg, A. and Oerlander, J., Physical training in old men, *Age Ageing* 9(3), 186–7, 1980.
149. Essen-Gustavsson, B. and Borges, O., Histochemical and metabolic characteristics of human skeletal muscle in relation to age, *Acta Physiol. Scand.* 126, 107–11, 1986.
150. Larsson, L. and Karlsson, J., Isometric and dynamic endurance as a function of age and skeletal muscle characteristics, *Acta Physiol. Scand.* 104, 129–36, 1978.
151. Reaburn, P. The lifetime athlete – Physical work capacities and skeletal muscle characteristics. Brisbane: University of Queensland; 1994.
152. de Souza, E.O., Tricoli, V., Paulo, A.C. et al., Multivariate analysis in the maximum strength performance, *Int. J. Sports Med.* 33(12), 970–4, 2012.
153. Brunner, F., Schmid, A., Sheikhzadeh, A., Nordin, M., Yoon, J. and Frankel, V., Effects of aging on Type II muscle fibers: A systematic review of the literature., *J. Aging and Phys. Activ.* 15(3), 336–48, 2007.
154. Deschenes, M.R., Effects of aging on muscle fibre type and size, *Sports Med.* 34(12), 809–24, 2004.
155. Cristea, A., Korhonen, M.T., Hakkinen, K. et al., Effects of combined strength and sprint training on regulation of muscle contraction at the whole-muscle and single-fibre levels in elite master sprinters, *Acta Physiol.* 193(3), 275–89, 2008.
156. Aniansson, A., Hedberg, M., Henning, G.B. and Grimby, G., Muscle morphology, enzymatic activity, and muscle strength in elderly men: A follow-up study, *Muscle Nerve* 9(7), 585–91, 1986.
157. Larsson, L., Morphological and functional characteristics of the ageing skeletal muscle in man: A cross-sectional study, *Acta Physiol. Scand.* 457, 1978.
158. Lexell, J., Taylor, C.C. and Sjostrom, M., What is the cause of the ageing atrophy? Total number, size and proportion of different fiber types studied in whole vastus lateralis muscle from 15- to 83-year-old men, *J. Neurol. Sci.* 84(2–3), 275–94, 1988.
159. Frontera, W.R., Meredith, C.N., O'Reilly, K.P., Knuttgen, H.G. and Evans, W.J., Strength conditioning in older men: Skeletal muscle hypertrophy and improved function, *J. Appl. Physiol.* 64(3), 1038–44, 1988.

160. Hortobagyi, T., Zheng, D., Weidner, M., Lambert, N.J., Westbrook, S. and Houmard, J.A., The influence of aging on muscle strength and muscle fiber characteristics with special reference to eccentric strength, *J. Gerontol. A- Biol. Med.* 50(6), B399–B406, 1995.
161. Blazevich, A., Effects of physical training and detraining, immobilisation, growth and aging on human fascicle geometry, *Sports Med.* 36, 1003–1017, 2006.
162. Brechue, W.F. and Abe, T., The role of FFM accumulation and skeletal muscle architecture in powerlifting performance, *Eur. J. Appl. Physiol.* 86(4), 327–36, 2002.
163. Thom, J.M., Morse, C.I., Birk, K.M. and Narici, M.V., Influence of muscle architecture on the torque and power velocity characteristics of young and elderly men, *Eur. J. Appl. Physiol.* 100, 613–9, 2007.
164. D'Antona, G., Lanfranconi, F., Pellegrino, M.A. et al., Skeletal muscle hypertrophy and structure and function of skeletal muscle fibres in male body builders, *J. Physiol.* 570(3), 611–27, 2006.
165. Krivickas, L.S., Suh, D., Wilkins, J., Hughes, V.A., Roubenoff, R. and Frontera, W.R., Age- and gender-related differences in maximum shortening velocity of skeletal muscle fibers, *Am. J. Phys. Med. Rehab.* 80, 447–55, 2001.
166. Moller, P., Bergstrom, J., Furst, P. and Hellstrom, K., Effect of aging on energy-rich phosphagens in human skeletal muscles, *Clin. Sci.* 58, 553–5, 1980.
167. McCully, K.K., Fielding, R.A., Evans, W.J., Leigh, J.S. Jr. and Posner, J.D., Relationships between in vivo and in vitro measurements of metabolism in young and old human calf muscles, *J. Appl. Physiol.* 75(2), 813–9, 1993.
168. Cartee, G.D., Influence of age on skeletal muscle glucose transport and glycogen metabolism, *Med. Sci. Sports Exerc.* 26(5), 577–85, 1994.
169. Meredith, C.N., Frontera, W.R., Fisher, E.C. et al., Peripheral effects of endurance training in young and old subjects, *J. Appl. Physiol.* 66(6), 2844–9, 1989.
170. Schalin-Jantti, C., Laurila, E., Lofman, M. and Groop, L.C., Determinants of insulin-stimulated skeletal muscle glycogen metabolism in man, *Eur. J. Clin. Invest.* 25(9), 693–8, 1995.
171. Kaczor, J.J., Ziolkowski, W., Antosiewicz, J., Hac, S., Tarnopolsky, M.A. and Popinigis, J., The effect of aging on anaerobic and aerobic enzyme activities in human skeletal muscle, *J. Gerontol. A- Med* 61(4), 339–44, 2006.
172. Steinhagen-Thiessen, E. and Hilz, H., The age-dependent decrease in creatine kinase and aldolase activities in human striated muscle is not caused by an accumulation of faulty proteins, *Mech. Ageing Dev.* 5, 447–57, 1996.
173. Borges, O. and Essen-Gustavsson, B., Enzyme activities in type I and II muscle fibres of human skeletal muscle in relation to age and torque development, *Acta Physiol. Scand.* 136(1), 29–36, 1989.
174. Lanza, I.R., Befroy, D.E. and Kent-Braun, J.A., Age-related changes in ATP-producing pathways in human skeletal muscle in vivo, *J. Appl. Physiol.* 99, 1736–44, 2005.
175. Grimby, G., Danneskiold-Samsoe, B., Hvid, K. and Saltin, B., Morphology and enzymatic capacity in arm and leg muscles in 78–81 year old men and women, *Acta Physiol. Scand.* 115(1), 125–34, 1982.
176. Pastoris, O., Boschi, F., Verri, M. et al., The effects of aging on enzyme activities and metabolite concentrations in skeletal muscle from sedentary male and female subjects, *Exp. Gerontol.* 35(1), 95–104, 2000.
177. Donaldson, S.K., Hermansen, L. and Bolles, L., Differential, direct effects of H^+ on Ca^{2+}-activated force of skinned fibers from the soleus, cardiac and adductor magnus muscles of rabbits, *Pflug. Arch. Eur. J. Phys.* 376(1), 55–65, 1978.
178. Parkhouse, W.S. and McKenzie, D.C., Possible contribution of skeletal muscle buffers to enhanced anaerobic performance: A brief review, *Med. Sci. Sports Exerc.* 16(4), 328–38, 1984.
179. Lacour, J.R., Bouvat, E. and Barthelemy, J.C., Post-competition blood lactate concentrations as indicators of anaerobic energy expenditure during 400-m and 800-m races, *Eur. J. Appl. Physiol. Occup. Physiol.* 61(3–4), 172–6, 1990.
180. Marsh, G.D., Paterson, D.H., Govindasamy, D. and Cunningham, D.A., Anaerobic power of the arms and legs of young and older men, *Exp. Physiol.* 84(3), 589–97, 1999.
181. Korhonen, M.T., Suominen, H. and Mero, A., Age and sex differences in blood lactate response to sprint running in elite master athletes, *Can. J. Appl. Physiol.* 30(6), 649–65, 2005.
182. Benelli, P., Ditroilo, M., Forte, R., De Vito, G. and Stocchi, V., Assessment of post competition peak blood lactate in male and female master swimmers aged 40–79 years and its relationship with swimming performance, *Eur. J. Appl. Physiol.* 99, 685–93, 2007.
183. Frassetto, L. and Sebastian, A., Age and systemic acid base equilibrium: Analysis of published data, *J. Gerontol. A- Med.* 51, B91–9, 1996.
184. Duffield, R., Dawson, B. and Goodman, C., Energy system contribution to 100-m and 200-m track running events, *J. Sci. Med. Sport* 7(3), 302–13, 2004.

185. Duffield, R., Dawson, B. and Goodman, C., Energy system contribution to 400-m and 800-m track running, *J. Sports Sci.* 23(3), 299–307, 2005.
186. Gastin, P.B., Energy system interaction and relative contribution during maximal exercise. *Sports Med.* 31(10), 725–41, 2001.
187. Hill, D.W., Energy system contributions in middle-distance running events, *J. Sports Sci.* 17(6), 477–83, 1999.
188. Hill, D.W. and Smith, J.C., Calculation of aerobic contribution during high intensity exercise, *Res. Q. Exerc. Sport.* 63(1), 85–8, 1992.
189. Babcock, M.A., Paterson, D.H. and Cunningham, D.A., Influence of ageing on aerobic parameters determined from a ramp test, *Eur. J. Appl. Physiol. Occup. Physiol.* 65(2), 138–43, 1992.
190. Babcock, M.A., Paterson, D.H. and Cunningham, D.A., Effects of aerobic endurance training on gas kinetics of older men, *Med. Sci. Sports Exerc.* 26(4), 447–52, 1994.
191. Babcock, M.A., Paterson, D.H., Cunningham, D.A. and Dickinson, J.R., Exercise on-transient gas exchange kinetics are slowed as a function of age, *Med. Sci. Sports Exerc.* 26(4), 440–6, 1994.
192. Berger, N., Rittweger, J., Kwiet, A. et al., Pulmonary O_2 uptake on-kinetics in endurance and sprint trained master athletes, *Int. J. Sports Med.* 32, 383–93, 2006.
193. DeLorey, D.S., Kowalchuck, J.M. and Paterson, D.H., Effect of age on O_2 uptake kinetics and the adaptation of muscle deoxygenation at the onset of moderate-intensity cycling exercise, *J. Appl. Physiol.* 97, 165–72, 2004.
194. DeLorey, D.S., Kowalchuk, J.M. and Paterson, D.H., The effect of age on VO_2 kinetics and the adaptation of muscle deoxygenation at exercise onset, *Med. Sci. Sports Exerc.* 35(5), S335, 2003.
195. Makrides, L., Heigenhauser, G.J.F. and Jones, N.L., High-intensity endurance training in 20- to 30- and 60- to 70-yr-old healthy men, *J. Appl. Physiol.* 69(5), 1792–8, 1990.

3 Energy Needs of Masters Athletes

Nuala M. Byrne and Andrew P. Hills

CONTENTS

3.1 INTRODUCTION

Throughout the majority of human history, population growth was very modest with world population not reaching 1 billion until around 1800 A.D. and 2 billion 125 years later [1]. However, from this point, population growth accelerated rapidly until the mid-1960s peaking at just over 2% per year, before decreasing to 1.1% per year in 2010 [2]. World population increased sevenfold between 1800 and 2011, and this period of substantially faster population growth coincided with global economic expansion. In 2011, an expected ~135 million births and 57 million deaths would equate with a net increase in the world population of 78 million people [1].

Importantly, however, population growth is consistent with both expansion and demographic transition. A decline in mortality has occurred alongside and generally preceded a decline in fertility such that a reduction in infant mortality has launched a baby boom generation that has aged alongside a concomitant reducing birth rate. As a result there has been a shift in life expectancy and an older average age of the world population. The UN Population Division projects an increase in the number of individuals aged 60 years or over from just under 800 million in 2011 (~11% of the world's population) to just over 2 billion in 2050 (~22% of the world's population). Furthermore, the proportion of those aged 80 years and over is projected to increase by 270% in this same time frame [3].

Age is a major risk factor for non-communicable diseases (NCDs) such as cardiovascular disease, cancer and diabetes. Furthermore, NCDs are currently responsible for roughly 60% of all deaths [4], and tend to have relatively high treatment and care costs [5]. These costs are likely to escalate as new medical technologies are introduced and access to health care becomes increasingly universal. Therefore, optimising healthy ageing must be a priority in order to mediate the clear economic burden that will fall upon all national health care systems as a consequence of the increased population longevity.

Edward Stanley, Earl of Derby (1826–1893), is quoted as saying, 'Those who think they have not time for bodily exercise will sooner or later have to find time for illness'. More recently, Dr Kenneth Cooper is quoted as noting, 'We do not stop exercising because we grow old—we grow old because we stop exercising'. A quote from an unknown author states, 'Obviously you can't change your genes, but you can give them a damn good run for their money'. From these insights we may propose that whilst exercise may not be the cure-all, along with other healthy lifestyle habits such as diet and stress management, regular exercise places us in the best position to age well.

Considerable epidemiological and clinical evidence supports the beneficial effects of a physically active lifestyle on numerous health parameters [6–9]. In a study of 2205 Swedish men aged 50 years, Byberg et al. reported a graded reduction in total mortality risk with increasing physical activity level [10]. High physical activity levels reduced mortality rate by 32% relative to low and 22% relative to medium physical activity levels. Furthermore, in those categorised as inactive, increasing physical activity was found to have the same impact on lowering mortality rate in the long term as smoking cessation [10]. Given the breadth and strength of such evidence, the American College of Sports Medicine concluded that physical activity should be one of the highest priorities for preventing and treating disease and disablement in older adults [11].

However, can we have too much of a good thing? Since the early 1900s there has been interest in determining if undertaking higher intensity or prolonged physical training into older age is also beneficial for longevity. A seminal 1916 study found Harvard oarsmen exceeded predicted longevity by 5.1 years [12] while other early studies showed a more modest advantage from lower intensity athletic endeavours [13]. More recently, Teramoto and Bungum investigated the association between long-term vigorous exercise training and survival rates by examining a series of studies on the mortality and longevity of elite athletes [14]. Elite endurance athletes and mixed-sports (aerobic and anaerobic) athletes were found to have greater longevity than the general population, with lower cardiovascular disease mortality the primary reason for their better survival rates. While inconsistent data was found from studies of power athletes, if athletes from all sports were considered collectively, longevity was greater in elite athletes than in the general population.

Although the precise mechanisms underlying the benefits of exercise on morbidity and mortality remain unclear [15], there is good evidence that both generally higher physical activity levels and regular exercise training for athletic performance improves longevity. A growing body of evidence in studies of rodents and primates also suggests that chronic caloric restriction, as long as it is nutritionally adequate, may improve longevity [16–18]. Whether the same benefits in terms of enhanced longevity are achieved when the energy imbalance is driven by marked increases in energy expenditure is less clear. Although beyond the scope of this review, the mechanisms through which physical activity, exercise and dietary intake impact on energy metabolism, weight regulation and lifespan is currently the focus of considerable research interest.

The previous two chapters have provided an excellent review of how ageing impacts both the body's physiological systems as well as nutritional needs and the capacity to perform exercise in older age. A key determinant of one's ability to perform physically demanding work is the maintenance of energy needs. However, in the previous half century the prevalence of unhealthy weight gain globally has increased markedly [19–26]. Whatever the primary causes, weight gain reflects an uncoupling of energy expenditure for activities of daily living from energy intake, resulting in a positive energy balance. Energy requirements for exercise training and performance need to be considered alongside the challenges of maintaining a healthy body weight within the current obesogenic environment. Therefore, the aim of this chapter is to examine the energy needs of masters athletes and older exercisers, factors that dictate energy requirements, and the estimation of energy requirements at an individual level.

3.2 ENERGY BALANCE REQUIREMENTS

3.2.1 Daily Energy Requirements

Estimated energy requirement (EER) is defined as the average dietary energy intake predicted to maintain energy balance in a healthy adult of a defined age, gender, weight, height and level of physical activity consistent with good health [27,28]. EERs are similar to *estimated average requirements* (EARs), the average daily amount of a particular nutrient that will maintain a specific biochemical or physiological function in half the healthy people of a given age and gender group—in that they are set at the average of the population's estimated requirements. While this level meets the requirements of 50% of the population, a proportion of the population who meet this target will consume less than is ideal for their health. *Recommended dietary allowances* (RDAs) represent the average daily amount of a nutrient considered adequate to meet the known nutrient needs of *nearly all* healthy people of a given age and gender group.

RDAs are set at the top end of a population's estimated requirement to ensure the needs of as many people as possible are met. However, without consideration of the energy density of foods consumed, it is possible to meet the EARs or RDAs for a given age and gender group but be in energy excess, and thus be at risk of gaining weight. Further, it is also possible to consume an energy-dense but nutritionally inadequate or unbalanced diet, and so meet the EER without meeting the EAR or the RDA for given nutrients. Consequently, there is no RDA for energy intake as this may lead to a considerable positive energy balance for some individuals. Because any amount consumed in excess of needs will result in weight (primarily fat) gain, there is considerable interest in approaches to accurately predict weight maintenance energy requirements for an individual at a body size and composition and level of physical activity consistent with long-term good health. The EER is based on body size and composition considered healthy for a given age and gender group, and as indicated by the Food and Agriculture Organization/World Health Organization/United Nations University (FAO/WHO/UNU) recommendations, would allow for *the maintenance of economically necessary and socially desirable physical activity* [28,29].

Inter-individual variance in energy needed to maintain weight stability is primarily dictated by differences in body size as well as the amount of movement performed [27]. In predicting the energy needs of the older athlete, it is important to consider the extent to which the EER prediction equations devised on the general population account for the amount of physical activity undertaken in training and competition.

3.2.2 Determining Daily Energy Requirements

Imbalances between energy intake and expenditure result in gains or losses of body tissues, predominantly fat, which determine changes in body weight [28]. Thus, energy balance or weight maintenance energy requirements can be determined during weight stability either by measuring an individual's energy intake or, alternatively, daily energy expenditure. Energy intake can be measured with high precision with participants housed in research facilities using carefully weighed foods coupled with energy content measured by bomb calorimetry of food and metabolic wastes. However, determining energy requirements from energy intake assessment under free-living conditions is less precise.

EER can be determined in weight-stable individuals using self-reported dietary energy intake. However, a number of issues impact on the utility of this approach. Firstly, day-to-day variability in energy intake is typically 20%–25% [30,31]; consequently the number of days of recorded dietary intake must be sufficient to minimise the effects of intra- and inter-individual variability [32–35]. Results of studies in a variety of populations suggest between 6 and 11 days of dietary intake measurements are required for a valid measurement of EER [36–38]. Using the multiple-pass 24-hour recall interview method, we have found that 8 days of dietary records were required to minimise the effect of random error (day-to-day variation in dietary intake) in a cohort of overweight and obese men and women [39].

A second important issue impacting the utility of dietary intake data is underreporting [40]. Ranging from 10% to 45%, underreporting tends to be greater among women than men [41], and is more pronounced among overweight and obese than lean individuals [42,43]. Underreporting also appears typical in athletic groups of all ages [44–49]. Clinical studies show weight loss in true under reporters when these participants were provided with a diet containing the amount of metabolisable energy they reported eating [50–52]. Furthermore, some elderly adults who report low energy intakes are not under-reporting but rather are under-eaters as evidenced by weight loss over time [53]. Consequently, the determination of weight maintenance energy requirements using self-reported dietary intake data is untenable in most individuals, including athletes. The Joint FAO/WHO/UNU Expert Consultation on energy and protein requirements adopted the principle of relying on estimates of energy expenditure rather than energy intake from dietary surveys to determine energy requirements of adults [29]. Thus, when the energy balance equation is maintained and an individual is weight-stable, the measure of total energy expenditure (TEE) provides the most appropriate estimate of energy requirements for a given body weight.

Humans constantly need to expend energy to perform physical work, to maintain body temperature and physiological concentration gradients and to transport, synthesise, degrade and replace small and large molecules that make up body tissue [28,29]. As outlined in more detail in Section 3.3, TEE is determined by the combined energy costs of basal metabolism (or resting energy expenditure [REE]), thermic effect of food (or diet-induced thermogenesis [DIT]), and thermic effect of physical activity (or activity energy expenditure [AEE]). During pregnancy and the growing years, additional energy is expended to synthesise new tissue (pregnancy) and for growth. The Institute of Medicine (IOM) EER prediction equations provided in Table 3.1 were derived from TEE of weight-stable cohorts measured by the criterion doubly labelled water (DLW) approach (described below) [28].

TABLE 3.1
Estimated Energy Requirements (EER) for Healthy Weight Men and Women Aged ≥19 Years

Men ≥19 Years in the Healthy Weight Range (Body Mass Index [BMI] ≥18.5 and <25 kg/m²)

EER (kcal/d) = 662 – [9.53 × age (y)] + PA × [15.91 × weight (kg) + 539.6 × height (m)]

$R^2 = 0.75$; SEE = 284.5

PA refers to physical activity level, which is categorised as sedentary (1.00), low active (1.11), active (1.25) and very active (1.48)

Women ≥19 Years and in the Healthy Weight Range (BMI ≥18.5 and <25 kg/m²)

EER (kcal/d) = 354 – [6.91 × age (y)] + PA × [9.36 × weight (kg) + 726 × height (m)]

$R^2 = 0.74$; SEE = 231.6

PA refers to physical activity level, which is categorised as sedentary (1.00), low active (1.12), active (1.27) and very active (1.45)

Source: Institute of Medicine. Panel on Macronutrients, Subcommittees on Upper Reference Levels of Nutrients Interpretation and Uses of Dietary Reference Intakes, Standing Committee on the Scientific Evaluation of Dietary Reference Intakes, *Dietary reference intakes for energy, carbohydrate, fiber, fat, fatty acids, cholesterol, protein, and amino acids (macronutrients)*, The National Academies Press, Washington, DC, 2005.

Note: Sedentary = no physical activity aside from that needed for independent living. Low active = 2.4–4.8 km/d at 3.2–4.6 km/h in addition to light activity associated with typical day-to-day life. Active = 4.8–16 km/d at 3.2–4.6 km/h in addition to light activity associated with typical day-to-day life. Very active = >16 km/d at 3.2–4.6 km/h in addition to light activity associated with typical day-to-day life.

As both REE and the energy cost of movement are heavily impacted by body size, both body weight and height positively impact on energy requirements. It is also evident that age negatively impacts daily energy requirements such that each year of age over 19 years is estimated to be associated with a reduction of 9.53 kcal/d in men and 6.91 kcal/d in women. This change may, in part, be due to age-related changes in body composition (as will be discussed in Section 3.4) that are not completely accounted for by the height and weight parameters in the equation. It is important to note however, that these equations were not developed on athletic cohorts. Therefore, the most active category (>16 km/d at 3.2–4.6 km/hour in addition to light activity associated with typical day-to-day life) may not be an appropriate representation of the energy needs of endurance athletes with high training and competition loads.

3.2.3 Upper Limits of Daily Energy Requirements for Athletes

There is great diversity in the amount of energy expended for training and competition depending on the mode of activity and level of performance, with endurance events commonly having the greatest energy demands over the duration of the event. The maximum performance in endurance activities depends on the availability and convertibility of energy [54]. It is widely recognised there is a ceiling or upper limit to TEE, and in humans this ceiling may be set by maximal daily energy intake [55,56]. In addition to maximal rates of food intake and digestion, Hammond and Diamond identify maximal sustainable energy expenditure is limited by rates of O_2 uptake and distribution, metabolite removal and energy utilisation by end-organs [57]. The most likely limiting factor is end-organ use-work levels that can be maintained by our musculature. Using estimates from factorial analyses, Brody found that heavy labour could increase TEE to approximately four times REE [58]. These values were confirmed with DLW studies showing that while the upper limit to sustainable TEE in the general population is 2.2–2.5 times REE, young well-trained athletes who consume large quantities of food while training and competing can maintain energy balance while expending 4–5 times REE [55,59]. Higher levels of daily energy expenditure are possible but not sustainable with negative energy balance and possibly negative nitrogen balance resulting in a loss of weight, the higher proportion of which over time will be lean body mass [55,60].

If we consider the EER prediction equations from Table 3.1, the highest EER possible for a 1.8 m, 35-year old male weighing 80 kg would be 3650 kcal/day. A 55-year old male of the same height and weight who also meets the 'high active' category would have a predicted EER of 3459 kcal/day. These values are much lower than the energy expenditures associated with a range of athletic endeavours. The DLW technique has enabled the investigation of energy expenditure during multi-day endurance cycle and running events plus treks in hostile environments (such as in Antarctica and climbing Mt. Everest) and in military exercises.

Westerterp et al. measured energy expenditure three times in four elite cyclists (69.2 ± 5.9 kg) during the 22-day Tour de France and found average daily TEE was 7000–8600 kcal/day or 3.6–5.3 times the REE (an index known as the physical activity level [PAL]) [61]. Over the 3826-km race, participants were reasonably weight-stable with body weight decreasing on average 1.4 kg. In another study, Rehrer et al. utilised DLW to measure TEE in five cyclists who completed the 6-day, 10-stage 883 km Tour of Southland [62]. The average TEE was 6550 kcal/day, but as this cohort were on average 14.6 kg heavier (and thus had a higher REE) than the cyclists measured by Westerterp et al., the average PAL was lower at 2.39 [61]. Fudge et al. employed a 7-day DLW protocol in nine elite Kenyan endurance runners (56.0 ± 3.4 kg) during a pre-competition training phase [63]. Weight loss was not statistically significant (0.3 ± 0.8 kg) and TEE was ~3500 kcal/day, with an average PAL of 2.3.

Hoyt et al. used DLW to measure 23 marines (79.8 ± 1.3 kg) during 11 days of severe cold-weather mountain training; the average TEE was 4924 kcal/day with a PAL of 2.8 ± 0.2 [64]. Reportedly, during the first 4 days of the exercise the marines were physically active for 17.93 ± 0.22 hours/day and during this time TEE was 7131 kcal/day with a PAL of 4.0 ± 0.2. However, during the 11 days there was a loss of body weight of –2.48 ± 0.25 kg. Similar TEE values have been reported in other military cohorts and weight loss is common [65,66]. Thus, although the energy expenditure is lower than seen in studies of athletes, energy intake is not well matched.

Finally, in possibly the most extreme test of human energy expenditure, a DLW study was undertaken in two men (89.9 kg, 48 years and 69.0 kg, 37 years) who pulled sledges initially weighing 222 kg for ~10 hours/day over 95 days in temperatures ranging from –10°C to –55°C, covering a distance of 2300 km across Antarctica [67]. The reported TEE in the first 50 days (multiple DLW doses were administered) was 8485 kcal/day and 6955 kcal/day for the heavier and lighter man, respectively. Because energy intake was on average 5090 kcal/day, both men lost >25% of body weight. The highest TEE values were 10,660 kcal/day and 11,640 kcal/day, recorded between the 20th and 30th days of the expedition during which time the sledges were pulled for 12 hours/day up hills of 50 m to >3000 m in altitude. PAL values reached 6–7, although these were not able to be sustained due to the rapid weight loss [60]. These are the highest values reported in the literature using DLW.

Such DLW studies provide us with objective gold standard data and a reality check of the highest levels of sustainable and short-term (in terms of days to months) levels of daily energy expenditure that are physiologically possible in athletes [55]. Any measurement tool that provides values beyond 4–5 PAL when the athlete is weight-stable, or greater than 6–7 PAL in any situation lasting more than a few days, is most certainly erroneous.

3.3 ASSESSING TOTAL DAILY ENERGY EXPENDITURE (TEE) AND ITS COMPONENTS

TEE of healthy, non-pregnant/lactating adults is comprised of three main components: basal metabolic rate (BMR) or REE; DIT, also termed thermic effect of feeding (TEF) and the energy expenditure associated with physical activity (PAEE) or AEE. Despite some differences between each of these paired terms, for simplicity they will be used interchangeably during this chapter. REE accounts for approximately 60%–80% (higher end for very sedentary individuals), DIT accounts for 5%–15%, and AEE accounts for 15%–30% (higher end for very active individuals) of TEE. When summing these mean values, a small percentage remains unaccounted for which may include the influences of drug-induced thermogenesis (e.g. smoking) and/or a thermoregulatory component (e.g. energy produced in response to cold) [68].

To effectively interpret the findings of research investigating the impact of ageing and chronic exercise training on TEE and its components, it is important to have a working knowledge of the strengths and weakness of different measurement methodologies. A brief review of these issues will be covered in the next section, and then a discussion of the impact of ageing and exercise training on TEE and its components will follow.

3.3.1 TEE

Traditionally, TEE has been measured in a metabolic chamber with REE, DIT and the energy cost of specific physical activities measured using respiratory exchange analysis with precision of a few percentage points. However, movement in such a setting is limited by the size of the chamber (typically equivalent to a small room), hence, unless exercise equipment is installed measures of 24-hour energy expenditure reflect a daily sedentary lifestyle, with energy above REE and DIT reflecting only small amounts of movement and spontaneous physical activity. Comparable precision in free-living situations was not possible until the DLW technique to assess TEE was devised by Lifson in 1955 and applied to humans in 1982 by Schoeller et al. [69]. The DLW technique is the gold-standard or criterion measure for assessing TEE in free-living situations [69–71].

3.3.1.1 The DLW Technique

Major advantages of the technique are that it is non-invasive and imposes minimal participant burden. This enables assessment of TEE in athletes under normal living and training conditions over a 7- to 21-day period (depending on the analysis approach). Two stable isotopes, deuterium (^{2}H) and oxygen-18 (^{18}O) are administered orally via a drink of water, and the elimination of the isotopes from the body is tracked by analysing daily urine samples [72–74]. The difference between the elimination rates of the two isotopes is equivalent to the rate of carbon dioxide production which can then be converted to average daily energy expenditure [75]. Ideally, the DLW protocol can be combined with measurement of REE and DIT via indirect calorimetry (or predicted using equations) to determine AEE by subtraction.

The major advantage of the DLW technique is that it provides an indication of TEE over a number of weeks. However, the technique is a gross measure of energy expenditure and provides an accurate measure of average daily energy expenditure and not information on the nature or types of activity or intensity and duration [76]. Furthermore, despite the ability to collect samples in the field with minimal participant burden, analysis of samples requires specialised laboratory-based equipment.

The DLW technique is commonly used to validate other techniques employed to quantify free-living energy expenditure, including physical activity questionnaires [77–80]. For a detailed overview of the DLW technique, readers are referred to an International Atomic Energy Agency publication [71]. Due to limitations associated with cost, availability and technical expertise, TEE and thus weight maintenance energy requirements are more routinely estimated using factorial approaches as discussed below [28,81,82].

Despite being the gold standard technique for the assessment of TEE in free-living situations, bladder retention can impact on the validity of the DLW approach [83] with consequent implications in the older individual, particularly when utilising urine samples [84]. It is important that water stored in the bladder is in complete equilibrium with body water – if not, the sample may represent an integrated sample collected over a previously indeterminate period [75]. Accuracy of TEE estimates can be undermined by errors associated with the timing of sample collection and determination of isotope equilibration [83], which is less of an issue in young individuals because the bladder is completely emptied after the first void before DLW urine collection [69,85,86] whereas in the elderly, voiding may be incomplete [87,88].

Individuals with a larger post-void retention volume present with the greatest potential error for the DLW technique. As outlined by Blanc et al., assuming a pre-void volume of 150 mL, then a post-void retention volume of 100 mL would introduce a 30% error in the isotope enrichment of the third post-dose void [83]. In a study of 987 ambulatory women aged 55–75 years, more than 10% were identified to have a post-void retention of 100 mL or greater [87]. It is unclear if the occurrence of post-void urine retention in older athletes is the same as for their less active peers.

3.3.1.2 The Factorial Method

FAO/WHO/UNU dietary energy requirement recommendations were based on the factorial method of estimating daily energy expenditure. TEE is calculated using information collected regarding time spent sleeping and in activities of daily living, transport, manual labour and recreation over 24-hour periods with physical intensity of effort also indicated. TEE is determined from the summed energy costs of all activity over the 24-hour period [81]. Despite the relative simplicity of the approach, Roberts and Dalall have outlined a range of theoretical problems which create uncertainty regarding the validity of predictions of energy requirements [89].

Importantly, it is not feasible to measure the energy cost and intensity of all activities performed during normal life and therefore considerable error is possible. For example, inter-individual non-accountable small body movement activities reportedly ranged from 100 to 800 kcal/day in one study [90], while energy expenditure of comparable activities such as sleeping, lying rest and sitting rest can vary by 5%–10% [91–94]. Furthermore, the same activity at the same intensity may have a different energy cost in different seasonal or environmental conditions [95].

The factorial method is employed in subjective approaches including direct observation, activity diaries and physical activity questionnaires, therefore the validity of these approaches is dependent on the ability of the individual to recall information on both duration and intensity retrospectively. The method can be used to assess TEE or AEE or exercise energy expenditure (ExEE) components [96,97]. Measurement of AEE will be covered briefly in Section 3.3.4, and readers are referred to a number of extended reviews of approaches to assess AEE [98–102].

Studies to compare the factorial method with DLW have produced mixed results. Recently, the accuracy of the factorial method to estimate energy needs of 16 young (22.1 ± 1.2 years) healthy-weight (20.4 ± 1.7 kg/m^2) Chinese women was compared with DLW measures [103]. Strong agreement was reported between factorial (7.46 ± 0.59 MJ/day) and DLW assessments (7.64 ± 0.49 MJ/day). In contrast, many other studies have reported significantly higher TEE values than predicted energy requirements based on the factorial method [104–109]. Some suggest there is no difference between methods in the elderly [110]. Roberts and Dallal [89] suggest that activities such as fidgeting are likely to be reduced in elderly cohorts such as that measured by Morio et al. [110], and proposed that the reduced fidgeting may explain the greater similarity between estimated and measured TEE. It is uncertain whether the same rationale applies in an elderly athletic cohort.

3.3.2 BMR and REE

BMR represents the minimal rate of metabolism necessary to sustain life, and is the energy requirement of a variety of essential cellular events. Assessment of BMR requires the participant to be measured 10–12 hours post-prandial, in a darkened room upon waking after 8 hours restful sleep. Commonly, the less stringent RMR or REE assessment is undertaken with the same fasting and restful sleep requirements, but the participant sleeps at home and then comes directly to the test facility by automobile early in the morning after waking. Sleeping metabolic rate (SMR) is commonly measured during an overnight stay in a metabolic chamber. BMR is slightly (5%) greater than SMR, and REE is a few percent points greater than BMR. The ability to measure REE directly is theoretically simple, but in practical terms can be quite complex to achieve with accuracy [111]. Because REE is the largest component of TEE considerable research has been dedicated to measuring REE and developing REE prediction equations.

From 1890 to 1925 there was considerable academic interest in indirect calorimetry and in 1924, the landmark BMR studies of DuBois were instrumental in establishing the use of the measure for the assessment of thyroid dysfunction [112]. A resurgence of clinical interest in the measure came in the 1970s, along with the development of new instruments suitable for bedside assessments and a consequent move away from BMR to measures of REE. Numerous prediction formulae have been developed based on descriptors of body size including FFM, body surface area or body weight and height. For convenience, the term REE will be used for the remainder of the chapter.

As metabolic rate increases with body mass (or weight), the simplest estimate of REE is made using the factor of 1 kcal/kg/hour. Thus for an individual weighing 80 kg, REE would be estimated as 1920 kcal/day (1 kcal × 80 kg × 24 hours). However, REE (kcal/day) expressed as a function of body weight is non-linear and is best described by the equation: REE = 73.3 × weight (kg)$^{0.74}$. Using a later equation proposed by Kleiber [113] (REE = 70.0 × weight (kg)$^{0.75}$), the REE of the 80-kg person would be estimated as 1872 kcal/day.

The surface law, defined by Rubner in the late 1800s, provided the basis for explaining differences in heat production based on body surface area (BSA) [68]. In a large study undertaken at the Mayo Clinic (Rochester, Minnesota), reference values for REE in relation to BSA were developed [114]. However, it was later realised that BSA alone could not explain heat production. In particular, per unit BSA infants and children have a much greater REE than adults (~30%), and with advancing years, REE decreases further. It was also realised that women have a lower REE than men, and that changing surface area by moving from outstretched to foetal position when measuring REE did not alter the measure appreciably [113,115–117]. Measurement of BSA is difficult [118] and prediction equations employing BSA are sufficiently inaccurate (as much as 20%) to invalidate their use with individual subjects [68].

As more reference standards for BMR became available, notable discrepancies between derived values became evident. Consequently, determining normalcy of REE relative to prediction formulae is difficult given discrepancies of more than 15%–20% in some cases, reflecting more than 2 standard deviations above or below the mean predicted value. Despite these limitations, REE predicted from BSA-derived formulae are still used in both clinical and research settings. Given the magnitude of the discrepancies the usefulness of this practice is debatable. A large proportion of the discrepancy between BSA-derived predictions is likely to be due to differences in the body composition of the populations studied [119]. The difference in REE per unit body weight between men and women can be explained on average by the greater proportion of body weight in women being composed of adipose tissue which has a lower oxygen utilisation, and thus metabolic rate, than other tissues [120,121]. Consequently, to account for differences in body composition, REE is commonly predicted in terms of fat-free mass (FFM) using the linear function: $\text{REE} = a + b \times \text{FFM}$; where a and b are the regression line intercept and slope, respectively.

Using the equation: REE = 370 + 21.6 × FFM (kg); an 80-kg person who is 10% body fat (FFM = 72 kg) will have an estimated REE of 1925 kcal/day. If the 80-kg person is 30% body fat (FFM = 56 kg) they will have an estimated REE of 1580 kcal/day.

Numerous prediction equations have been developed over the years, and the constant a is usually positive. Therefore, the calculated metabolic rate per unit FFM decreases in the larger individual [68]. Wang et al. evaluated 15 descriptive REE-FFM linear regression equations and found the positive intercept ranged from 186 to 662 kcal/day (779–2770 kJ/day) and slopes varied from 19.7 to 24.5 kcal/kg FFM/day [119]. When REE in adult humans is plotted against FFM, a linear relationship is observed within the FFM range of ~40–80 kg. Given the non-zero intercept of this relationship, an unfeasible consequence is that a component of REE remains (~1675 kJ/day) when there is no FFM. Furthermore, this non-zero intercept implies that subjects with a small FFM have a relatively high REE compared with those with a large FFM. While many studies have demonstrated the variance in REE can be significantly predicted from FFM (for example, [122–128]; R^2 0.53–0.88), there remains a meaningful amount of the variance unexplained. Moreover, the resulting standard error of the estimate may be of a size that limits the utility of the prediction equation.

In order to explain some of the variance in REE unexplained by FFM, FM has been found to add significantly more predictive power than using FFM alone [129–131]. This is particularly the case in studies where the population measured displayed heterogeneity in FM. Consequently, numerous formulae have been derived using multiple regression analysis in which both FFM and FM are entered as independent variables, resulting with the linear function: $\text{REE} = a + b \times \text{FFM} + c \times \text{FM}$.

For example, in the study of 213 adults heterogeneous in body composition, Nelson et al. [129] found that REE was best explained by the following equation:

$$\text{REE (kJ/day)} = (1114 \pm 218) + (904 \pm 3.9 \times \text{FFM}) +$$
$$(13.2 \pm 3.7 \times \text{FM})\ [R^2 = 0.743;\ \text{SEE} = 174\ \text{kJ/day}]$$

Applying this to the 80-kg person with 72-kg FFM and 8-kg FM, REE would be predicted to equate 7728 ± 174 kJ/day (1840 ± 41 kcal/day). The 80-kg person with 56-kg FFM and 24-kg FM would have a predicted REE from this equation of 6493 ± 174 kJ/day (1546 ± 41 kcal/day).

While FFM is a strong predictor of REE, and addition of FM to the prediction model can reduce the predictive error, it has been understood for some time that there remains variance unaccounted for when considering body composition simply as two compartments, and that better differentiating FFM into organ tissues and skeletal muscle provides better estimates of REE [68,132]. New technology for the assessment of body composition in terms of organs and tissue masses is enabling a better understanding of the differences in REE between cohorts and within individuals over time, or with weight change [133].

Both athletic status and age may impact on these predictions, but in opposing ways. A decrease of 13%–20% in RMR has been reported between the ages of 30 and 80 years [134]. However, research also indicates that regular athletic training may result in a higher REE per unit FFM tissue [135], although with a few days detraining this effect may be negated [136]. Whether regular exercise training can reverse or ameliorate the ageing-related reduction in REE and ultimately TEE is a topic of some debate, and will be discussed in more detail below.

3.3.3 DIT

The thermic effect of food or DIT is the increase in energy expenditure above REE after the ingestion of food and is comprised of an obligatory component which includes the processes of digestion, absorption and storage of nutrients, and a facultative component which is linked with the neural stimulation of processes regulating chewing and swallowing [137]. Measurement of DIT is complex as it is relatively small in magnitude and requires stringent assessment protocols with participants sitting or lying semi-recumbent for 3 to 8 hours, during which indirect calorimetry measures are taken continuously [99,138,139]. There are many differences between measurement protocols, including the use of either a ventilated hood or respiratory chamber to measure energy expenditure to a single meal or number of meals across a day, the duration over which the thermogenic response is measured, the baseline used to calculate the net thermogenic response to a meal and differences in the meals provided to participants. Even under well-controlled conditions, DIT may be highly variable with reports of between-day variation between 4.2% and 41.2% [140–144]. Given the difficulty and inconvenience of measurement, DIT is commonly assumed to equate to 10% TEE, and thus 10% EER during weight stability.

In absolute terms, DIT increases with increased energy consumption simply as a function of the increased energy to be consumed. However, the degree to which the thermogenic response per unit energy processed is modifiable (i.e. increased or decreased efficiency of food/drink consumption) is unclear. There is some evidence that DIT may reduce in chronically undernourished individuals, such that when energy intake is increased, the thermogenic response to the meal is profligate [145–150].

3.3.4 Physical Activity and AEE

Physical activity is a global term traditionally defined as bodily movement resulting from contraction of skeletal muscle leading to a substantial increase in energy expenditure above resting levels. Physical activity can be categorised according to context or setting, and broadly encompasses exercise, sports and physical activities done as part of daily living, occupation, leisure and active transportation [151,152]. *Exercise*, a sub-component of physical activity, is commonly defined as planned, structured and repetitive movement with the intention of promoting or maintaining one or more components of physical fitness [153].

Energy expenditure associated with exercise training and competition will be referred to in this chapter as ExEE. AEE is the sum of energy expended in the performance of all daily physical activity, including both structured exercise (ExEE) and non-exercise activities (obligatory physical activities such as postural maintenance and the activities of daily living which is referred to as non-exercise activity thermogenesis [NEAT]) [100]. AEE is a function both of the total amount of physical movement as well as the efficiency, or energy cost, per unit of that movement. There are numerous ways AEE, ExEE and NEAT may be measured, but this is beyond the scope of this chapter therefore readers are referred to other reviews [98–102].

The extent to which ageing can alter the energy cost of movement (exercise or movement economy) has been the topic of considerable research. Similarly, the ability of regular exercise training to minimise the age-related changes has been examined particularly with regards to maintenance of normal function and mobility in the ageing population. However, there is considerably less research into comparisons between energy cost of movement in masters athletes and age-matched inactive peers, or comparably active younger cohorts. In the next section we will examine the evidence available, and try to examine the independent effects of ageing and exercise training on TEE and its components.

3.4 EFFECT OF AGEING AND EXERCISE TRAINING ON COMPONENTS OF TEE

When considered on a population level, TEE including the three major components reportedly decreases with age [154–157]. Research studies have consistently demonstrated that both REE and TEE decline with age after early adulthood [158–167]. There has been considerable interest in determining the degree to which the alterations in energy metabolism that accompany ageing are as a consequence of the ageing process *per se*, or subsequent to reductions in physical activity and lean mass that are often seen in older adults.

While free-living TEE measured by DLW demonstrates a drop after 40 years of age [28], in studies employing whole-body calorimeter protocols in which sedentary activity protocols are standardised, 24-hour energy expenditure does not differ between young and old adults [168,169]. Consequently, reduced TEE may be attributed, in part, to reduced intentional and spontaneous physical activity in old age in free-living individuals. However, if the energy cost per unit movement relative to weight is not decreased [170], the main mechanisms for the reduction in TEE on a population level is likely to be due to reduced movement as well as reduced body weight.

In research studies undertaken with physically active older adults, there is evidence that in addition to the increased energy expenditure associated with participation in a given activity, regular aerobic exercise in older adults may also contribute to increases in TEE [171] and its components including RMR, DIT and NEAT [172,173]. However, the extent to which increased expenditures in components of TEE are true increases, or part of the carry-over effect of the training session is poorly understood, particularly in the case of highly trained older adults.

The age-related declines in TEE are reported to parallel an increase in body fat mass, suggesting that changes in body composition may be important [155]. There is a positive association between fat-free mass and energy expenditure but a negative association of fat mass with energy expenditure [155]. Roberts et al. have speculated that the increase in body fat mass may help promote a decrease in energy expenditure for physical activity [89,174]. In National Health and Nutrition Examination Survey (NHANES) III, in those over 70 years, increased BMI or body fat was associated with limitations in functional living activities such as carrying groceries, suggesting that increasing body fat may influence energy expenditure through impairment of daily activities [175]. However, Westerterp and Meijer and co-workers [176,177] have reported that the decline in physical activity energy expenditure with age is most strongly predicted by age itself and not by body composition, indicating an effect of ageing on expenditure independent of the quantity of lean tissue and fat mass.

Importantly, maximal oxygen consumption is recognised to decline progressively with age [178–180], and while lifelong endurance training does not stop the decline in VO_{2max} with ageing, vigorous training is important to attenuate the decline [181]. These observations suggest that some parallel changes in fitness, AEE and body composition with age are most likely an inevitable consequence of the ageing process, probably due to underlying hormonal and biochemical changes in skeletal muscle and the cardiovascular system rather than a cumulative consequence of long-term inactivity [89,174]. However, even though the effects of exercise training on energy balance in particularly older adults may be small, it is important to recognise that there are additional positive effects of exercise on cardiovascular and bone health and prevention of falls and frailty. As for the components of TEE discussed below, there are a limited number of published studies on masters athletes, and the elderly participants in training studies may not well represent masters athletes.

3.4.1 REE

A longitudinal study of men documented a decline in REE with age of 1%–2% per decade [182], which equates with an average reduction in REE of 400 kJ/day (~95 kcal/day) between 20 and 70 years of age [174,182]. Because FFM commonly accounts for over one-half of the observed inter-individual variation in REE [183], age-related sarcopenia (or loss of lean body mass or FFM) is a likely candidate for the reduced REE in older adults [184–186]. There is some evidence from cross-sectional studies that even after adjusting for body composition, REE remains ~5% lower in older compared with younger adults [170,187–191]. However, not all research concurs, with as many studies finding that the age-related decline is completely explained by the differences in FFM [185,192–194].

One reason for this apparent discrepancy between studies is the aforementioned difference in the components of FFM. Because body composition is often simply defined by the two-compartment model—variations in the metabolic rates of the individual tissues that make up FFM (e.g. organs versus skeletal muscle) are not taken into consideration [133]. FFM is commonly lost with age; however more of the tissue lost is skeletal muscle than organ tissue, particularly in males [195]. As organ tissue is more metabolically active at rest than skeletal muscle [68], the preferential loss of skeletal muscle would result in a higher energy metabolism per unit of remaining FFM tissue. Bosy-Westphal et al. found no effect of age on REE when organ sizes within the FFM (assessed by magnetic resonance imaging) were taken into account [158].

A lower REE in older adults, even after accounting for organ tissue separately from skeletal muscle tissue, this suggests a reduced metabolic demand of the organ and/or skeletal tissues Kutsuzawa et al. reported no effect of age on forearm muscle energy metabolism assessed by 31P-magnetic resonance spectroscopy, suggesting no effect of age on REE beyond that due to the loss of different body tissues (with their different resting metabolic rates) [196]. Some contrasting evidence comes from Willis et al. who reported a significant age-associated decline in cerebral glucose metabolism which is indicative of brain energy expenditure as glucose is the primary metabolic fuel of this tissue [197]. However, the change in cerebral glucose metabolism was estimated to decrease 5 g/day between ages 20 and 70 years on average, and would result in an estimated decrease in REE of only 125 kJ/day (~30 kcal/day). Collectively, these findings suggest that even if REE is lower in the elderly compared with young adults even after appropriately accounting for body composition changes associated with ageing, the difference is so small that it can be considered insignificant [174].

In addition to the primary FFM-related effects on reduced REE, smaller reductions in REE have been related to declines in physical activity and age-associated reductions in exercise volume and energy intake [168,190,198]. Numerous studies have assessed the effect of endurance training on REE in young adults, but relatively less research has been undertaken in older individuals. In the former group, there is consistent evidence that REE is elevated in endurance-trained individuals [166,199,200] and for up to 2 days post-exercise after aerobic and resistance exercise in previously inactive adults [136,201,203].

Individuals who regularly participate in aerobic exercise have higher body composition-adjusted REE than those who are sedentary, at least in part, because of increased sympathetic tone [204–207]. Energy flux (the absolute level of energy intake and expenditure under conditions of energy balance) is higher in adults who exercise regularly than in individuals who are sedentary. When adults who have been exercising regularly reduce physical activity, they experience a decrease in energy flux and REE [208]. The decrease in REE is accompanied by decreases in plasma catecholamines, suggesting sympathetic involvement [208]. Bell et al. have shown that high energy flux is a factor contributing to increased β-adrenergic receptor stimulation of REE [207].

In one of the few studies to examine the influence of regular aerobic exercise on RMR in older men, Poehlman et al. reported that REE adjusted for body composition was not statistically different between older (~60 years) (1570 ± 173 kcal/day) and younger runners (~24 years) (1656 ± 137 kcal/day) or sedentary individuals (1728 ± 137 kcal/day) [190]. However, older sedentary men had a significantly lower REE (1397 ± 190 kcal/day) compared to the other three groups. Despite being cross-sectional, the findings from this study suggest that regular participation in aerobic activities such as running may attenuate the age-related decline in REE.

Similar findings have been reported in older women. For example, Van Pelt et al. studied active and sedentary older (~60 years) and younger (~30 years) women and found that REE adjusted for body composition was not statistically different between older (1368 ± 24 kcal/day) and younger women runners (1416 ± 48 kcal/day) or sedentary women (1368 ± 48 kcal/day) [209]. However, as for men in the study by Poehlman et al. [190], older sedentary women had a significantly lower REE (1248 ± 48 kcal/day) compared to the other groups. Accordingly, cross-sectional findings suggest that participation in regular aerobic exercise may attenuate the age-related decline in REE in both men and women. However, the cause of this decline is unclear. In contrast, other studies have found no correlation between REE and aerobic power [210–215].

There is some evidence that in men who are able to maintain an exercise volume and/or energy intake at levels similar to that of young physically active men, REE does not decline. For example, Sullo et al. reported a positive correlation between aerobic power and REE in masters athletes [216]. This finding is consistent with reports of increased REE in cross-sectional studies in resistance-trained young men [217] and women [218] compared with age-matched sedentary controls, and the increase in RMR after resistance training in older men reported in longitudinal studies [219,220]. High volumes of exercise therefore may help to preserve muscle mass (and REE) and buffer the commonly observed increase in body fat with age [221]. Ballor and Poehlman suggested that increased REE may be influenced by increased food flux, increased activity of various enzymatic reactions, the replacement of glycogen stores, repair of exercise-induced trauma and the increased concentration of metabolic hormones [218].

3.4.2 DIT

DIT may decline with advancing chronological age. However, the impact of any decline in the smallest component of energy expenditure is unclear. DIT is difficult to measure, and has a high day-to-day variability. There is also confusion regarding any potential decline in DIT being the result of primary or secondary ageing. Some studies report a decrease in the thermic effect of feeding in older age [222–225], while other studies report no change [188,226–229].

Ageing is often associated with decreases in food intake that will have an automatic reduction on DIT. However, this is not evidence of a change in efficiency of the processing of nutrients, but rather a decrease in the amount of nutrient to be processed. A rationale provided for the different findings of various studies is that DIT may not decline with ageing *per se*, but that some studies may have confounded age with factors that decrease thermic effect of feeding independent of ageing, such as obesity and/or digestive problems that limit nutrient absorption [227].

To avoid the potential concern that meal size might influence differences in DIT between young and older individuals, Melanson et al. measured the thermic effect of feeding at three levels of energy intake [227]. There was no significant difference in DIT between the age groups, and mean post-prandial values for energy expenditure above initial fasting values were actually slightly higher in the older group than the young group.

Other cross-sectional data suggest that an age-related decline in DIT is secondary to ageing. For example, Visser et al. examined DIT for 180 min following a mixed ~300-kcal meal in 103 older women and men (~73 years) and 56 younger women and men (~25 years) [229]. No difference was found between the younger (27.5 ± 6.0 kcal/180 min) and older (26.5 ± 6.2 kcal/180 min) women. However, in men, DIT was 18% lower in older (30.1 ± 6.5 kcal/180 min) vs. younger (36.8 ± 8.1 kcal/180 min) individuals. As for other components of energy expenditure, body composition differences should be accounted for when considering relationships between ageing and DIT.

In addition to body composition, differences in daily physical activity levels between younger and older adults may influence DIT. Poehlman et al. examined DIT for 180 min following a mixed, 10-kcal/kg fat-free mass meal in active and sedentary, older (~60 years) and younger (~24 years) men [190]. DIT adjusted for body composition was greater for younger (77.0 ± 3.7 kcal/180 min) and older runners (69.8 ± 7.0 kcal/180 min) compared to sedentary younger (53.1 ± 4.0 kcal/180 min) and older (51.5 ± 6.9 kcal/180 min) individuals.

Contrasting earlier views regarding the nature of DIT and exercise include some research that reports a higher DIT in trained individuals [230] while other research suggests a lower DIT effect in trained athletes vs. untrained individuals [231]. Sullo et al. reported a higher mean DIT in athletes with higher levels of aerobic power but the differences were not statistically significant [216].

3.4.3 AEE and NEAT

Regular participation in physical activity and exercise has numerous potential benefits. Along with the increase in energy expenditure as a function of increased physical activity participation, improvements in fitness and a consequent increase in activity levels across the rest of the day may also occur. However, there are some data to suggest that participation in regular aerobic exercise may decrease activity during non-exercising periods in older adults [232,233].

In a study of 11 healthy, 56–78-year-old men and women, Goran and Poehlman examined the influence of an 8-week aerobic cycling program on TEE assessed by DLW [232]. The cycling program consisted of three sessions per week with 150–300 kcal expended per session. While TEE did not change significantly, daily physical activity separate to the cycling session decreased by 62% following the 8-week intervention. This suggests that the cycling intensity, (~85% of aerobic capacity at the end of the intervention), may have been too vigorous for the older adults and contributed to a reduction in activity during the balance of the day because of fatigue.

Meijer et al. examined the influence of moderate-intensity aerobic exercise in combination with resistance training on activity counts over 12 weeks in 15 men and women (59 years) [233]. At 12 weeks, older adults spent less time being active on days they participated in structured aerobic activities. Unlike the study by Goran and Poehlman [232] where exercise was performed in the morning, training was undertaken in the afternoon with the anticipation of overcoming the effect of structured exercise earlier in the day decreasing daily activity.

In contrast, Hunter et al. studied the effect of a 26-week resistance training program REE, TEE and AEE in 61- to 77-year-old men and women [171]. Body composition (four-compartment model), strength, REE, TEE (DLW) and AEE (TEE – REE + DIT) were evaluated before and after the intervention. Both muscular strength (36%) and fat-free mass (2 kg) significantly increased while body weight did not change. TEE (12%) increased significantly, and AEE (30%) approached significance ($P = 0.06$). The TEE increase remained significant even after adjustment for the energy expenditure of the resistance training. The increase in TEE occurred as a result of increases in both REE and physical activity. This was a longer intervention, so it is uncertain if the same effect on NEAT may have been noted earlier in the intervention.

Withers et al. compared REE, TEE and activity-related energy expenditure (AEE) of chronically active and chronically inactive women ranging in age between 49 and 70 years of age [234]. They reported that the chronically active older women had increased REE, TEE and AEE. Furthermore, they found an almost identical AEE adjusted for the estimated energy expenditure of the planned training sessions, indicating no reduction in NEAT as a consequence of the exercise training.

In summary, improvements in cardiorespiratory fitness as a function of training in healthy older adults may not result in an increase in TEE because of a compensatory decline in physical activity across the remainder of the day [230,232,233]. However, to date we are not aware of any published studies on compensatory behaviours in masters athletes. It is also important to mention that in the relatively small number of energy expenditure studies on chronically trained older athletes, a key question is the representativeness of the participants.

As outlined in Section 3.3, AEE is the sum of energy expended in the performance of all daily physical activity and is a consequence of the total amount of movement performed (a function of duration, intensity and type) and the energy costs per unit movement (exercise or movement economy). The energy cost of ambulation in older adults is elevated as compared with young, healthy adults [235,236], and may be attributed to differences in body composition, cardiorespiratory fitness and muscular strength [237,238]. Furthermore, in previously untrained older women, strength training can improve efficiency of undertaking activities of daily living [239].

Few studies are available to examine the differential effects of chronic exercise training and ageing on movement economy. Quinn et al. investigated the relationship that age has on factors affecting running economy in competitive distance runners [240]. Running, step rate, lactate threshold, VO_{2max}, muscle strength and endurance, flexibility, power and body composition was measured in sub-elite distance runners in three group: young (18–39 years), masters (40–59 years) and older adults (> 60 years). The older group was significantly lower than in the young and masters groups in VO_{2max}, flexibility, power and upper body strength. However, there were no differences in the slopes of the running economy regression lines among age groups. The results from this cross-sectional analysis suggest that age-related declines in running performance are associated with declines in maximal and sub-maximal cardiorespiratory variables and declines in strength and power, not due to declines in running economy.

3.5 SUMMARY

There is a paucity of information regarding the energy needs of the masters athlete. Consequently, to gain some understanding the energy needs of this cohort we have attempted to combine the literature pertaining to both younger athletes and the ageing adult. As mentioned in Section 3.2, to predict the energy needs of the masters athlete, it is important to consider the extent to which the EER prediction equations devised on the general older population account for the amount of physical activity undertaken in training and competition. It is likely that even in the most dedicated masters athlete, ageing will still have an impact on components of TEE.

The available evidence suggests that regular exercise in older individuals maintains FFM and limits the reductions in maximal aerobic power and muscular strength, which collectively limits reductions in REE. Further, age does not appear to alter efficiency of nutrient processing, and therefore DIT, in well-functioning older adults with DIT being comparable with younger adults. However, absolute reductions in DIT are evident in any cohort if habitual dietary intake is reduced. It is clear that the efficiency of movement (movement economy) changes with ageing. However, in older adults who are functioning well enough to perform in masters competitions, these changes are likely to have a small effect, if any, on TEE. What is more likely is that over time the energy costs of performing physical work and the ability to recover between training sessions will reduce the amount of training undertaken, the AEE and thus TEE, and therefore energy needs.

Readers interested in a number of recent reviews focused on energy balance and weight control in relation to both sports performance and general health are directed to [241,242].

3.6 PRACTICAL IMPLICATIONS FOR SPORTS MEDICINE PROFESSIONALS, CLINICIANS, COACHES AND MASTERS ATHLETES

- Maintenance of muscular strength and aerobic capacity is paramount in older individuals. Ensuring that these components of physical fitness are maintained will prevent or at least minimise the rate of decline of each of the components of TEE and TEE itself.

- The amount of energy expended through exercise is very easily compensated for by reductions in non-exercise activity thermogenesis (NEAT) or modifications to activities of daily living. It is important that exercise is seen as an additional component in the day and not a substitute for usual activities.
- The energy expended through exercise is even more easily compensated for by injudicious consumption of 'rewarding' foods. While the cardiorespiratory and strength benefits of the exercise may still be realised, this is a sure way of causing a positive energy balance and a possible path to undesirable fat gain.

3.7 FUTURE RESEARCH DIRECTIONS

Despite considerable research into human energy requirements, determining the energy needs for an individual to achieve weight stability remains a challenge. This challenge is largely due to the inaccuracies of field-based methods of measuring energy intake, and the time frame over which measurement is needed to accurately reflect habitual energy intake and/or expenditure. This challenge becomes more complex when accounting for the additional energy needs of regular exercise training and competition, alongside proposed reductions in basal energy requirements that may accompany ageing. Unfortunately, the master athlete is an underrepresented cohort in terms of studies focused on determining energy requirements. Future research needs to be undertaken, where possible using gold-standard methodologies, to better profile the energy requirements of exercise training and competition. This research should ideally also consider the magnitude of alteration in energy requirements where fat loss or lean mass gains are a focus of the training program to optimise athletic performance. Arguably this research is needed in athletes of all age groups, but is particularly important in the ageing athlete.

REFERENCES

1. Bloom, D.E., 7 Billion and counting, *Science* 333(6042), 562–9, 2011.
2. Lee, R., The outlook for population growth, *Science* 333(6042), 569–73, 2011.
3. United National Department of Economic and Social Affairs, Population Ageing and the Non-communicable Diseases, http://www.un.org/en/development/desa/population/publications/factsheets/index.shtml, accessed 3 February 2014.
4. World Health Organization, *World Health Organization, 2008–2013 Action Plan for the Global Strategy for the Prevention and Control of Noncommunicable Diseases*, August 2011.
5. World Health Organization, *World Health Organization, Global Status Report on Noncommunicable Diseases 2010*, August 2011.
6. Allen, J. and Morelli, V., Aging and exercise, *Clin. Geriatr. Med.* 27(4), 661–71, 2011.
7. Lanza, I.R., Short, D.K., Short, K.R. et al., Endurance exercise as a countermeasure for aging, *Diabetes* 57(11), 2933–42, 2008.
8. Morelli, V., Fatigue and chronic fatigue in the elderly: Definitions, diagnoses, and treatments, *Clin. Geriatr. Med.* 27(4), 673–86, 2011.
9. Zoorob, R.J., Kihlberg, C.J., and Taylor, S.E., Aging and disease prevention, *Clin. Geriatr. Med.* 27(4), 523–39, 2011.
10. Byberg, L., Melhus, H., Gedeborg, R. et al., Total mortality after changes in leisure time physical activity in 50 year old men: 35 year follow-up of population based cohort, *BMJ* 338, 2009.
11. Nelson, M.E., Rejeski, W.J., Blair, S.N. et al., Physical activity and public health in older adults: Recommendation from the American College of Sports Medicine and the American Heart Association, *Med. Sci. Sports Exerc.* 39(8), 1435–45, 2007.
12. Andersen, W.G., Further studies on the longevity of Yale athletes, *Med. Times* 44, 75–6, 1916.
13. Hill, A.B., Cricket and its relation to the duration of life, *Lancet* 2, 949–50, 1927.
14. Teramoto, M. and Bungum, T.J., Mortality and longevity of elite athletes, *J. Sci. Med. Sport* 13(4), 410–6, 2010.
15. Denvir, M.A. and Gray, G.A., Run for your life: Exercise, oxidative stress and the ageing endothelium, *J. Physiol.* 587(17), 4137–8, 2009.

16. Speakman, J.R. and Mitchell, S.E., Caloric restriction, *Mol. Aspects Med.* 32(3), 159–221, 2011.
17. Vitousek, K.M., Gray, J.A., and Grubbs, K.M., Caloric restriction for longevity: I. Paradigm, protocols and physiological findings in animal research, *Eur. Eat. Disord. Rev.* 12(5), 279–99, 2004.
18. Vitousek, K.M., Manke, F.P., Gray, J.A., and Vitousek, M.N., Caloric restriction for longevity: II. The systematic neglect of behavioural and psychological outcomes in animal research, *Eur. Eat. Disord. Rev.* 12(6), 338–60, 2004.
19. Popkin, B.M., Adair, L.S., and Ng, S.W., Global nutrition transition and the pandemic of obesity in developing countries, *Nut. Rev.* 70(1), 3–21, 2012.
20. Giskes, K., van Lenthe, F., Avendano-Pabon, M., and Brug, J., A systematic review of environmental factors and obesogenic dietary intakes among adults: Are we getting closer to understanding obesogenic environments? *Obes. Rev.* 12(5), 95–106, 2011.
21. Ng, S.W., Zaghloul, S., Ali, H.I., Harrison, G., and Popkin, B.M., The prevalence and trends of overweight, obesity and nutrition-related non-communicable diseases in the Arabian Gulf States, *Obes. Rev.* 12(1), 1–13, 2011.
22. Doak, C.M., Wijnhoven, T.M.A., Schokker, D.F., Visscher, T.L.S., and Seidell, J.C., Age standardization in mapping adult overweight and obesity trends in the WHO European Region, *Obes. Rev.* 13(2), 174–91, 2012.
23. Xi, B., Liang, Y., He, T. et al., Secular trends in the prevalence of general and abdominal obesity among Chinese adults, 1993–2009, *Obes. Rev.* 13(3), 287–96, 2012.
24. Lahti-Koski, M., Seppänen-Nuijten, E., Männistö, S. et al., Twenty-year changes in the prevalence of obesity among Finnish adults, *Obes. Rev.* 11(3), 171–6, 2010.
25. Baskin, M.L., Ard, J., Franklin, F., and Allison, D.B., Prevalence of obesity in the United States, *Obes. Rev.* 6(1), 5–7, 2005.
26. International Obesity Task Force, Obesity the Global Epidemic, http://www.iaso.org/iotf/obesity/obesitytheglobalepidemic/, accessed 1 February 2014.
27. Brooks, G.A., Butte, N.F., Rand, W.M., Flatt, J.-P., and Caballero, B., Chronicle of the Institute of Medicine physical activity recommendation: How a physical activity recommendation came to be among dietary recommendations, *Am. J. Clin. Nutr.* 79(5), 921S–30, 2004.
28. Institute of Medicine, Panel on Macronutrients, Panel on the Definition of Dietary Fiber, Subcommittee on Upper Reference Levels of Nutrients, Subcommittee on Interpretation and Uses of Dietary Reference Intakes, and the Standing Committee on the Scientific Evaluation of Dietary Reference Intakes, *Dietary Reference Intakes for Energy, Carbohydrate, Fiber, Fat, Fatty Acids, Cholesterol, Protein, and Amino Acids*, The National Academies Press, Washington, DC, 2005.
29. World Health Organization, the Food and Agriculture Organization of the United Nations, and the United Nations University, *Energy and Protein Requirements*, World Health Organization, Geneva, 1985.
30. Black, A. and Cole, T., Within- and between-subject variation in energy expenditure measured by the doubly-labelled water technique: Implications for validating reported dietary energy intake, *Eur. J. Clin. Nutr.* 54(5), 386–94, 2000.
31. Black, A.E., Critical evaluation of energy intake using the Goldberg cut-off for energy intake: Basal metabolic rate. A practical guide to its calculation, use and limitations, *Int. J. Obes.* 24(9), 1119–30, 2000.
32. Block, G. and Hartman, A.M., Issues in reproducibility and validity of dietary studies, *Am. J. Clin. Nutr.* 50(5), 1133–8, 1989.
33. Guyatt, G., Walter, S., and Norman, G., Measuring change over time: Assessing the usefulness of evaluative instruments, *J. Chronic Dis.* 40(2), 171–8, 1987.
34. Potosky, A., Block, G., and Hartman, A., The apparent validity of diet questionnaires is influenced by number of diet-record days used for comparison, *J. Am. Diet. Assoc.* 90(6), 810–3, 1990.
35. Spiegelman, D., McDermott, A., and Rosner, B., Regression calibration method for correcting measurement-error bias in nutritional epidemiology, *Am. J. Clin. Nutr.* 65(4), 1179S–86, 1997.
36. Nelson, M., Black, A., Morris, J., and Cole, T., Between- and within-subject variation in nutrient intake from infancy to old age: Estimating the number of days required to rank dietary intakes with desired precision, *Am. J. Clin. Nutr.* 50(1), 155–67, 1989.
37. Basiotis, P.P., Welsh, S.O., Cronin, F.J., Kelsay, J.L., and Mertz, W., Number of days of food intake records required to estimate individual and group nutrient intakes with defined confidence, *J. Nutr.* 117(9), 1638–41, 1987.
38. Palaniappan, U., Cue, R.I., Payette, H., and Gray-Donald, K., Implications of day-to-day variability on measurements of usual food and nutrient intakes, *J. Nutr.* 133(1), 232–5, 2003.
39. Jackson, K.A., Byrne, N.M., Magarey, A.M., and Hills, A.P., Minimizing random error in dietary intakes assessed by 24-h recall, in overweight and obese adults, *Eur. J. Clin. Nutr.* 62(4), 537–43, 2008.

40. Hill, R. and Davies, P., The validity of self-reported energy intake as determined using the doubly labelled water technique, *Br. J. Nutr.* 85(4), 415–30, 2001.
41. Johnson, R., Goran, M., and Poehlman, E., Correlates of over- and underreporting of energy intake in healthy older men and women, *Am. J. Clin. Nutr.* 59(6), 1286–90, 1994.
42. Prentice, A.M., Black, A.E., Coward, W.A. et al., High levels of energy expenditure in obese women, *Br. Med. J.* 292(6526), 983–7, 1986.
43. Lichtman, S., Pisarska, K., Berman, E. et al., Discrepancy between self-reported and actual caloric intake and exercise in obese subjects, *N. Engl. J. Med.* 327(27), 1893–8, 1992.
44. Drenowatz, C., Eisenmann, J.C., Carlson, J.J., Pfeiffer, K.A., and Pivarnik, J.M., Energy expenditure and dietary intake during high-volume and low-volume training periods among male endurance athletes, *Appl. Physiol. Nutr. Metab.* 37(2), 199–205, 2012.
45. Fudge, B.W., Westerterp, K.R., Kiplamai, F.K. et al., Evidence of negative energy balance using doubly labelled water in elite Kenyan endurance runners prior to competition, *Br. J. Nutr.* 95(1), 59–66, 2006.
46. Hill, R.J. and Davies, P.S., Energy intake and energy expenditure in elite lightweight female rowers, *Med. Sci. Sports Exerc.* 34(11), 1823–9, 2002.
47. Edwards, J.E., Lindeman, A.K., Mikesky, A.E., and Stager, J.M., Energy balance in highly trained female endurance runners, *Med. Sci. Sports Exerc.* 25(12), 1398–404, 1993.
48. Sundgot-Borgen, J., Prevalence of eating disorders in elite female athletes, *Int. J. Sport Nutr.* 3(1), 29–40, 1993.
49. Bingham, S.A., Limitations of the various methods for collecting dietary intake data, *Ann. Nutr. Metab.* 35(3), 117–27, 1991.
50. Mertz, W., Tsui, J., Judd, J. et al., What are people really eating? The relation between energy intake derived from estimated diet records and intake determined to maintain body weight, *Am. J. Clin. Nutr.* 54(2), 291–5, 1991.
51. Pannemans, D.L.E. and Westerterp, K.R., Estimation of energy intake to feed subjects at energy balance as verified with doubly labelled water—a study in the elderly, *Eur. J. Clin. Nutr.* 47(7), 490–6, 1993.
52. Seale, J., Energy expenditure measurements in relation to energy requirements, *Am. J. Clin. Nutr.* 62(5), 1042S–6, 1995.
53. Shahar, D.R., Yu, B., Houston, D.K. et al., Misreporting of energy intake in the elderly using doubly labeled water to measure total energy expenditure and weight change, *J. Am Coll. Nutr.* 29(1), 14–24, 2010.
54. Costill, D., Water and electrolyte requirements during exercise, *Clin. Sports Med.* 3(3), 639–48, 1984.
55. Cooper, J., Nguyen, D., Ruby, B., and Schoeller, D., Maximal sustained levels of energy expenditure in humans during exercise, *Med. Sci. Sports Exerc.* 43(12), 2359–67, 2011.
56. Kirkwood, J., Minireview. A limit to metabolisable energy intake in mammals and birds, *Comp. Biochem. Physiol. A Comp. Physiol.* 75(1), 1–3, 1983.
57. Hammond, K. and Diamond, J., Maximal sustained energy budgets in humans and animals, *Nature* 386(6624), 457–62, 1997.
58. Brody, S., *Bioenergetics of Growth*, Reinhold, New York, 1945.
59. Westerterp, K.R., Limits to sustainable human metabolic rate, *J. Exp. Biol.* 204(18), 3183–7, 2001.
60. Stroud, M., The nutritional demands of very prolonged exercise in man, *Proc. Nutr. Soc.* 57(1), 55–61, 1998.
61. Westerterp, K.R., Saris, W.H., van Es, M., and ten Hoor, F., Use of the doubly labeled water technique in humans during heavy sustained exercise, *J. Appl. Physiol.* 61(6), 2162–7, 1986.
62. Rehrer, N., Hellemans, I., Rolleston, A., Rush, E., and Miller, B., Energy intake and expenditure during a 6-day cycling stage race, *Scand. J. Med. Sci. Sports* 20(4), 609–18, 2010.
63. Fudge, B., Westerterp, K., Kiplamai, F. et al., Evidence of negative energy balance using doubly labelled water in elite Kenyan endurance runners prior to competition, *Br. J. Nutr.* 95(1), 59–66, 2006.
64. Hoyt, R.W., Jones, T.E., Stein, T.P. et al., Doubly labeled water measurement of human energy expenditure during strenuous exercise, *J. Appl. Physiol.* 71(1), 16–22, 1991.
65. Forbes-Ewan, C.H., Morrissey, B.L., Gregg, G.C., and Waters, D.R., Use of doubly labeled water technique in soldiers training for jungle warfare, *J. Appl. Physiol.* 67(1), 14–8, 1989.
66. Jones, P.J., Jacobs, I., Morris, A., and Ducharme, M.B., Adequacy of food rations in soldiers during an arctic exercise measured by doubly labeled water, *J. Appl. Physiol.* 75(4), 1790–7, 1993.
67. Stroud, M., Ritz, P., Coward, W. et al., Energy expenditure using isotope-labelled water ($^2H_2{}^{18}O$), exercise performance, skeletal muscle enzyme activities and plasma biochemical parameters in humans during 95 days of endurance exercise with inadequate energy intake, *Eur. J. Appl. Physiol. Occup. Physiol.* 76(3), 243–52, 1997.

68. Elia, M., Organ and tissue contribution to metabolic rate, in *Energy Metabolism: Tissue Determinants and Cellular Corollaries*, Kinney, J.M. and Tucker, H.N., Eds, Raven, New York, 1992, pp. 61–80.
69. Schoeller, D.A. and van Santen, E., Measurement of energy expenditure in humans by doubly labeled water method, *J. Appl. Physiol.* 53(4), 955–9, 1982.
70. Schoeller, D.A. and Webb, P., Five-day comparison of the doubly labeled water method with respiratory gas exchange, *Am. J. Clin. Nutr.* 40(1), 153–8, 1984.
71. International Atomic Energy Agency, Assessment of body composition and total energy expenditure in humans using stable isotope techniques. Human Health Series, 2009, http://www-pub.iaea.org/MTCD/publications/PubDetails.asp?pubId=7982, accessed 2 February 2014.
72. Schoeller, D.A., Measurement of energy expenditure in free-living humans by using doubly labeled water, *J. Nutr.* 118(11), 1278–89, 1988.
73. Schoeller, D.A., Insights into energy balance from doubly labeled water, *Int. J. Obes.* 32(Suppl 7), S72–5, 2008.
74. Speakman, J.R. and Thomson, S.C., Validation of the labeled bicarbonate technique for measurement of short-term energy expenditure in the mouse, *Z. Emahrungswiss.* 36(4), 273–7, 1997.
75. Speakman, J.R., The history and theory of the doubly labeled water technique, *Am. J. Clin. Nutr.* 68(4), 932S–8S, 1998.
76. Ainslie, P., Reilly, T., and Westerterp, K., Estimating human energy expenditure: A review of techniques with particular reference to doubly labelled water, *Sports Med.* 33(9), 683–98, 2003.
77. Conway, J.M., Seale, J.L., Jacobs, D.R., Jr., Irwin, M.L., and Ainsworth, B.E., Comparison of energy expenditure estimates from doubly labeled water, a physical activity questionnaire, and physical activity records, *Am. J. Clin. Nutr.* 75(3), 519–25, 2002.
78. Neilson, H.K., Robson, P.J., Friedenreich, C.M., and Csizmadi, I., Estimating activity energy expenditure: How valid are physical activity questionnaires? *Am. J. Clin. Nutr.* 87(2), 279–91, 2008.
79. Westerterp, K.R., Assessment of physical activity: A critical appraisal, *Eur. J. Appl. Physiol.* 105(6), 823–8, 2009.
80. Westerterp, K.R. and Plasqui, G., Physical activity and human energy expenditure, *Curr. Opin. Clin. Nutr. Metab. Care* 7(6), 607–13, 2004.
81. Bouchard, C., Tremblay, A., Leblanc, C., Lortie, G., Savard, R., and Theriault, G., A method to assess energy expenditure in children and adults, *Am. J. Clin. Nutr.* 37(3), 461–7, 1983.
82. Heymsfield, S., Harp, J., Rowell, P., Nguyen, A., and Pietrobelli, A., How much may I eat? Calorie estimates based upon energy expenditure prediction equations, *Obes. Rev.* 7(4), 361–70, 2006.
83. Blanc, S., Colligan, A.S., Trabulsi, J. et al., Influence of delayed isotopic equilibration in urine on the accuracy of the (2)H(2)(18)O method in the elderly, *J. Appl. Physiol.* 92(3), 1036–44, 2002.
84. Ritz, P., Johnson, P., and Coward, W., Measurements of ^{2}H and ^{18}O in body water: Analytical considerations and physiological implications, *Br. J. Nutr.* 72(1), 3–12, 1994.
85. Ravussin, E., Harper, I.T., Rising, R., and Bogardus, C., Energy expenditure by doubly labeled water: Validation in lean and obese subjects, *Am. J. Physiol.* 261, E402–9, 1991.
86. Schoeller, D.A., Ravussin, E., Schutz, Y., Acheson, K.J., Baertschi, P., and Jequier, E., Energy expenditure by doubly labeled water: Validation in humans and proposed calculation, *Am. J. Physiol.* 250, R823–30, 1986.
87. Huang, A.J., Brown, J.S., Boyko, E.J. et al., Clinical significance of postvoid residual volume in older ambulatory women, *J. Am. Geriatr. Soc.* 59(8), 1452–8, 2011.
88. Negro, C.L.A. and Muir, G.H., Chronic urinary retention in men: How we define it, and how does it affect treatment outcome, *BJU Int.*, 110(11), 1590–4, 2012.
89. Roberts, S.B. and Dallal, G.E., Energy requirements and aging, *Public Health Nutr.* 8(7a), 1028–36, 2005.
90. Ravussin, E., Lillioja, S., Anderson, T., Christin, L., and Bogardus, C., Determinants of 24-hour energy expenditure in man. Methods and results using a respiratory chamber, *J. Clin. Invest.* 78(6), 1568–78, 1986.
91. Duncan, R., Variations in resting metabolic rates of men in Antarctica, *Eur. J. Appl. Physiol. Occup. Physiol.* 57(4), 514–8, 1988.
92. Garby, L., Metabolic adaptation to decreases in energy intake due to changes in the energy cost of low energy expenditure regimen, *World Rev. Nutr. Diet.* 61, 173–208, 1990.
93. Plasqui, G., Kester, A.D.M., and Westerterp, K.R., Seasonal variation in sleeping metabolic rate, thyroid activity, and leptin, *Am. J. Physiol.* 285(2), E338–43, 2003.
94. Treuth, M.S., Hunter, G.R., and Williams, M., Effects of exercise intensity on 24-h energy expenditure and substrate oxidation, *Med. Sci. Sports Exerc.* 28(9), 1138–43, 1996.

95. Garby, L., Lammert, O., and Nielsen, E., Changes in energy expenditure of light physical activity during a 10 day period at 34 degrees C environmental temperature, *Eur. J. Clin. Nutr.* 44(3), 241–4, 1990.
96. Neilson, H.K., Robson, P.J., Friedenreich, C.M., and Csizmadi, I., Estimating activity energy expenditure: How valid are physical activity questionnaires? *Am. J. Clin. Nutr.* 87(2), 279–91, 2008.
97. Spurr, G.B., Dufour, D.L., Reina, J.C., and Haught, T.A., Daily energy expenditure of women by factorial and heart rate methods, *Med. Sci. Sports Exerc.* 29(9), 1255–62, 1997.
98. Byrne, N.M., Shultz, S.P., and Hills, A.P., Field assessment of physical activity and energy expenditure among athletes, in *Nutritional Assessment of Athletes*, 2nd ed., CRC Press, Boca Raton, FL, 2010, pp. 183–212.
99. Donahoo, W., Levine, J., and Melanson, E., Variability in energy expenditure and its components, *Curr. Opin. Clin. Nutr. Metab. Care* 7(6), 599–605, 2004.
100. Levine, J., Melanson, E.L., Westerterp, K.R., and Hill, J.O., Measurement of the components of nonexercise activity thermogenesis, *Am. J. Physiol. Endocrinol. Metab.* 281(4), E670–5, 2001.
101. Schutz, Y., Weinsier, R.L., and Hunter, G.R., Assessment of free-living physical activity in humans: An overview of currently available and proposed new measures, *Obes. Res.* 9(6), 368–79, 2001.
102. Westerterp, K. and Plasqui, G., Physical activity and human energy expenditure, *Curr. Opin. Clin. Nutr. Metab. Care* 7(6), 607–13, 2004.
103. Liu, J., Piao, J., Sun, R., Tian, Y., and Yang, X., Evaluation of the factorial method for determination of energy expenditure in 16 young adult women living in China, *Biomed. Environ. Sci.* 24(4), 357–63, 2011.
104. Jones, P., Martin, L., Su, W., and Boyd, N., Canadian recommended nutrient intakes underestimate true energy requirements in middle-aged women, *Can. J. Pub. Health* 88(5), 314–9, 1997.
105. Martin, L., Su, W., Jones, P., Lockwood, G., Tritchler, D., and Boyd, N., Comparison of energy intakes determined by food records and doubly labeled water in women participating in a dietary-intervention trial, *Am. J. Clin. Nutr.* 63(4), 483–90, 1996.
106. Roberts, S., Energy expenditure and the development of early obesity, *Ann. N. Y. Acad. Sci.* 699, 18–25, 1993.
107. Roberts, S., Heyman, M., Evans, W., Fuss, P., Tsay, R., and Young, V., Dietary energy requirements of young adult men, determined by using the doubly labeled water method, *Am. J. Clin. Nutr.* 54(3), 499–505, 1991.
108. Sawaya, A., Saltzman, E., Fuss, P., Young, V., and Roberts, S., Dietary energy requirements of young and older women determined by using the doubly labeled water method, *Am. J. Clin. Nutr.* 62(2), 338–44, 1995.
109. Sawaya, A., Tucker, K., Tsay, R. et al., Evaluation of four methods for determining energy intake in young and older women: Comparison with doubly labeled water measurements of total energy expenditure, *Am. J. Clin. Nutr.* 63(4), 491–9, 1996.
110. Morio, B., Ritz, P., Verdier, E., Montaurier, C., Beaufrere, B., and Vermorel, M., Critical evaluation of the factorial and heart-rate recording methods for the determination of energy expenditure of free-living elderly people, *Br. J. Nutr.* 78(5), 709–22, 1997.
111. Gallagher, D., Belmonte, D., Deurenberg, P. et al., Organ-tissue mass measurement allows modeling of REE and metabolically active tissue mass, *Am. J. Physiol.* 275(2 Pt 1), E249–58, 1998.
112. Kinney, J.M. and Tucker, H.N., eds., *Energy Metabolism: Tissue Determinants and Cellular Corollaries*, Raven, New York, 1992.
113. Kleiber, M., *The Fire of Life*, Krieger Publishing Co., New York, 1975.
114. Boothby, W.M., Berkson, J., and Dunn, H.L., Studies of the energy metabolism of normal individuals: A standard for basal metabolism, with a nomogram for clinical application, *Am. J. Physiol.* 116, 468–84, 1936.
115. Aub, J.C. and Du Bois, E.F., Clinical metabolism of old men, *Arch. Int. Med.* 19, 823–31, 1917.
116. Benedict, F.G., *Vital energetics. A study in comparative metabolism*, Carnegie Institute of Washington No. 503, Washington, DC, 1938.
117. Benedict, F.G., Sherman, H.C., Campbell, H.L., and Zmachinsky, A., Basal metabolism of rats in relation to old age and exercise during old age: Three figures, *J. Nutr.* 14(2), 179–98, 1937.
118. Sendroy, J. and Cecchini, L.P., Determination of human body surface area from height and weight, *Am. J. Physiol.* 7, 1–12, 1954.
119. Wang, Z., Heshka, S., Gallagher, D., Boozer, C.N., Donald, P.K., and Heysmfield, S.B., Resting energy expenditure-fat-free mass relationship: New insights provided by body composition modeling, *Am. J. Physiol.* 279(3), E539–45, 2000.
120. Cunningham, J.J., Body composition and resting metabolic rate: The myth of feminine metabolism, *Am. J. Clin. Nutr.* 36(4), 721–6, 1982.

121. Webb, P., Energy expenditure and fat-free mass in men and women, *Am. J. Clin. Nutr.* 34(9), 1816–26, 1981.
122. Heshka, S., Yang, M.U., Wang, J., Burt, P., and Pi-Sunyer, F.X., Weight loss and change in resting metabolic rate, *Am. J. Clin. Nutr.* 52(6), 981–6, 1990.
123. Jensen, M.D., Braun, J.S., Vetter, R.J., and Marsh, H.M., Measurement of body potassium with a whole-body counter: Relationship between lean body mass and resting energy expenditure, *Mayo Clin. Proc.* 63(9), 864–8, 1988.
124. Ravussin, E. and Bogardus, C., Relationship of genetics, age, and physical fitness to daily energy expenditure and fuel utilization, *Am. J. Clin. Nutr.* 49(5 Suppl), 968–75, 1989.
125. Ravussin, E., Burnand, B., Schutz, Y., and Jequier, E., Twenty-four-hour energy expenditure and resting metabolic rate in obese, moderately obese, and control subjects, *Am. J. Clin. Nutr.* 35(3), 566–73, 1982.
126. Ravussin, E., Lillioja, S., Anderson, T.E., Christin, L., and Bogardus, C., Determinants of 24-hour energy expenditure in man. Methods and results using a respiratory chamber, *J. Clin. Invest.* 78(6), 1568–78, 1986.
127. Weigle, D.S., Sande, K.J., Iverius, P.H., Monsen, E.R., and Brunzell, J.D., Weight loss leads to a marked decrease in nonresting energy expenditure in ambulatory human subjects, *Metabolism* 37(10), 930–6, 1988.
128. Cunningham, J.J., Body composition as a determinant of energy expenditure: A synthetic review and a proposed general prediction equation, *Am. J. Clin. Nutr.* 54(6), 963–9, 1991.
129. Nelson, K.M., Weinsier, R.L., Long, C.L., and Schutz, Y., Prediction of resting energy expenditure from fat-free mass and fat mass, *Am. J. Clin. Nutr.* 56(5), 848–56, 1992.
130. Hoffmans, M., Pfeifer, W.A., Gundlach, B.L., Nijkrake, H.G., Oude Ophuis, A.J., and Hautvast, J.G., Resting metabolic rate in obese and normal weight women, *Int. J. Obes.* 3(2), 111–8, 1979.
131. Garby, L., Garrow, J.S., Jorgensen, B. et al., Relation between energy expenditure and body composition in man: Specific energy expenditure in vivo of fat and fat-free tissue, *Eur. J. Clin. Nutr.* 42(4), 301–5, 1988.
132. Byrne, N.M., Weinsier, R.L., Hunter, G.R. et al., Influence of distribution of lean body mass on resting metabolic rate after weight loss and weight regain: Comparison of responses in white and black women, *Am. J. Clin. Nutr.* 77(6), 1368–73, 2003.
133. Heymsfield, S.B., Thomas, D., Bosy-Westphal, A., Shen, W., Peterson, C.M., and Muller, M.J., Evolving concepts on adjusting human resting energy expenditure measurements for body size, *Obes, Rev.* 13(11), 1001–14, 2012.
134. Poehlman, E.T., Berke, E.M., Joseph, J.R., Gardner, A.W., Katzman-Rooks, S.M., and Goran, M.I., Influence of aerobic capacity, body composition, and thyroid hormones on the age-related decline in resting metabolic rate, *Metabolism* 41(8), 915–21, 1992.
135. Carlsohn, A., Scharhag-Rosenberger, F., Cassel, M., and Mayer, F., Resting metabolic rate in elite rowers and canoeists: Difference between indirect calorimetry and prediction, *Ann. Nutr. Metab.* 58(3), 239–44, 2011.
136. Hunter, G.R., Byrne, N.M., Gower, B.A., Sirikul, B., and Hills, A.P., Increased resting energy expenditure after 40 minutes of aerobic but not resistance exercise, *Obesity* 14(11), 2018–25, 2006.
137. Diamond, P. and LeBlanc, J., Hormonal control of postprandial thermogenesis in dogs, *Am. J. Physiol.* 253(5 Pt 1), E521–9, 1987.
138. Scott, C. and Devore, R., Diet-induced thermogenesis: Variations among three isocaloric meal-replacement shakes, *Nutrition* 21(7–8), 874–7, 2005.
139. Piers, L., Soares, M., Makan, T., and Shetty, P., Thermic effect of a meal. 1. Methodology and variation in normal young adults, *Br. J. Nutr.* 67(2), 165–75, 1992.
140. Dabbech, M., Aubert, R., Apfelbaum, M., and Boulier, A., Reproducible measurement of postprandial energy expenditure in young healthy males, *Am. J. Cin. Nutr.* 60(6), 849–54, 1994.
141. Weststrate, J., Resting metabolic rate and diet-induced thermogenesis: A methodological reappraisal, *Am. J. Cin. Nutr.* 58(5), 592–601, 1993.
142. Houde-Nadeau, M., de Jonge, L., and Garrel, D.R., Thermogenic response to food: Intra-individual variability and measurement reliability, *J. Am. Coll. Nutr.* 12(5), 511–6, 1993.
143. Piers, L.S., Soares, M.J., Maken, T., and Shetty, P.S. Thermic effect of a meal. 1. Methodolodgy and variation in normal young adults, *Br. J. Nutr.* 67(2), 165–75, 1992.
144. Armellini, F., Zamboni, M., Mino, A., Bissoli, L., Micciolo, R., and Bosello, O., Postabsorptive resting metabolic rate and thermic effect of food in relation to body composition and adipose tissue distribution, *Metabolism* 49(1), 6–10, 2000.

145. Moukaddem, M., Boulier, A., Apfelbaum, M., and Rigaud, D., Increase in diet-induced thermogenesis at the start of refeeding in severely malnourished anorexia nervosa patients, *Am. J. Clin. Nutr.* 66(1), 133–40, 1997.
146. Vaisman, N., Rossi, M.F., Corey, M., Clarke, R., Goldberg, E., and Pencharz, P.B., Effect of refeeding on the energy metabolism of adolescent girls who have anorexia nervosa, *Eur. J. Clin. Nutr.* 45(11), 527–37, 1991.
147. Van Wymelbeke, V., Brondel, L., Marcel Brun, J., and Rigaud, D., Factors associated with the increase in resting energy expenditure during refeeding in malnourished anorexia nervosa patients, *Am. J. Clin. Nutr.* 80(6), 1469–77, 2004.
148. Winter, T.A., The effects of undernutrition and refeeding on metabolism and digestive function, *Curr. Opin. Clin. Nutr. Metab. Care* 9(5), 596–602, 2006.
149. Piers, L., Soares, M., Kulkarni, R., and Shetty, P., Thermic effect of a meal. 3. Effect of dietary supplementation in chronically undernourished human subjects, *Br. J. Nutr.* 67(2), 187–94, 1992.
150. Piers, L., Soares, M., and Shetty, P., Thermic effect of a meal. 2. Role in chronic undernutrition, *Br. J. Nutr.* 67(2), 177–85, 1992.
151. Caspersen, C.J., Powell, K.E., and Christenson, G.M., Physical activity, exercise, and physical fitness: Definitions and distinctions for health-related research, *Public Health Rep.* 100(2), 126–31, 1985.
152. US Department of Health and Human Services, *Physical Activity and Health: A Report of the Surgeon General*. Atlanta (GA): US Department of Health and Human Services, Centers for Disease Control and Prevention, National Center for Chronic Disease Prevention and Health Promotion, http://www.cdc.gov/nccdphp/sgr/pdf/sgrfull.pdf, accessed 3 February 2014.
153. US Department of Health and Human Services, *Physical Activity Guidelines Advisory Committee Report*, Washington, DC, ODPHP Publication No. U0049. 2008 (cited 2010 Sep 24), http://www.health.gov/paguidelines/Report/pdf/CommitteeReport.pdf, accessed 3 February 2014.
154. Elia, M., Obesity in the elderly, *Obesity* 9(11S), 244S–8S, 2001.
155. Roberts, S.B. and Dallal, G.E., Effects of age on energy balance, *Am. J. Clin. Nutr.* 68(4), 975S–9S, 1998.
156. Black, A., Coward, W., Cole, T., and Prentice, A., Human energy expenditure in affluent societies: An analysis of 574 doubly-labelled water measurements, *Eur. J. Clin. Nutr.* 50(2), 72–92, 1996.
157. Roberts, S., Energy requirements of older individuals, *Eur. J. Clin. Nutr.* 50(Suppl 1), S112–7; discussion S7–8, 1996.
158. Bosy-Westphal, A., Eichhorn, C., Kutzner, D., Illner, K., Heller, M., and Muller, M.J., The age-related decline in resting energy expenditure in humans is due to the loss of fat-free mass and to alterations in its metabolically active components, *J. Nutr.* 133(7), 2356–62, 2003.
159. Elia, M., Ritz, P., and Stubbs, R.J., Total energy expenditure in the elderly, *Eur. J. Clin. Nutr.* 54(Suppl 3), S92–S103, 2000.
160. Henry, C.J., Mechanisms of changes in basal metabolism during ageing, *Eur. J. Clin. Nutr.* 54(Suppl 3), S77–91, 2000.
161. Meunier, N., Beattie, J.H., Ciarapica, D. et al., Basal metabolic rate and thyroid hormones of late-middle-aged and older human subjects: The ZENITH study, *Eur. J. Clin. Nutr.* 59(S2), S53–7, 2005.
162. Poehlman, E.T., Energy expenditure and requirements in aging humans, *J. Nutr.* 122(11), 2057–65, 1992.
163. Poehlman, E.T., Energy intake and energy expenditure in the elderly, *Am. J. Hum. Biol.* 8, 199–206, 1996.
164. Poehlman, E.T., Arciero, P.J., and Goran, M.I., Endurance exercise in aging humans: Effects on energy metabolism, *Exerc. Sport. Sci. Rev.* 22, 251–84, 1994.
165. Poehlman, E.T., Goran, M.I., Gardner, A.W. et al., Determinants of decline in resting metabolic rate in aging females, *Am. J. Physiol.* 264(3 Pt 1), E450–5, 1993.
166. Poehlman, E.T. and Horton, E.S., Regulation of energy expenditure in aging humans, *Annu. Rev. Nutr.* 10, 255–75, 1990.
167. Poehlman, E.T., Toth, M.J., and Gardner, A.W., Changes in energy balance and body composition at menopause: A controlled longitudinal study, *Ann. Intern. Med.* 123(9), 673–5, 1995.
168. Vaughan, L., Zurlo, F., and Ravussin, E., Aging and energy expenditure, *Am. J. Clin. Nutr.* 53(4), 821–5, 1991.
169. Ortega, R., Andres, P., Redondo, M., Zamora, M., Lopez-Sobaler, A., and Encinas-Sotillos, A., Dietary assessment of a group of elderly Spanish people, *Int. J. Food Sci. Nutr.* 46(2), 137–44, 1995.
170. Visser, M., van der Horst, A., de Groot, L.C.P.G.M., Deurenberg, P., and van Staveren, W.A., Energy cost of physical activities in healthy elderly women, *Metabolism* 44(8), 1046–51, 1995.
171. Hunter, G.R., Wetzstein, C.J., Fields, D.A., Brown, A., and Bamman, M.M., Resistance training increases total energy expenditure and free-living physical activity in older adults, *J. Appl. Physiol.* 89(3), 977–84, 2000.

172. Starling, R.D., Energy expenditure and aging: Effects of physical activity, *Int. J. Sport Nutr. Exerc. Metab.* 11 (Suppl), S208–17, 2001.
173. Starling, R.D., Toth, M.J., Carpenter, W.H., Matthews, D.E., and Poehlman, E.T., Energy requirements and physical activity in free-living older women and men: A doubly labeled water study, *J. Appl. Physiol.* 85(3), 1063–9, 1998.
174. Roberts, S.B. and Rosenberg, I., Nutrition and aging: Changes in the regulation of energy metabolism with aging, *Physiol. Rev.* 86(2), 651–67, 2006.
175. Davison, K.K., Ford, E.S., Cogswell, M.E., and Dietz, W.H., Percentage of body fat and body mass index are associated with mobility limitations in people aged 70 and older from NHANES III, *J. Am. Geriatr. Soc.* 50(11), 1802–9, 2002.
176. Meijer, E.P., Westerterp, K.R., and Verstappen, F.T., Effect of exercise training on physical activity and substrate utilization in the elderly, *Int. J. Sports Med.* 21(7), 499–504, 2000.
177. Westerterp, K.R. and Meijer, E.P., Physical activity and parameters of aging: A physiological perspective, *J. Gerontol. A Biol. Sci. Med. Sci.* 56(Suppl 2), 7–12, 2001.
178. Astrand, P.O., Bergh, U., and Kilbom, A., A 33-yr follow-up of peak oxygen uptake and related variables of former physical education students, *J. Appl. Physiol.* 82(6), 1844–52, 1997.
179. Astrand, I., Astrand, P.O., Hallback, I., and Kilbom, A., Reduction in maximal oxygen uptake with age, *J. Appl. Physiol.* 35(5), 649–54, 1973.
180. von Dobeln, W., Astrand, I., and Bergstrom, A., An analysis of age and other factors related to maximal oxygen uptake, *J. Appl. Physiol.* 22(5), 934–8, 1967.
181. Grimsmo, J., Arnesen, H., and Maehlum, S., Changes in cardiorespiratory function in different groups of former and still active male cross-country skiers: A 28–30-year follow-up study, *Scand. J. Med. Sci. Sports* 20(1), e151–61, 2010.
182. Keys, A., Taylor, H.L., and Grande, F., Basal metabolism and age of adult man, *Metabolism* 22(4), 579–87, 1973.
183. Weinsier, R.L., Schutz, Y., and Bracco, D., Reexamination of the relationship of resting metabolic rate to fat-free mass and to the metabolically active components of fat-free mass in humans, *Am. J. Clin. Nutr.* 55(4), 790–4, 1992.
184. Tzankoff, S.P. and Norris, A.H., Longitudinal changes in basal metabolism in man, *J. Appl. Physiol.* 45(4), 536–9, 1978.
185. Tzankoff, S.P. and Norris, A.H., Effect of muscle mass decrease on age-related BMR changes, *J. Appl. Physiol.* 43(6), 1001–6, 1977.
186. Welle, S. and Nair, K.S., Relationship of resting metabolic rate to body composition and protein turnover, *Am. J. Physiol.* 258(6 Pt 1), E990–8, 1990.
187. Pannemans, D.L. and Westerterp, K.R., Energy expenditure, physical activity and basal metabolic rate of elderly subjects, *Br. J. Nutr.* 73(4), 571–81, 1995.
188. Fukagawa, N.K., Bandini, L.G., and Young, J.B., Effect of age on body composition and resting metabolic rate, *Am. J. Physiol.* 259(2 Pt 1), E233–8, 1990.
189. Klausen, B., Toubro, S., and Astrup, A., Age and sex effects on energy expenditure, *Am. J. Clin. Nutr.* 65(4), 895–907, 1997.
190. Poehlman, E.T., Melby, C.L., and Badylak, S.F., Relation of age and physical exercise status on metabolic rate in younger and older healthy men, *J. Gerontol.* 46(2), B54–8, 1991.
191. Roberts, S., Fuss, P., Heyman, M., and Young, V., Influence of age on energy requirements, *Am. J. Clin. Nutr.* 62(5), 1053S–8, 1995.
192. Roubenoff, R., Hughes, V.A., Dallal, G.E. et al., The effect of gender and body composition method on the apparent decline in lean mass-adjusted resting metabolic rate with age, *J. Gerontol. A Biol. Sci. Med. Sci.* 55(12), M757–M60, 2000.
193. Speakman, J.R. and Westerterp, K.R., Associations between energy demands, physical activity, and body composition in adult humans between 18 and 96 y of age, *Am. J. Clin. Nutr.* 92(4), 826–34, 2010.
194. Cunningham, J.J., A reanalysis of the factors influencing basal metabolic rate in normal adults, *Am. J. Clin. Nutr.* 33(11), 2372–4, 1980.
195. Iannuzzi-Sucich, M., Prestwood, K.M., and Kenny, A.M., Prevalence of sarcopenia and predictors of skeletal muscle mass in healthy, older men and women, *J. Gerontol. A Biol. Sci. Med. Sci.* 57(12), M772–7, 2002.
196. Kutsuzawa, T., Shioya, S., Kurita, D., Haida, M., and Yamabayashi, H., Effects of age on muscle energy metabolism and oxygenation in the forearm muscles, *Med. Sci. Sports Exerc.* 33(6), 901–6, 2001.
197. Willis, M.W., Ketter, T.A., Kimbrell, T.A. et al., Age, sex and laterality effects on cerebral glucose metabolism in healthy adults, *Psychiatry Res.* 114(1), 23–37, 2002.

198. De Lorenzo, A., Andreoli, A., Bertoli, S., Testolin, G., Oriani, G., and Deurenberg, P., Resting metabolic rate in Italians: Relation with body composition and anthropometric parameters, *Acta Diabetol.* 37(2), 77–81, 2000.
199. Poehlman, E.T., Arciero, P.J., Melby, C.L., and Badylak, S.F., Resting metabolic rate and postprandial thermogenesis in vegetarians and nonvegetarians, *Am. J. Clin. Nutr.* 48(2), 209–13, 1988.
200. Poehlman, E.T., Melby, C.L., Badylak, S.F., and Calles, J., Aerobic fitness and resting energy expenditure in young adult males, *Metabolism* 38(1), 85–90, 1989.
201. Dolezal, B.A., Potteiger, J.A., Jacobsen, D.J., and Benedict, S.H., Muscle damage and resting metabolic rate after acute resistance exercise with an eccentric overload, *Med. Sci. Sports Exerc.* 32(7), 1202–7, 2000.
202. Lawson, S., Webster, J.D., Pacy, P.J., and Garrow, J.S., Effect of a 10-week aerobic exercise programme on metabolic rate, body composition and fitness in lean sedentary females, *Br. J. Clin. Pract.* 41(4), 684–8, 1987.
203. Osterberg, K.L. and Melby, C.L., Effect of acute resistance exercise on postexercise oxygen consumption and resting metabolic rate in young women, *Int. J. Sport Nutr. Exerc. Metab.* 10(1), 71–81, 2000.
204. Bell, C., Petitt, D.S., Jones, P.P., and Seals, D.R., Influence of adiposity on tonic sympathetic support of resting metabolism in healthy adults, *Int. J. Obes. Relat. Metab. Disord.* 27(11), 1315–8, 2003.
205. Bell, C., Seals, D.R., Monroe, M.B. et al., Tonic sympathetic support of metabolic rate is attenuated with age, sedentary lifestyle, and female sex in healthy adults, *J. Clin. Endocrinol. Metab.* 86(9), 4440–4, 2001.
206. Poehlman, E.T. and Danforth, E., Jr., Endurance training increases metabolic rate and norepinephrine appearance rate in older individuals, *Am. J. Physiol.* 261(2 Pt 1), E233–9, 1991.
207. Bell, C., Day, D.S., Jones, P.P. et al., High energy flux mediates the tonically augmented beta-adrenergic support of resting metabolic rate in habitually exercising older adults, *J. Clin. Endocrinol. Metab.* 89(7), 3573–8, 2004.
208. Bullough, R.C., Gillette, C.A., Harris, M.A., and Melby, C.L., Interaction of acute changes in exercise energy expenditure and energy intake on resting metabolic rate, *Am. J. Clin. Nutr.* 61(3), 473–81, 1995.
209. Van Pelt, R.E., Jones, P.P., Davy, K.P. et al., Regular exercise and the age-related decline in resting metabolic rate in women, *J. Clin. Endocrinol. Metab.* 82(10), 3208–12, 1997.
210. Schulz, L.O., Nyomba, B.L., Alger, S., Anderson, T.E., and Ravussin, E., Effect of endurance training on sedentary energy expenditure measured in a respiratory chamber, *Am. J. Physiol.* 260(2 Pt 1), E257–61, 1991.
211. Davis, J.R., Tagliaferro, A.R., Kertzer, R., Gerardo, T., Nichols, J., and Wheeler, J., Variations of dietary-induced thermogenesis and body fatness with aerobic capacity, *Eur. J. Appl. Physiol. Occup. Physiol.* 50(3), 319–29, 1983.
212. LeBlanc, J., Mercier, P., and Samson, P., Diet-induced thermogenesis with relation to training state in female subjects, *Can. J. Physiol. Pharmacol.* 62(3), 334–7, 1984.
213. Gilbert, J.A., Misner, J.E., Boileau, R.A., Ji, L.L., and Slaughter, M.H., Lower thermic effect of a meal post-exercise in aerobically trained and resistance-trained subjects, *Med. Sci. Sports Exerc.* 23(7), 825–30, 1991.
214. Broeder, C.E., Burrhus, K.A., Svanevik, L.S., and Wilmore, J.H., The effects of either high-intensity resistance or endurance training on resting metabolic rate, *Am. J. Clin. Nutr.* 55(4), 802–10, 1992.
215. Broeder, C.E., Burrhus, K.A., Svanevik, L.S., and Wilmore, J.H., The effects of aerobic fitness on resting metabolic rate, *Am. J. Clin. Nutr.* 55(4), 795–801, 1992.
216. Sullo, A., Cardinale, P., Brizzi, G., Fabbri, B., and Maffulli, N., Resting metabolic rate and post-prandial thermogenesis by level of aerobic power in older athletes, *Clin. Exp. Pharmacol. Physiol.* 31(4), 202–6, 2004.
217. Poehlman, E.T., Gardner, A.W., Ades, P.A. et al., Resting energy metabolism and cardiovascular disease risk in resistance-trained and aerobically trained males, *Metabolism* 41(12), 1351–60, 1992.
218. Ballor, D.L. and Poehlman, E.T., Resting metabolic rate and coronary-heart-disease risk factors in aerobically and resistance-trained women, *Am. J. Clin. Nutr.* 56(6), 968–74, 1992.
219. Pratley, R., Nicklas, B., Rubin, M. et al., Strength training increases resting metabolic rate and norepinephrine levels in healthy 50- to 65-yr-old men, *J. Appl. Physiol.* 76(1), 133–7, 1994.
220. Campbell, W.W., Crim, M.C., Young, V.R., and Evans, W.J., Increased energy requirements and changes in body composition with resistance training in older adults, *Am. J. Clin. Nutr.* 60(2), 167–75, 1994.
221. Brochu, M., Starling, R.D., Ades, P.A., and Poehlman, E.T., Are aerobically fit older individuals more physically active in their free-living time? A doubly labeled water approach, *J. Clin. Endocrinol. Metab.* 84(11), 3872–6, 1999.

222. Golay, A., Schutz, Y., Meyer, H.U. et al., Glucose-induced thermogenesis in nondiabetic and diabetic obese subjects, *Diabetes* 31(11), 1023–8, 1982.
223. Morgan, J.B. and York, D.A., Thermic effect of feeding in relation to energy balance in elderly men, *Ann. Nutr. Metab.* 27(1), 71–7, 1983.
224. Schutz, Y., Bessard, T., and Jequier, E., Diet-induced thermogenesis measured over a whole day in obese and nonobese women, *Am. J. Clin. Nutr.* 40(3), 542–52, 1984.
225. Vansant, G., Van Gaal, L., Van Acker, K., and De Leeuw, I., Importance of glucagon as a determinant of resting metabolic rate and glucose-induced thermogenesis in obese women, *Metabolism* 40(7), 672–5, 1991.
226. Das, S.K., Moriguti, J.C., McCrory, M.A. et al., An underfeeding study in healthy men and women provides further evidence of impaired regulation of energy expenditure in old age, *J. Nutr.* 131(6), 1833–8, 2001.
227. Melanson, K.J., Saltzman, E., Vinken, A.G., Russell, R., and Roberts, S.B., The effects of age on postprandial thermogenesis at four graded energetic challenges: Findings in young and older women, *J. Gerontol. A Biol. Sci. Med. Sci.* 53(6), B409–14, 1998.
228. Poehlman, E.T., Viers, H.F., and Detzer, M., Influence of physical activity and dietary restraint on resting energy expenditure in young nonobese females, *Can. J. Physiol. Pharmacol.* 69(3), 320–6, 1991.
229. Visser, M., Deurenberg, P., van Staveren, W.A., and Hautvast, J.G., Resting metabolic rate and diet-induced thermogenesis in young and elderly subjects: Relationship with body composition, fat distribution, and physical activity level, *Am. J. Clin. Nutr.* 61(4), 772–8, 1995.
230. Hill, J.O., Heymsfield, S.B., McMannus, C., 3rd, and DiGirolamo, M., Meal size and thermic response to food in male subjects as a function of maximum aerobic capacity, *Metabolism* 33(8), 743–9, 1984.
231. Poehlman, E.T., Melby, C.L., and Badylak, S.F., Resting metabolic rate and postprandial thermogenesis in highly trained and untrained males, *Am. J. Clin. Nutr.* 47(5), 793–8, 1988.
232. Goran, M.I. and Poehlman, E.T., Endurance training does not enhance total energy expenditure in healthy elderly persons, *Am. J. Physiol.* 263(5 Pt 1), E950–7, 1992.
233. Meijer, E., Goris, A., Wouters, L., and Westerterp, K., Physical inactivity as a determinant of the physical activity level in the elderly, *Int. J. Obes. Relat. Metab. Disord.* 25(7), 935–9, 2001.
234. Withers, R.T., Smith, D.A., Tucker, R.C., Brinkman, M., and Clark, D.G., Energy metabolism in sedentary and active 49- to 70-yr-old women, *J. Appl. Physiol.* 84(4), 1333–40, 1998.
235. Voorrips, L.E., Vanacker, T., Deurenberg, P., and Vanstaveren, W.A., Energy expenditure at rest and during standardized activities—a comparison between elderly and middle-aged women, *Am. J. Clin. Nutr.* 58(1), 15–20, 1993.
236. Hausdorff, J.M., Nelson, M.E., Kaliton, D. et al., Etiology and modification of gait instability in older adults: A randomized controlled trial of exercise, *J. Appl. Physiol.* 90(6), 2117–29, 2001.
237. Havemannies, A., Vaniperen, C., and Deurenberg, P., Energy expenditure at rest and during activities—a comparison between young and elderly women, *Am. J. Hum. Biol.* 8(3), 383–8, 1996.
238. Fiser, W.M., Hays, N.P., Rogers, S.C. et al., Energetics of walking in elderly people: Factors related to gait speed, *J. Gerontol. A Biol. Sci. Med. Sci.* 65A(12), 1332–7, 2010.
239. Hunter, G.R., Treuth, M.S., Weinsier, R.L. et al., The effects of strength conditioning on older women's ability to perform daily tasks, *J. Am. Geriatr. Soc.* 43(7), 756–60, 1995.
240. Quinn, T.J., Manley, M.J., Aziz, J., Padham, J.L., and MacKenzie, A.M., Aging and factors related to running economy, *J. Strength Cond. Res.* 25(11), 2971–9, 2011.
241. Ramage, S., Farmer, A., Apps Eccles, K., and McCarger, L., Healthy strategies for successful weight loss and weight maintenance: A systematic review, *Appl. Physiol. Nutr. Metab.* 39(1), 1–20, 2014.
242. Sundgot-Borgen, J., Meyer, N.L., Lohman, T.G. et al., How to minimise the health risks to athletes who compete in weight-sensitive sports review and position statement on behalf of the Ad Hoc Research Working Group on Body Composition, Health and Performance, under the auspices of the IOC Medical Commission, *Br. J. Sports Med.* 47(16), 1012–22, 2013.

4 Carbohydrate Needs of Masters Athletes

Gregory R. Cox

CONTENTS

4.1 INTRODUCTION

The importance of carbohydrate as a substrate for exercise has formed a cornerstone of sports nutrition advice for the past four decades [1]. New information has emerged throughout this period which has changed our understanding of the needs of athletes and the advice provided to them regarding their daily training carbohydrate intake and competition carbohydrate strategies [2]. For endurance athletes, the availability of carbohydrate as a substrate for the working muscle and the central nervous system is well known and subsequently reflected in sports nutrition guidelines. Although not as widely acknowledged, carbohydrate availability is also likely to influence an athlete's performance of intermittent, high-intensity exercise of shorter duration and repeated explosive exercise activities [3,4]. And finally, success in skill sports that require high-level cognitive tasks and complex motor skills are also likely to be affected by carbohydrate availability, as carbohydrate is the most important fuel for the central nervous system. Carbohydrate is therefore an important component of any athlete's diet, regardless of age. While the importance of carbohydrate is widely acknowledged in younger athletes, little if any empirical research has examined the carbohydrate needs of older exercisers in general and masters athletes in particular. In this chapter we will review current principles for dietary carbohydrate instruction and provide practical strategies in the context of masters athletes.

4.2 CARBOHYDRATE METABOLISM DURING EXERCISE

It is well known that carbohydrate from both blood glucose and muscle glycogen is an important fuel for contracting muscle during exercise [5,6]. Glucose (or glycogen) is utilised by active muscle via either anaerobic glycolysis or aerobic metabolism (oxidative phosphorylation). The relative contribution of carbohydrate as an energy substrate for the muscle is influenced primarily by the exercise intensity and to a lesser degree by exercise duration, the preceding diet, substrate availability during exercise, training status and environmental conditions [7,8]. A useful summary of such effects, both in relation to intensity and duration of exercise, is presented in the work of Romijn and others [9]. As the intensity of exercise increases, both energy expenditure and the contribution of carbohydrate to work production increases [9]. Older sedentary adults oxidise less fat than their younger counterparts during endurance exercise when exercising at the same absolute or relative exercise intensity [10]. Furthermore, carbohydrate oxidation is higher than young adults exercising at the same absolute intensity, but lower than young adults at the same relative intensity [10]. However, in response to a short-term endurance training programme, older men and women can increase fat oxidation and decrease carbohydrate oxidation as commonly observed in younger people [11]. In fact, the favoured skeletal muscle adaptations that occur in response to endurance training in young people are also observed in sedentary older men and women [12–14].

As muscle glycogen stores decline during prolonged exercise, blood glucose becomes more important as a source of carbohydrate for the contracting muscle [15]. Furthermore, the contracting muscle competes with the brain for circulating glucose, as the brain relies predominantly on glucose as a substrate. In essence, carbohydrate is a critical fuel for the majority of the activities undertaken by athletes, yet older healthy subjects have a reduced capacity for muscle glycogen storage compared to younger subjects [16]. Of note, endurance training has been shown to improve glucose tolerance, increase muscle glycogen storage capacity and skeletal muscle transporter (GLUT-4) activity in older previously sedentary subjects to a similar extent to that of younger subjects [12,17]. In fact, researchers investigating glucose tolerance in young and older athletes and sedentary men reported that masters athletes have similar glucose tolerance to that of both younger untrained and younger trained males, whereas the older untrained males had a twofold greater area under the glucose curve [18,19].

While maximal oxygen uptake capacity (VO_{2max}) in masters athletes declines with age, the progression of this decline is less compared to that of their sedentary elderly counterparts [20]. Of interest, the decline in VO_{2max} is further minimised in masters athletes who maintain training intensity and remain competitive [21]. In fact, a direct relationship exists between maximal aerobic capacity and *in vivo* insulin action in elderly males [22]. Furthermore, undertaking an endurance training programme results in a significant improvement in VO_{2max} in sedentary older men and women [13].

Despite a lower VO_{2max}, high-performance masters athletes are able to compete alongside non-elite younger athletes. This has been attributed to the fact that endurance-trained masters runners attain a blood lactate threshold at a higher percentage of their VO_{2max}, although they possess the same absolute VO_2 and running velocity as younger runners [23]. This increased ability to maintain a higher percentage of VO_{2max} in the masters runners was revealed in a follow-up study which showed higher activities of succinate dehydrogenase and β-hydroxyacl-CoA dehydrogenase in the masters runners compared to similarly performed younger runners [24]. See Chapters 14 and 15 for a detailed discussion of the physiology and nutrition needs of the older endurance and ultra-endurance athlete, respectively.

4.3 CARBOHYDRATE INTAKE OF MASTERS ATHLETES

Little is known about the daily carbohydrate intakes or competition intakes of masters athletes despite considerable research investigating daily carbohydrate intakes of younger athletes [25]. Many studies investigating the dietary habits of athletes have included, by virtue of the athlete cohort, masters athletes. Not surprisingly, endurance-trained male and female athletes consume higher daily carbohydrate intakes compared to non-endurance athletes, with male athletes consuming more carbohydrate than female athletes [25]. A study of female masters runners and cyclists reported an average daily carbohydrate intake of 269 grams, which is similar to that reported for non-endurance female athletes, but slightly lower than that reported for endurance-trained younger females [25,26]. Currently, there is little evidence to suggest that the daily carbohydrate intake of masters athletes of either gender is different to that of younger athletes although descriptive research is needed in this area.

4.4 CARBOHYDRATE INTAKE GUIDELINES FOR ATHLETES

A fundamental difference in the dietary requirement between an athlete of any age and their sedentary counterparts is that athletes must consume adequate energy and carbohydrate to meet the demands of both training and competition [27]. Despite overwhelming support for the acute benefits of consuming carbohydrate before, during and after exercise, the benefits of chronic high-carbohydrate diets on the performance of subsequent exercise are less clear. Only a small number of studies have attempted to investigate the cumulative benefits of implementing appropriate nutritional strategies to facilitate daily exercise performance and recovery of muscle energy stores. While several of these studies have found benefits to the performance of an exercise task or reduced symptoms associated with overreaching following a period of training on a high-carbohydrate intake [28–31], others have found no evidence in support of improved subsequent performance [32–35].

One important methodological consideration in these studies is how well the high-carbohydrate diet was able to enhance *carbohydrate availability* during daily training sessions. Researchers have either failed to mention when the additional carbohydrate was consumed throughout the day [36], or have required subjects in the higher carbohydrate group to consume the additional carbohydrate outside of scheduled exercise times [28–30,33,34]. Only in the studies by de Sousa et al. and Cox et al. did subjects in the higher carbohydrate group consume the additional carbohydrate during daily training sessions to promote high carbohydrate availability [31,35]. Moreover, no study to date has examined the effect of carbohydrate availability and timing during training in masters athletes or older exercisers.

The International Olympic Committee consensus meeting on Nutrition for Sport in 2010 provided clarity on this issue as well as the opportunity to incorporate new concepts into earlier sports nutrition guidelines [2,37]. These guidelines highlight specific daily carbohydrate intake strategies which are thought, at least in younger athletes, to support daily performance and enhance recovery between training sessions. Key points relating to carbohydrate intake for athletes within this recent consensus statement are given in Table 4.1.

The end result of the consensus statement was the development of new carbohydrate intake guidelines which reflect these recent advancements in our understanding of carbohydrate as a substrate for exercise (Table 4.2). It should be duly noted that daily carbohydrate needs are not static, but rather reflect changes in daily, weekly or seasonal changes in exercise within a periodised training programme. Thus, an athlete's daily carbohydrate intake should be modified throughout the training year accordingly.

The interpretation of these guidelines into individual dietary prescription should consider the athlete's overall daily energy requirements, body mass and body composition goals, and specific training volume and intensity as well as athlete feedback from daily training outcomes and competition performances. While daily carbohydrate requirements are likely to be similar for masters athletes [38], interpretation of modern-day carbohydrate intake guidelines should consider the unique physiological and metabolic characteristics of older exercisers and masters athletes as previously noted in Section 4.2 [2]. Of specific note, fat-free mass decreases in sedentary elderly populations [39]. This shift is also evident in male masters athletes when matched to younger, similarly trained and performed athletes [24]. However, in a study of female athletes, no difference in fat-free mass

TABLE 4.1
Key Points of the 2010 Consensus Meeting of the International Olympic Committee on Nutrition for Sport regarding Carbohydrate

- A key recommendation was to change the *qualitative* terminology used to describe the carbohydrate content of an athlete's diet. This was an extension of previous guidelines to change the *quantitative* descriptions of carbohydrate intake – specifically, that carbohydrate guidelines be provided in grams relative to an athlete's body mass (g/kg) rather than its contribution to total energy intake (% energy) [37].
- The update recommended that we replace generic descriptions of 'high carbohydrate diets' or 'low carbohydrate diets' with a more specific consideration of the interaction between the amount of carbohydrate consumed, the timing of its consumption in relation to exercise and individual activity patterns during daily training and competition. Hence, the term *carbohydrate availability*. An adequate supply of carbohydrate substrate for the muscle and central nervous system before and during exercise achieved by an adequate daily carbohydrate intake, strategically timed before and during exercise promotes *high carbohydrate availability*. Alternatively, commencing daily training with depleted or limited carbohydrate fuel sources by means of a reduced daily carbohydrate intake or withholding carbohydrate before exercise promotes *low carbohydrate availability*. This approach promotes the concept of manipulating carbohydrate intake to reflect daily exercise loads while strategically timing carbohydrate intake around daily exercise (i.e. dietary periodisation). For instance, an endurance athlete with a relatively low intake of carbohydrate on a rest day or during a reduced training phase would be considered to have adequate carbohydrate availability, assuming a higher carbohydrate intake is achieved on days/periods of higher volume and intensity training.
- Practical implications of novel strategies that exist to enhance glycogen storage post-exercise such as the use of high molecular weight glucose polymers, co-ingestion of large amounts of caffeine and prior creatine loading should be considered before implementing into an athlete's diet. For example, reliance of glucose polymers reduces the nutrient density of the diet and may impair the athlete's ability to meet other nutritional goals that are of greater importance to health and performance. Furthermore, side effects associated with the intake of large doses of caffeine (e.g. disruption to sleep) or creatine loading (e.g. weight gain) may limit routine use of such strategies.
- When carbohydrate intake is suboptimal post exercise for refuelling, adding protein to a meal/snack will enhance glycogen storage [40].
- While the GI of carbohydrate foods incorporated within the pre-exercise meal are often considered, further research is needed before systematic manipulation of the pre-exercise meal GI can be recommended.
- The amount and type of carbohydrate recommended during exercise has been expanded in light of recent findings regarding the benefits of carbohydrate mouth rinsing [41] and the use of multiple transportable carbohydrates [42] during exercise.
- While strategies that promote training with low carbohydrate availability during exercise appear to enhance cellular adaptations to endurance exercise [43], there are several disadvantages associated with train-low techniques [2].

was observed between older and younger athletes [44]. Given that daily carbohydrate intake guidelines are based on grams per kilogram body mass, an adjustment may be required when interpreting current recommendations given the lower fat-free mass in some but not all masters athletes. The extent to which current recommendations might be modified should reflect the individual morphological characteristics of the older athlete or exerciser. Furthermore, the training history of masters athletes should be considered when interpreting carbohydrate intake guidelines given that age and training status alters carbohydrate metabolism [10–13]. Older, relative newcomers to masters competition may have higher requirements for carbohydrate to that of lifelong-trained masters athletes. Carbohydrate intake guidelines should be modified accordingly to reflect the current training status and previous training history of masters athletes.

Masters athletes are encouraged to adjust their daily carbohydrate intakes by adopting eating patterns in which meals/snacks providing carbohydrate and other important nutrients are placed strategically around daily exercise or training sessions. This means that additional carbohydrate

TABLE 4.2
Summary of Guidelines for Carbohydrate Intake for Athletes

	Situation	Carbohydrate Targets	Comments on Type and Timing of Carbohydrate Intake
Daily needs for fuel and recovery: These general recommendations should be fine-tuned with individual consideration of total energy needs, specific training needs and feedback from training performance			
Light	• Low-intensity or skill-based activities	3–5 g/kg of athlete's body mass per day	• Timing of intake may be chosen to promote speedy refuelling, or to provide fuel intake around training sessions in the day. Otherwise, as long as total fuel needs are provided, the pattern of intake may simply be guided by convenience and individual choice. • Protein- and nutrient-rich carbohydrate foods or meal combinations will allow the athlete to meet other acute or chronic sports nutrition goals.
Moderate	• Moderate exercise programme (i.e. ~1 hour/day)	5–7 g/kg/day	
High	• Endurance programme (e.g. moderate-to-high intensity exercise of 1–3 hours/day)	6–10 g/kg/day	
Very high	• Extreme commitment (i.e. moderate-to-high-intensity exercise of >4–5 hours/day)	8–12 g/kg/day	
Acute fuelling strategies: These guidelines promote high carbohydrate availability to promote optimal performance in competition or key training sessions			
General fuelling up	• Preparation for events <90 minutes exercise	7–12 g/kg per 24 hours as for daily fuel needs	• Athletes may choose compact carbohydrate-rich sources that are low in fibre/residue and easily consumed to ensure that fuel targets are met, and to meet goals for gut comfort or lighter 'racing weight'.
Carbohydrate loading	• Preparation for events >90 minutes of sustained/intermittent exercise	36–48 hours of 10–12 g/kg per 24 hours	
Speedy refuelling	• <8-hour recovery between two fuel-demanding sessions	1.0–1.2 g/kg/hour for first 4 hours then resume daily fuel needs	• There may be benefits in consuming small regular snacks. • Compact carbohydrate-rich foods and drinks may help to ensure fuel targets are met.
Pre-event fuelling	• Before exercise > 60 minutes	1–4 g/kg consumed 1–4 hours before exercise	• The timing, amount and type of carbohydrate foods and drinks should be chosen to suit the practical needs of the event and individual preferences/experiences. • Choices high in fat/protein/fibre may need to be avoided to reduce risk of gastrointestinal issues during the event. • Low GI choices may provide a more sustained source of fuel for situations where carbohydrate cannot be consumed during exercise.
During brief exercise	• <45 minutes	Not needed	
During sustained high-intensity exercise	• 45–75 minutes	Small amounts including mouth rinse	• A range of drinks and sports products can provide easily consumed carbohydrate.

(continued)

TABLE 4.2 (Continued)
Summary of Guidelines for Carbohydrate Intake for Athletes

	Situation	Carbohydrate Targets	Comments on Type and Timing of Carbohydrate Intake
During endurance exercise including stop-and-start sports	• 1.0–2.5 hours	30–60 g/hour	• Opportunities to consume foods and drinks vary according to the rules and nature of each sport. • A range of everyday dietary choices and specialised sports products ranging in form from liquid to solid may be useful. • The athlete should practice to find a refuelling plan that suits their individual goals including hydration needs and gut comfort.
During ultra-endurance exercise	• >2.5–3.0 hours	Up to 90 g/hour	• As above. • Higher hourly intakes of carbohydrate are associated with better performance. • Products containing multiple transportable carbohydrates (glucose: fructose mixtures) will achieve high rates of oxidation of carbohydrate consumed during exercise.

Source: Adapted from Burke, L.M. et al., *J. Sports Sci.* 29(Suppl 1), 17–27, 2011.

containing food and fluid is automatically consumed around daily training sessions or competitions, allowing total nutrient and energy intake to reflect a change in the fuel cost of the athlete's exercise commitments. Table 4.3 outlines various practical strategies which may assist masters athletes to implement current carbohydrate intake guidelines.

4.5 CARBOHYDRATE NEEDS OF ATHLETES DURING RECOVERY BETWEEN TRAINING SESSIONS

More competitive masters athletes are likely to undertake two or even three workouts per day during periods throughout a competitive year. To maximise training performance, refuelling, physical and physiological adaptation and health, masters athletes need to implement appropriate carbohydrate recovery nutrition practices (Table 4.2). Both the duration and intensity of the training session or competition event along with the timing of the next scheduled exercise session will dictate how much glycogen is used and the speed at which it needs to be replaced.

The most important dietary factor affecting muscle glycogen storage is the amount of carbohydrate consumed following exercise [37]. However, in the absence of an adequate carbohydrate intake, co-ingestion of protein can enhance muscle glycogen resynthesis in the early hours of recovery [40]. This has practical significance for sports nutrition professionals when planning post-exercise snacks for habitually low-energy intake consumers. A well-timed carbohydrate-rich snack (providing 1–1.2 g/kg body mass) post-exercise will promote high rates of muscle glycogen resynthesis in the early recovery period [45], with sufficient carbohydrate intake required (7–10 g/kg body mass) throughout the subsequent 24 hours [46]. Thus, eating a carbohydrate-rich snack soon after exercise is most important when there are only 4–8 hours of recovery between exercise sessions, but less concerning when there is a longer recovery time (12 hours or more). And finally, while a diet based on high glycaemic index (GI) foods promotes greater muscle glycogen resynthesis over 24 hours [47], a moderate-low GI diet would be advised for older exercises and masters athletes with impaired

TABLE 4.3
Considerations for an Appropriate Carbohydrate Intake

- Plan daily carbohydrate intake to reflect changes in daily training intensity and volume. Total carbohydrate intake should reflect daily activity patterns. Plan to eat additional carbohydrate at meals or add an extra snack when undertaking high-volume or increased intensity training, or when preparing for an endurance event. The opposite is true for reduced training days or rest days.
- Special consideration should be given to older men and women with relatively low energy intakes, particularly in times where higher carbohydrate intakes are warranted.
- For masters athletes engaged in non-endurance events, the focus should be on timing carbohydrate intake strategically around training or competition to ensure adequate carbohydrate availability during exercise, not increasing daily carbohydrate intake *per se*.
- To support quality and/or extended training sessions consume carbohydrate before, during and after sessions to increase carbohydrate availability. This will ensure fuel is available during the session when it is needed most, and further aid recovery of muscle glycogen stores between training sessions.
- If masters athletes are unsure of daily carbohydrate requirements, or are trying to juggle daily training performance while reducing body fat levels, they should consult a sports nutrition professional for an individualised nutrition plan.
- It is common for masters athletes to incorporate overseas travel with an international event. Masters athletes should be reminded of their specific needs for carbohydrate in preparation for the event and during actual competition. Athletes may need to plan ahead and incorporate new carbohydrate foods to meet daily carbohydrate requirements particularly when travelling to exotic locations. Travelling with a small supply of staple carbohydrate foods that can be easily prepared, added to meals or provide a nutritious carbohydrate snack is an excellent option when travelling to remote locations were food quality and safety may be an issue.

Nutrient-Dense Whole Grain Carbohydrate-Rich Foods

- In general, when daily carbohydrate needs are increased, nutrient-dense whole grain carbohydrate foods or recipe ideas should form the basis of each meal. When carbohydrate requirements are more modest, incorporate recipe ideas and food choices that make carbohydrate a component of a meal, whereby the carbohydrate content can be easily adjusted to reflect reduced fuel requirements.
- Given that nutrient intakes in elderly populations can be lower than that reported for younger adults, masters athletes and older exercisers should chose high-quality, nutrient-dense carbohydrate foods when permissible.
- Select whole grain breakfast cereals that have less added sugar (i.e. where sugar is not listed within the first few ingredients) and that are higher in fibre. Toasted mueslis are high in fat and energy-dense compared with natural, untoasted muesli and lighter-style blends of cereal flakes with dried fruits and other ingredients. Rolled oats are a great example of a whole grain, nutrient-dense, low-sugar carbohydrate-rich breakfast cereal when served with milk and an added banana for sweetness.
- Whole grain breads, wraps, pita breads, bagels, rolls, crumpets, damper and fruit bread are all great examples of carbohydrate-rich, nutrient-dense options. Where possible, select whole grain options where the seeds are visible. If you are trying to reduce carbohydrate intake at a meal when carbohydrate needs are modest, chose thin-sliced breads and lower carbohydrate wraps. Reading food labels will provide you with information about the amount of carbohydrate contained in a serving. For instance, pita breads and mountain breads offer a great low-carbohydrate alternative to pre-made pizza bases.
- When fuel needs are high, consider meal choices and recipes where rice, pasta, noodles or couscous are the main ingredient (rice in risottos or paella, pasta bake or combination rice, etc.). When carbohydrate needs are more modest, select recipes in which staple carbohydrates are a component of the dish (e.g. pasta sheets in a lasagna). Incorporating rice, pasta, noodles, couscous or quinoa as a side dish offers the greatest flexibility to scale the amount of carbohydrate included in the meal.
- Legumes such as kidney beans, lentils, chick peas, broad beans or baked beans can be used easily in pasta sauces and casseroles to replace some or all of the meat, fish or chicken. Including a bean salad at lunch or a minestrone soup at dinner provides an excellent alternative to boost carbohydrate intake.

(*continued*)

TABLE 4.3 (Continued)
Considerations for an Appropriate Carbohydrate Intake

- Starchy vegetables such as potatoes, sweet potatoes and corn also offer a variety of options to assist in increasing total carbohydrate at meals. While other vegetables, particularly salad vegetables, are good sources of fibre as well as some vitamins and minerals, they contain small amounts of carbohydrate. When carbohydrate needs are more modest, including a side salad with a pasta dish or adding additional vegetables to a stir-fry is a great way to maintain a lower carbohydrate intake at a meal.
- While fruit is variable in its carbohydrate content, including a variety of fruit at meals and snacks offers a nutritious way to increase daily carbohydrate intake. Bananas, apples, pears and mangoes to name a few are higher-carbohydrate fruit choices, while strawberries, blueberries and watermelon contain less carbohydrate.
- Milk and yogurt – sweetened and unsweetened varieties – provide an alternative option to increase daily carbohydrate intake at meals and snacks. Unsweetened varieties with added fruit provide your most nutritious choice, while sweetened varieties of yogurt, milk and custards provide a more compact carbohydrate choice.

High-Sugar Foods Should Be Used Strategically

- Sugar or higher-sugar-containing foods and fluids offer a convenient, compact, low-fibre option to increase daily carbohydrate intake when fuelling requirements are high. There are specific situations in sports (i.e. carbohydrate loading), where these lower nutrient carbohydrate choices offer an advantage over nutrient-dense, bulky, whole grain carbohydrate choices. However, sugar and sugar-rich foods and fluids should accompany but not dominate your total carbohydrate intake.
- During periods of high daily training or when carbohydrate loading for an endurance event where high intakes of bulky whole grain carbohydrate food choices cause gastrointestinal discomfort, including compact, carbohydrate-rich foods offer an advantage to meeting daily fuel needs.
- When weight loss is desired and total energy intake is low, reducing sugar intake by avoiding highly refined options (i.e. confectionery, sugary drinks, added sugar) will allow room for higher-quality nutrient-dense carbohydrate foods.
- Apart from times when a carbohydrate drink is specifically required to assist performance during daily training sessions or competition, stick to water as the major form of fluid intake.

Carbohydrate Intake and Dental Hygiene

- Sports drinks, soft drinks, cordials and juice all have the potential to be erosive to teeth.
- The frequent intake of acidic drinks such as sports drinks (pH ~3–4) during training and competition can lead to dental erosion. Limit this pattern to situations where it actually fuels sports performance, rather than times when you are sedentary and not training.
- Avoid brushing your teeth immediately after using sugary, low-pH drinks as this may further accelerate the damaged caused by sipping on sugary drinks during extended training sessions or endurance competitions.
- Manufacturers are investigating ways to increase the pH of sports drinks or adding calcium to reduce enamel erosion.

glucose tolerance. Table 4.4 provides a range of suitable carbohydrate-rich recovery options to promote muscle glycogen resynthesis post-exercise.

4.6 IS THERE A BENEFIT TO TRAINING WITH LOW CARBOHYDRATE AVAILABILITY?

In past years, much of the focus regarding carbohydrate in an athlete's diet has been in the provision of a substrate to support daily training performance, health and well-being, competition performance or recovery between exercise sessions. These strategies are clearly articulated in recent carbohydrate intake guidelines for athletes as previously highlighted in this chapter. However, recent studies manipulating muscle glycogen content (i.e. carbohydrate availability) with exercise in both young trained and untrained subjects have fuelled debate about the benefits of training under conditions of low carbohydrate availability [43]. Findings from these studies have shown that compared with high muscle glycogen content, an acute endurance exercise bout or routine daily training

TABLE 4.4
Post-Exercise Carbohydrate Recovery Issues and Snack Ideas

- Small, frequent snacks and meals over the day are as effective to promote muscle glycogen storage over 24 hours compared to larger meals consumed less often.
- The amount and type of food and/or fluid consumed immediately following exercise should be considered within the athlete's daily meal plan. The type, duration and intensity of exercise undertaken, the timing of the next meal and/or training session, the amount of carbohydrate consumed during exercise and the tolerance for intake by the athlete will influence the post-exercise recovery snack.
- Low-nutrient carbohydrate snacks (i.e. refined carbohydrate foods and fluids), while offering a compact source of carbohydrate, should not provide the cornerstone for post-exercise nutrition recovery.
- Glycogen storage is impaired by muscle damage, either through direct body contact and bruising or through eccentric loading. This has relevance to masters athletes playing contact sports or activities with high eccentric loading such as running.

Recovery Snacks Providing Carbohydrates (40–50 g) and Protein (>10 g)

- 250–350 ml of liquid meal supplement, milk shake, or fruit smoothie with added yogurt
- 500 ml of flavoured low-fat milk
- 60 g (1.5–2 cups) of breakfast cereal with 1/2 cup of low-fat milk
- Sandwich or crackers with cheese, meat, chicken or tinned fish filling + piece of fruit
- 1 cup of fruit salad + 200 g tub fruit-flavoured yogurt or custard
- 200 g tub fruit-flavoured yogurt or 300 ml of flavoured milk + a cereal, muesli or granola bar
- 4 wholegrain crackers + cottage cheese and tomato + a banana

throughout a chronic exercise block commenced with low carbohydrate availability results in an increase in adaptive responses favouring fat metabolism [48]. In an earlier study that employed a bilateral leg design, untrained young subjects achieved greater training-induced metabolic adaptations and exercise endurance in the leg trained with a protocol promoting depleted glycogen stores than the contra-lateral leg which undertook the same volume of training in a glycogen-recovered state [49]. This study has led to the *train low, compete high* model of periodisation of carbohydrate availability: limiting carbohydrate during training to enhance the training response, then restoring fuel status for optimal competition performance. It should be noted that training with low muscle glycogen content in this study comprised only 50% of the total training load throughout the intervention period [49].

Although the findings have significant scientific merit and possible application for exercise programs targeting metabolic improvements and health outcomes, there are some concerns in applying the technique to athletes of any age who are regularly engaged in physical training. In fact, studies in trained populations have failed to find any enhancement of performance gains from the *two a day training* model of low glycogen training [50,51] or training in fasted/water-fed state with reduced daily carbohydrate intake [35] over conventional training and nutritional support even when there was evidence of enhancement of the metabolic adaptations associated with training [48,49]. Furthermore, several disadvantages are associated with train-low techniques including an impairment of the ability to train at high intensities and a possible increase in the risk of injury or illness while undertaking strenuous daily training with low carbohydrate availability [48]. And finally, skeletal muscle protein balance has been shown to be lower during exercise under conditions of low carbohydrate compared with high carbohydrate availability [52], which may have more significance for masters athletes given the age-related loss of fat-free mass [21].

In real life, athletes manipulate availability carbohydrate availability via combinations of dietary practices both in training and competition. Some workouts are likely to be undertaken with low carbohydrate availability (e.g. the second or third session of a heavy training day, early morning training sessions undertaken before breakfast, training during a period of energy restriction for weight loss) while others are undertaken with adequate carbohydrate support (e.g. quality sessions scheduled during lower volume periods, sessions undertaken after a meal or when carbohydrate is consumed throughout training). Based on current evidence, masters athletes should focus on good carbohydrate availability for sessions requiring high intensity or high levels of technique and skill, while noting that high carbohydrate availability is less important during lower-intensity workouts or non-specific conditioning sessions. This may require strategic thinking and planning on behalf of the athlete as not all athletes report the intake of carbohydrate during and after daily workouts to promote high carbohydrate availability when warranted [53].

4.7 CARBOHYDRATE LOADING FOR COMPETITION

A goal of pre-competition eating is to prepare the body's carbohydrate stores in anticipation of the fuel needs of the event. In short, high-intensity events (i.e. track running, swimming, rowing, explosive team sports such as basketball, power sports such as weight lifting and combat sports) which rely on muscle carbohydrate stores as a fuel are unlikely to exhaust normal muscle glycogen stores. Hence, a day of rest in combination with a normal dietary intake will sufficiently elevate carbohydrate stores to meet the demands of exercise in these athlete groups. However, in situations where masters athletes are required to play multiple games or compete several times throughout the day, or play strenuous team sports that extend beyond 60 minutes, increasing carbohydrate stores by employing a higher carbohydrate diet may be warranted. Furthermore, the fuel demands of many endurance and ultra-endurance events are greater than the muscle's normal glycogen stores, as evidenced by competitors in marathons, road cycling races and Ironman triathlons experiencing exhaustion due to muscle glycogen depletion. For these athletes, combining adequate rest with a suitably adjusted carbohydrate intake specific to their individual needs will carbohydrate load or super-compensate glycogen stores before competition.

The early protocols developed by Scandinavian researchers in the 1960s demonstrated that muscle glycogen stores were doubled in response to a dietary technique involving a 3-day depletion phase (low carbohydrate + training) followed by a 3-day loading phase (taper plus high carbohydrate intake) [1]. The so-called *depletion method* for carbohydrate loading was found to prolong the time that race pace could be sustained, delaying fatigue or producing a faster race time [54]. Subsequent carbohydrate loading protocols have shown that no depletion phase is required [55], and high-carbohydrate eating strategies with adequate rest employed for as little as 24–36 hours result in a similar elevation of muscle glycogen stores above normal resting values in trained athletes [56]. In a comprehensive review, Hawley and colleagues concluded that undertaking a carbohydrate loading protocol prior to exercise improves endurance by ~20% compared to a low-to-moderate carbohydrate diet. Furthermore, exercise performance is increased by ~2%–3% after carbohydrate loading when subjects are required to complete a fixed distance or workload of >90 min [57]. Of interest, carbohydrate loading does not appear to enhance exercise performance of high-intensity exercise lasting ~60 min [58].

While an early study suggested that young female athletes could not load muscle glycogen stores to a similar extent to that of male athletes [59], a follow-up study revealed that when total energy and carbohydrate intake were adequately increased, female athletes' muscle glycogen stores were similarly elevated [60]. The earlier report was an artefact of a habitually low reported energy intake in the female athlete group. This has practical significance for female masters athletes due to lower than expected reported energy and carbohydrate intakes in this group [26]. And finally, while athletes typically increase fibre-rich carbohydrate foods (i.e. pasta) to increase daily carbohydrate intake leading into competition, such a dietary regimen increases gastrointestinal discomfort compared to a diet where carbohydrate intake is increased with a lower-fibre, compact-liquid carbohydrate drink [61]. Table 4.5 outlines key practical considerations for athletes when carbohydrate loading for competition.

TABLE 4.5
Practical Suggestions and Examples of Suitable Food Choices That Provide Carbohydrates for Various Situations in Sports

Carbohydrate Loading

- Total food intake should be reduced leading into competition to reflect a taper in training. The number of days which carbohydrate intake is increased leading into competition should reflect the likely carbohydrate requirements for the event and opportunities to consume carbohydrate while exercising.
- To consume adequate carbohydrate and maintain fibre at a normal intake, compact, refined carbohydrate foods and fluids as listed in Table 4.6 should be included.
- While it is common practice for athletes to increase fluid intake in the days leading into competition, unlike carbohydrate, the body is not capable of fluid loading (long-term). Athletes are reminded to avoid drinking more than their daily fluid losses while preparing for competition.
- The food suggestions and volumes required to supercompensate muscle glycogen stores are specific to carbohydrate loading and should not be misinterpreted to reflect everyday eating habits or strategies. Athletes may need to include foods when carbohydrate loading that they would otherwise avoid on normal training days to ensure daily carbohydrate intake is sufficiently increased.

Pre-Competition Meal Suggestions

Above all considerations, the amount and types of food included at the pre-event meal should be familiar to the athlete and reflect strategies trialled in the daily training environment.

Early Morning Competition Start

Choices need to be simple and easy to consume 1.5–2 hours before the start of competition to avoid eating at 2–3 a.m. For athletes who are too nervous to eat or find it difficult to eat on the morning of competition, including a pre-bedtime snack the night before will reduce the requirement at the pre-event meal. Furthermore, a liquid meal supplement may be better tolerated in these athletes compared to solid foods.

Suitable pre-event meal options for early morning competition starts include

- Cooked oats + low-fat milk with honey + glass of fruit juice
- Toasted muffin/s or crumpet/s + jam or honey + banana with 300–600 ml of sports drink
- 1–2 Pancakes with syrup + liquid meal supplement
- 400–600 ml of sports drink + sports bar

Late Competition Start

A normal schedule of meals should be consumed before the pre-competition meal when the event start time is scheduled for later in the day. Timing of pre-race meal can be varied to suit athlete preference (1–3 hours pre-event). High-fibre food choices (i.e. salads) that provide little carbohydrate should be used sparingly. Water should be consumed to thirst in addition to fluid listed to top-up fluid intake.

Suitable pre-event meal options for early morning competition starts include

- Roll/s, wrap/s or sandwich/es + 400–600 ml of sports drink
- Pasta with tomato or low-fat sauce + glass of fruit juice
- Toasted sandwich + glass of flavoured milk
- Toast with jam or honey + 1/2–1 sports bar + 300–600 ml of sports drink
- Liquid meal supplement + a sports bar

Fuelling during Competition

Before making a final decision on the amount of carbohydrate needed to support performance during exercise, it is important to consider the possible interaction that may exist with strategies that acutely promote increased carbohydrate availability immediately before exercise (i.e. carbohydrate loading and pre-exercise meal).

Events lasting less than 45 minutes such as power sports, swimming, rowing, canoeing, track and field events and 10-km running races are unlikely to either provide opportunity or benefit from ingesting carbohydrate during exercise.

High-intensity Endurance Events of 45–75 minutes (i.e. Sprint Distance Triathlon, Half Marathon, Soccer, Basketball)
Small amounts of carbohydrate from a sports drink or even a mouth rinse if practical and tolerated and water as required.

(*continued*)

TABLE 4.5 (Continued)
Practical Suggestions and Examples of Suitable Food Choices That Provide Carbohydrates for Various Situations in Sports

High-Intensity Endurance Events 90–150 minutes (i.e. Olympic Distance Triathlon, Marathon, Adventure Race)

The goal is to consume 30–60 g of carbohydrate/hour. Water should be consumed to thirst in addition to fluid listed to top-up fluid intake. Suitable hourly options include

- 200–300 ml of a sports drink ± sport gel (25 g CHO per gel)
- 200–300 ml of cola soft drink ± sports gel (25 g CHO)

Endurance Events > 2.5–3 h (i.e. Marathon Or Ultra-Marathon, Ocean Marathon Paddle, Open Water Swimming Event, Adventure Race, Road Cycling Event)

The amount of carbohydrate consumed can be titrated up to 90 g of carbohydrate/hour. For ultra-endurance races a variety of tastes (sweet and savoury) should be included to avoid flavour fatigue and the amount of carbohydrate consumed reflect the nature of the event and specific requirements of the athlete. Lower intake rates are suggested when the intensity (i.e. pace) is low, with hourly intakes increased to reflect an increased intensity of exercise. The combination of solid versus liquid forms of carbohydrate should be modified to reflect the intensity of exercise and the duration of the event. When high rates of carbohydrate intake are required (60–90 g/hour), formulated sports products made with a 2:1 ratio of glucose:fructose will enhance intestinal absorption of carbohydrate and fluid. Water should be consumed to thirst in addition to fluid listed to top-up fluid intake. Athletes are suggested to rehearse competition intake strategies as high rates of carbohydrate intake during competition may cause gastrointestinal discomfort and distress. Athletes are encouraged to modify their intake of carbohydrate as dictated by feelings of gastrointestinal comfort during the event, particularly in hot, humid competition environments.

Carbohydrate target 50–60 g per hour

- 400 ml of sports drink + 1 × sport gel (~25 g carbohydrate per gel)
- 2 × sport gels (~25 g carbohydrate per gel)
- 500 ml of sports drink + banana
- 300 ml of sports drink + sports bar
- 500 ml of cola drink
- 40 g of jelly confectionery or sports confectionery + cereal bar or granola bar

Carbohydrate target 70–90 g per hour

- 400 ml of sports drink + 2 × sport gels (~25 g carbohydrate per gel)
- 300 ml of sports drink + 1 × sport gel (~25 g carbohydrate per gel) + sandwich (sweet or savoury spread)
- 600 ml of cola drink + 1/2 sports bar (~40 g carbohydrate per bar)
- 60 g chocolate bar + sandwich (sweet or savoury spread) ± sports gel (~25 g carbohydrate per gel)
- 250 ml of liquid meal supplement + cereal bar, muesli bar or granola bar
- 600 ml of sports drink + 50 g of dried fruit and nut mix + 20 g packet of savoury crisps

4.8 THE PRE-COMPETITION MEAL

Carbohydrate-rich foods and drinks consumed in the 4 hours before an endurance event have a role in fine-tuning competition preparation by enhancing muscle glycogen stores (if they have not been fully loaded since the last exercise session) and restoring liver glycogen stores (for morning training or competition undertaken after an overnight fast). An early study by Coyle and Coggan demonstrated that a carbohydrate meal consumed 4 hours prior to exercise resulted in a 42% elevation in muscle glycogen at the beginning of the session [62]. The same researchers also observed a decline in blood glucose, a suppression of the normally observed rise in free fatty acid levels and increased carbohydrate oxidation in the first hour of exercise following the ingestion of a pre-exercise carbohydrate meal. Although these metabolic perturbations may exist for up to 6 hours following a carbohydrate meal [63], as long as sufficient carbohydrate is consumed there is a net increase in carbohydrate availability during exercise.

Compared with an overnight fast, intake of a substantial amount of carbohydrate (~100–300 g) 2–4 hours before exercise has been shown to increase cycling endurance and enhance endurance cycling performance [64–67]. In a much publicised study, Foster and others found a decrease in exercise capacity following ingestion of 75 g of carbohydrate 30 min before an endurance cycling task in male and female students [68]. The majority of subjects demonstrated a transient decline in serum glucose at the onset of exercise when fed the carbohydrate prior to exercise. It has been suggested that the amount of carbohydrate consumed pre-exercise, the timing of the meal, increased sensitivity to insulin and low-moderate exercise intensity are risk factors in individuals susceptible to displaying symptoms of hypoglycaemia at the onset of exercise following a pre-exercise carbohydrate meal or snack [69]. Thus, older athletes exercising at lower intensities maybe more susceptible than their younger counterparts.

More recently, in a series of related studies which explored this issue systematically, researchers found no differences in the decline of blood glucose during exercise or prevalence of blood glucose levels indicative of hypoglycaemia (<3.5 mmol·L^{-1}) when varying the amount of carbohydrate consumed 45 min before exercise (20–200 g) or the intensity of exercise (55%–90% VO_{2max}) performed in the subsequent exercise bout [70,71]. A change in timing of 75 g of carbohydrate (15–75 min) before exercise has been shown to cause a difference in blood glucose concentrations at the onset of exercise [72], with the later feeding times (45 and 75 min) being associated with greater prevalence of blood glucose levels below 3.5 mmol·L^{-1}. Of note, differences were self-corrected within 10 min of the start of exercise and no differences were observed in exercise performance between trials. These findings suggest that while transient hypoglycaemia may occur in some individuals following pre-exercise carbohydrate meal, it is has no effect on subsequent exercise performance.

Current guidelines for the pre-competition meal (see Table 4.2) suggest carbohydrate intakes of 1–4 grams per kilogram of body mass at least 60 min before exercise (most cases 2–3 hours prior to exercise). The timing of the meal, the amount of carbohydrate consumed and the overall composition of the meal or snack should be familiar to the athlete to minimise gastrointestinal discomfort and meet the unique nutrition and practical challenges of the event. Table 4.5 outlines key practical considerations that relate to the pre-competition meal.

4.9 CARBOHYDRATE INTAKE DURING COMPETITION AND QUALITY TRAINING SESSIONS

The beneficial effect of consuming carbohydrate throughout endurance exercise (>90 min duration) on endurance capacity and performance is a consistent and reproducible finding [73,74]. It appears to offer a further performance benefit to that of providing a pre-exercise meal alone [75]. While it is often overlooked, carbohydrate intake during exercise has also been shown to increase endurance capabilities within intermittent exercise protocols that replicate team sport activities [4]. The amount of carbohydrate associated with performance benefits seems to vary according to the duration of exercise, which suggests that several mechanisms may be responsible for the performance enhancement [76]. Possible mechanisms of action include an attenuation in central fatigue, better maintenance of carbohydrate oxidation rates, muscle glycogen sparing, changes in muscle metabolite levels and maintenance of blood glucose concentrations [76]. It is important to consider these mechanisms as this will influence the recommendations regarding the amount and pattern of feeding carbohydrate during competition. The latest guidelines for carbohydrate, as outlined in Table 4.2, take into account recent findings which have further extended our knowledge regarding the benefits of consuming carbohydrate during exercise.

There is now considerable evidence that in situations when a high-power output is required over durations of ~45–75 min, frequent mouth rinsing or intake of very small amounts of carbohydrate can enhance performance by 2%–3% in younger athletes [77]. Assuming appropriate nutritional strategies are undertaken to normalise muscle glycogen stores before the event, the availability of muscle glycogen is not limiting to exercise performance in such situations. Recent evidence, at least in younger athletes, suggests that the benefits from consuming small amounts of carbohydrate or rinsing the mouth with carbohydrate-containing fluids is explained by an intriguing hypothesis that the central nervous system can sense the presence of carbohydrate via receptors in the mouth and oral space, promoting an enhanced sense of well-being and improved pacing within competitive events [41]. Currently, there are conflicting reports as to whether the provision of carbohydrate (as a mouth rinse or actual intake) during high-intensity endurance exercise offers a further performance benefit to that of ingesting a pre-exercise meal alone [78,79]. Therefore, it is important to consider the overall nutrient and carbohydrate requirements of the athlete when making recommendations regarding training and competition carbohydrate intake strategies for such training sessions or competitive events.

In sports which feature more than ~3 hours of sustained moderate–high intensity exercise the muscle becomes increasingly reliant on carbohydrate from exogenous carbohydrate sources as muscle glycogen stores become depleted. Peak rates of exogenous carbohydrate in the form of single transportable carbohydrate are capped at ~1.1 $g \cdot min^{-1}$ [80,81]. In a series of related studies, ingestion of multiple transportable carbohydrates (i.e. glucose + fructose) increases peak oxidation rates of exogenous carbohydrate to as much as 1.75 $g \cdot min^{-1}$ and results in improved endurance performance in younger athletes [82]. It appears that the rate of exogenous carbohydrate oxidation (namely glucose) is most likely limited by the rate of absorption from the small intestine into the systemic circulation [42], although a high habitual carbohydrate intake may increase this capacity [35]. These findings have been incorporated into updated guidelines for carbohydrate intake during exercise (Table 4.2), which need to be translated into competition practices according to the likely requirements for carbohydrate, opportunities provided by each event, gastrointestinal tolerance and the experience of individual athletes both young and old (Table 4.5). It is prudent to remind athletes that a tailored nutrition plan based on current carbohydrate and fluid intake recommendations for endurance events has been shown to outperform an ad hoc athlete approach [83].

4.10 CONCLUSION

There is little evidence to currently suggest that the carbohydrate intake guidelines for masters athletes and older exercises should be modified from recently updated guidelines for younger athletes. As with other athlete populations, these guidelines should be interpreted to reflect the unique requirements (e.g. training vs. competition; training volume, intensity, duration, frequency and type of exercise; body composition and health status) of each individual masters athlete.

4.11 IMPLICATIONS FOR SPORTS MEDICINE PROFESSIONALS AND CLINICIANS

- Consideration should be given to the age-related decline in fat-free mass which is observed in masters athletes when interpreting current carbohydrate intake guidelines.
- Despite a high GI diet accelerating muscle glycogen resynthesis, a low-to-moderate GI diet should be encouraged given the increased likelihood of decreased glucose sensitivity in older athletes.
- Nutrient-dense carbohydrate foods should be promoted, particularly in older athletes with decreased daily energy intakes and/or requirements.
- Sports medicine professionals and clinicians should be familiar with current carbohydrate intake guidelines during exercise given the recent advancements made over the past 10 years.

4.12 IMPLICATIONS FOR MASTERS ATHLETES AND COACHES

Masters athletes and older exercisers should equip themselves with sufficient dietary knowledge or seek the professional guidance of a sports nutrition professional to adjust daily carbohydrate intake to reflect daily exercise patterns and promote high carbohydrate availability for key exercise sessions. By way of example, a female masters endurance cyclist or runner (55 kg, 60 years of age training once daily for around 45–90 min of actual exercise, would have approximate carbohydrate needs of 220–275 g per day. As ample time is available between training sessions to recover muscle glycogen stores, there would be little need to schedule extra snacks or consume specially formulated carbohydrate-dense sports foods to promote recovery of muscle glycogen stores before the following day's training session. In contrast, a 80-kg, well-muscled male crossfit masters athlete (45 years of age) undertaking twice daily strenuous training totalling 90–120 min is likely to require 480–560 g of carbohydrate daily, paying particular attention to the timing of carbohydrate intake around high-quality workouts and training sessions scheduled closely together. Athletes interested in checking their daily carbohydrate intake or planning their carbohydrate intake to reflect estimated daily requirements should refer to Table 4.6.

TABLE 4.6
Carbohydrate Content of Typically Consumed Carbohydrate Foods and Fluids

Carbohydrate Food	Amount for 30 g Carbohydrate
Breads and Cereals	
Wheat biscuit cereal	45 g (3 biscuits)
Flake/bubble breakfast cereal	45 g (1 cup)
Mixed whole grain cereal with added fruit	45 g (3/4 cup)
Toasted or natural muesli	60 g (1/2 cup) toasted, (2/3 cup) natural
Rolled oats, raw	50 g (1/2 cup)
Rolled oats, raw, on milk	30 g (1/3 cup) oats + 3/4 cup of milk (200 ml)
Bread, mixed grain, whole meal or white	2 regular slices (40 g)
Bread roll, mixed grain, whole meal or white	1 medium roll (80 g)
Pita, Lebanese bread and wraps	Approximately 1 pita or wrap (60–70 g)
English muffin	1 muffin (~60 g)
Bars, Crackers and Cakes	
Commercial cereal or muesli bar	1–2 bars (varies according to brand)
Rice cakes	4 rice cakes (~40 g)
Crispbreads	4 crispbreads (~50 g)
Café-style muffin	1 muffin (~80 g)
Pancakes	2 medium (~70 g)
Scones	1 medium-sized scone (~70 g)
Fruit cake	Medium slice (~60 g)
Croissant	1 large (~75 g)
Pasta, Rice and Noodles	
Rice, boiled	2/3 cup (120 g)
Pasta or noodles, boiled	3/4 cup (120 g)
Couscous	2/3 cup (100 g)
Creamed rice	1/2 cup (120 g)
Fruit	
Bananas	1.5 medium-to-large bananas
Oranges and other medium-sized fruit	1–2 large, depending on piece of fruit
Mangoes, apples, pears and other large fruit	1 large piece of fruit
Grapes	1 cup

(continued)

TABLE 4.6 (Continued)
Carbohydrate Content of Typically Consumed Carbohydrate Foods and Fluids

Carbohydrate Food	Amount for 30 g Carbohydrate
Strawberries and blueberries	Approximately 2 punnets or 2 cups
Melon	2–3 cups
Canned fruit, in natural juice	1 cup
Carbohydrate-Rich Vegetables and Legumes	
Potatoes, sweet potato	2 medium
Corn	1 large cob
Lentils, kidney beans and the like	1.5 cups
Canned baked beans	1 cup
Dairy Products	
Milk	2 cups (500 ml)
Flavoured milk	1.5 cups (400 ml)
Custard	3/4 cup (200 g)
Non-sugar sweetened or natural yogurt	1.5 cups (2 × 200 g tubs)
Flavoured fruit yogurt	3/4 cup (1 × 200 g tub)
Ice cream	1 cup (150 g) will vary according to brand
Surgary Food Items	
Sugar, jams, syrups and honey	1.5–2 tbsps
Chocolate and chocolate bars	50 g
Jubes/jelly confectionary	40 g
Carbohydrate-Containing Drinks	
Fruit juice, unsweetened	300–500 ml depending on fruit
Soft drink (not diet) and flavoured mineral water	375 ml can
Sweetened iced tea	500 ml
Cordial	300 ml (large glass)
Sports Foods and Fluids	
Sports drink (e.g. 6% carbohydrate)	500 ml
Liquid meal supplement powder	50 g (typical serving size varies between 40–60 g)
Sports bar	3/4–1 typical bar (~50 g)
Sports gel	1–1.5 gels depending on brands
Sports confectionery	6 pieces

4.13 FUTURE RESEARCH DIRECTIONS

Our understanding of the daily carbohydrate intakes of masters athletes is currently lacking and requires further investigation. Furthermore, while the effect of increasing carbohydrate availability for an acute exercise bout is now more clearly understood for younger trained athletes, specific studies investigating the effects of increased carbohydrate availability by elevating pre-exercise muscle glycogen stores and consuming carbohydrate during exercise are lacking in masters athletes and older exercises.

REFERENCES

1. Ahlborg, B., Bergstrom, J., Brohult, J. et al., Human muscle glycogen content and capacity for prolonged exercise after different diets, *Forsvarsmedicin*. 3(Suppl 1), 85–99, 1967.
2. Burke, L.M., Hawley, J.A., Wong, S.H. and Jeukendrup, A.E., Carbohydrates for training and competition, *J. Sports Sci*. 29(Suppl 1), 17–27, 2011.

3. Slater, G. and Phillips, S.M., Nutrition guidelines for strength sports: Sprinting, weightlifting, throwing events and bodybuilding, *J. Sports Sci.* 29(Suppl 1), 67–77, 2011.
4. Phillips, S.M., Sproule, J. and Turner, A.P., Carbohydrate ingestion during team games exercise: Current knowledge and areas for future investigation, *Sports Med.* 41(7), 559–85, 2011.
5. Coyle, E.F., Substrate utilization during exercise in active people, *Am. J. Clin. Nutr.* 61(Suppl 4), 968–79, 1995.
6. O'Brien, M.J., Viguie, C.A., Mazzeo, R.S. and Brooks, G.A., Carbohydrate dependence during marathon running, *Med. Sci. Sports. Exerc.* 25(9), 1009–17, 1993.
7. Hargreaves, M., Exercise physiology and metabolism, in *Clinical Sports Nutrition*, L. Burke and V. Deakin, eds., McGraw Hill, North Ryde, Australia, 2010, 1–9.
8. Hargreaves, M., Carbohydrates and exercise. *J. Sports Sci.* 9, 17–28, 1991.
9. Romijn, J.A., Coyle, E.F., Sidossis, L.S. et al., Regulation of endogenous fat and carbohydrate metabolism in relation to exercise intensity and duration, *Am. J. Physiol.* 265(3 Pt 1), E380–91, 1993.
10. Sial, S., Coggan, A.R., Carroll, R., Goodwin, J. and Klein, S., Fat and carbohydrate metabolism during exercise in elderly and young subjects, *Am. J. Physiol.* 271(6 Pt 1), E983–9, 1996.
11. Sial, S., Coggan, A.R., Hickner, R.C. and Klein, S., Training-induced alterations in fat and carbohydrate metabolism during exercise in elderly subjects, *Am. J. Physiol.* 274(5 Pt 1), E785–90, 1998.
12. Cox, J.H., Cortright, R.N., Dohm, G.L. and Houmard, J.A., Effect of aging on response to exercise training in humans: Skeletal muscle GLUT-4 and insulin sensitivity, *J. Appl. Physiol.* 86(6), 2019–25, 1999.
13. Coggan, A.R., Spina, R.J., King, D.S. et al., Skeletal muscle adaptations to endurance training in 60- to 70-yr-old men and women, *J. Appl. Physiol.* 72(5), 1780–6, 1992.
14. Coffey, V.G. and Hawley, J.A., The molecular bases of training adaptation, *Sports Med.* 37(9), 737–63, 2007.
15. Costill, D.L., Carbohydrates for exercise: Dietary demands for optimal performance, *Int. J. Sports Med.* 9(1), 1–18, 1988.
16. Meredith, C.N., Frontera, W.R., Fisher, E.C. et al., Peripheral effects of endurance training in young and old subjects, *J. Appl. Physiol.* 66(6), 2844–9, 1989.
17. Hughes, V.A., Fiatarone, M.A., Fielding, R.A. et al., Exercise increases muscle GLUT-4 levels and insulin action in subjects with impaired glucose tolerance, *Am. J. Physiol.* 264(6 Pt 1), E855–62, 1993.
18. Seals, D.R., Hagberg, J.M., Allen, W.K. et al., Glucose tolerance in young and older athletes and sedentary men, *J. Appl. Physiol.* 56(6), 1521–5, 1984.
19. Pratley, R.E., Hagberg, J.M., Rogus, E.M. and Goldberg, A.P., Enhanced insulin sensitivity and lower waist-to-hip ratio in master athletes, *Am. J. Physiol.* 268(3 Pt 1), E484–90, 1995.
20. Rogers, M.A., Hagberg, J.M., Martin, W.H., 3rd, Ehsani, A.A. and Holloszy, J.O., Decline in VO_{2max} with aging in master athletes and sedentary men, *J. Appl. Physiol.* 68(5), 2195–9, 1990.
21. Pollock, M.L., Foster, C., Knapp, D., Rod, J.L. and Schmidt, D.H., Effect of age and training on aerobic capacity and body composition of master athletes, *J. Appl. Physiol.* 62(2), 725–31, 1987.
22. Hollenbeck, C.B., Haskell, W., Rosenthal, M. and Reaven, G.M., Effect of habitual physical activity on regulation of insulin-stimulated glucose disposal in older males, *J. Am. Geriatr. Soc.* 33(4), 273–7, 1985.
23. Allen, W.K., Seals, D.R., Hurley, B.F., Ehsani, A.A. and Hagberg, J.M., Lactate threshold and distance-running performance in young and older endurance athletes, *J. Appl. Physiol.* 58(4), 1281–4, 1985.
24. Coggan, A.R., Spina, R.J., Rogers, M.A. et al., Histochemical and enzymatic characteristics of skeletal muscle in master athletes, *J. Appl. Physiol.* 68(5), 1896–1901, 1990.
25. Burke, L.M., Cox, G.R., Cummings, N.K. and Desbrow, B., Guidelines for daily carbohydrate intake: Do athletes achieve them? *Sports Med.* 31(4), 267–99, 2001.
26. Beshgetoor, D. and Nichols, J.F., Dietary intake and supplement use in female master cyclists and runners, *Int. J. Sport. Nutr. Exerc. Metab.* 13(2), 166–72, 2003.
27. Tarnopolsky, M.A., Gibala, M., Jeukendrup, A.E. and Phillips, S.M., Nutritional needs of elite endurance athletes. Part 1: Carbohydrate and fluid requirements, *Eur. J. Sport Sci.* 5(1), 3–14, 2005.
28. Achten, J., Halson, S.L., Moseley, L. et al., Higher dietary carbohydrate content during intensified running training results in better maintenance of performance and mood state, *J. Appl. Physiol.* 96(4), 1331–40, 2004.
29. Kirwan, J.P., Costill, D.L., Mitchell, J.B. et al., Carbohydrate balance in competitive runners during successive days of intense training, *J. Appl. Physiol.* 65(6), 2601–06, 1988.
30. Simonsen, J.C., Sherman, W.M., Lamb, D.R. et al., Dietary carbohydrate, muscle glycogen and power output during rowing training, *J. Appl. Physiol.* 70(4), 1500–05, 1991.
31. de Sousa, M.V., Madsen, K., Simoes, H.G. et al., Effects of carbohydrate supplementation on competitive runners undergoing overload training followed by a session of intermittent exercise, *Eur. J. Appl. Physiol.* 109(3), 507–16, 2010.

32. Vogt, M., Puntschart, A., Howald, H. et al., Effects of dietary fat on muscle substrates, metabolism and performance in athletes, *Med. Sci. Sports. Exerc.* 35(6), 952–60, 2003.
33. Sherman, W.M., Doyle, J.A., Lamb, D.R. and Strauss, R.H., Dietary carbohydrate, muscle glycogen and exercise performance during 7 d of training, *Am. J. Clin. Nutr.* 57(1), 27–31, 1993.
34. Lamb, D.R., Rinehardt, K.F., Bartels, R.L., Sherman, W.M. and Snook, J.T., Dietary carbohydrate and intensity of interval swim training, *Am. J. Clin. Nutr.* 52(6), 1058–63, 1990.
35. Cox, G.R., Clark, S.A., Cox, A.J. et al., Daily training with high carbohydrate availability increases exogenous carbohydrate oxidation during endurance cycling, *J. Appl. Physiol (1985).* 109(1), 126–34, 2010.
36. Costill, D.L., Flynn, M.G., Kirwan, J.P. et al., Effects of repeated days of intensified training on muscle glycogen and swimming performance, *Med. Sci. Sports Exerc.* 20(3), 249–54, 1988.
37. Burke, L.M., Kiens, B. and Ivy, J.L., Carbohydrates and fat for training and recovery, *J. Sports Sci.* 22(1), 15–30, 2004.
38. Tarnopolsky, M.A., Nutritional consideration in the aging athlete, *Clin. J. Sport Med.* 18(6), 531–8, 2008.
39. Forbes, G.B. and Reina, J.C., Adult lean body mass declines with age: Some longitudinal observations, *Metabolism.* 19(9), 653–63, 1970.
40. Betts, J.A. and Williams, C., Short-term recovery from prolonged exercise: Exploring the potential for protein ingestion to accentuate the benefits of carbohydrate supplements, *Sports Med.* 40(11), 941–59, 2010.
41. Chambers, E.S., Bridge, M.W. and Jones, D.A., Carbohydrate sensing in the human mouth: Effects on exercise performance and brain activity, *J. Physiol.* 587(Pt 8), 1779–94, 2009.
42. Shi, X., Summers, R.W., Schedl, H.P. et al., Effects of carbohydrate type and concentration and solution osmolality on water absorption, *Med. Sci. Sports Exerc.* 27(12), 1607–15, 1995.
43. Baar, K. and McGee, S., Optimizing training adaptations by manipulating glycogen, *Eur. J. Sports Sci.* 8(2), 97–106, 2008.
44. Ryan, A.S., Nicklas, B.J. and Elahi, D., A cross-sectional study on body composition and energy expenditure in women athletes during aging, *Am. J. Physiol.* 271(5 Pt 1), E916–21, 1996.
45. Ivy, J.L., Katz, A.L., Cutler, C.L., Sherman, W.M. and Coyle, E.F., Muscle glycogen synthesis after exercise: Effect of time of carbohydrate ingestion, *J. Appl. Physiol.* 64(4), 1480–5, 1988.
46. Burke, L.M., Collier, G.R., Beasley, S.K. et al., Effect of coingestion of fat and protein with carbohydrate feedings on muscle glycogen storage, *J. Appl. Physiol.* 78(6), 2187–92, 1995.
47. Burke, L.M., Collier, G.R. and Hargreaves, M., Muscle glycogen storage after prolonged exercise: Effect of the glycemic index of carbohydrate feedings, *J. Appl. Physiol.* 75(2), 1019–23, 1993.
48. Hawley, J.A. and Burke, L.M., Carbohydrate availability and training adaptation: Effects on cell metabolism, *Exerc. Sport Sci. Rev.* 38(4), 152–60, 2010.
49. Hansen, A.K., Fischer, C.P., Plomgaard, P. et al., Skeletal muscle adaptation: Training twice every second day vs. training once daily, *J. Appl. Physiol.* 98(1), 93–9, 2005.
50. Yeo, W.K., Paton, C.D., Garnham, A.P. et al., Skeletal muscle adaptation and performance responses to once a day versus twice every second day endurance training regimens, *J. Appl. Physiol.* 105(5), 1462–70, 2008.
51. Hulston, C.J., Venables, M.C., Mann, C.H. et al., Training with low muscle glycogen enhances fat metabolism in well-trained cyclists, *Med. Sci. Sports Exerc.* 42(11), 2046–55, 2010.
52. Howarth, K.R., Phillips, S.M., MacDonald, M.J. et al., Effect of glycogen availability on human skeletal muscle protein turnover during exercise and recovery, *J. Appl. Physiol.* 109(2), 431–8, 2010.
53. Burke, L.M., Slater, G., Broad, E.M. et al., Eating patterns and meal frequency of elite Australian athletes, *Int. J. Sport Nutr. Exerc. Metab.* 13(4), 521–38, 2003.
54. Karlsson, J. and Saltin, B., Diet, muscle glycogen and endurance performance, *J. Appl. Physiol.* 31(2), 203–6, 1971.
55. Sherman, W.M., Costill, D.L., Fink, W.J. and Miller, J.M., Effect of exercise-diet manipulation on muscle glycogen and its subsequent utilization during performance, *Int. J. Sports Med.* 2(2), 114–8, 1981.
56. Bussau, V.A., Fairchild, T.J., Rao, A., Steele, P. and Fournier, P.A., Carbohydrate loading in human muscle: An improved 1 day protocol, *Eur. J. Appl. Physiol.* 87(3), 290–5, 2002.
57. Hawley, J.A., Schabort, E.J., Noakes, T.D. and Dennis, S.C., Carbohydrate-loading and exercise performance. An update, *Sports Med.* 24(2), 73–81, 1997.
58. Hawley, J.A., Palmer, G.S. and Noakes, T.D., Effects of 3 days of carbohydrate supplementation on muscle glycogen content and utilisation during a 1-h cycling performance, *Eur. J. Appl. Physiol. Occup. Physiol.* 75(5), 407–12, 1997.
59. Tarnopolsky, M.A., Atkinson, S.A., Phillips, S.M. and MacDougall, J.D., Carbohydrate loading and metabolism during exercise in men and women, *J. Appl. Physiol.* 78(4), 1360–8, 1995.

60. Tarnopolsky, M.A., Zawada, C., Richmond, L.B. et al., Gender differences in carbohydrate loading are related to energy intake, *J. Appl. Physiol.* 91(1), 225–30, 2001.
61. Lamb, D.R., Snyder, A.C. and Baur, T.S., Muscle glycogen loading with a liquid carbohydrate supplement, *Int. J. Sport Nutr.* 1(1), 52–60, 1991.
62. Coyle, E.F., Coggan, A.R., Hemmert, M.K., Lowe, R.C. and Walters, T.J., Substrate usage during prolonged exercise following a preexercise meal, *J. Appl. Physiol.* 59(2), 429–33, 1985.
63. Montain, S.J., Hopper, M.K., Coggan, A.R. and Coyle, E.F., Exercise metabolism at different time intervals after a meal, *J. Appl. Physiol.* 70(2), 882–8, 1991.
64. Wright, D.A., Sherman, W.M. and Dernbach, A.R., Carbohydrate feedings before, during, or in combination improve cycling endurance performance, *J. Appl. Physiol.* 71(3), 1082–8, 1991.
65. Schabort, E.J., Bosch, A.N., Weltan, S.M. and Noakes, T.D., The effect of a preexercise meal on time to fatigue during prolonged cycling exercise, *Med. Sci. Sports Exerc.* 31(3), 464–71, 1999.
66. Sherman, W.M., Brodowicz, G., Wright, D.A. et al., Effects of 4 h preexercise carbohydrate feedings on cycling performance, *Med. Sci. Sports Exerc.* 21(5), 598–604, 1989.
67. Neufer, P.D., Costill, D.L., Flynn, M.G. et al., Improvements in exercise performance: Effects of carbohydrate feedings and diet, *J. Appl. Physiol.* 62(3), 983–8, 1987.
68. Foster, C., Costill, D.L. and Fink, W.J., Effects of preexercise feedings on endurance performance, *Med. Sci. Sports.* 11(1), 1–5, 1979.
69. Kuipers, H., Fransen, E.J. and Keizer, H.A., Pre-exercise ingestion of carbohydrate and transient hypoglycemia during exercise, *Int. J. Sports Med.* 20(4), 227–31, 1999.
70. Achten, J. and Jeukendrup, A.E., Effects of pre-exercise ingestion of carbohydrate on glycaemic and insulinaemic responses during subsequent exercise at differing intensities, *Eur. J. Appl. Physiol.* 88(4–5), 466–71, 2003.
71. Jentjens, R.L., Cale, C., Gutch, C. and Jeukendrup, A.E., Effects of pre-exercise ingestion of differing amounts of carbohydrate on subsequent metabolism and cycling performance, *Eur. J. Appl. Physiol.* 88(4–5), 444–52, 2003.
72. Moseley, L., Lancaster, G.I. and Jeukendrup, A.E., Effects of timing of pre-exercise ingestion of carbohydrate on subsequent metabolism and cycling performance, *Eur. J. Appl. Physiol.* 88(4–5), 453-8, 2003.
73. Temesi, J., Johnson, N.A., Raymond, J., Burdon, C.A. and O'Connor, H.T., Carbohydrate ingestion during endurance exercise improves performance in adults, *J. Nutr.* 141(5), 890–7, 2011.
74. Cermak, N.M. and van Loon, L.J., The use of carbohydrates during exercise as an ergogenic aid, *Sports Med.* 43(11), 1139–55, 2013.
75. Colombani, P.C., Mannhart, C. and Mettler, S., Carbohydrates and exercise performance in non-fasted athletes: A systematic review of studies mimicking real-life, *Nutr. J.* 12, 16, 2013.
76. Karelis, A.D., Smith, J.W., Passe, D.H. and Peronnet, F., Carbohydrate administration and exercise performance: What are the potential mechanisms involved?, *Sports Med.* 40(9), 747–63, 2010.
77. Jeukendrup, A.E. and Chambers, E.S., Oral carbohydrate sensing and exercise performance, *Curr. Opin. Clin. Nutr. Metab. Care.* 13(4), 447–51, 2010.
78. Lane, S.C., Bird, S.R., Burke, L.M. and Hawley, J.A., Effect of a carbohydrate mouth rinse on simulated cycling time-trial performance commenced in a fed or fasted state, *Appl. Physiol. Nutr. Metab.* 38(2), 134–9, 2013.
79. Beelen, M., Berghuis, J., Bonaparte, B. et al., Carbohydrate mouth rinsing in the fed state: Lack of enhancement of time-trial performance, *Int. J. Sport. Nutr. Exerc. Metab.* 19(4), 400–9, 2009.
80. Jentjens, R.L., Moseley, L., Waring, R.H., Harding, L.K. and Jeukendrup, A.E., Oxidation of combined ingestion of glucose and fructose during exercise, *J. Appl. Physiol.* 96(4), 1277–84, 2004.
81. Jentjens, R.L., Venables, M.C. and Jeukendrup, A.E., Oxidation of exogenous glucose, sucrose and maltose during prolonged cycling exercise, *J. Appl. Physiol.* 96(4), 1285–91, 2004.
82. Jeukendrup, A.E., Carbohydrate and exercise performance: The role of multiple transportable carbohydrates, *Curr. Opin. Clin. Nutr. Metab. Care.* 13(4), 452–7, 2010.
83. Hottenrott, K., Hass, E., Kraus, M. et al., A scientific nutrition strategy improves time trial performance by approximately 6% when compared with a self-chosen nutrition strategy in trained cyclists: A randomized cross-over study, *Appl. Physiol. Nutr. Metab.* 37(4), 637–45, 2012.

5 Fat Needs in Masters Athletes

Nathan A. Johnson and Stephen R. Stannard

CONTENTS

5.1 INTRODUCTION

The oxidation of glucose and fatty acids provides almost all energy requirements at rest and during sub-maximal exercise. Although the rate of energy supply (adenosine triphosphate [ATP] resynthesis) from fat oxidation is insufficient to meet the high energetic demands of short duration sprint-type activities, fatty acids from stored triglycerides are available in essentially unlimited supply. The ability to rely on fatty acid oxidation and spare the relatively limited body glucose reserves is viewed as important for the optimisation of endurance exercise performance. Indeed, the adaptive response to endurance training is characterised by an enhanced capacity for oxidative metabolism including fat oxidation.

There is a history of research examining strategies to promote fat oxidation during exercise. However, in contrast to the clear dietary carbohydrate recommendations for endurance athletes, the abundant body reserves and the implicated role of fat in cardiovascular disease mean that dietary fat requirements for the young athlete are less clear. Indeed, the requirements for the masters athlete are even less clear. Despite a lack of research examining fat metabolism in older exercisers, and especially the masters athlete, it is suggested that the capacity for fat oxidation is reduced with age [1]. The purpose of this chapter is to firstly overview fat metabolism and the role of fat in endurance exercise, to then critically examine the effect of ageing on fat metabolism and the implications for the masters athlete, then finally to provide practical recommendations for promoting fat oxidation whilst maximising endurance performance in the masters athlete, including dietary fat needs.

5.2 FAT METABOLISM

Fatty acids are stored in the body as triacylglycerols, more commonly referred to as triglycerides. Triglycerides comprise three fatty acid chains of repeated carbon and hydrogen units which typically vary in length from 16 to 22 carbon atoms and are attached to a glycerol backbone. These hydrophobic compounds accumulate as droplets mainly in specialised fat cells in adipose tissue, and are the body's preferential energy store. The adipose tissue comprises the large subcutaneous compartment and the smaller visceral (intra-abdominal) adipose tissue as shown in Figure 5.1a.

Glycogen storage, the alternate means of storing energy, is limited because glycogen is hydrophilic. This limited storage is likely an evolutionary consequence of the trade-off to sustain sufficient glucose fuel for central nervous system function and locomotion while at the same time avoiding excessive body weight (1 gram of glycogen is associated with 3–4 grams of water *in vivo*). Furthermore, the energy density of fat, some 2.25 times greater than carbohydrate, is such that even in a lean adult there are enough triglycerides in adipose tissue to exclusively sustain the equivalent energy demand of over 20 marathons. In contrast, muscle and liver glycogen reserves could sustain just one marathon [2,3].

Assessment of skeletal muscle by electron microscopy has shown that droplets of triglyceride, known as intramyocellular triglyceride (IMTG), can accumulate within the muscle cell (see Figure 5.1a). While the available energy potential of IMTG is significantly lower than adipose tissue reserves, it is similar to that of muscle glycogen [3]. Nevertheless, being close to the muscle contractile machinery, IMTG is seen as an important fuel source for exercise metabolism [4]. A small amount of triglyceride can also be found in liver cells.

Unlike glucose (the form of carbohydrate the body can use as a fuel), which may be oxidised soon after ingestion of carbohydrate-containing foods, fat oxidation is almost exclusively from the release and subsequent cell oxidation of fatty acids from the body's reserves. Replenishment of the body's net triglyceride stores, which includes body fat, occurs mainly from the ingestion of dietary lipids in the form of saturated fats (from foods such as meat, dairy products, eggs, nuts and plant oils) and unsaturated fats (from foods such as fish, seeds and oils). The liver can also contribute to this via generation of fatty acids from partially metabolised carbohydrate (lipogenesis); this process increases particularly when excess carbohydrate has been ingested [5].

Digestion of dietary lipids involves the breakdown of triglyceride to constituent fatty acids or diacylglycerols by pancreatic (and to a lesser extent stomach) enzymes. These small molecules can be absorbed across the intestine, re-esterified, and then released as triglycerides in chylomicrons (a lipoprotein) into the circulation. However, medium chain triglycerides (MCTs) with fatty acid chain lengths of 6 to 12 carbons can enter the circulation directly through the hepatic portal vein.

Fatty acids for storage in adipose cells are derived from circulating free fatty acids (FFAs) or from very low density lipoproteins (VLDLs) or chylomicrons which are broken down by the lipoprotein lipase at the blood capillary wall (endothelium) prior to uptake by the cell. Once inside the cell these can be combined (esterified) with glycerol to form triglycerides. The process of esterification is encouraged when circulating insulin levels are elevated. Conversely, in order to be used for oxidation, fatty acids must be released from their triglyceride stores and enter the circulation for distribution (Figure 5.1a).

The initial step in the breakdown of fatty acids from triglycerides is termed lipolysis and is under the control of a hormone-sensitive lipase (HSL) in the adipose cell (Figure 5.1b) [6]. The rate of adipose lipolysis is dependent on HSL activity which is increased by adrenalin, growth hormone and glucagon but inhibited by insulin. As a result, conditions which promote high insulin levels, such as ingestion of dietary carbohydrate, may lead to the general storage of fatty acids whilst the hormonal

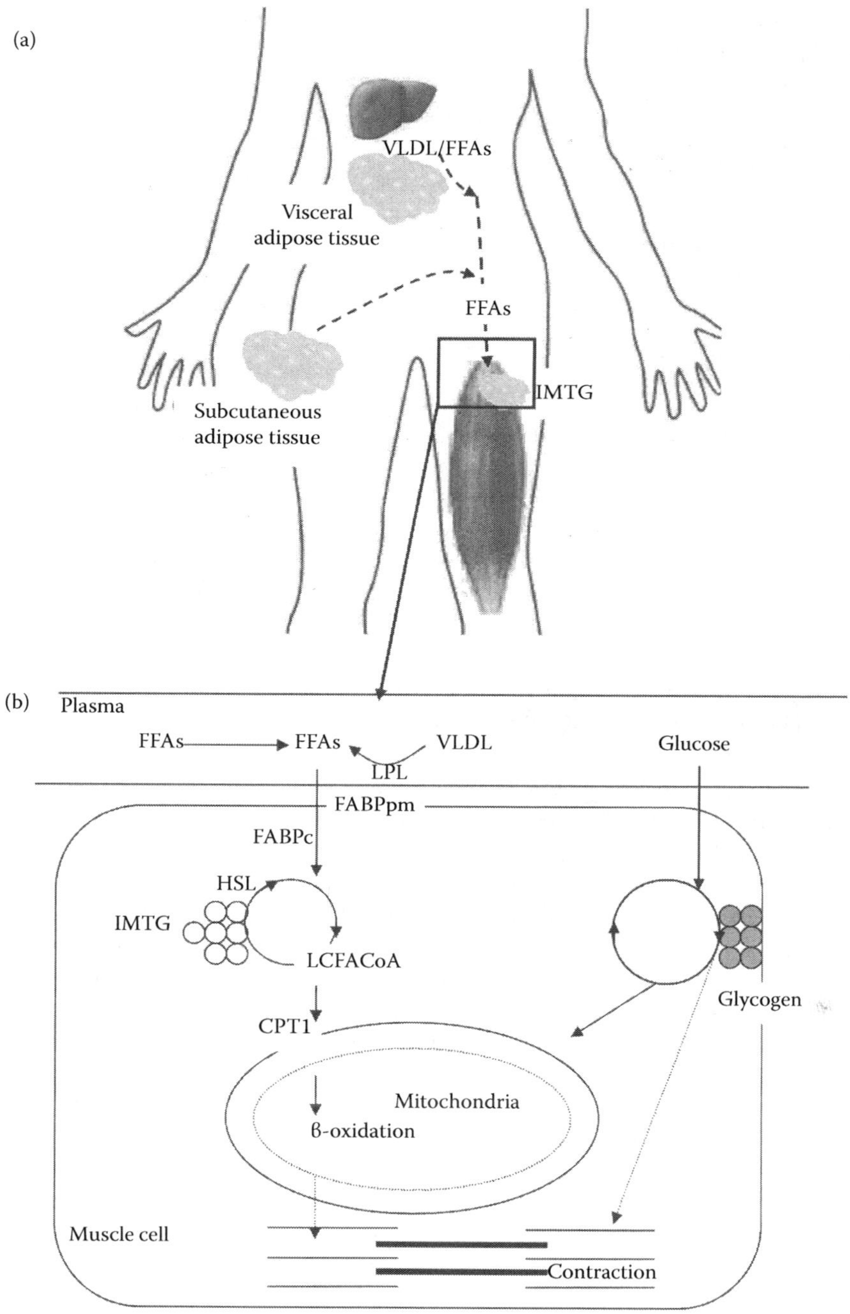

FIGURE 5.1 Human fat metabolism. (a) Fat is stored as triglyceride in subcutaneous and visceral adipose tissue, and as IMTG; to be used for oxidation FFAs from adipose tissue or liver VLDLs must be released and enter the circulation for distribution. (b) Fatty acid transport into and within the muscle is via FABPs; inside the muscle cell fatty acids become activated to LCFACoA. These LCFACoAs and those from HSL-induced IMTG lipolysis can be directed to energy production through conversion to a fatty acyl carnitine compound and transported across the mitochondrial membranes. The initial step is controlled by CPT. LCFACoAs are then broken down through β-oxidation and are metabolized in the tricarboxylic acid cycle for ATP resynthesis via mitochondrial respiration. CPT = carnitine palmitoyltransferase, FABPc = FABP cytoplasmic, FABPpm = FABP plasma membrane, FFA = free fatty acid, HSL = hormone-sensitive lipase, IMTG = intramyocellular triglyceride, LCFACoA = long-chain fatty acyl coenzyme A, VLDL = very low density lipoprotein.

response to stressors, including exercise or low carbohydrate intake, promote fatty acid and glycerol release into the circulation [7].

The delivery of FFAs to muscle cells is a function of both lipolysis and blood flow to the muscle. It was earlier believed that fatty acid transport from the circulation into the muscle cell was a passive process because a positive linear relationship existed between the plasma FFA concentration and fatty acid use [8]. However, fatty acid transport is now thought to be largely (facilitated) protein-mediated [9] with some passive non-protein-mediated contribution [10,11].

Fatty acid binding proteins (FABPs) within the plasma membrane, FABPpm and FAT/CD36, are thought to be responsible for the capture of circulating long-chain fatty acids and their transport into the cell. Fatty acid trafficking in the muscle may be controlled by a cytoplasmic FABP (FABPc) (Figure 5.1b) [12]. Muscle contraction and/or insulin stimulate the movement of FAT/CD36 from the intracellular compartment to the plasma membrane to promote fatty acid uptake [13–15]. Despite the facilitative role of FABPpm and FAT/CD36, fatty acid uptake into the muscle cell is encouraged when the fatty acid concentration gradient between the blood and cell is increased [16,17].

After entering the cell, fatty acids become activated to long-chain fatty acyl coenzyme A (LCFACoA), an intermediate between the processes of lipid synthesis (as IMTG or phospholipids) and fatty acid oxidation (Figure 5.1b). Whether LCFACoAs are directed to oxidation or storage is dictated by their availability and the muscle cell's energy needs (Figure 5.1b). For instance, there is a bias towards a reduction in the IMTG pool during the initial stages (0–2 h) of prolonged exercise when the oxidation of fatty acids by the muscle may exceed their delivery to the cell [18]. Conversely, raising FFAs levels under resting conditions by interventions such as low-carbohydrate/high-fat diets [19], starvation [20] or artificial lipid-heparin infusion [19] increases the concentration gradient and subsequent fatty acid uptake and IMTG formation.

Fatty acids are stored as IMTG by attachment to glycerol derived from the breakdown of glucose metabolism within the cell. HSL is also present in skeletal muscle tissue and promotes the release of fatty acids from stored IMTG in response to adrenalin [21,22] or muscle contraction [23] and is inhibited by insulin [24]. LCFACoA from IMTG lipolysis, and/or from direct uptake into the cell, can be directed to energy production by oxidation in the mitochondria of the cell. This involves the brief conversion to a fatty acyl carnitine compound and transport across the mitochondrial membranes, the initial step of which is controlled by the enzyme carnitine palmitoyltransferase (CPT). LCFACoAs are then broken down into smaller acetyl CoA units by a process termed β-oxidation (Figure 5.1b). Like the products of glucose breakdown, these products can then be metabolised in the tricarboxylic acid cycle and subsequently (with oxygen) contribute to ATP resynthesis via the electron transport chain (cell respiration). The rate of this is partly controlled by mitochondrial enzymes such as citrate synthase, succinate dehydrogenase (tricarboxylic acid cycle) and cytochrome C oxidase (electron transport chain).

5.3 THE ROLE OF FAT IN EXERCISE METABOLISM

5.3.1 Measurement Techniques

Respiratory gas collection and analysis has contributed significantly to the fundamental understanding of both exercise metabolism and the effect of regular exercise training. This non-invasive technique for measuring metabolic rate and fuel selection has shown that whole-body fat oxidation increases with both duration and intensity of exercise, but is reduced at intensities close to the maximal aerobic capacity (VO_{2max}). However, these insights are limited to a whole-body level and are insensitive to the relative contributions of body fat (adipose, IMTG and liver) and glucose (liver and muscle) reserves.

The application of needle biopsy/biochemical assessment of muscle tissue and the use of isotope tracer techniques has informed knowledge of the importance of fuel selection and utilisation in skeletal muscle. The tracer technique involves the intravenous infusion of a stable or radioactive isotope-labelled fuel substrate. The subsequent plasma concentration and the plasma isotope enrichment obtained under steady state conditions is used as an index of the rate of substrate release (termed rate of appearance [Ra]) or use (uptake, termed rate of disappearance [Rd]). For example, FFA release can be determined by isotope-labelled fat infusion (typically ^{14}C or ^{13}C palmitate) and whole-body lipolysis measured when undertaken in combination with glycerol ($^{2}H_5$) infusion. When combined with VO_2 and respiratory exchange ratio (RER), the oxidation of circulating FFAs can be quantified by measuring the rate of appearance of carbon label appearing in the expiratory gas (e.g. $^{13}CO_2$ or $^{14}CO_2$). Together, these techniques have shown that under resting conditions the release of fatty acids from adipose tissue exceeds their oxidation by the body tissues, a 'futile-cycling' which is believed to partly allow for an oversupply of circulating FFAs to buffer large changes in energy use (such as which occurs at the onset of exercise).

Studies in young lean adults have shown that the splanchnic bed accounts for ~40% of circulating FFA uptake in the fasted state, which is higher than that of the muscles (~15%–20%) [25,26]. These fatty acids are oxidised by the liver, the heart, and other tissues in the splanchnic bed or converted to ketones [27,28]. There is also significant re-esterification of adipose-derived FFAs back to triglycerides in the liver [29] which can remain in the liver triglyceride pool or be exported in the blood as VLDLs.

5.3.2 Energy Contributions of Fat during Exercise

During exercise, an increase in adipose lipolysis promoted by elevated blood adrenalin [30] and associated lower insulin levels [31], together with a reduction in futile cycling [32], increases the circulating FFA availability [33]. When combined with changes to blood flow distribution during exercise, the majority of FFAs are directed to the contracting musculature [34]. Although the precise contribution remains unclear, whole-body fat use reflects the oxidation of both these circulating FFAs and fatty acids from IMTG in both young [18,34–37] and older [1] exercisers. It is thought that liver VLDL-derived fatty acids can also be oxidised by skeletal muscle [38], but the consensus is that the contribution of these to metabolism during exercise is trivial [39,40] and that acute exercise does not reduce liver triglyceride levels in lean adults [41].

Through observation of a decline in RER it has long been known that the relative contribution of fat to whole-body metabolism increases with duration of exercise [42]. This coordinated response is enabled partly by hormonal changes which alter the rate of lipolysis, and also by direct down-regulation of glucose oxidation within the contracting muscle with exercise duration. This shift from glucose toward an increased reliance on fat is seen as a positive (rapid) adaption which spares dwindling glucose supply and therefore helps delay fatigue. Evidence of this benefit can be seen in the significantly faster glycogen depletion and earlier fatigue during prolonged exercise when nicotinic acid is ingested to blunt FFA release and fat oxidation [43,44]. This change in whole-body fuel selection with exercise duration occurs simultaneously with a progressive increase in the plasma FFA concentration [45] and is explained partly by the increased uptake and oxidation of these in muscle [34]. However, the tracer technique shows clearly that FFA uptake and oxidation cannot account for the total whole-body rate of fat oxidation measured with indirect calorimetry [34,45]. Therefore, it is now accepted that IMTG oxidation explains the remainder of this fat use, and its contribution is greatest early in exercise when the adipose-derived FFA concentration is relatively low [34,46–49].

Energy expenditure from fuel oxidation (VO_2) increases linearly with increasing exercise intensity to VO_{2max}. The observed close matching of glucose oxidation to work-rate mainly reflects the use of muscle glycogen [34,37,50–52]. During moderate to vigorous exercise at ~45%–85% of the VO_{2max} (typical of most endurance exercise), muscle glycogen oxidation provides the major contribution to carbohydrate metabolism (~40%–65%) with a lesser contribution from liver glucose (~5%–15%) [34,37].

Using tracer measurements in young trained cyclists, both the Romijn (24 ± 2 years) and van Loon (22 ± 1 years) groups showed that the increase in fat oxidation with exercise intensity is enabled partly by an increase in FFA delivery due to an increased adipose lipolysis and muscle blood flow and also by non-FFA (IMTG) oxidation [34,37]. As shown in Figure 5.2, FFA and IMTG oxidation increase as a function of exercise intensity, at least until ~65% VO_{2max}, but are reduced during vigorous exercise (~70%–85% VO_{2max}).

Overall, depending on factors including nutritional and training status, fat oxidation contributes ~55%–20% of total metabolism from 50% to 85% of the VO_{2max} and peak absolute fat oxidation rate occurs between ~50%–65% VO_{2max} (Figure 5.2) [37,53]. By demonstrating that the rate of adipose lipolysis at 85% VO_{2max} was similar to that at 65% VO_{2max} [34], and that the rate of fat oxidation during vigorous exercise (85% VO_{2max}) was only partly elevated by artificially maintaining (lipid-heparin infusion) FFA supply [54], Romijn and colleagues proved that fat oxidation in the muscle is directly inhibited at high intensities of endurance exercise. Similar detailed investigations have not been performed in older exercisers or masters athletes.

The factors which control the changes in fat oxidation with exercise duration and intensity remain debated. Certainly, increased (spatial) recruitment of glycolysis-dependent motor units as more muscular tension is required explain in part the reduced proportional reliance on fat as exercise intensity increases. However, the results of Romijn et al. highlight that enhancing fat oxidation is not simply a matter of increasing lipolysis and FFA supply to the muscle [54]. A potential site of control of fat oxidation may occur at the level of cell (mediated) fatty acid uptake. Interventions which increase fat uptake and oxidation (e.g. obesity [55], high-fat diet [19], starvation [20] and lipid-heparin infusion [19]) are often associated with increased FABP activity [56], and animal models do suggest a dependence on FABPs for fatty acid uptake and oxidation [57].

Whether this is a limiting site in humans is yet to be substantiated. CPT-I activity is rate-limiting in cell fat oxidation, but at present the precise factors controlling the increase in CPT-I activity from rest to low- and moderate-intensity exercise, and its decrease during high-intensity exercise, remain unclear. The absolute rate at which fatty acids can be used to fuel exercise is ultimately a function of the muscle cell mitochondria content and associated oxidative enzymes responsible for fatty acid oxidation. That mitochondrial content is heavily influenced by chronic contractile activity, but within the bounds of genetics, practically means that enhancement of the maximal capacity for fat use for an individual is a function of endurance exercise training.

Many of the metabolic alterations to exercise persist into the post-exercise period. Muscle glucose uptake and glycogen synthase activity are elevated for several hours to promote glycogen

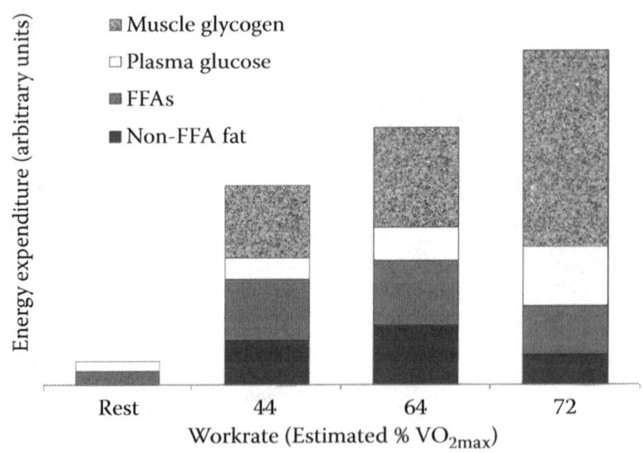

FIGURE 5.2 Energy expenditure and contribution of fuel substrates to metabolism at rest and with exercise of increasing intensity in young men. FFA = free fatty acids; non-FFA - presumed intramyocellular triglyceride (IMTG); VO_{2max} = maximal aerobic power. Results show that FFA and IMTG oxidation increase as a function of exercise intensity but are reduced during vigorous (>70% VO_{2max}) exercise. (Adapted from van Loon, L.J.C. et al., *J. Physiol.* 536(1), 295–304, 2001.)

replenishment [58], and the enhanced insulin-mediated glucose uptake in muscle after exercise [59] is amplified if more glycogen has been used during the exercise bout [60]. During this time whole-body fat oxidation is also elevated and helps sustain energy requirements during recovery [61,62]. This higher lipolysis and fat oxidation is influenced by the exercise dose (intensity and duration) [63,64] and may largely reflect higher IMTG oxidation, the concentration of which can reduce in the post-exercise period [65]. This shift towards fat use reflects the physiological impetus to replenish glycogen after exercise [66] and is sufficient to enable some glycogen repletion when strenuous exercise is followed by even low dietary carbohydrate intake [67] or starvation [68].

5.3.3 Adaptations with Exercise Training

Regular exercise (training) is associated with cardiovascular and muscular adaptations which further promote the maintenance of homeostasis in response to the strain incurred by an acute exercise bout. This often includes an increase in the capacity for oxygen consumption (VO_{2max}) and closely linked increase in maximal cardiac output [69].

The adaptive response to training is also characterised by a greater contribution of fatty acids and a 'sparing' of glucose to the fuel mix at a given absolute work-rate [70] which is revealed as a reduction in the RER in both young [71,72] and older [73] cohorts who undergo exercise training. Given the limited capacity to store muscle glycogen and the importance of glycogen for optimal performance, the improved ability to use non-glucose fuel during exercise is an important metabolic adaptation to enhance endurance capacity. The observations of glucose and glycogen sparing subsequent to artificial FFA elevation [74–76], and the accelerated glycogen loss observed when plasma FFA availability is restricted [43], are evidence that glycogen can be spared if fat availability and oxidation is increased during exercise. This adaptation is not restricted to a greater contribution of fat to the exercise fuel mix at the same absolute work-rate, but also means that the maximal rate at which fat can be oxidised is increased.

Practically, these changes enhance endurance performance by allowing the same intensity of exercise to be sustained for longer or a higher absolute work-rate (higher power output or speed) to be sustained at the same glucose cost. In the specific case of masters athletes, events are sometimes deliberately shorter (e.g. 25-km cycling time trial) than the associated open endurance races (40-km time trial). The alternate and more common situation is that there is only one (set) distance for an event and, generally speaking, masters athletes take longer to complete that distance. In particular, the older masters athlete might take 50% longer and as a consequence (1) will move relatively slower and thus a greater proportion of fuel is likely to be fat, and (2) towards the end of their event there will be a greater reliance upon fat compared with faster, younger fellow competitors.

Interestingly, the higher fat use after endurance training is not accounted for by improved adipose FFA release and oxidation in either young [72] or older [73] exercisers, which makes sense given that training blunts the lipolytic hormone response to exercise [30,77]. That is, after training circulating insulin may be higher [78,79] and blood glycerol and FFAs are lower at the same absolute exercise intensity [71,72,79]. Given that a requirement for FFA uptake by the muscle is the concentration gradient between the plasma and cell [17], these changes would favour lower FFA uptake and oxidation during exercise. However, both cross-sectional and intervention studies suggest that higher storage and oxidation of IMTG may largely explain the higher fat oxidation seen with endurance training [18,71,72]. These adaptations are viewed as a positive training effects because fatty acids from IMTG are readily available inside the muscle close to the mitochondria [4], and unlike circulating fats, need not first be released from their remote depots, transported in the circulation and then diffused/transported into the muscle cell before oxidation [34].

Following endurance training, the ability to rely more heavily on fat oxidation at a higher metabolic rate is primarily due to changes in the muscle. The structure and biochemistry of muscle adapts to chronic exercise with increases in capillarisation, volume of mitochondria [69] and capacity of mitochondrial enzymes for oxidative metabolism [80,81]. Given that the maximum rate of myocellular fatty acid oxidation during muscle contraction is dictated by the activities of both fat-handling proteins and oxidative enzymes, these adaptations not only contribute to improvements in maximal aerobic capacity, but also to a greater capacity for the muscle uptake and oxidation of fatty acids [38,82,83].

Endurance training also results in a greater potential for fat metabolism at numerous points in the passage of fatty acids from release to oxidation, including an increase in the content of FABPpm [84] and the activities of palmityl-coenzyme-A (CoA) synthase, CPT-I (transport across inner mitochondrial membrane) and palmityl-CoA dehydrogenase [85], and reduces the percentage of fatty acids that are recycled [34]. Nevertheless, when muscle and liver glycogen stores are replete and/or insulin and blood glucose is elevated, lipid uptake and oxidation in trained muscle is inhibited just as it is in untrained muscle. The increased capacity for lipid uptake, handling and oxidation in endurance-trained persons is only employed when needed, such as when exercise becomes prolonged or dietary carbohydrate intake is insufficient.

In summary:

- Fatty acids are stored as triglycerides in adipose tissue and muscle cells, and are the major energy reserve in the human body.
- The release of fatty acids from triglyceride droplets for energy use in tissues (including muscle) is under hormonal control, and the rate of this is higher under conditions which lead to low levels of insulin and raised adrenalin and growth hormone notably exercise, fasting and low-carbohydrate diets.
- The uptake of adipose-derived free fatty acids from the blood into muscle and/or the release of muscle triglyceride (IMTG) fatty acids increase during exercise.
- The higher rate of fat oxidation in exercise is largely explained by both adipose and IMTG oxidation in the mitochondria of skeletal muscle.
- The rate of fat oxidation increases with exercise intensity, but is then reduced during vigorous exercise.
- By acting as an adjunct/alternative energy source, fat oxidation can spare limited glycogen, thereby promoting fatigue resistance and potentially enhancing endurance exercise performance.
- The contribution of fat to metabolism increases with duration of exercise.
- Regular endurance training is associated with an increased reliance on fat oxidation at the same exercise intensity, and the maximal capacity for fat oxidation during exercise is largely dictated by the concentration of mitochondria and mitochondrial enzymes in muscle.
- Although these phenomena have been largely studied in young adult cohorts, there is no reason to suggest that these basic principles of metabolism do not apply to masters athletes.

5.4 FAT METABOLISM IN THE OLDER INDIVIDUAL

5.4.1 Changes That May Affect Fat Metabolism in Older Individuals

It is well documented that endurance exercise performance is reduced with age, although behavioural factors including a reduction in training volume and motivation contribute to this [86]. The relative impact of direct physiological changes in explaining this phenomenon are difficult to gauge, but age-related decreases in VO_{2max} and associated velocity at lactate threshold likely account for some of this decrement [86]. Early reports of an age-related decline in VO_{2max} were attributed to cardiovascular factors whereas peripheral adaptations were suggested to be relatively well preserved [87].

Both longitudinal and cross-sectional investigations, including those in which factors such as training volume were matched, have since confirmed that the loss of aerobic power with age closely reflects a decrease in maximal cardiac output and associated maximal heart rate [88–90] and possibly a reduction in blood flow to the active muscles [91]. Importantly, although regular training may lessen the rate of decline in endurance performance, this age-related reduction in aerobic power is independent of training status [92]. The evidence for peripheral factors contributing to declining endurance performance with age is more contentious.

The following sections discuss the evidence for a possible age-related change in fat oxidation. It should be highlighted firstly that, by definition, a reduction in VO_{2max} itself dictates that the maximal rate of fuel oxidation is reduced with age, and subsequently that exercise at the same percentage of VO_{2max} will likely expend energy (fat and/or glucose oxidation) at a slower rate. This means, for instance, that whilst a highly trained masters endurance athlete may be able to sustain 80% of VO_{2max} for a marathon, the age-related decline in VO_{2max} dictates that this athlete will move slower and thus oxidise fuel more slowly and, assuming no change in the economy/efficiency of movement, will burn fat at a lesser rate.

5.4.2 Fat Metabolism at Rest in Older Individuals

Most studies confirm that in healthy sedentary older people the whole-body rate of fat oxidation at rest, including in response to feeding [93], declines with age [94,95]. Although it is difficult to clearly delineate the influence of changes in body composition and habitual activity levels in this phenomenon [94], the absolute reduction if fat oxidation appears to be largely a function of reduced energy expenditure (metabolic rate). This can be partly attributed to the well-established decline with age in lean body mass [96]. However, the effect of energy expenditure on the rate of fat metabolism can also exist independent of body composition [93]. For instance, measurements taken over 24 h in a whole-body calorimetry chamber showed that sleeping fat oxidation was lower in older (~65 years) versus young (~25 years) females and that this was related to the amount of fat-free mass and energy balance, whilst total 24-h fat oxidation was correlated with energy balance and energy expenditure [97].

Whether there is an independent age-related change in the process of fat oxidation is more contentious. Although there is little evidence to suggest that there is a shift in resting proportional substrate selection (indicated by RER) under resting conditions with age [93], there is evidence that the adipose tissue is less responsive to lipolysis in older individuals [98]. For example, at the same level of beta-adrenergic stimulation, middle-aged subjects (53 ± 2 years) were shown to have both blunted adipose FFA release and fatty acid oxidation when compared with young adults (25 ± 2 years) [99]. This has also been shown *in vitro* in fat cells from older adults which had been isolated and exposed to hormonal stimulation [100]. However, there is conflicting evidence as to whether this manifests as a reduced rate of FFA release at the whole-body level (*in vivo*) under resting conditions. For instance, using the tracer technique, Klein and colleagues found a similar the rate of adipose lipolysis (FFA Ra) during fasting in older and young individuals, although this was significantly lower in the older cohort when expressed relative to the amount of fat mass (the older individuals had more body fat) [101]. In contrast, a higher FFA Ra has been observed in older men and women at rest despite reduced energy expenditure [102,103] and this was coupled with a tendency for higher 'non-oxidative FFA disposal' [102].

5.4.3 Effects of Exercise on Fat Metabolism in Older Individuals

There is some evidence that regular exercise may impact on ageing-related changes in resting fat metabolism. For instance, the reduction in fat oxidation (as a function of lower metabolic rate) in sedentary older individuals (50–78 years) was not evident in those who ran at least three times per week [93]. However, despite a lifetime participation in exercise training and no difference in percentage body fatness or fat-free mass (FFM), fat oxidation at rest was lower in older (50–69 years) versus younger (18–29 years) female athletes, all of whom participated in at least 12 h/week of training [104].

Regular exercise training in previously sedentary older and younger individuals was associated with an increase in basal fat oxidation [105]. However, the increase in basal fat oxidation during training may only be a transient effect of negative fat balance [106]. Although these findings show that exercise may modify resting fat oxidation in older active individuals, there is little evidence to suggest an inherent change in basal fat metabolism independent of energy expenditure. It must also be remembered that skeletal muscle fatty acid oxidation only accounts for a small fraction of the whole-body fat oxidation under resting conditions [25,26].

It has been argued that the age-related reduction in the rate of fat oxidation extends to exercise. In their seminal study using the tracer technique, Sial and co-workers compared fat metabolism during exercise in older (73 ± 2 years) and young (26 ± 2 years) active untrained men and women who were matched for both gender and FFM [1]. During prolonged exercise performed at the same absolute intensity, fat oxidation was lower in older exercisers and associated with a lower adipose FFA release [1]. This result was interpreted as evidence that the ability to use fat during exercise declines with age perhaps due to age-related deconditioning and/or ageing itself. The researchers also suggested that, because the lipolytic rate was not limiting factor, this phenomenon must reflect a reduced capacity for fat oxidation in the peripheral (muscle) tissues of older exercisers [1]. Cross-sectional studies have supported this suggestion by showing a reduction in muscle oxidative enzymes citrate synthase, cytochrome C oxidase and enzymes specific to fat oxidation (β-hydroxyacyl-CoA dehydrogenase) in sedentary older versus younger adults [107,108]. Accordingly, maximal oxygen extraction by the muscle ([a-v]O_2 difference) has been argued to decline with age and there is some evidence of a reduction in maximal [a-v]O_2 difference in masters athletes [89].

However, as discussed previously, comparing the metabolic response to exercise on the basis of absolute intensity can be misleading, because as a consequence of the reductions in VO_{2max} with age, older exercisers must work at a higher percentage of VO_{2max} to perform at the same level (work-rate) as younger individuals. Working at a higher percentage of VO_{2max} directly influences both metabolism and performance. For instance, older men were shown to oxidize more fat than older women during exercise at the same relative intensity (45% VO_{2max}) which could simply be accounted for by the higher work-rate and thus greater rate of energy expenditure in the males [109]. In the investigation by Sial et al., the contribution of fat to energy expenditure was similar at the same relative intensity in older versus younger individuals during exercise, although it was associated with a lower rate of adipose FFA release [1].

Taken together, this suggests that the rate of fat oxidation during exercise may be reduced with age, but this is likely a result of a reduction in work-rate associated with the decline in aerobic capacit rather than an age-related alteration in the ability of the muscle to use fat during exercise. While the sensitivity of fat tissue to lipolysis may be altered with age, this has little practical significance because adipose lipolysis generally does not appear to limit fat oxidation during exercise.

Notably, the potential confounding effect of differences in training status between age groups in the above studies cannot be excluded, and the apparent differences in metabolism and muscle adaptations may disappear when attempts are made to tightly control for exercise training and fitness levels. For instance, in studies which have more closely matched masters and younger athletes for performance level and/or habitual training volume, the reduction in maximal [a-v]O_2 difference and [a-v]O_2 difference at the same percentage of VO_{2max} with age was prevented in the masters athletes [88,90]. Similarly, the age-related decrease in the content of type 1 muscle fibres appears to be ameliorated in masters athletes in most [91,110] but not all [87] studies. Furthermore, muscle biopsies taken from the gastrocnemius muscles of previously trained older men showed that succinate dehydrogenase (SDH) and citrate synthase activity, as well as capillary density and capillary to fibre ratio, were better maintained in those who continued as masters athletes versus those who were less fit or had become untrained [111]. In fact Coggan and colleagues suggested that masters athletes may have superior muscle adaptations which potentially preserve endurance performance in the face of declining cardiovascular capacity. The Coggan group found that despite having lower VO_{2max} (11%), fibre type distribution was no different but SDH and β-hydroxyacyldehdrogenase were ~25%–30% higher in the masters athletes (63 ± 2 years) versus younger controls (26 ± 1 years) who had similar 10-km running time and purported training volume [110]. Again caution should be taken before accepting this suggestion because in order to sustain the same level of performance, the age-related reduction in VO_{2max} means that masters athletes would need to train harder to sustain the same work rate. That is, the skeletal muscle of masters athletes would essentially be 'fitter' than a performance-matched younger person.

Importantly, the general adaptive response to exercise training in older individuals, including the adaptations in muscle, seems to mirror that seen in younger cohorts. It is notable that muscles such as the diaphragm, for which extraneous confounders such as a reduction in habitual activity/training can be excluded, maintain their characteristics with age [87]. Sial and others gave 16 wk of endurance training to previously sedentary older (26 ± 2 years) men and women, which involved cycling at ~60%–80% VO_{2max} and a progressive increase in volume to a target of 45-min sessions on 5 d per week. The results showed that, in addition to a mean 21% increase in VO_{2max}, fat oxidation was significantly increased during exercise at the same absolute intensity after training. Using tracer isotopes, the researchers showed that neither the adipose FFA release (FFA Ra) or FFA uptake (FFA Rd) were altered by the endurance training, suggesting that the increase in fat oxidation with training reflected higher non-FFA oxidation (IMTG) and associated peripheral adaptations permitting higher fatty acid oxidation [73].

This finding is entirely consistent with the adaptations normally seen in younger research cohorts and discussed previously in this chapter. Van Aggel-Leijssen et al. also showed that obese men aged 40–43 years experienced a significant increase in the rate of fat oxidation during exercise at 50% of pre-training VO_{2max} which was not accounted for by enhanced adipose lipolysis and/or plasma FFA oxidation [98]. Similarly, Coggan et al. confirmed that these adaptations to an endurance training program in older men and women were associated with significant increases in muscle capillarisation and activities of muscle citrate synthase, SDH and β-hydroxyacyldehdrogenase [112]. Strangely, one of the few studies to actually directly examine fatty acid oxidation in muscle tissue which had been isolated and incubated in palmitate failed to find a difference in maximal fatty acid oxidative capacity between sedentary and trained older men [103].

In conclusion, there is strong evidence that fatty acid oxidation may be altered at rest in older individuals but this predominantly reflects a decline in metabolic rate, in part, as a consequence of reduced activity levels and altered body composition. While there are some data to suggest that the rate of fat oxidation is reduced during exercise with age, it is difficult to isolate ageing effects *per se* from potential confounding influences of anthropometry and training status/habitual activity levels. Critically, there are limited data regarding the effect of age of fat metabolism in the older exerciser. However, the weight of available evidence suggests that there is no inherent reduction in the capacity for fat oxidation in the masters athlete when differences in training volume and fitness are excluded. Older exercises appear to adapt to endurance training with muscle mitochondrial enzyme increases and an increased reliance on fat (likely IMTG) at the same exercise intensity in the same manner as younger exercisers. With this in mind, it is highly likely that training and dietary strategies which modulate fat utilisation in younger athletes will also apply to the masters endurance athletes.

5.5 DIETARY AND EXERCISE RECOMMENDATIONS FOR MASTERS ATHLETES

5.5.1 Short-Term Strategies to Alter Fat Metabolism and Performance

Several strategies have been trialled in experimental studies on younger athletes which aim to increase endurance exercise performance by acutely increasing fat availability and oxidation rate. These include high fat feeding, MCT ingestion, caffeine ingestion, L-carnitine ingestion and intravenous fat infusion. In general, dietary macronutrient alteration via a high fat pre-event meal does not improve endurance performance [113]. However, benefits have been shown with longer low-carbohydrates/high-fat diets and are discussed later. In light of the overall lack of compelling ergogenic effects on fat metabolism and performance demonstrated from the other strategies, a thorough examination of these is unwarranted.

Briefly, the effect of liquid MCTs on metabolism and performance has been examined in small experimental studies. Unlike long-chain fatty acids (which represent the majority of dietary fatty acids), the shorter fatty acid chain length (6–10) of MCTs allows them to be rapidly digested and enter the circulation. This potentially provides an 'immediate' exogenous form of fat for metabolism, in a similar way as that observed with glucose ingestion. However, the majority of research shows that the contribution of MCTs to exercise energy expenditure is very low (<10%) [106,114] and does not appear to alter glycogen use [115]. Most notably, their usefulness appears to be limited by the capacity to digest MCTs without gastrointestinal upset and the sole study to show a performance benefit of the strategy employed a high MCT dose [109] which was beyond the tolerable levels of most studies (<30g/h).

Ingestion of caffeine is known to stimulate lipolysis which may [116] or may not [104] enhance FFA oxidation and reduce glycogen use. Rather than increasing FFA availability, the (endurance) performance benefit of caffeine use is thought to reflect other factors including nervous system stimulation and/or reduction of biochemical fatiguing effects in muscle [117]. Nevertheless, associated increases in exercise intensity as a function of caffeine administration (or any other pharmacologic ergogenic aids for that matter) may indeed result in increased rates of carbohydrate and possibly fat oxidation. See Chapter 11 for a more detailed discussion of the ergogenic effects of caffeine.

Because of its role in enabling long-chain fatty acids to pass into the mitochondria, L-carnitine supplementation is often touted as a means of enhancing fat oxidation. In reality, the availability of carnitine even in supplement form is low, and because the urinary threshold for excretion is low, little enters the muscle [118]. Though there is some dissonance in regard to exercise performance, the weight of evidence does not favour dietary carnitine supplementation [102]. Nevertheless, there is recent evidence of a direct effect of longer term supplemental carnitine on both intramuscular concentration and fuel selection [119].

Finally, fat oxidation is significantly increased when fat is intravenously infused with heparin during exercise [74]. The increased fat oxidation appears to be associated with reduced reliance on glycogen [75] and plasma glucose [76]. Although this result clearly demonstrates the efficacy of strategies aimed at increasing fat use to enhance endurance performance, fat infusion is impractical and potentially dangerous for athletes of all ages.

5.5.2 Longer-Term Strategies to Enhance Fat Metabolism and Endurance Performance

Over 80 years have passed since the Scandinavian physiologists Christensen and Hansen first highlighted the interaction between the dietary availability of fuels, subsequent fuel use and exercise performance. These researchers demonstrated that a high-carbohydrate diet increased glucose oxidation during exercise and promoted optimal endurance performance in healthy young men [42]. In contrast, although five days of low-carbohydrate, high-fat intake increased the reliance on fat oxidation, this also resulted in early fatigue and/or the onset of hypoglycaemia during endurance exercise [42].

Some 25 years ago, there was scientific interest in the possible positive effects of a high-fat training diet on endurance exercise performance. This was underpinned by the well-known study of Phinney and others who observed significant increases in the fat-handling enzymes of the *vastus lateralis* and maintained sub-maximal endurance in cyclists who continued training on a high-fat diet [120]. A number of more recent performance-based studies were not able to support the idea that a period of high-fat diet during training produced improved endurance performance [121–123]. This was despite consistent reports that such diets increased fat oxidation rates during sub-maximal exercise. Many of these studies tended to be, unlike the Phinney study, short-term dietary interventions of less than 10-d so probably did not provide enough stimulus duration to enable appropriate adaptive effects at the muscle level. At the same time, the low carbohydrate intake likely reduced muscle glycogen storage and performance was unlikely to be enhanced as a result.

Indeed some of the longer-duration intervention studies did show performance benefits [93,124,125]. Furthermore, the performance tests used (2–3 h) in most studies did not reflect the very long duration of some athletic events, such as elite road race cycling and Ironman triathlon. Only two studies, those of Rowlands and Hopkins [126] and Carey et al. [123] have investigated the impact of a high-fat training diet on 5-h endurance performance. The former research employed a 2-wk high-fat diet and an 11.5-d high-fat diet followed by a 2.5-d carbohydrate load compared with a 2-wk high-carbohydrate diet. Rowlands and Hopkins observed a tendency towards improved cycling power output at the end of the trial with high fat followed by 2.5-d carbohydrate load, but the overall performance improvement was not statistically significant [126]. These results are very similar to the shorter dietary intervention study by Carey et al., where the high-fat diet/carbohydrate load tended to improve performance but not statistically [123].

The above studies, together with the studies of Burke and others [122] and Lambert [124,125] suggest that high-fat training diets potentially improve endurance performance in well-trained persons, but more likely when supplemented with carbohydrate in the days immediately prior to competition. However, more research is necessary to fully gauge the impact of a high-fat training diet on ultra-endurance performance, particularly that reflecting events such as Ironman in which the number of masters competitors is usually greater than in the younger age groups.

Invasive research techniques have enabled a greater understanding of the metabolic responses to altered dietary macronutrient intakes at rest and during exercise. The early response to reduced dietary carbohydrate high-fat intake involves a rapid shift in whole-body substrate metabolism away from carbohydrate oxidation at the expense of non-carbohydrate substrate, including fatty acids. This is associated with a decline in the plasma insulin concentration and a marked increase in FFA release from adipose tissue [5,127]. These changes are largely a result of dietary carbohydrate restriction rather than the increase in fat consumption [5].

Several investigations have shown that these responses to either low-carbohydrate, high-dietary fat [128–131] or complete absence of all macronutrient consumption through fasting [20,132] also increase IMTG levels. Despite an increase in their release and oxidation, plasma FFAs cannot account for the elevated rate of fat metabolism evident following low CHO/high-fat feeding [133,134] and the higher-fat oxidation during exercise therefore appears to reflect both higher FFA and IMTG oxidation [133,135]. Rapid biochemical changes also occur within the muscle to promote fat oxidation and spare glucose use at rest [136] and during exercise. These include increases in the activities of carnitine palmitoyltransferase [137] β-hydroxyacyl-CoA dehydrogenase [138] and rapid changes in enzymes which reduce glycogen use, such as pyruvate dehydrogenase kinase [127] and lactate dehydrogenase (LDH) [139].

5.5.3 Manipulating Timing of Food Intake during Training to Improve Fat Oxidation

As previously discussed, the metabolic response to a low-carbohydrate diet is similar to that of a high-fat diet, indicating that the metabolic effect of a high-fat diet is most likely driven by the lack of dietary carbohydrate. Indeed, the metabolic profile following a water-only fast is very similar to that of a very-low-carbohydrate, high-fat diet [140]. Therefore, in theory at least, undertaking training in a fasted state, when carbohydrate status is reduced, should mimic the effect of training with a high-fat diet, and thereby potentiate the effect of training on the ability of muscles to utilize fat.

A series of studies investigating a fed versus fasted training regime have shown potential advantages of training in an overnight fasted state [141–143]. In general, these studies have shown that fasted training enables the trained muscle to store more glycogen and also have a relatively better oxidative and fat-handling capacity. However, despite this increased potential to utilise fat during exercise, significant increases in fat oxidation during sub-maximal exercise were not observed even when exercise became prolonged [141,143]. A longer training period or a more stressful period of daily fasting may be required for this to occur. Similar to the high-fat diet training studies, perhaps a longer exercising duration may reveal an advantage to this training strategy.

5.5.4 Effect of Gender on Fat Metabolism during Exercise

Research evidence conclusively shows gender-related differences in substrate utilization during exercise [144,145]. In general, these data show that females utilise a proportionally greater rate of fat for the same relative exercise intensity as males. There is also some suggestion that females show a greater reliance upon IMTG, rather than circulating FFAs [145]. Plausible reasons for these findings include increased body fatness in females. However, the difference in fuel selection persists even when body fatness is accounted for. Despite this increased reliance upon fat during sub-maximal exercise, it is not sensible to extrapolate this to conclude that females require proportionally more fat in their diet. This is because, as previously mentioned, body fat stores are likely more than sufficient to cover this small increase in fat demand.

Perhaps of more interest to training athletes, Stannard et al., were able to show that females responded differently to overnight fasted training than males [142]. Indeed, the trained muscles of females did not increase their oxidative capacity with fasted training; rather, the trend was for the other direction. Whether this observation could be extrapolated to conclude that a high-fat training diet has the same effects is only conjecture, but the possibility remains intriguing. More recently, Maher and others showed that, when matched for age and VO_{2max} per kilogram of fat mass, females exhibited a greater mitochondrial protein content for key enzymes of fat metabolism than males [146]. Therefore, it is possible that males are more sensitive than females for diet-induced modulations of fat metabolism because the muscles of females are already more suited to fat metabolism in the first place. Whether or not these gender-related substrate preferences transition through the ageing process is unknown. Sensibly however, we can speculate that reductions in testosterone in men and oestrogen in women may bring about more similar responses through menopause and the later years.

5.5.5 Health Implications of Training on High-Fat Diets and Dietary Recommendations

It seems reasonable to suggest that the fat requirements of masters athletes, to fuel their training and competition needs at least, are proportionally higher than younger athletes with similar competitive goals. However, whether or not masters athletes therefore require more fat in their diet should be questioned. Fat can be derived either from food or from the release of stored fats and most athletes have sufficient fat stores to sustain their fat requirements during even the most prolonged exercise events exercise, and so do not need to increase fat intake. There is little doubt the same probably applies to older athletes. However, if a greater reliance upon fat oxidation *is* required during an event, then it would seem sensible that any training diet strategy would include approaches to improve fat oxidation for the same intensity of exercise. Regular exercise training is the primary stimulus for this, and may include (for males at least), replacing some dietary carbohydrate with fat or protein, or occasionally exercising in the overnight-fasted or carbohydrate-deplete state.

Importantly, at the population level, ageing is a primary risk factor for heart disease and type 2 diabetes. These conditions remain two of the most important causes of morbidity and mortality in the Western world. Both of these non-communicable diseases are associated with a high-fat diet at a population level, though this could be through the temporal association of ageing with increasing adiposity and the fact that a high-fat diet is separately associated with obesity. Despite evidence that sufficient levels of physical activity can to some extent counter the health risk of a high-fat diet, an element of risk with such a diet will remain, especially for those masters competitors who are new to sport or non-elite. Although the level of saturation of fatty acids in the diet modulate health-related effects, prescribing a diet higher in fat should therefore be exercised with caution because some education is required by the athlete to know how to avoid food high in saturated and transaturated fat. That an already increased level of risk of heart disease will exist in the older age groups, even those physically active, should strengthen this recommendation. In this context it should be highlighted that the metabolic responses to low-carbohydrate, high-fat diets are driven largely by the low carbohydrate rather than augmented fat intake. With appropriate knowledge and food availability, there is little evidence to suggest that a higher-(non-trans-, mono-, or poly-unsaturated) fat diet accompanied by adequate carbohydrate and lean protein sources cannot provide the basis for a successful training diet, provided there is no prolonged caloric surplus.

5.5.6 Training Practices for Maximising Fat Oxidation and Performance

Practically, not all training sessions can be conducted in a carbohydrate-deplete state, and indeed intense (including interval) training, which has in part the primary aim of cardiovascular remodelling, may not be possible. Therefore, recommendations concerning high-fat training diets and training in a fasted state should emphasise that such a practice should be part of a training regime; the training regime should not be built around that practice.

A common misconception amongst athletes and coaches is that, because endurance events are performed at relatively low intensities where rates of fat oxidation are near-maximal (the fat-burning zone), training should be done at these intensities. However, this 'long slow distance' approach will in fact only provide greater *endurance* at these intensities. Indeed to be able to go faster the athlete must produce more power and this requires recruitment of the larger, more carbohydrate-reliant motor units for the same cadence or movement patterns. What must be done is to increase the oxidative capacity of the muscle fibres comprising these larger motor units, to enable them to be less fatiguable. This can only be done with more intense exercise training. For more detailed discussions on training for both endurance and ultra-endurance events in masters athletes, see Chapters 14 and 15.

Demonstration of the potency of exercise intensity in the adaptive response can be seen in recent data from studies involving young trained and untrained adults. These clearly show that training involving repeated (5–8 times), short bursts of maximal or supra-maximal exercise (10–30 s) increases maximal aerobic capacity and muscle oxidative enzymes to an equivalent level to that seen with traditional aerobic exercise training regimes (~300 min per wk) [147,148]. These findings are remarkable given the low amount of weekly energy expenditure achieved with this high-intensity interval training (~200–500 kcal) versus traditional exercise programs (~1200–3300 kcal per wk) representing a possible 70%–90% reduction in weekly time commitment [149] and highlight the importance of incorporating vigorous exercise into training programs.

5.6 CONCLUSIONS

Fat provides a significant proportion of the energy requirements for endurance exercise. This contribution increases with exercise duration. Although there is limited research in older exercisers, critical appraisal of the existing literature suggests that the ability to oxidise fat during exercise is not inherently altered with age, when influences such as energy expenditure are accounted for. Because an increased reliance on fat potentially spares limited glycogen and glucose reserves and therefore enhances exercise performance, there has been particular interest in strategies to enhance fat use.

In light of the limited evidence to support their use, MCTs, caffeine and L-carnitine supplementation cannot be recommended for the purpose of enhancing fat oxidation and performance in athletes of any age, although there is a paucity of such studies in masters athletes. More evidence may, in the future, support supplementation with L-carnitine. However, there is increasing evidence that low-carbohydrate/high-fat diets or overnight fasting during training increase the activity of muscle fat oxidation enzymes and fat oxidation (FFAs and/or IMTG) during exercise. However, these benefits are often not statistically significant and there has been no examination of this in strategy in masters athletes. Importantly, the increased fat oxidation evident with such interventions likely reflects the use of body fat stores as a result of carbohydrate restriction. As such, given the potential health risks masters athletes should be discouraged from augmenting dietary saturated fats with the misconception that this increases fat use.

Ultimately peripheral (muscle) adaptations (including mitochondrial volume) dictate the capacity for fat oxidation, and these increase with regular training similarly in both young and older exercisers. In fact, masters athletes have been shown to have similar (or perhaps even higher) levels of mitochondrial enzymes and capillaries in muscle to younger training-matched counterparts. With this in mind, training should be targeted at maximising peripheral adaptations and the incorporation of high-intensity training over 'long slow distance' emphasised.

5.7 IMPLICATIONS FOR SPORTS MEDICINE PROFESSIONALS AND CLINICIANS

- Endurance athletes are often aware of the importance of fat as a fuel for exercise metabolism and may seek dietary and/or training strategies to maximise fat oxidation and performance for prolonged exercise events. This may be particularly the case for masters athletes, for whom events can take longer and therefore necessitate a greater reliance on fat.
- There is good evidence that the rate of fat oxidation at rest is reduced with age, but despite some studies showing a reduction of fat oxidation during exercise in older individuals, the evidence is not compelling. In this context, the masters athlete may be expected to respond to training and dietary interventions aimed at promoting fat oxidation similarly to younger individuals in whom most research has been conducted.
- Fat oxidation is from the release and oxidation of fatty acids from stored triglyceride reserves. Therefore strategies, including dietary change, primarily affect the rate of fat oxidation by altering the release and/or oxidation of these stored fats. As a result, low-carbohydrate, high-fat diets or fasting can increase fat oxidation.
- Recommendations for such dietary approaches should be titrated against the potential increase in cardiovascular disease risk of high-fat diets in older individuals, especially for those with a personal or family history of heart disease or with coronary artery disease risk factors.

5.8 IMPLICATIONS FOR MASTERS ATHLETES AND COACHES

- Short-term high-fat, low-carbohydrate intake prior to competition provides no advantage to endurance exercise performance and appears to be detrimental to performance because it compromises glycogen status.
- Lower carbohydrate training diets, especially if more than 10 d, may improve endurance performance especially when dietary carbohydrate is re-introduced in the days prior to self-paced exercise performance. Because the body doesn't distinguish between fat from food and body-fat stores, similar adaptations can be found with training in the overnight fasted state which raises fat availability. However, reduced carbohydrate availability in either of these cases would reduce the capacity to undertake high-intensity training so therefore these strategies should form part of, not the basis of, an exercise training program.
- Other strategies to augment fat oxidation and improve exercise performance have been trialled, including caffeine, L-carnitine and medium-chain triglyceride ingestion. There is no consensus that these improve performance by positively affecting fat metabolism.
- It is more likely that training/diet strategies will be of greater benefit to males than premenopausal females because of the already elevated rates of fat oxidation in these women.
- Regular endurance exercise training increases the capacity for fat oxidation, meaning that the trained individual can exercise for longer before fatigue or sustain a higher intensity for the same glycogen cost. All athletes should be counselled that the best way to improve the capacity for fat oxidation and performance is by regular training.

5.9 FUTURE RESEARCH DIRECTIONS

In light of the limited and conflicting current evidence, there is a clear need for more research studies examining the interaction between ageing and exercise in the masters athlete. These studies should

- Compare fat oxidation between older and younger individuals at the same absolute and relative exercise intensities.
- Aim to reduce potentially confounding influences of differences in habitual training status and fitness level between cohorts.
- Examine the potential benefit of low-carbohydrate training diets (and the possible benefit of ergogenic aids such as L-carnitine supplementation) in older individuals, including masters athletes. This is warranted given that the demands of masters events often necessitate a greater reliance on fat during exercise but most available research has been conducted in young cohorts.
- Examine changes in fuel selection during exercise following menopause in female masters athletes, and the subsequent effect on exercise performance. Some research has been done to investigate the impact of hormone replacement therapy (HRT) on fuel selection during exercise [150], though no difference between those post-menopausal women with or without HRT was noted. It is thus too early to understand whether differences in dietary fat requirements exist or might be important to postmenopausal women master athletes for optimal performance.

REFERENCES

1. Sial, S., Coggan, A.R., Carroll, R., Goodwin, J. and Klein, S., Fat and carbohydrate metabolism during exercise in elderly and young subjects, *Am. J. Physiol. Endocrinol. Metab.* 271(6), E983–9, 1996.
2. Behnke, A.R. and Wilmore, J.H., *Evaluation and Regulation of Body Build and Composition*, Prentice-Hall, New Jersey, 1959.
3. Johnson, N.A., Stannard, S.R. and Thompson, M.W., Muscle triglyceride and glycogen in endurance exercise: Implications for performance, *Sports. Med.* 34(3), 151–64, 2004.
4. Hoppeler, H., Luthi, P., Claassen, H., Weibel, E.R. and Howald, H., The ultrastructure of the normal human skeletal muscle. A morphometric analysis on untrained men, women and well-trained orienteers, *Pflugers Archiv.* 344(3), 217–32, 1973.
5. Schwarz, J.M., Neese, R.A., Turner, S., Dare, D. and Hellerstein, M.K., Short-term alterations in carbohydrate energy intake in humans. Striking effects on hepatic glucose production, de novo lipogenesis, lipolysis, and whole-body fuel selection, *J. Clin. Invest.* 96(6), 2735–43, 1995.
6. Kather, H., Bieger, W., Michel, G., Aktories, K. and Jakobs, K.H., Human fat cell lipolysis is primarily regulated by inhibitory modulators acting through distinct mechanisms, *J. Clin. Invest.* 76(4), 1559–65, 1985.
7. Klein, S., Sakurai, Y., Romijn, J.A. and Carroll, R.M., Progressive alterations in lipid and glucose metabolism during short-term fasting in young adult men, *Am. J. Physiol.* 265(5 Pt 1), E801–6, 1993.
8. Issekutz, B., Jr., Bortz, W.M., Miller, H.I. and Paul, P., Turnover rate of plasma FFA in humans and in dogs, *Metabolism* 16(11), 1001–9, 1967.
9. Hamilton, J.A. and Kamp, F., How are free fatty acids transported in membranes? Is it by proteins or by free diffusion through the lipids?, *Diabetes* 48(12), 2255–69, 1999.
10. Zakim, D., Thermodynamics of fatty acid transfer, *J. Membr. Biol.* 176(2), 101–9, 2000.
11. Schaffer, J.E., Fatty acid transport: The roads taken, *Am. J. Physiol. Endocrinol. Metab.* 282(2), E239–46, 2002.
12. Van der Vusse, G.J. and Renneman, R.S., Lipid metabolism in muscle, in *Handbook of Physiology. Section 12: Exercise: Regulation and Integration of Multiple Systems*, L.B. Rowell and J.T. Shepherd, eds., American Physiological Society, New York, 1996, pp. 952–94.

13. Bonen, A., Muscle contractile activity increases fatty acid metabolism and transport and FAT/CD36, *Am. J. Physiol.* 276(4 Pt 1), E642–9, 1999.
14. Turcotte, L.P., Petry, C., Kiens, B. and Richter, E.A., Contraction-induced increase in V_{max} of palmitate uptake and oxidation in perfused skeletal muscle, *J. Appl. Physiol.* 84(5), 1788–94, 1998.
15. Luiken, J.J., Dyck, D.J., Han, X.X. et al., Insulin induces the translocation of the fatty acid transporter FAT/CD36 to the plasma membrane, *Am. J. Physiol. Endocrinol. Metab.* 282(2), E491–5, 2002.
16. Glatz, J.F. and van der Vusse, G.J., Cellular fatty acid-binding proteins: Their function and physiological significance, *Progr. Lipid Res.* 35(3), 243–82, 1996.
17. Van der Vusse, G.J. and Roemen, T.H., Gradient of fatty acids from blood plasma to skeletal muscle in dogs, *J. Appl. Physiol.* 78(5), 1839–43, 1995.
18. Watt, M.J., Heigenhauser, G.J.F. and Spriet, L.L., Intramuscular triacylglycerol utilization in human skeletal muscle during exercise: Is there a controversy? *J. Appl. Physiol.* 93(4), 1185–95, 2002.
19. Bachmann, O.P., Dahl, D.B., Brechtel, K. et al., Effects of intravenous and dietary lipid challenge on intramyocellular lipid content and the relation with insulin sensitivity in humans, *Diabetes* 50(11), 2579–84, 2001.
20. Stannard, S.R., Thompson, M.W., Fairbairn, K., Huard, B., Sachinwalla, T. and Thompson, C.H., Fasting for 72 h increases intramyocellular lipid content in non-diabetic, physically-fit men, *Am. J. Physiol. Endocrinol. Metab.* 283, E1185–91, 2002.
21. Watt, M.J., Stellingwerff, T., Heigenhauser, G.J.F. and Spriet, L.L., Effect of plasma adrenaline on hormone-sensitive lipase at rest and during moderate exercise in human skeletal muscle, *J. Physiol.* 550(1), 325–32, 2003.
22. Langfort, J., Ploug, T., Ihlemann, J., Saldo, M., Holm, C. and Galbo, H., Expression of hormone-sensitive lipase and its regulation by adrenaline in skeletal muscle, *Biochem. J.* 340(Pt 2), 459–65, 1999.
23. Miller, W.C., Epinephrine-activation of heparin-nonreleasable lipoprotein lipase in 3 skeletal muscle fiber types of the rat, *Biochem. Biophys. Res. Com.* 164(2), 615–9, 1989.
24. Yost, T.J., Froyd, K.K., Jensen, D.R. and Eckel, R.H., Change in skeletal muscle lipoprotein lipase activity in response to insulin/glucose in non-insulin-dependent diabetes mellitus, *Metabolism* 44(6), 786–90, 1995.
25. Jensen, M.D., Gender differences in regional fatty-acid metabolism before and after meal ingestion, *J. Clin. Invest.* 96(5), 2297–303, 1995.
26. Meek, S.E., Nair, K.S. and Jensen, M.D., Insulin regulation of regional free fatty acid metabolism, *Diabetes* 48(1), 10–4, 1999.
27. Havel, R.J., Kane, J.P., Balasse, E.O., Segel, N. and Basso, L.V., Splanchnic metabolsim of free fatty acids and production of triglycerides of very low density lipoproteins in normotriglyceridemic and hypertriglyceridemic humans, *J. Clin. Invest.* 49(11), 2017–35, 1970.
28. Wolfe, B.M., Havel, J.R., Marliss, E.B., Kane, J.P., Seymour, J. and Ahuja, S.P., Effects of a 3-day fast and of ethanol on splanchnic metabolism of FFA, amino-acids, and carbohydrates in healthy young men, *J. Clin. Invest.* 57(2), 329–40, 1976.
29. Klein, S., Peters, E.J., Holland, O.B. and Wolfe, R.R., Effect of short-term and long-term beta-adrenergic-blockade on lipolysis during fasting in humans, *Am. J. Physiol.* 257(1), E65–73, 1989.
30. Stallknecht, B., Lorentsen, J., Enevoldsen, L.H. et al., Role of the sympathoadrenergic system in adipose tissue metabolism during exercise in humans, *J. Physiol.* 536, 283–94, 2001.
31. Kjaer, M., Engfred, K., Fernandes, A., Secher, N.H. and Galbo, H., Regulation of hepatic glucose production during exercise in humans: Role of sympathoadrenergic activity, *Am. J. Physiol.* 265(2 Pt 1), E275–83, 1993.
32. Wolfe, R.R., Klein, S., Carraro, F. and Weber, J.M., Role of triglyceride-fatty acid cycle in controlling fat metabolism in humans during and after exercise, *Am. J. Physiol.* 258(2 Pt 1), E382–9, 1990.
33. Wolfe, R.R., Klein, S., Carraro, F. and Weber, J.M., Role of triglyceride fatty-acid cycle in controlling fat-metabolism in humans during and after exercise, *Am. J. Physiol.* 258(2), E382–9, 1990.
34. Romijn, J.A., Coyle, E.F., Sidossis, L.S. et al., Regulation of endogenous fat and carbohydrate metabolism in relation to exercise intensity and duration, *Am. J. Physiol.* 265(3 Pt 1), E380–91, 1993.
35. Ahlborg, G., Felig, P., Hagenfel, L., Hendler, R. and Wahren, J., Substrate turnover during prolonged exercise in man: Splanchnic and leg metabolism of glucose, free fatty-acids, and amino-acids, *J. Clin. Invest.* 53(4), 1080–90, 1974.
36. Burguera, B., Proctor, D., Dietz, N., Guo, Z.K., Joyner, M. and Jensen, M.D., Leg free fatty acid kinetics during exercise in men and women, *Am. J. Physiol. Endocrinol. Metab.* 278(1), E113–7, 2000.
37. van Loon, L.J.C., Greenhaff, P.L., Teodosiu, D.C., Saris, W.H.M. and Wagenmakers, A.J.M., The effects of increasing exercise intensity on muscle fuel utilisation in humans, *J. Physiol.* 536(1), 295–304, 2001.

38. Kiens, B., Skeletal muscle substrate utilization during submaximal exercise in man: Effect of endurance training, *J. Physiol.* 469, 459–78, 1993.
39. Helge, J.W., Watt, P.W., Richter, E.A., Rennie, M.J. and Kiens, B., Fat utilization during exercise: Adaptation to a fat-rich diet increases utilization of plasma fatty acids and very low density lipoprotein-triacylglycerol in humans, *J. Physiol.* 537(Pt 3), 1009–20, 2001.
40. Sondergaard, E., Rahbek, I., Sorensen, L.P. et al., Effects of exercise on VLDL-triglyceride oxidation and turnover, *Am. J. Physiol. Endocrinol. Metab.* 300(5), E939–44, 2011.
41. Johnson, N.A., van Overbeek, D., Chapman, P.G., Thompson, M.W., Sachinwalla, T. and George, J., Effect of prolonged exercise and pre-exercise dietary manipulation on hepatic triglycerides in trained men, *Eur. J. Appl. Physiol.* 112(5), 1817–25, 2011.
42. Christensen, E.H. and Hansen, O., Arbeitsfahigkeit und Emahrung., *Scand. Arch. Physiol.* 81, 160–71, 1939.
43. Bergstrom, J., Hultman, E., Jorfeldt, L., Pernow, B. and Wahren, J., Effect of nicotinic acid on physical working capacity and on metabolism of muscle glycogen in man, *J. Appl. Physiol.* 26(2), 170–6, 1969.
44. Pernow, B. and Saltin, B., Availability of substrates and capacity for prolonged heavy exercise in man, *J. Appl. Physiol.* 31(3), 416–22, 1971.
45. Havel, R.J., Pernow, B. and Jones, N.L., Uptake and release of free fatty acids and other metabolites in the legs of exercising men, *J. Appl. Physiol.* 23(1), 90–9, 1967.
46. van Loon, L.J., Greenhaff, P.L., Constantin-Teodosiu, D., Saris, W.H. and Wagenmakers, A.J., The effects of increasing exercise intensity on muscle fuel utilisation in humans, *J. Physiol.* 536(Pt 1), 295–304, 2001.
47. Watt, M.J., Heigenhauser, G.F., Dyck, D.J. and Spriet, L.L., Intramuscular triacylglycerol, glycogen and acetyl group metabolism during 4 h of moderate exercise in man, *J. Physiol.* 541(3), 969–78, 2002.
48. Essen, B., Intramuscular substrate utilization during prolonged exercise, *Ann. N.Y. Acad. Sci.* 301, 30–44, 1977.
49. Essen, B., Hagenfeldt, L. and Kaijser, L., Utilization of blood-borne and intramuscular substrates during continuous and intermittent exercise in man, *J. Physiol.* 265(2), 489–506, 1977.
50. Bergstrom, J., Hermansen, L., Hultman, E. and Saltin, B., Diet, muscle glycogen and physical performance, *Acta. Physiol. Scand.* 71(2), 140–50, 1967.
51. Bergstrom, J. and Hultman, E., A study of the glycogen metabolism during exercise in man, *Scand. J. Clin. Lab. Invest.* 19(3), 218–28, 1967.
52. Hultman, E. and Nilsson, L.H., Liver glycogen in man. Effect of different diets and muscular exercise, in *Muscle Metabolism During Exercise*, B. Pernow and B. Saltin, eds., Plenum Press, New York, 1971, pp. 143–51.
53. Jones, N.L., Heigenhauser, G.J., Kuksis, A., Matsos, C.G., Sutton, J.R. and Toews, C.J., Fat metabolism in heavy exercise, *Clin. Sci.* 59(6), 469–78, 1980.
54. Romijn, J.A., Coyle, E.F., Sidossis, L.S., Zhang, X.J. and Wolfe, R.R., Relationship between fatty acid delivery and fatty acid oxidation during strenuous exercise, *J. Appl. Physiol.* 79(6), 1939–45, 1995.
55. Rosenbaum, M., Hirsch, J., Murphy, E. and Leibel, R.L., Effects of changes in body weight on carbohydrate metabolism, catecholamine excretion, and thyroid function, *Am. J. Clin. Nutr.* 71(6), 1421–32, 2000.
56. Turcotte, L.P., Srivastava, A.K. and Chiasson, J.L., Fasting increases plasma membrane fatty acid-binding protein (FABP(PM)) in red skeletal muscle, *Mol. Cell. Biochem.* 166(1–2), 153–8, 1997.
57. Binas, B., Danneberg, H., McWhir, J., Mullins, L. and Clark, A.J., Requirement for the heart-type fatty acid binding protein in cardiac fatty acid utilization, *FASEB J.* 13(8), 805–12, 1999.
58. Richter, E.A., Garetto, L.P., Goodman, M.N. and Ruderman, N.B., Muscle glucose metabolism following exercise in the rat: Increased sensitivity to insulin, *J. Clin. Invest.* 69(4), 785–93, 1982.
59. Bogardus, C., Ravussin, E., Robbins, D.C., Wolfe, R.R., Horton, E.S. and Sims, E.A.H., Effects of physical-training and diet therapy on carbohydrate-metabolism in patients with glucose- intolerance and non-insulin-dependent diabetes-mellitus, *Diabetes* 33(4), 311–8, 1984.
60. Zachwieja, J.J., Costill, D.L., Pascoe, D.D., Robergs, R.A. and Fink, W.J., Influence of muscle glycogen depletion on the rate of resynthesis, *Med. Sci. Sports Exerc.* 23(1), 44–8, 1991.
61. van Loon, L.J., Koopman, R., Stegen, J.H., Wagenmakers, A.J., Keizer, H.A. and Saris, W.H., Intramyocellular lipids form an important substrate source during moderate intensity exercise in endurance-trained males in a fasted state, *J. Physiol.* 553, 611–25, 2003.
62. Kuo, C.C., Fattor, J.A., Henderson, G.C. and Brooks, G.A., Lipid oxidation in fit young adults during postexercise recovery, *J. Appl. Physiol.* 99(1), 349–56, 2005.
63. Warren, A., Howden, E.J., Williams, A.D., Fell, J.W. and Johnson, N.A., Postexerise fat oxidation: Effect of exercise duration, intensity and modality, *Int. J. Sport Nutr. Exerc.Metab.* 19, 607–23, 2009.

64. Al Mulla, N., Simonsen, L. and Bulow, J., Post-exercise adipose tissue and skeletal muscle lipid metabolism in humans: The effects of exercise intensity, *J. Physiol.* 524(3), 919–28, 2000.
65. Kiens, B. and Richter, E.A., Utilization of skeletal muscle triacylglycerol during postexercise recovery in humans, *Am. J. Physiol.* 275(2 Pt 1), E332–7, 1998.
66. Richter, E.A., Derave, W. and Wojtaszewski, J.F., Glucose, exercise and insulin: Emerging concepts, *J. Physiol.* 535(Pt 2), 313–22, 2001.
67. Bergstrom, J., Hermansen, L., Hultman, E. and Saltin, B., Diet, muscle glycogen and physical performance, *Acta Physiol. Scand.* 71(2), 140–50, 1967.
68. Maehlum, S. and Hermansen, L., Muscle glycogen concentration during recovery after prolonged severe exercise in fasting subjects, *Scand. J. Clin. Lab. Invest.* 38(6), 557–60, 1978.
69. Hoppeler, H., Howald, H., Conley, K. et al., Endurance training in humans: Aerobic capacity and structure of skeletal muscle, *J. Appl. Physiol.* 59(2), 320–7, 1985.
70. Holloszy, J.O., Biochemical adaptations in muscle, *J. Biol. Chem.* 242(9), 2278–82, 1967.
71. Hurley, B.F. and Seals, D.R., Muscle triglyceride utilization during exercise: Effect of training, *J. Appl. Physiol.* 60(2), 562–7, 1986.
72. Martin, W.H., 3rd, Dalsky, G.P., Hurley, B.F. et al., Effect of endurance training on plasma free fatty acid turnover and oxidation during exercise, *Am. J. Physiol.* 265(5 Pt 1), E708–14, 1993.
73. Sial, S., Coggan, A.R., Hickner, R.C. and Klein, S., Training-induced alterations in fat and carbohydrate metabolism during exercise in elderly subjects, *Am. J. Physiol. Endocrinol. Metab.* 274(5), E785–90, 1998.
74. Costill, D.L., Coyle, E., Dalsky, G., Evans, W., Fink, W. and Hoopes, D., Effects of elevated plasma FFA and insulin on muscle glycogen usage during exercise, *J. Appl. Physiol.* 43(4), 695–9, 1977.
75. Rennie, M.J., Winder, W.W. and Holloszy, J.O., A sparing effect of increased plasma fatty acids on muscle and liver glycogen content in the exercising rat, *Biochem. J.* 156(3), 647–55, 1976.
76. Hargreaves, M., Kiens, B. and Richter, E.A., Effect of increased plasma free fatty acid concentrations on muscle metabolism in exercising men, *J. Appl. Physiol.*. 70(1), 194–201, 1991.
77. Green, H.J., Jones, S., Ball-Burnett, M., Smith, D., Livesey, J. and Farrance, B., Early muscular and metabolic adaptations to prolonged exercise training in humans, *J. Appl. Physiol.* 70(5), 2032–8, 1991.
78. Coggan, A.R., Swanson, S.C., Mendenhall, L.A., Habash, D.L. and Kien, C.L., Effect of endurance training on hepatic glycogenolysis and gluconeogenesis during prolonged exercise in men, *Am. J. Physiol.* 268(3 Pt 1), E375–83, 1995.
79. Winder, W.W., Hickson, R.C., Hagberg, J.M., Ehsani, A.A. and McLane, J.A., Training-induced changes in hormonal and metabolic responses to submaximal exercise, *J. Appl. Physiol.* 46(4), 766–71, 1979.
80. Gollnick, P.D., Armstrong, R.B., Saltin, B., Saubert, C.W.t., Sembrowich, W.L. and Shepherd, R.E., Effect of training on enzyme activity and fiber composition of human skeletal muscle, *J. Appl. Physiol.* 34(1), 107–11, 1973.
81. Holloszy, J.O. and Coyle, E.F., Adaptations of skeletal muscle to endurance exercise and their metabolic consequences, *J. Appl. Physiol.* 56(4), 831–8, 1984.
82. Henriksson, J. and Reitman, J.S., Time course of changes in human skeletal muscle succinate dehydrogenase and cytochrome oxidase activities and maximal oxygen uptake with physical activity and inactivity, *Acta Physiol. Scand.* 99(1), 91–7, 1977.
83. Turcotte, L.P., Richter, E.A. and Kiens, B., Increased plasma FFA uptake and oxidation during prolonged exercise in trained vs untrained humans, *Am. J. Physiol. Endocrinol. Metab.* 262(25), E791–9, 1992.
84. Kiens, B., Kristiansen, S., Jensen, P., Richter, E.A. and Turcotte, L.P., Membrane associated fatty acid binding protein (FABPpm) in human skeletal muscle is increased by endurance training, *Biochem. Biophys. Res. Com.* 231(2), 463–5, 1997.
85. Spina, R.J., Chi, M.M., Hopkins, M.G., Nemeth, P.M., Lowry, O.H. and Holloszy, J.O., Mitochondrial enzymes increase in muscle in response to 7–10 days of cycle exercise, *J. Appl. Physiol.* 80, 2250–4., 1996.
86. Reaburn, P. and Dascombe, B., Endurance performance in masters athletes, *Eur. Rev. Aging Phys. Act.* 5(1), 31–42, 2008.
87. Grimby, G. and Saltin, B., The aging muscle, *Clin. Physiol.* 3(3), 209–18, 1983.
88. Fuchi, T., Iwaoka, K., Higuchi, M. and Kobayashi, S., Cardiovascular changes associated with decreased aerobic capacity and aging in long-distance runners, *Eur. J. Appl. Physiol.* 58(8), 884–9, 1989.
89. Rivera, A.M., Pels, A.E., Sady, S.P., Sady, M.A., Cullinane, E.M. and Thompson, P.D., Physiological factors associated with the lower maximal oxygen-consumption of master runners, *J. Appl. Physiol.* 66(2), 949–54, 1989.
90. Hagberg, J.M., Allen, W.K., Seals, D.R., Hurley, B.F., Ehsani, A.A. and Holloszy, J.O., A hemodynamic comparison of young and older endurance athletes during exercise, *J. Appl. Physiol.* 58(6), 2041–6, 1985.

91. Klitgaard, H., Mantoni, M., Schiaffino, S. et al., Function, morphology and protein expression of aging skeletal muscle—a cross-sectional study of elderly men with different training backgrounds, *Acta Physiol. Scand.* 140(1), 41–54, 1990.
92. Trappe, S.W., Costill, D.L., Vukovich, M.D., Jones, J. and Melham, T., Aging among elite distance runners: A 22-yr longitudinal study, *J. Appl. Physiol.* 80(1), 285–90, 1996.
93. Hoppeler, H., Billeter, R., Horvath, P.J., Leddy, J.J. and Pendergast, D.R., Muscle structure with low- and high-fat diets in well-trained male runners, *Int. J. Sports Med.* 20(8), 522–6, 1999.
94. Nagy, T.R., Goran, M.I., Weinsier, R.L., Toth, M.J., Schutz, Y. and Poehlman, E.T., Determinants of basal fat oxidation in healthy Caucasians, *J. Appl. Physiol.* 80(5), 1743–8, 1996.
95. Callesescandon, J., Arciero, P.J., Gardner, A.W., Bauman, C. and Poehlman, E.T., Basal fat oxidation decreases with aging in women, *J. Appl. Physiol.* 78(1), 266–71, 1995.
96. Brunner, F., Schmid, A., Sheikhzadeh, A., Nordin, M., Yoon, J. and Frankel, V., Effects of aging on type II muscle fibers: A systematic review of the literature, *J. Aging Phys. Act.* 15(3), 336–48, 2007.
97. Levadoux, E., Morio, B., Montaurier, C. et al., Reduced whole-body fat oxidation in women and in the elderly, *Int. J. Obes.* 25(1), 39–44, 2001.
98. Dillon, N., Chung, S., Kelly, J. and Omalley, K., Age and beta adrenoceptor-mediated function, *Clin. Pharmacol. Therap.* 27(6), 769–72, 1980.
99. Blaak, E.E., van Baak, M.A. and Saris, W.H.M., Beta-adrenergically stimulated fat oxidation is diminished in middle-aged compared to young subjects, *J. Clin. Endocrinol. Metab.* 84(10), 3764–9, 1999.
100. Lonnqvist, F., Nyberg, B., Wahrenberg, H. and Arner, P., Catecholamine-induced lipolysis in adipose tissue of the elderly, *J. Clin. Invest.* 85(5), 1614–21, 1990.
101. Klein, S., Young, V.R., Blackburn, G.L., Bistrian, B.R. and Wolfe, R.R., Palmitate and glycerol kinetics during brief starvation in normal weight young adult and elderly subjects, *J. Clin. Invest.* 78(4), 928–33, 1986.
102. Heinonen, O.J., Carnitine and physical exercise, *Sports Med.* 22(2), 109–32, 1996.
103. Bonadonna, R.C., Groop, L.C., Simonson, D.C. and Defronzo, R.A., Free fatty acid and glucose metabolism in human aging—evidence for operation of the Randle cycle, *Am. J. Physiol.* 266(3), E501–9, 1994.
104. Conway, K.J., Orr, R. and Stannard, S.R., Effect of a divided caffeine dose on endurance cycling performance, postexercise urinary caffeine concentration, and plasma paraxanthine, *J. Appl. Physiol.* 94(4), 1557–62, 2003.
105. Solomon, T.P.J., Sistrun, S.N., Krishnan, R.K. et al., Exercise and diet enhance fat oxidation and reduce insulin resistance in older obese adults, *J. Appl. Physiol.* 104(5), 1313–9, 2008.
106. Massicotte, D., Peronnet, F., Brisson, G.R. and Hillairemarcel, C., Oxidation of exogenous medium chain free fatty acids during prolonged exercise—comparison with glucose, *J. Appl. Physiol.* 73(4), 1334–9, 1992.
107. Rooyackers, O.E., Adey, D.B., Ades, P.A. and Nair, K.S., Effect of age on in vivo rates of mitochondrial protein synthesis in human skeletal muscle, *Proc. Nat. Acad. Sci.* 93(26), 15364–9, 1996.
108. Coggan, A.R., Spina, R.J., King, D.S. et al., Histochemical and enzymatic comparison of the gastrocnemius muscle of young and elderly men and women, *J. Gerontol.* 47(3), B71–6, 1992.
109. Van Zyl, C.G., Lambert, E.V., Hawley, J.A., Noakes, T.D. and Dennis, S.C., Effects of medium-chain triglyceride ingestion on fuel metabolism and cycling performance, *J. Appl. Physiol.* 80(6), 2217–25, 1996.
110. Coggan, A.R., Spina, R.J., Rogers, M.A. et al., Histochemical and enzymatic characteristics of skeletal muscle in master athletes, *J. Appl. Physiol.* 68(5), 1896–901, 1990.
111. Trappe, S.W., Costill, D.L., Fink, W.J. and Pearson, D.R., Skeletal muscle characteristics among distance runners: A 20-yr follow-up study, *J. Appl. Physiol.* 78(3), 823–9, 1995.
112. Coggan, A.R., Spina, R.J., King, D.S. et al., Skeletal muscle adaptations to endurance training in 60 yr old to 70 yr old men and women, *J. Appl. Physiol.* 72(5), 1780–6, 1992.
113. Kiens, B., Diet and training in the week before competition, *Can. J. Appl. Physiol.* 26, S56–63, 2001.
114. Jeukendrup, A.E., Saris, W.H.M., Schrauwen, P., Brouns, F. and Wagenmakers, A.J.M., Metabolic availability of medium chain triglycerides coingested with carbohydrates during prolonged exercise, *J. Appl. Physiol.* 79(3), 756–62, 1995.
115. Horowitz, J.F., Mora-Rodriguez, R., Byerley, L.O. and Coyle, E.F., Preexercise medium-chain triglyceride ingestion does not alter muscle glycogen use during exercise, *J. Appl. Physiol.* 88(1), 219–25, 2000.
116. Ivy, J.L., Costill, D.L., Fink, W.J. and Lower, R.W., Influence of caffeine and carbohydrate feedings on endurance performance, *Med. Sci. Sports Exerc.* 11(1), 6–11, 1979.
117. Jacobson, T.L., Febbraio, M.A., Arkinstall, M.J. and Hawley, J.A., Effect of caffeine co-ingested with carbohydrate or fat on metabolism and performance in endurance-trained men, *Exp. Physiol.* 86(1), 137–44, 2001.

118. Brass, E.P., Supplemental carnitine and exercise, *Am. J. Clin. Nutr.* 72(2), 618S–23S, 2000.
119. Wall, B.T., Stephens, F.B., Constantin-Teodosiu, D., Marimuthu, K., Macdonald, I.A. and Greenhaff, P.L., Chronic oral ingestion of L-carnitine and carbohydrate increases muscle carnitine content and alters muscle fuel metabolism during exercise in humans, *J. Physiol.* 589(4), 963–73, 2011.
120. Phinney, S.D., Bistrian, B.R., Evans, W.J., Gervino, E. and Blackburn, G.L., The human metabolic response to chronic ketosis without calorie restriction: Preservation of submaximal exercise capability with reduced carbohydrate oxidation, *Metabolism* 32(8), 769–76, 1983.
121. Burke, L., Fat adaptation and glycogen restoration for prolonged cycling—recent studies from the Australian Institute of Sport, *Aust. J. Nutr. Diet.* 58(Suppl 1), S23–7, 2001.
122. Burke, L.M., Angus, D.J., Cox, G.R. et al., Effect of fat adaptation and carbohydrate restoration on metabolism and performance during prolonged cycling, *J. Appl. Physiol.* 89(6), 2413–21, 2000.
123. Carey, A.L., Staudacher, H.M., Cummings, N.K. et al., Effects of fat adaptation and carbohydrate restoration on prolonged endurance exercise, *J. Appl. Physiol.* 91(1), 115–22, 2001.
124. Lambert, E.V., Goedecke, J.H., van Zyl, C. et al., High-fat diet versus habitual diet prior to carbohydrate loading: Effects on exercise metabolism and cycling performance, *Int. J. Sport Nutr. Exerc. Metab.* 11(2), 209–25, 2001.
125. Lambert, E.V., Speechly, D.P., Dennis, S.C. and Noakes, T.D., Enhanced endurance in trained cyclists during moderate intensity exercise following 2 weeks adaptation to a high-fat diet, *Eur. J. Appl. Physiol.* 69(4), 287–93, 1994.
126. Rowlands, D.S. and Hopkins, W.G., Effects of high-fat and high-carbohydrate diets on metabolism and performance in cycling, *Metabolism* 51(6), 678–90, 2002.
127. Peters, S.J., Harris, R.A., Wu, P., Pehleman, T.L., Heigenhauser, G.J. and Spriet, L.L., Human skeletal muscle PDH kinase activity and isoform expression during a 3-day high-fat/low-carbohydrate diet, *Am. J. Physiol. Endocrinol. Metab.* 281(6), E1151–8, 2001.
128. Jansson, E. and Kaijser, L., Effect of diet on the utilization of blood-borne and intramuscular substrates during exercise in man, *Acta Physiol. Scand.* 115(1), 19–30, 1982.
129. Starling, R.D., Trappe, T.A., Parcell, A.C., Kerr, C.G., Fink, W.J. and Costill, D.L., Effects of diet on muscle triglyceride and endurance performance, *J. Appl. Physiol.* 82(4), 1185–9, 1997.
130. Decombaz, J., Schmitt, B., Ith, M. et al., Postexercise fat intake repletes intramyocellular lipids but no faster in trained than in sedentary subjects, *Am. J. Physiol. Reg. Integr. Comp. Physiol.* 281(3), R760–9, 2001.
131. Larson-Meyer, D.E., Newcomer, B.R. and Hunter, G.R., Influence of endurance running and recovery diet on intramyocellular lipid content in women: A 1H NMR study, *Am. J. Physiol. Endocrinol. Metab.* 282(1), E95–106, 2002.
132. Wietek, B.M., Machann, J., Mader, I. et al., Muscle type dependent increase in intramyocellular lipids during prolonged fasting of human subjects: A proton MRS study, *Horm. Metab. Res.* 36(9), 639–44, 2004.
133. Zderic, T.W., Davidson, C.J., Schenk, S., Byerley, L.O. and Coyle, E.F., High-fat diet elevates resting intramuscular triglyceride concentration and whole body lipolysis during exercise, *Am. J. Physiol. Endocrinol. Metab.* 286(2), E217–25, 2004.
134. Helge, J.W., Watt, P.W., Richter, E.A., Rennie, M.J. and Kiens, B., Fat utilization during exercise: Adaptation to a fat-rich diet increases utilization of plasma fatty acids and very low density lipoprotein-triacylglycerol in humans, *J. Physiol.* 537(Pt 3), 1009–20, 2001.
135. Johnson, N.A., Stannard, S.R., Mehalski, K. et al., Intramyocellular triacylglycerol in prolonged cycling with high- and low-carbohydrate availability, *J. Appl. Physiol.* 94, 1365–72, 2003.
136. Peters, S.J., St Amand, T.A., Howlett, R.A., Heigenhauser, G.J. and Spriet, L.L., Human skeletal muscle pyruvate dehydrogenase kinase activity increases after a low-carbohydrate diet, *Am. J. Physiol.* 275(6 Pt 1), E980–6, 1998.
137. Fisher, E.C., Evans, W.J. and Phinney, S., Changes in skeletal muscle metabolism induced by a eucaloric ketogenic diet., in *Biochemistry of Exercise*, H. G. Knuttgen, J. A. Vogel, and J. Poortmans, eds., Human Kinetics, Champaign, IL., 1983, pp. 497–501.
138. Helge, J.W. and Kiens, B., Muscle enzyme activity in humans: Role of substrate availability and training, *Am. J. Physiol.* 272(5 Pt 2), R1620–4, 1997.
139. Putman, C.T., Spriet, L.L., Hultman, E. et al., Pyruvate dehydrogenase activity and acetyl group accumulation during exercise after different diets, *Am. J. Physiol.* 265(5 Pt 1), E752–60, 1993.
140. Klein, S. and Wolfe, R.R., Carbohydrate restriction regulates the adaptive response to fasting, *Am. J. Physiol. Endocrinol. Metab.* 262(25), E631–6, 1992.

141. Nybo, L., Pedersen, K., Christensen, B., Aagaard, P., Brandt, N. and Kiens, B., Impact of carbohydrate supplementation during endurance training on glycogen storage and performance, *Acta Physiol.* 197(2), 117–27, 2009.
142. Stannard, S.R., Buckley, A.J., Edge, J.A. and Thompson, M.W., Adaptations to skeletal muscle with endurance exercise training in the acutely fed versus overnight-fasted state, *J. Sci. Med. Sport* 13(4), 465–9, 2010.
143. Van Proeyen, K., Szlufcik, K., Nielens, H., Ramaekers, M. and Hespel, P., Beneficial metabolic adaptations due to endurance exercise training in the fasted state, *J. Appl. Physiol.* 110(1), 236–45, 2011.
144. Tarnopolsky, M.A., Atkinson, S.A., Phillips, S.M. and Macdougall, J.D., Carbohydrate loading and metabolism during exercise in men and women, *J. Appl. Physiol.* 78(4), 1360–8, 1995.
145. Mittendorfer, B., Horowitz, J.F. and Klein, S., Effect of gender on lipid kinetics during endurance exercise of moderate intensity in untrained subjects, *Am. J. Physiol. Endocrinol. Metab.* 283(1), E58–65, 2002.
146. Maher, A.C., Akhtar, M., Vockley, J. and Tarnopolsky, M.A., Women have higher protein content of beta-oxidation enzymes in skeletal muscle than men, *Plos One* 5(8), 2010.
147. Babraj, J.A., Vollaard, N.B., Keast, C., Guppy, F.M., Cottrell, G. and Timmons, J.A., Extremely short duration high intensity interval training substantially improves insulin action in young healthy males, *BMC. Endocr. Disord.* 9(1), 3, 2009.
148. Gibala, M.J., Little, J.P., van Essen, M. et al., Short-term sprint interval versus traditional endurance training: Similar initial adaptations in human skeletal muscle and exercise performance, *J. Physiol.* 575(3), 901–11, 2006.
149. Burgomaster, K.A., Howarth, K.R., Phillips, S.M. et al., Similar metabolic adaptations during exercise after low volume sprint interval and traditional endurance training in humans, *J. Physiol.* 586(1), 151–60, 2008.
150. Johnson, L.G., Kraemer, R.R., Kraemer, G.R. et al., Substrate utilization during exercise in postmenopausal women on hormone replacement therapy, *Eur. J. Appl. Physiol.* 88(3), 282–7, 2002.

6 Protein Needs of Masters Athletes

Mark A. Tarnopolsky

CONTENTS

6.1 INTRODUCTION

For hundreds and perhaps thousands of years there have been many opinions put forth regarding the optimal dietary protein intake required to support maximal athletic performance. There is some evidence that Olympic athletes in ancient Greek times were encouraged to consume large amounts of meat to support muscle function. It is currently well known that carbohydrate and fat provides most of the energy for muscle metabolism during exercise [1]. For decades, many endurance athletes focused their nutrition on a high carbohydrate intake with little regard for the quality and quantity of protein. During this period, there remained the belief that high amounts of dietary protein were required to promote optimal muscle mass accretion during strength/resistance exercise. Certainly, the anecdotes of body builders and power lifters eating huge amounts of protein and the fact that the nutrition supplement industry is hugely invested in the sale of various protein supplements attest to this belief. Exclusive of protein supplements, we have found that body builders traditionally have protein intakes at approximately three times national dietary recommended intake levels in spite of a requirement that was only marginally above that of sedentary individuals [2].

It has become apparent that the belief that protein requirements for endurance athletes are no different to those of sedentary individuals, and that body builders/resistance athletes need massive amounts of protein, are not correct [2]. Indeed, the answer lies somewhere in the middle. For example, there is no strong evidence that protein intakes above 1.7 g/kg/day will enhance muscle or strength gains during resistance exercise training [2,3]. Conversely, although carbohydrate and fat supply most of the energy during endurance exercise, high-performance endurance athletes training on a daily basis may have protein intake levels (~1.6 g/kg/day) that are nearly twice those recommended for sedentary individuals [2].

The question regarding dietary protein requirements for masters athletes becomes even more complex given the fact that older adults do have changes in protein metabolism which could impact on these requirements. For example, athletes over the age of 65 years may start to experience a loss of muscle mass called sarcopenia and/or could have co-existent medical conditions that could further interact with exercise-induced protein needs to make dietary protein requirements even more challenging to estimate [4]. In addition to the interactive effect of ageing, there is also evidence that the timing of nutrition, independent of absolute daily protein intake, can influence protein balance and ultimately requirements [5].

The purpose of this chapter is to evaluate dietary protein requirements for masters athletes in the context of the known data regarding the influence of different modes of exercise on protein metabolism and the resultant effect on dietary protein intake. The chapter will divide exercise broadly into 'resistance' or 'endurance' to refer to exercise modes at the opposite end of the contraction pattern/intensity spectrum. Most of the studies have used running or cycling as models of endurance sports and weightlifting as a model of a resistance activity. Consideration will also be given to the timing of nutrient intake relative to exercise and to sex differences in metabolism and their respective influences on protein requirements. Most of the work on dietary protein requirements has been done using younger men (18–25 years) and older but healthy non-athletic adults (>65 years), so there is a degree of extrapolation required to interpolate the results to those masters athletes older than 25–35 years. It is hoped this review will provide the athlete, coaches and sport scientists with the necessary tools to integrate all of the scientific data into practical advice when providing sport nutrition counselling to a specific masters athlete.

6.2 OVERVIEW OF PROTEIN METABOLISM AND INFLUENCE OF EXERCISE

Proteins are biomolecules composed of amino acids that provide either structural or regulatory functions in the body. Examples of structural proteins would include dystrophin for muscle and collagen for bone with examples of regulatory proteins including enzymes (myosin ATPase) and carrier molecules (albumin, ferritin). Each of the 20 amino acids contains an amino ($-NH_2$) and carboxylic acid ($-COOH$) group with each amino acid having a different radical component. Of the 20 amino acids in humans, there are nine that are considered essential (histidine, isoleucine, leucine, lysine, methionine, phenylalanine, threonine, tryptophan and valine, with arginine being considered conditionally essential). The essential or indispensible amino acid terminology refers to the fact that these cannot be synthesised in the human body and must be obtained from the diet. Given the importance of proteins to the structure and function of the human body, it is understandable that a severe deficiency of dietary protein could lead to structural or functional compromise such as seen in victims of severe starvation. Although severe deficits are not seen in the developed world, more subtle deficiencies may certainly compromise some degree of biological function that may be more apparent for athletes of any age who are stressing their body through exercise. Examples of sub-optimal protein intake could be an attenuation of physiological adaptations (mitochondrial and/or capillary biogenesis) or the development of conditions such as hypoferritinaemia, anaemia or increased risk of infection.

Perhaps the best way to consider dietary protein requirements is in the context of nutrient deficiency (as described above)/accommodation/adaptation and nutrient excess. The term *accommodation* refers to adaptive changes in the body's reutilisation and distribution of amino acids within the body through continued turnover (synthesis and breakdown) under situations of sub-optimal protein intake where the body is trying to preserve critical proteins. Under such situations of accommodation, cellular structure and function could be compromised, especially under situations of further physiological stress such as superimposed infection or injury. The concept of *adaptation* refers to a protein intake that keeps the body in an optimal state of amino acid flux to maintain structural and functional proteins with some buffer to handle additional metabolic stress such as infection, injury, racing or very heavy training. The final concept of importance along the spectrum is that of *nutrient excess* where the protein intake is excessive and possibly even toxic [6].

Protein is broken down in the human body through three main pathways; the lysosomal (cathepsin) and non-lysosomal (calpain and ubiquitin) pathways. The lysosomal pathway involves a process termed autophagy where proteins are broken down by proteolytic enzymes such as cathepsin within the lysosomes. In general, autophagy is activated in the fasting state and inhibited in the fed state [7]. There is an increase in autophagy in skeletal muscle following exercise which may be required to remove damaged organelles and proteins possibly activated by oxidative stress and signalling through p38 mitrogen activated protein (MAP) kinase [8]. There seems to be an attenuation of autophagy with ageing that may lead to the accumulation of macromolecular damage in older adults [9,10]. However, the influence of acute or chronic exercise on these processes in older adults is unclear at this point. The non-lysosomal pathways in human skeletal muscle include the ATP-dependent ubiquitin pathway [11] and the calcium-activated neutral protease pathway (calpain) [12]. Both of these pathways have been shown to be activated following various types of exercise in humans [13,14], and there is likely a chronic elevation of the ubiquitin proteosome pathway in association with age-associated sarcopenia and immobilisation [11,15]. However, the quantitative contribution of these are still in question. There is a net increase in skeletal muscle protein breakdown for approximately 36 h after a single acute bout of resistance exercise [16], which is more prominent in untrained verses trained men [17]; yet, the basal steady-state level of protein breakdown appears to be increased following training in the fed state [18].

Although fat and carbohydrate are the predominant fuels used by skeletal muscle during exercise, it is known that skeletal muscle has the ability to oxidise eight amino acids (alanine, asparagine, aspartate, glutamate, isoleucine, leucine, lysine and valine) [19]. It appears that the branch chain amino acids (isoleucine, leucine and valine) are predominately oxidised during an acute bout of endurance exercise with leucine being quantitatively the most important [20]. An acute bout of endurance exercise leads to an increase in leucine oxidation that lasts for a couple of hours post-exercise [21–23]. In contrast, acute resistance exercise does not increase leucine oxidation in humans [24], and therefore this mechanism would not likely influence protein requirements in those participating in resistance exercise. In general, leucine oxidation is lower in women verses men during endurance exercise [21], and this fact may have an impact on their protein requirements (see below).

The increase in leucine oxidation during endurance exercise is mediated by increased activity of the rate-limiting enzyme called branched-chain oxo-acid dehydrogenase (BCKD) [23]. Following endurance exercise training, there is an increase in the total amount of BCKD protein and total activity; however, the activation of the BCKD complex and resultant leucine oxidation is attenuated at the same absolute and relative exercise intensity [23]. From a protein requirement perspective, the higher total amount and activity of BCKD after training could increase protein requirements given that highly trained athletes of any age usually exercise at higher intensities or for longer periods of time and could oxidise quantitatively more leucine over a 24-h period compared to sedentary people [23].

Protein synthesis is a complex process whereby a cellular signal (stretch, energy charge, heat, oxidative stress, etc.) is detected, often by phosphorylation or dephosphorylation of protein kinases, which leads to activation of transcription factors that in turn initiate RNA transcription from the DNA template. The specific RNA is translated into a growing polypeptide chain through the process of translation by ribosomes that are part of the rough endoplasmic reticulum or free in the cytosol. The translation process of initiation, elongation and termination ultimately results in polypeptide chain that is reflective of the gene encoded in the DNA. There are multiple fates for the polypeptide (protein) that may include a number of post-translational modifications (phosphorylation, glycosylation) or organisation into complexes through protein-protein interactions (dimeric, hetero-trimeric, etc.).

It is well known that endurance exercise training leads predominately to an increase in mitochondrial proteins [23], and resistance exercise training leads to skeletal muscle hypertrophy through an increase in myofibrillar proteins [3,25]. In younger adults, we and others have shown that the mRNA transcriptome pattern is very different for resistance and endurance exercise [26]; yet mixed muscle protein synthetic rates appear to be similarly elevated following either endurance [27] or resistance activity [16]. Mixed muscle protein synthesis is elevated by about 3 to 4 h post-resistance exercise and persists for approximately 72 h before returning to baseline [16]. Following a period of resistance exercise training, there is an increase in the basal rate of mixed muscle protein synthesis with an attenuation of each individual increase (pulse amplitude) of the acute response in myofibrillar protein synthesis still showing increases even after resistance exercise training [17]. More recent studies separating out the various sub-fractions of muscle have shown that acute resistance exercise activates both myofibrillar and mitochondrial fractions whereas endurance exercise only stimulates mitochondrial protein synthesis [28].

Given that all of the aforementioned work has been completed in younger men, it is important to consider the influence of both ageing and gender-based differences on protein metabolism before considering the influence of these metabolic changes upon protein requirements.

6.3 EFFECT OF AGEING ON PROTEIN METABOLISM AND THE RESPONSE TO FEEDING

The loss of muscle mass with ageing (0.5%–1.5%/year between 50 and 85 years) is a multi-factorial process including oxidative stress, mitochondrial dysfunction, protein metabolism alterations, inflammation and a loss of alpha motor neurons [29–31]. The activation of satellite cells is attenuated in response to a single bout of resistance exercise in older adults [32], and this attenuation is associated with greater myostatin expression, most evident in type II fibers [33]. As a consequence of the apparent satellite cell impairment, nutritional (i.e. creatine monohydrate supplementation) and exercise training strategies that enhance satellite cell recruitment [34,35] may be of some benefit in older athletes completing resistance exercise.

From an endurance exercise perspective, lower mitochondrial enzyme activity and mitochondrial transcriptome pattern and higher oxidative stress are associated with ageing, at least in older non-athletes [36–38]. These processes may be linked in that oxidative stress *per se* can lead to mitochondrial DNA, lipid and protein damage that can alter the structure and function of the mitochondria. The lower mitochondrial capacity [36,37] and impaired conductive blood flow [39] are important factors contributing to the age-associated reduction of VO_{2max}. Although VO_{2max} does decline with ageing, older master's endurance athletes can have VO_{2max} values equivalent to sedentary young individuals and significantly higher than sedentary older adults [40,41]. Unfortunately, there is no research to date evaluating how human ageing can influence the nutrient needs of masters athletes in relationship to the known biological changes described above. It is likely that the age-associated decline in aerobic capacity will limit the volume and intensity of endurance exercise in older adults and thus attenuate any exercise induced increases in dietary protein requirements (see below).

Most of the research into the effects of ageing on protein turnover has focused on measurements of muscle protein synthesis in relation to resistance exercise. Initially, it appeared that there was a definite age-associated reduction in the basal level of skeletal muscle sarcoplasmic, myofibrillar and mitochondrial protein synthesis in sedentary older adults [42,43]. This apparent reduction in protein synthesis may contribute to the age-associated decline in both muscle mass and strength [44]. It is likely that chronological age, physical activity status and nutritional status influence the results regarding the influence of ageing on protein metabolism. For example, some research groups have not found a reduction in the basal rate of protein synthesis in older adults when subjects were testing in the post-absorptive state [45–49]. Consistently however, older and younger adults do show a similar increase in myofibrillar and mixed muscle protein synthesis rates (~150%) following acute resistance exercise training [50].

A generally accepted finding in older adults is the process of anabolic resistance where the normal stimulation of net protein balance following exercise + protein (amino acids) is blunted as compared to younger adults [45–49]. There is greater retention of amino acids in younger verses older adults at lower levels of amino acid ingestion [45]. However, with adequate amounts of essential amino acids the blunting of amino acid uptake is not seen in older adults [49]. Furthermore, it appears that the essential amino acid, leucine is most critical of the amino acids in restoring the anabolic resistance in older adults to that of younger adults [46]. Our research group has recently found that 20 g of whey protein was more effective than 20 g of casein in stimulating muscle protein synthesis following a single bout of resistance exercise in older healthy but inactive older adults [51]. The greater stimulation of protein synthesis with whey protein is likely due to the higher leucine content of the whey protein (~2 g leu/20 g whey) and the rapid absorption of the whey vs. casein [52,53]. My colleague, Dr. Stuart Phillips, has also shown that older adults get an even greater enhancement of muscle protein synthesis with 40 vs. 20 g of whey protein [51], in contrast to younger adults who appear to have a plateau of the stimulatory effect at 20 g of whey protein.

Although leucine is an essential component of the anabolic benefit in younger and older adults performing resistance exercise [46], adding leucine (6.25 g) to whey (18.75 g) was not superior to whey alone (25 g) in sustaining post-exercise protein synthesis [54]. Consequently, there may be a plateau in leucine that is already achieved by 25 g of whey and additional leucine is not required. From a practical food perspective, milk appears to be a viable 'natural' alternative for athletes vs. a whey supplement since milk contains a mixture of both whey and casein. As another food alternative, a single serving of 4 oz of lean beef resulted in a similar increase in muscle protein synthesis in both older and younger adults [49]. The strength of the data supports that milk or whey proteins are the most potent in stimulating muscle anabolism; however, it is likely that other proteins such as eggs with equivalent biological value as milk may be equally effective as anabolic agents.

It is well known that the consumption of carbohydrates in the immediate post-exercise (both endurance and resistance) period is associated with enhanced glycogen re-synthesis as compared to a 2-h delay [55,56], and an analogous finding has been reported with the early post-exercise consumption of amino acids/protein following resistance exercise [57]. Timing of nutrient delivery was further highlighted by a study showing that immediate pre-exercise protein and carbohydrate supplementation was more effective at stimulating protein synthesis versus the same supplement given post-exercise [58]. The consumption of carbohydrate and protein and leucine following 30 minutes of activities of daily living exercises lead to a greater stimulation of muscle protein synthesis and a net positive balance versus carbohydrate (CHO) feeding alone in both younger and older adults. [59]. In contrast, another study found that 50 g of CHO did not further enhance net protein balance at rest or after resistance exercise when added to 25 g of whey protein [60]. A potential advantage of including carbohydrate in a post-exercise meal is that it also leads to an increase in insulin that can enhance glycogen re-synthesis in both resistance [61] and endurance exercise [55].

From a practical perspective, the fact that adding carbohydrate to a protein source was not deleterious to the anabolic effects of the post-exercise protein feeding is important in that a much expanded repertoire of foods can be consumed. For example, protein balance was more positive in post-menopausal women receiving protein and carbohydrate verses a placebo consumed following resistance exercise [62]. Another study in older adults found that a supplement containing 10 g protein + 7 g carbohydrate + 3 g fat provided immediately after resistance exercise, as compared to a 2-h delay, resulted in greater muscle mass and strength gains after 12 weeks of resistance exercise training [5]. Another very important practical suggestion is based upon the finding that a rapid bolus of 25 g of whey protein was superior to 10 × 2.5 g pulses in stimulating muscle protein synthesis in young men following resistance exercise [63].

Taken together, the above data suggest that older adults are less responsive to a given amount of protein at lower intakes (<20 g). However, similar rates of net protein accretion can be achieved in older as compared to younger adults with adequate amounts (20–40 g) of high-quality protein (i.e. milk, beef, whey, egg white) consumed following resistance exercise. The timing of nutrient delivery in relation to an exercise bout is important for optimal stimulation of protein retention and it is prudent for masters athletes performing resistance exercise to consume at least 20 g of high biological value protein as rapidly as possible within 30 min of a training session with or without carbohydrates. For the masters athlete training for endurance sports it would be recommended that the protein suggestions would be similar with the inclusion of carbohydrates (30–50 g as a function of weight) to restore muscle glycogen content.

6.4 EFFECT OF SEX DIFFERENCES ON EXERCISE METABOLISM

Several studies have examined the influence of sex on metabolic fuel selection during endurance exercise [1,20,21,23,64–68]. The consensus is that women oxidise proportionately more fat and less carbohydrate compared to men during endurance exercise [1,20,21,23,64–68]. A lower dependence on carbohydrate metabolism should lead to a lesser reliance on amino acid/protein oxidation with a minimal impact upon dietary protein requirements. We found that young men, but not women, showed greater 24-h urinary urea excretion over a 24-h period that included a 15.5-km treadmill run, as compared to a rest day [1]. We [21] and others [20,21,69] found that women oxidised proportionately less leucine as compared to men during endurance cycling. The lesser leucine oxidation observed for women during endurance exercise was not affected by 31 days of endurance exercise training [23]. We used nitrogen balance to show that the well-trained young men and women required more dietary protein than the amount suggested by Canadian dietary intake guidelines [21]. The fact that exercise had a more negative effect on nitrogen balance in men vs. women in the latter study implied that both genders required more dietary protein during endurance exercise training as compared to sedentary individuals. However, the men were quantitatively more affected by exercise training [21]. Several of our subsequent studies have shown that 17-β-estradiol is the main factor that mediates the gender differences in metabolism (and likely the attenuation of the effect of exercise training upon protein requirements) [70,71]. Consequently, dietary protein requirements for pre-menopausal/eumenorrheic women are likely to be less impacted by exercise (~15%–25% less) as compared to post-menopausal/amenorrheic women.

6.5 METHODS FOR DETERMINING PROTEIN REQUIREMENTS

Nitrogen balance (NBAL) is the traditional method used to determine athlete protein requirements. Nitrogen balance measures of all protein sources that enter the body and all sources of excreted nitrogen [72]. Proteins contain ~16% nitrogen by weight; consequently, NBAL is equal to total nitrogen intake (N_{IN}) minus total nitrogen excretion (N_{OUT} = urine + faeces + sweat + miscellaneous [i.e. menstrual loss, hair, semen and skin]). NBAL is positive during periods of net anabolism and negative during catabolic states. The estimated safe protein intake is determined by feeding subjects different amounts of protein and measuring NBAL at each level. Regression analysis is then used to determine the intake required for a zero balance and a safety factor (often + 2 standard deviation [SD]) is added to account for inter-individual variability. It is also important to consider the biological value of the dietary protein for a protein requirement calculated from high biological value proteins (i.e. egg white and milk) would be less (~15%) than for estimates based on a mixed diet containing protein sources of lower biological value (i.e. grains, soy) [52].

A concern with NBAL-derived requirements is that they may under-estimate the protein requirement for 'optimal' function given that the body attempts to compensate for lower protein intakes by increasing the efficiency of amino acid re-utilisation and reducing amino acid flux. The latter metabolic state may not be optimal for high-performance training or competition. For example, a sub-optimal protein intake may be achieved by compromising a physiologically relevant process such as attenuating the up-regulation after mitochondrial enzymes after endurance exercise training or limiting the accretion of myofibrillar protein after resistance training.

Given the concerns that NBAL does not give specific details on the regulation of protein metabolism, researchers have used amino acid tracer methodology to get a better understanding of protein turnover during exercise [73]. Using the terminology coined by the late Vernon Young [6,73], *accommodation* is a state where NBAL is achieved through a reduction in a physiologically relevant process and can be reflected in a lower protein synthesis. An example of *adaptation* would be the protein intake level that would provide for optimal myofibrillar protein synthesis during resistance exercise training while providing a safety margin for times of stress (i.e. infection, increased training). Finally, dietary *protein excess* would be an intake where amino acids showed an exponential increase in oxidation and protein synthesis plateaued with higher protein intakes. From protein turnover data taken at various protein intake levels, the optimal dietary protein intake for a given athlete of any age would be that where amino acid oxidation exponentially increases and protein synthesis plateaus.

The true gold standard for the determination of athlete protein requirements would be to start a large group of sedentary individuals on a long-term exercise training program after randomly allocating them to a variety of protein intakes and measuring important physiological outcome variables that are reflective of adaptation (i.e. VO_{2max}, muscle mass/strength). In addition to the high cost and the fact that few of these subjects would ever become well-trained or high-level athletes, there would be an infinite number of variables that would influence the requirements including genetic capacity, exercise intensity and duration, protein quality, energy balance, timing of nutrient delivery, macronutrient distribution and gender/menstrual cycle/menopause. Given these issues, our understanding of protein requirements for athletes of all ages has come from NBAL and isotopic tracer turnover studies in small groups of men and women under various exercise conditions (early training, cross-sectional studies in athletes/controls). Unfortunately, most of the studies have been in young men and women with only one exception where middle-aged male runners were specifically studied [74]. To date, specific requirements for masters athletes have not been established in randomised trials. Thus, I will attempt to extrapolate from data in young athletes in combination with the known biology of ageing and its influence on protein turnover.

6.6 PROTEIN REQUIREMENTS DURING RESISTANCE EXERCISE TRAINING IN OLDER ADULTS

Based on the aforementioned theoretical data, it is important to determine the actual protein requirements for older adults and whether they are higher for masters athletes performing resistance exercise training. In younger adults, the protein requirements for very highly trained body builders was only minimally elevated above that recommended for sedentary males [2] in spite of the self perception that a very high protein intake was required to promote muscle hypertrophy. Even with very high training volumes in the early adaptive period in previously untrained men, we found that dietary protein intakes were twice that of the Canadian and US recommended intake of 0.8 g/kg/day (i.e. 1.6 g/kg/day) [3,25]. Furthermore, in young men performing resistance exercise and training for university level team sports (rugby, American football), the maximal recommended protein intake was still in this range (~1.6 g/kg/day) [3]. Consequently, for young healthy men completing even very strenuous exercise, the maximal dietary protein intake is ~1.6 g/kg/day and likely lower if strategies such as consuming high biological value proteins and/or consuming protein shortly after a work-out are employed. Even with some degree of anabolic resistance in older adults, it is very unlikely that masters athletes would attain the intensity and/or volume of activity seen in the highly trained body builders or university athletes described above. Consequently, the value of 1.6 g/kg/day would also represent a maximal protein intake for serious masters athletes performing or training in resistance activities.

Dr. Wayne Campbell has completed several studies evaluating protein requirements in resistance-trained older adults (>55 years) [75–79]. His group reported that older adults consuming a meat-containing mixed diet showed greater increase in type II muscle fibre size as compared with those consuming a lacto-ovo (dairy and egg) vegetarian diet during resistance exercise training [76]. More recently, the same research group also showed that when the dietary protein intake was 'clamped' between 1.03–1.17 g/kg/day, the gains in muscle mass and strength after a period of resistance training were similar for the groups of older adults consuming a beef containing diet verses a lacto-ovo vegetarian diet [79]. The latter is not surprising since egg-white protein has a very high biological value. At the molecular level, this research group has clearly shown that when older adults consume sub-optimal levels of protein (0.5 g/kg/day) versus an adequate amount (1.2 g/kg/day), there are alterations in mRNA transcript abundance directionally supportive of adverse metabolic, functional and structural components that would favour sarcopenia [80]. Taken together, the above data suggest that older adults completing resistance-type exercise should ensure the dietary protein intake is between 1.0 and 1.2 g/kg/day and that the sources of protein should include those with high biological value (egg white, milk, beef, fish). The masters athlete who is doing intensive and large-volume training should not exceed a dietary protein requirement of >1.6 g/kg/day. For more details regarding suggested nutritional and training recommendations in masters strength and power athletes, see Chapter 17.

6.7 PROTEIN REQUIREMENTS FOR ENDURANCE ATHLETES

Based upon the studies published to date, it is possible to provide some general guidelines for younger (18–30 years) male endurance athletes in three categories: recreational athletes (low-moderate intensity), moderately trained and high-performance endurance athletes. It is important to consider that the suggested requirements are better considered as suggestions and it is important they be applied with due consideration of the important determinants of nutrient timing, protein quality, training status, exercise intensity (frequency/intensity/duration), gender and menstrual status and dietary energy and CHO intake. Unfortunately, some researchers have rendered strong opinions stating that endurance exercise has no impact upon dietary protein requirements without considering the above factors [81,82]. The fact that most athletes get enough protein in their habitual diet is insufficient justification to discount that endurance exercise has an influence on protein requirements for athletes. The latter point is particularly relevant for masters athletes who may be on an energy-restricted diet that in itself can compromise body protein balance.

Several papers and reviews have found/concluded that even low- to moderate-intensity endurance exercise does have an impact upon protein (PRO) requirements, and if energy intake is adequate there is an increase in the utilisation of amino acids [81,83–86]. For example, NBAL was achieved with a protein intake of 1.0 g/kg/day in young males performing low–moderate physical activity (2 bouts × 90 minutes @ 50% of VO_{2max}/day) [87]. The consumption of protein beyond these estimated requirements resulted in higher leucine oxidation in males performing moderate endurance exercise [22,28], indicating a *nutrient excess* state. One study evaluated leucine oxidation, protein, carbohydrate fat and energy balance over a 24-h period in young men performing low–moderate-intensity exercise (90 minutes @ 45%–50% VO_{2max}) who consumed a higher (2.5 g PRO/kg/day) and lower (1.0 g PRO/kg/day) protein intake. Protein balance was slightly negative on the 1.0-g/kg/day diet, positive on the 2.5-g/kg/day diet, with fat oxidation and CHO storage higher on the 2.5-g PRO/kg/day diet [89].

Three studies have examined protein requirements in moderate- to well-trained endurance athletes using NBAL [21,74,90]. One study measured NBAL in young (27 years, VO_{2max} = 65 mL/kg/minutes) and middle-aged (52 years, VO_{2max} = 55 mL/kg/minute) athletic men randomised to three protein intakes (0.61, 0.92 and 1.21 g PRO/kg/day), and found an estimated safe protein intake of 1.26 g PRO/kg/day [74]. Of importance to this current chapter and to the entire book was the fact that the latter study did not find a difference in the estimated requirements for the younger and middle-aged masters athletes [74]. Our group measured NBAL in endurance-trained young men (VO_{2max} = 59 mL/kg/minute) and women (VO_{2max} = 55 mL/kg/minute) adapted to the then Canadian Recommended Daily Intake of ~0.86 g PRO/kg/day for a 10-day period and we found that they were in negative NBAL [21]. Finally, another study reported that moderately endurance-trained men and women were in slightly negative NBAL (women = –0.22; men = –3.95 g/day) [90]. Taken together, these three studies suggest that PRO intakes at ~1.0 g/kg/day were not adequate to meet the needs of the most of men and women training at this level of exercise volume/intensity. Two of the above studies found a more negative NBAL in the men [21,90], a finding that is consistent with the gender differences in metabolism described earlier in this chapter.

There have also been three studies evaluating PRO requirements in high-performance endurance athletes using NBAL [2,91–93]. Our group has measured all routes of N excretion (including faeces) and included a sedentary control group and found that high-performance male endurance athletes (mean VO_{2max} = 76.2 mL/kg/minute, ~12 hours/week training volume) required a protein intake of 1.6 g PRO/kg/day as compared to a value of 0.86 g PRO/kg/day for the sedentary men [2]. Another research group measured NBAL in five young well-trained endurance runners and a found safe PRO intake of 1.49 g PRO/kg/day [93]. Finally, a laboratory-based simulated Tour de France cycling study found protein requirement of 1.5–1.8 g/kg/day in well-trained male cyclists (VO_{2max} = 65.1 mL/kg/minute) [91,92].

In summary, the above data suggest that low-intensity recreational endurance exercise does not alter dietary PRO requirements beyond those for the general population. Moderate-intensity endurance athletes require only modestly higher dietary protein intakes (~1.2 g PRO/kg/day, ~50% increase) over that recommended for the general population (~0.8 g PRO/kg/day) and the maximal protein requirement for the very well-trained athlete is about 1.6 g PRO/kg/day. Although much less work has been done with women, the above-mentioned protein requirements are likely to be 15%–20% lower for women as compared with men. For more details regarding suggested nutritional and training recommendations in masters endurance and ultra-endurance athletes, see Chapters 14 and 15, respectively.

6.8 CONCLUSIONS/PRACTICAL SUGGESTIONS

Low- and moderate-intensity endurance exercise does not have a major impact upon dietary protein requirements. However, high volumes and intensities of endurance exercise training can elevate dietary protein requirements to ~1.6 g PRO/kg/day. It is very unlikely that older masters athletes (>55 years) would achieve the exercise volumes/intensity to elevate protein requirements to the 1.6-g/kg/day level and there is no evidence that higher levels of protein would be of any advantage to either athletic performance or health.

In general, older adults have some degree of anabolic resistance to the stimulatory effects of amino acid/protein ingestion. However, this can be overcome by timing the ingestion of food in the early post-exercise period and by consuming foods with high biological value such as milk, egg white, cheese and yoghurt. In addition, it would be reasonable for the athlete to consume the nutrition rapidly (within a 5- or 10-min period) to maximise the bolus effect of the amino acids on plasma concentrations. Most young, middle-aged and older adults are likely to have an adequate protein intake at levels of ~1.2 g/kg/day with habitual resistance exercise training. At the initiation of a vigorous exercise program, or during a period of increased metabolic demands (i.e. a training camp or intensified training), there is a temporary elevation in dietary protein needs likely to ~1.4 g/kg/day but not likely to ever exceed 1.6 g/kg/day. In spite of these marginally elevated protein requirements, there is no need for specific dietary supplements when the masters athlete is consuming a mixed diet providing adequate energy with 10%–15% of macronutrient energy coming from protein. As an example for a high-performance athlete, an energy intake of ~3500 kcal/day would provide ~125 g PRO/day or ~1.7 g/kg/day.

Establishing dietary protein requirements for masters athletes may seem unnecessary if all athletes had ideal eating patterns and stable training/injuries/racing. As any coach or athlete knows, the ideal situation of long-term stability is rarely achieved in all situations. For example, we have reported huge ranges in dietary protein intakes by young athletes [2,21,70] and we and others have reported that ~10% of male and 20% of female athletes have protein intakes below those for sedentary individuals [21,94,95], and even more who are not achieving the modest suggestions in this chapter and other review articles [96,97]. Readers interested in protein metabolism and ageing are directed to a number of recent reviews [98,99].

6.9 IMPLICATIONS FOR SPORTS MEDICINE PROFESSIONALS AND CLINICIANS

Clinicians should be aware of the unique protein requirements of masters athletes and not simply assume that exercise of any type has no impact whatsoever upon dietary protein requirements. Physicians should have some idea of the requirements presented in the chapter and be in a position to refer athletes to a sport nutritionist/dietician to evaluate the specific dietary intake and make recommendations if the diet is failing to meet the protein intake needs of the individual masters athlete. The clinician should evaluate the specific needs of the individual athlete with respect to age, menstrual cycle/phase, training status, training intensity/volume/racing and habitual dietary intake to determine the specific protein requirements by considering factors such as protein quality, energy intake, timing of nutrition in relation to exercise and co-ingestion of carbohydrate to counsel athletes appropriately.

6.10 IMPLICATIONS FOR MASTERS ATHLETES AND COACHES

The bottom-line estimated recommendations for protein nutrition from the aforementioned review of the literature for masters athletes and coaches are the following (summary in Table 6.1):

- High-performance/top sport masters male endurance athletes should consume 1.6–1.7 g PRO/kg/day, high-performance amenorrheic and post-menopausal women 1.4–1.6 g PRO/kg/day and high-performance pre-menopausal/eumenorrheic female masters athletes should strive for 1.2–1.4 g PRO/kg/day.
- Recreational-endurance- and resistance-exercise-training masters athletes may need a transient (~3–4 months) increase in protein intake to ~1.4 g PRO/kg/day during the initial adaptive phase of a training program and during significant increases in the intensity, frequency and/or duration of an exercise program. However, most athletes consuming a well-balanced diet will have a sufficient protein intake at ~1.2 g/kg/day.
- In general, proteins with high biological value (egg white, milk products, meats, fish) can lower the recommended protein intakes by about 10%–15% versus a mixed protein source (give some examples please). Furthermore, the consumption of meat and dairy protein sources enhances resistance and endurance adaptations and helps to preserve muscle mass during periods of intentional weight loss as compared to soy-based proteins or mixed protein sources.

TABLE 6.1
Protein Requirements for Athletes

Target Group	Suggested Protein Intake (g/kg/day)
1. Sedentary men and women	0.8 (women)–0.9 (men)
Endurance Sports	
2. Top sport young male athletes	1.6–1.7
3. Top-level male and post-menopausal masters athletes	1.4–1.6
4. Top-level eumenorrheic masters athletes	1.2–1.4
5. Recreational athletes	1.2
Resistance Sports[a]	
6. Power sports (rugby, football)	1.4–1.7 (masters–younger)
7. Resistance training (early phase–few months)	1.4–1.7 (masters–younger)
8. Resistance training (adapted phase/maintenance)	1.0–1.2

[a] We do not have definitive data in women doing resistance exercise but it is likely that the above suggestions are 10%–20% lower.

TABLE 6.2
Practical Suggestions to Maximize Protein Retention

- Eat a variety of high-quality proteins (milk and milk products [casein and whey], egg whites, lean meat and fish).
- Consume protein (20–40 g) as soon as possible after a work-out.
- The post-exercise meal should be consumed rapidly.
- Consume an energy intake adequate to meet the demands of training.
- A pre-exercise protein and carbohydrate supplement is likely as effective as an immediate one for resistance training (use what feels best and is convenient).
- Pre- and during exercise carbohydrate supplements (gels, sport drink) will attenuate amino acid oxidation during exercise and will likely promote greater net protein retention during hard training sessions.
- Eating several smaller meals and snacks during the day is likely to allow an athlete to attain both energy and protein requirements versus eating only two or three meals a day.

- The consumption of a high-quality protein (~15 g women; ~20 g men and up to 40 g in older adults [>65 years]) with or without carbohydrate (15–25 g) within the first 30 minutes post-exercise will promote nitrogen retention and is likely to enhance the gains made during resistance exercise training. For tips on maximising protein retention see Table 6.2.
- It is better to consume post-exercise nutrition as a bolus (i.e. <5 min) vs. a slower/pulsed intake to maximise the peak amino acid concentration in blood.

6.11 FUTURE RESEARCH DIRECTIONS

Although we have a general idea of the suggested protein requirements for masters athletes, there remain many interesting directions for future investigation, including the following considerations:

- Does the timing of post-exercise protein/carbohydrate nutrition enhance the benefits from endurance exercise training on mitochondrial biogenesis?
- Are dietary protein requirements altered during recovery from a sports injury?
- What is the effect of menopause on dietary protein requirements in female masters athletes?

REFERENCES

1. Tarnopolsky, L.J., MacDougall, J.D., Atkinson, S.A., Tarnopolsky, M.A. and Sutton, J.R., Gender differences in substrate for endurance exercise, *J. Appl. Physiol.* 68(1), 302–8, 1990.
2. Tarnopolsky, M.A., MacDougall, J.D. and Atkinson, S.A., Influence of protein intake and training status on nitrogen balance and lean body mass, *J. Appl. Physiol.* 64(1), 187–93, 1988.
3. Tarnopolsky, M.A. et al., Evaluation of protein requirements for trained strength athletes, *J. Appl. Physiol.* 73(5), 1986–95, 1992.
4. Safdar, A. et al., Aberrant mitochondrial homeostasis in the skeletal muscle of sedentary older adults, *PloS one* 5(5), e10778, 2010.
5. Esmarck, B. et al., Timing of postexercise protein intake is important for muscle hypertrophy with resistance training in elderly humans, *J. Physiol.* 535(Pt 1), 301–11, 2001.
6. Young, V.R. and Bier, D.M., A kinetic approach to the determination of human amino acid requirements, *Nutr. Rev.* 45(10), 289–98, 1987.
7. Moresi, V. et al., Histone deacetylases 1 and 2 regulate autophagy flux and skeletal muscle homeostasis in mice, *Proc. Nat. Acad. Sci. USA* 109(5), 1649–54, 2012.
8. McClung, J.M., Judge, A.R., Powers, S.K. and Yan, Z., p38 MAPK links oxidative stress to autophagy-related gene expression in cachectic muscle wasting, *AM. J. Physiol.Cell Physiol.* 298(3), C542–49, 2010.
9. Masiero, E. et al., Autophagy is required to maintain muscle mass, *Cell Metab.* 10(6), 507–15, 2009.
10. Wu, J.J. et al., Mitochondrial dysfunction and oxidative stress mediate the physiological impairment induced by the disruption of autophagy, *Aging (Albany NY)* 1(4), 425–37, 2009.

11. Gomes, M.D., Lecker, S.H., Jagoe, R.T., Navon, A. and Goldberg, A.L., Atrogin-1, a muscle-specific F-box protein highly expressed during muscle atrophy, *Proc. Nat. Acad. Sci. USA* 98(25), 14440–5, 2001.
12. Verburg, E., Murphy, R.M., Richard, I. and Lamb, G.D., Involvement of calpains in Ca^{2+}-induced disruption of excitation-contraction coupling in mammalian skeletal muscle fibers, *Am. J. Physiol. Cell Physiol.* 296(5), C1115–22, 2009.
13. Belcastro, A.N., Shewchuk, L.D. and Raj, D.A., Exercise-induced muscle injury: A calpain hypothesis, *Mol. Cell. Biochem.* 179(1–2), 135–45, 1998.
14. Stupka, N., Tarnopolsky, M.A., Yardley, N.J. and Phillips, S.M., Cellular adaptation to repeated eccentric exercise-induced muscle damage, *J. Appl. Physiol.* 91(4), 1669–78, 2001.
15. Combaret, L. et al., Skeletal muscle proteolysis in aging, *Curr. Opin.Clin. Nutr. Metab. Care* 12(1), 37–41, 2009.
16. Phillips, S.M., Tipton, K.D., Aarsland, A., Wolf, S.E. and Wolfe, R.R., Mixed muscle protein synthesis and breakdown after resistance exercise in humans, *Am. J. Physiol.* 273(1 Pt 1), E99–107, 1997.
17. Phillips, S.M., Tipton, K.D., Ferrando, A.A. and Wolfe, R.R., Resistance training reduces the acute exercise-induced increase in muscle protein turnover, *Am. J. Physiol.* 276(1 Pt 1), E118–24, 1999.
18. Phillips, S.M. et al., Resistance-training-induced adaptations in skeletal muscle protein turnover in the fed state, *Can. J. Physiol. Pharmacol.* 80(11), 1045–53, 2002.
19. Goldberg, A.L. and Chang, T.W., Regulation and significance of amino acid metabolism in skeletal muscle, *Fed. Proc.* 37(9), 2301–7, 1978.
20. Lamont, L.S., McCullough, A.J. and Kalhan S.C., Gender differences in leucine, but not lysine, kinetics, *J. Appl. Physiol.* 91(1), 357–62, 2001.
21. Phillips, S.M., Atkinson, S.A., Tarnopolsky, M.A. and MacDougall, J.D., Gender differences in leucine kinetics and nitrogen balance in endurance athletes, *J. Appl. Physiol.* 75(5), 2134–41, 1993.
22. Bowtell, J.L. et al., Modulation of whole body protein metabolism, during and after exercise, by variation of dietary protein, *J. Appl. Physiol.* 85(5), 1744–52, 1998.
23. McKenzie, S. et al., Endurance exercise training attenuates leucine oxidation and BCOAD activation during exercise in humans, *Am. J. Physiol. Endocrinol. Metab.* 278(4), E580–7, 2000.
24. Tarnopolsky, M.A. et al., Whole body leucine metabolism during and after resistance exercise in fed humans, *Med. Sci. Sports Exerc.* 23(3), 326–33, 1991.
25. Lemon, P.W., Tarnopolsky, M.A., MacDougall, J.D. and Atkinson, S.A., Protein requirements and muscle mass/strength changes during intensive training in novice bodybuilders, *J. Appl. Physiol.* 73(2), 767–75, 1992.
26. Mahoney, D.J. et al., Gene expression profiling in human skeletal muscle during recovery from eccentric exercise, *Am. J. Physiol. Regul. Integr. Comp. Physiol.* 294(6), R1901–10, 2008.
27. Howarth, K.R., Moreau, N.A., Phillips, S.M. and Gibala, M.J., Coingestion of protein with carbohydrate during recovery from endurance exercise stimulates skeletal muscle protein synthesis in humans, *J. Appl. Physiol.* 106(4), 1394–1402, 2009.
28. Wilkinson, S.B. et al., Differential effects of resistance and endurance exercise in the fed state on signalling molecule phosphorylation and protein synthesis in human muscle, *J. Physiol.* 586(Pt 15), 3701–17, 2008.
29. Doherty, T.J., Invited review: Aging and sarcopenia, *J. Appl. Physiol.* 95(4), 1717–27, 2003.
30. Doherty, T.J., Vandervoort, A.A., Taylor, A.W. and Brown W.F., Effects of motor unit losses on strength in older men and women, *J. Appl. Physiol.* 74(2), 868–74, 1993.
31. Lexell, J., Taylor, C.C. and Sjostrom, M., What is the cause of the ageing atrophy? Total number, size and proportion of different fiber types studied in whole vastus lateralis muscle from 15- to 83-year-old men, *J. Neurol. Sci.* 84(2–3), 275–94, 1988.
32. Dreyer, H.C., Blanco, C.E., Sattler, F.R., Schroeder, E.T. and Wiswell, R.A., Satellite cell numbers in young and older men 24 hours after eccentric exercise, *Muscle Nerve* 33(2), 242–53, 2006.
33. McKay, B.R., Ogborn, D.I., Bellamy, L.M., Tarnopolsky, M.A. and Parise, G., Myostatin is associated with age-related human muscle stem cell dysfunction, *FASEB J.* 26(6), 2509–21, 2012.
34. Mackey, A.L. et al., Enhanced satellite cell proliferation with resistance training in elderly men and women, *Scand. J. Med. Sci. Sports* 17(1), 34–42, 2007.
35. Olsen, S. et al., Creatine supplementation augments the increase in satellite cell and myonuclei number in human skeletal muscle induced by strength training, *J. Physiol.* 573(Pt 2), 525–34, 2006.
36. Parise, G., Brose, A.N. and Tarnopolsky, M.A., Resistance exercise training decreases oxidative damage to DNA and increases cytochrome oxidase activity in older adults, *Exp. Gerontol.* 40(3), 173–80, 2005.
37. Parise, G., Phillips, S.M., Kaczor, J.J. and Tarnopolsky, M.A., Antioxidant enzyme activity is up-regulated after unilateral resistance exercise training in older adults, *Free Radic. Biol. Med.* 39(2), 289–95, 2005.

38. Lemon, P.W. and Yarasheski, K.E., Feasibility of sweat collection by whole body washdown in moderate to high humidity environments, *Int. J. Sports Med.* 6(1), 41–3, 1985.
39. Hepple, R.T., Hagen, J.L., Krause, D.J. and Jackson, C.C., Aerobic power declines with aging in rat skeletal muscles perfused at matched convective O2 delivery, *J. Appl. Physiol.* 94(2), 744–51, 2003.
40. Coggan, A.R. et al., Histochemical and enzymatic characteristics of skeletal muscle in master athletes, *J. Appl. Physiol.* 68(5), 1896–1901, 1990.
41. Rogers, M.A., Hagberg, J.M., Martin, W.H., 3rd, Ehsani, A.A. and Holloszy, J.O., Decline in VO_{2max} with aging in master athletes and sedentary men, *J. Appl. Physiol.* 68(5), 2195–99, 1990.
42. Rooyackers, O.E., Adey, D.B., Ades, P.A. and Nair, K.S., Effect of age on in vivo rates of mitochondrial protein synthesis in human skeletal muscle, *Proc. Nat. Acad. Sci. USA.* 93(26), 15364–69, 1996.
43. Balagopal, P., Rooyackers, O.E., Adey, D.B., Ades, P.A. and Nair, K.S., Effects of aging on in vivo synthesis of skeletal muscle myosin heavy-chain and sarcoplasmic protein in humans, *Am. J. Physiol.* 273(4 Pt 1), E790–800, 1997.
44. Proctor, D.N., Balagopal, P. and Nair, K.S., Age-related sarcopenia in humans is associated with reduced synthetic rates of specific muscle proteins, *J. Nutr.* 128(2 Suppl), 351S–355S, 1998.
45. Katsanos, C.S., Kobayashi, H., Sheffield-Moore, M., Aarsland, A. and Wolfe, R.R., Aging is associated with diminished accretion of muscle proteins after the ingestion of a small bolus of essential amino acids, *Am. J. Clin. Nutr.* 82(5), 1065–73, 2005.
46. Katsanos, C.S., Kobayashi, H., Sheffield-Moore, M., Aarsland, A. and Wolfe, R.R., A high proportion of leucine is required for optimal stimulation of the rate of muscle protein synthesis by essential amino acids in the elderly, *Am. J. Physiol. Endocrinol. Metab.* 291(2), E381–7, 2006.
47. Paddon-Jones, D., Sheffield-Moore, M., Katsanos, C.S., Zhang, X.J. and Wolfe R.R., Differential stimulation of muscle protein synthesis in elderly humans following isocaloric ingestion of amino acids or whey protein, *Exp. Gerontol.* 41(2), 215–19, 2006.
48. Paddon-Jones, D. et al., Amino acid ingestion improves muscle protein synthesis in the young and elderly, *Am. J. Physiol. Endocrinol. Metab.* 286(3), E321–28, 2004.
49. Symons, T.B. et al., Aging does not impair the anabolic response to a protein-rich meal, *Am. J. Clin. Nutr.* 86(2), 451–56, 2007.
50. Hasten, D.L., Pak-Loduca, J., Obert, K.A. and Yarasheski, K.E., Resistance exercise acutely increases MHC and mixed muscle protein synthesis rates in 78–84 and 23–32 yr olds, *Am. J. Physiol. Endocrinol. Metab.* 278(4), E620–6, 2000.
51. Yang, Y. et al., Resistance exercise enhances myofibrillar protein synthesis with graded intakes of whey protein in older men, *Br. J. Nutr.* 108(10), 1780–8, 2012.
52. Phillips, S.M., Tang, J.E. and Moore, D.R., The role of milk- and soy-based protein in support of muscle protein synthesis and muscle protein accretion in young and elderly persons, *J. Am. Coll. Nutr.* 28(4), 343–54, 2009.
53. Tang, J.E., Moore, D.R., Kujbida, G.W., Tarnopolsky, M.A. and Phillips, S.M., Ingestion of whey hydrolysate, casein, or soy protein isolate: Effects on mixed muscle protein synthesis at rest and following resistance exercise in young men, *J. Appl. Physiol.* 107(3), 987–92, 2009.
54. Churchward-Venne, T.A. et al., Supplementation of a suboptimal protein dose with leucine or essential amino acids: Effects on myofibrillar protein synthesis at rest and following resistance exercise in men, *J. Physiol.* 59(Pt 11), 2751–65, 2012.
55. Ivy, J.L., Katz, A.L., Cutler, C.L., Sherman, W.M. and Coyle, E.F., Muscle glycogen synthesis after exercise: Effect of time of carbohydrate ingestion, *J. Appl. Physiol.* 64(4), 1480–5, 1988.
56. Roy, B.D., Tarnopolsky, M.A., MacDougall, J.D., Fowles, J. and Yarasheski, K.E., Effect of glucose supplement timing on protein metabolism after resistance training, *J. Appl. Physiol.* 82(6), 1882–8, 1997.
57. Tipton, K.D. and Wolfe, R.R., Protein and amino acids for athletes, *J. Sports Sci.* 22(1), 65–79, 2004.
58. Tipton, K.D. et al., Timing of amino acid-carbohydrate ingestion alters anabolic response of muscle to resistance exercise, *Am. J. Physiol. Endocrinol. Metab.* 281(2), E197–206, 2001.
59. Koopman, R. et al., Co-ingestion of protein and leucine stimulates muscle protein synthesis rates to the same extent in young and elderly lean men, *Am. J. Clin. Nutr.* 84(3), 623–32, 2006.
60. Staples, A.W. et al., Carbohydrate does not augment exercise-induced protein accretion versus protein alone, *Med. Sci. Sports Exerc.* 43(7), 1154–61, 2011.
61. Roy, B.D., Fowles, J.R., Hill, R. and Tarnopolsky, M.A., Macronutrient intake and whole body protein metabolism following resistance exercise, *Med. Sci. Sports Exerc.* 32(8), 1412–8, 2000.
62. Holm, L. et al., Postexercise nutrient intake enhances leg protein balance in early postmenopausal women, *J. Gerontol. A Biol. Sci. Med. Sci.* 60(9), 1212–8, 2005.

63. West, D.W. et al., Rapid aminoacidemia enhances myofibrillar protein synthesis and anabolic intramuscular signaling responses after resistance exercise, *Am. J. Clin. Nutr.* 94(3), 795–803, 2011.
64. Friedlander, A.L. et al., Training-induced alterations of carbohydrate metabolism in women: Women respond differently from men, *J. Appl. Physiol.* 85(3), 1175–86, 1998.
65. Horton, T.J., Pagliassotti, M.J., Hobbs, K. and Hill, J.O., Fuel metabolism in men and women during and after long-duration exercise, *J. Appl. Physiol.* 85(5), 1823–32, 1998.
66. Melanson, E.L. et al., Effect of exercise intensity on 24-h energy expenditure and nutrient oxidation, *J. Appl. Physiol.* 92(3), 1045–52, 2002.
67. Tarnopolsky, M.A., Atkinson, S.A., Phillips, S.M. and MacDougall, J.D., Carbohydrate loading and metabolism during exercise in men and women, *J. Appl. Physiol.* 78(4), 1360–8, 1995.
68. Tarnopolsky, M.A. et al., Postexercise protein-carbohydrate and carbohydrate supplements increase muscle glycogen in men and women, *J. Appl. Physiol.* 83(6), 1877–83, 1997.
69. Lamont, L.S., McCullough, A.J. and Kalhan, S.C., Gender differences in the regulation of amino acid metabolism, *J. Appl. Physiol.* 95(3), 1259–65, 2003.
70. Hamadeh, M.J., Devries, M.C. and Tarnopolsky, M.A., Estrogen supplementation reduces whole body leucine and carbohydrate oxidation and increases lipid oxidation in men during endurance exercise, *J. Clin. Endocrinol. Metab.* 90(6), 3592–9, 2005.
71. Maher, A.C., Akhtar, M. and Tarnopolsky, M.A., Men supplemented with 17beta-estradiol have increased beta-oxidation capacity in skeletal muscle, *Physiol. Genomics* 42(3), 342–7, 2010.
72. Pellet, P.L., Protein requirements in humans, *Am. J. Clin. Nutr.* 51(5), 723–37, 1990.
73. Young, V.R., Bier, D.M. and Pellett, P.L., A theoretical basis for increasing current estimates of the amino acid requirements in adult man, with experimental support, *Am. J. Clin. Nutr.* 50(1), 80–92, 1989.
74. Meredith, C.N., Zackin, M.J., Frontera, W.R. and Evans, W.J., Dietary protein requirements and body protein metabolism in endurance-trained men, *J. Appl. Physiol.* 66(6), 2850–6, 1989.
75. Campbell, W.W., Synergistic use of higher-protein diets or nutritional supplements with resistance training to counter sarcopenia, *Nutr. Rev.* 65(9), 416–22, 2007.
76. Campbell, W.W. et al., Effects of an omnivorous diet compared with a lactoovovegetarian diet on resistance-training-induced changes in body composition and skeletal muscle in older men, *Am. J. Clin. Nutr.* 70(6), 1032–9, 1999.
77. Campbell, W.W. et al., Effects of resistance training and chromium picolinate on body composition and skeletal muscle in older men, *J. Appl. Physiol.* 86(1), 29–39, 1999.
78. Campbell, W.W. and Leidy, H.J., Dietary protein and resistance training effects on muscle and body composition in older persons, *J. Am. Coll. Nutr.* 26(6), 696S–703S, 2007.
79. Dohm, G.L. et al., Adaptation of protein metabolism to endurance training. Increased amino acid oxidation in response to training, *Biochem. J.* 164(3), 705–8, 1977.
80. Thalacker-Mercer, A.E., Fleet, J.C., Craig, B.A., Carnell, N.S. and Campbell, W.W., Inadequate protein intake affects skeletal muscle transcript profiles in older humans, *Am. J. Clin. Nutr.* 85(5), 1344–52, 2007.
81. Millward, D.J., Bowtell, J.L., Pacy, P. and Rennie, M.J., Physical activity, protein metabolism and protein requirements, *Proc. Nutr. Soc.* 53(1), 223–40, 1994.
82. Rennie, M.J. and Tipton, K.D., Protein and amino acid metabolism during and after exercise and the effects of nutrition, *Ann. Rev. Nutr.* 20, 457–83, 2000.
83. Todd, K.S., Butterfield, G.E. and Calloway, D.H., Nitrogen balance in men with adequate and deficient energy intake at three levels of work, *J. Nutr.* 114(11), 2107–18, 1984.
84. Young, V.R. and Torun, B., Physical activity: Impact on protein and amino acid metabolism and implications for nutritional requirements, *Prog. Clin. Biol. Res.* 77, 57–85, 1981.
85. Butterfield, G.E. and Calloway, D.H., Physical activity improves protein utilization in young men, *Br. J. Nutr.* 51(2), 171–84, 1984.
86. Torun, B., Scrimshaw, N.S. and Young, V.R., Effect of isometric exercises on body potassium and dietary protein requirements of young men, *Am. J. Clin. Nutr.* 30(12), 1983–93, 1977.
87. el-Khoury, A.E. et al., Moderate exercise at energy balance does not affect 24-h leucine oxidation or nitrogen retention in healthy men, *Am. J. Physiol.* 273(2 Pt 1), E394–407, 1997.
88. Forslund, A.H. et al., Effect of protein intake and physical activity on 24-h pattern and rate of macronutrient utilization, *Am. J. Physiol.* 276(5 Pt 1), E964–76, 1999.
89. Forslund, A.H. et al., The 24-h whole body leucine and urea kinetics at normal and high protein intakes with exercise in healthy adults, *Am. J. Physiol.* 275(2 Pt 1), E310–20, 1988.
90. Lamont, L.S., Patel, D.G. and Kalhan, S.C., Leucine kinetics in endurance-trained humans, *J. Appl. Physiol.* 69(1), 1–6, 1990.

91. Brouns, F. et al., Eating, drinking, and cycling. A controlled Tour de France simulation study, Part II. Effect of diet manipulation, *Int. J. Sports Med.* 10(Suppl 1), S41–8, 1989.
92. Brouns, F. et al., Eating, drinking, and cycling. A controlled Tour de France simulation study, Part I, *Int. J. Sports Med.* 10(Suppl 1), S32–40, 1989.
93. Friedman, J.E. and Lemon, P.W., Effect of chronic endurance exercise on retention of dietary protein, *Int. J. Sports Med.* 10(2), 118–23, 1989.
94. Deuster, P.A. et al., Nutritional survey of highly trained women runners, *Am. J. Clin. Nutr.* 44(6), 954–62, 1986.
95. Roy, B.D., Luttmer, K., Bosman, M.J. and Tarnopolsky, M.A., The influence of post-exercise macronutrient intake on energy balance and protein metabolism in active females participating in endurance training, *Int. J. Sport Nutr. Exerc. Metab.* 12(2), 172–88, 2002.
96. Tarnopolsky, M., Protein requirements for endurance athletes, *Nutr.* 20(7–8), 662–8, 2004.
97. Tipton, K.D. and Witard, O.C., Protein requirements and recommendations for athletes: Relevance of ivory tower arguments for practical recommendations, *Clin. Sports Med.* 26(1), 17–36, 2007.
98. Burd, N., Gorissen, S.H. and van Loon, L.J.C., Anabolic resistance of muscle protein synthesis with aging, *Exerc. Sport Sci. Rev.* 41(3), 169–73, 2013.
99. Dickinson, J.M., Volpi, E. and Rasmussen, B.B., Exercise and nutrition to target protein synthesis impairments in aging skeletal muscle, *Exerc. Sport Sci. Rev.* 41(4), 216–23, 2013.

7 Vitamin Needs of Masters Athletes

Jeanick Brisswalter

CONTENTS

7.1 INTRODUCTION

Over the last decade the participation of masters athletes in competitive events has increased, particularly in long-distance events [1–3]. For participants in these events, matching energy intake and expenditure is critical to maintain health and performance. The proportions of carbohydrate, fat and protein must be optimised according to recommendations to provide enough calories to sustain the energy requirements of competiton or training and for recovery. In addition, endurance athletes must include adequate vitamins and mineral intakes in their diets to maintain healthy immune function [4,5]. However, vitamin and mineral intakes may be sufficient in the diets of endurance athletes who have a high energy intake [6]. This would make it unnecessary to use vitamin and mineral supplements.

The potential benefits of supplement use in athletes are thus questionable. Some studies indicate no benefits, while others highlight potential negative side effects of vitamin supplementation [7]. Nevertheless, supplement use is common among athletes. For example, Knez and Peake reported that compared with recommended dietary intakes for the general population, both male and female ironman triathletes met or exceeded these values for all vitamins and minerals, except vitamin D [8]. However, over 60% of athletes reported using vitamin supplements. Among supplements, those containing vitamin C (97.5%), vitamin E (78.3%) and multivitamins (52.2%) appeared to be the most commonly used [8].

In masters athletes, ageing is accompanied by an increase in free radical production with a concomitant decrease in the enzymatic defence mechanisms [9]. This combination favours oxidative stress. It could therefore be important to monitor levels of antioxidant micronutrients in an ageing population of older exercisers. All the more-so for masters athletes, who are doubly exposed to oxidative stress as a result of ageing and exercise, both inducing oxidative stress and possibly potentiating each other's effects. In this context, optimal levels of antioxidant vitamins and minerals may help to negate the effects of free radicals, could improve muscle recovery and possibly slow the effects of ageing. Few studies have tested the effect of micronutritional supplements on muscle recovery in masters athletes with the majority of available data relating to older sedentary subjects [10,11]. These studies, in general, do not agree on the effects isolated or combined supplements for vitamins C, B, E, carotenoids or selenium have on immune function in older subjects.

7.2 OXIDATIVE STRESS AND EXERCISE

Oxidative stress is defined as an excess of free radicals leading to a tissue state not compatible with cellular homeostasis [12]. Free radicals, which induce oxidative stress, have an unpaired electron on an oxygen atom [13]. This is why they are often referred to as reactive oxygen species (ROS). Due to their extreme reactivity, they are short-lived (between a few nanoseconds and a few seconds, depending on the molecule). Among all the radical species likely to be formed in cells, a select group, known as primary radicals, play a particular physiological role. The reaction of these primary radicals with chemical compounds within the cell produces other free radicals, or secondary radicals.

Primary radicals produced in the human body are derived from oxygen by one-electron reductions. This produces, for example, the superoxide anion and the hydroxyl radical, or the nitrous oxide radical [12]. Other oxygen-derived species, including singlet oxygen (1O2), hydrogen peroxide (H_2O_2) and nitroperoxide (ONOOH), are not free radicals. However, these molecules are as reactive as free radicals and can be precursors of radicals [13]. All free radicals and their precursors are collectively known as ROS.

ROS can be formed in the mitochondria of skeletal muscles [14]. Exercise causes oxygen consumption to rise 10- to 20-fold over resting levels. This increase in oxygen consumption is particularly marked during long-duration exercise [15]. The direct consequence of increased in oxygen consumption is increased oxygen flux of up to 100 or 200 times the flux measured in resting subjects [16]. As a result, the flow of electrons in the mitochondria also increases [16]. This can lead to transformation of between 1% and 5% of the oxygen into ROS. Thus, superoxide radical production can be amplified as the intensity of respiration increases to compensate for physical effort [17].

ROS production can also be increased by the ischaemia-reperfusion phenomenon [18]. A temporary decrease in blood flow (ischaemia) and/or oxygen supply can occur in the active muscles during exercise. This happens when muscle contractions are too intense, or when an individual reaches their maximum oxygen consumption level. The ischaemic tissues will only be reoxygenated through renewed blood flow (reperfusion) once the exercise and muscle contractions are discontinued. Ischaemia-reperfusion is not only known to induce excessive ROS production, but has also been shown to contribute to the extent of exercise-induced tissue damage [19].

Another major source of oxygen-derived free radicals is the inflammatory response. In this context, radicals are produced directly by activated phagocytic cells through a process known as the oxidative burst [20]. The superoxide generated by membrane-bound nicotinamide adenine dinucleotide phosphate-oxidase (NADPH) produces very powerful oxidants such as the hydroxyl radical and (H_2O_2) which are released into the extracellular space or into the phagosome (vesicle formed around a particle absorbed by phagocytosis) [21]. The H_2O_2 formed by this process is converted into hypochloric acid (HOCl) and chloramines, which are even more powerful oxidants. They are used by phagocytes to ensure thorough cleansing of the injured tissues [22].

In conclusion, during exercise, oxidative stress is increased during aerobic activites and can also be increased by inflammatory processes related to muscle damage. This effect could be potentiated by ageing.

7.3 OXIDATIVE STRESS AND AGEING

The free radical theory of ageing hypothesises that oxygen-derived free radicals are responsible for age-related damage to cells and tissues [9]. It appears that oxidation of proteins, and the system responsible for repair and degradation of oxidised proteins are key to the changes to cellular function during ageing [9]. Oxidative damage to biomolecules induced by radical species produced by the mitochondria could be exacerbated by reduced antioxidant capacities. Thus, the increase in oxidative stress with normal ageing appears to be a consequence of both increased free radical production and inadequate antioxidant defences [23]. In a normal situation these factors are balanced against each other. But, when excess free radicals are generated through either ageing and/or exercise, the natural cellular antioxidant defences may be overwhelmed, leading to oxidation and further cellular dysfunction [24].

7.4 ANTIOXIDANT CAPACITY

Antioxidants are substances which, even present in minute amounts, inhibit or delay oxidation of substrates including fat, carbohydrate and protein. Endogenous antioxidant defences are both non-enzymatic (e.g. nutritional factors, including vitamins and phenols) and enzymatic (e.g. the superoxide dismutases [SOD], the glutathione peroxidases [GSHPx] and catalase). In normal conditions, the endogenous antioxidant defences are balanced against production of ROS. With oxidative stress, antioxidants must be provided in large quantities through the diet [25].

Nutritional antioxidants use various mechanisms and are found in various cellular compartments, but they are mainly free radical scavengers [26]. Their activity can be summarised in the following three actions: (1) they directly neutralise free radicals, (2) they reduce peroxide concentrations and repair oxidised membranes and (3) they quench iron to decrease production of reactive oxygen species [27]. An estimate of the body's antioxidant defences can be obtained by measuring plasma antioxidant levels (micronutrients, enzymes, other antioxidants). In the following sections, the major dietary antioxidants are discussed in more detail.

7.4.1 VITAMIN C

Vitamin C is the major water-soluble antioxidant. It acts as the first line of defence against free radicals in whole blood and plasma. It is a powerful inhibitor of lipid peroxidation and regenerates vitamin E in lipoproteins and membranes. Plasma vitamin C concentrations have been shown to strongly inversely correlate to plasma isoprostanes [28] that are validated specific markers of oxidative damage to cellular lipids [29] and lipid peroxidation [30]. Chronic vitamin C treatment can reduce high levels of isoprostanes in animal models [31], while a combination of vitamin C and α-tocopherol (vitamin E) is particularly effective in inhibiting oxidation [31].

Excellent food sources of vitamin C include broccoli, bell peppers, parsley, Brussels sprouts, cauliflower, lemon juice, strawberries, mustard greens, kiwifruit, papaya, kale, cabbage, romaine lettuce, turnip greens, oranges, cantaloupe, summer squash, grapefruit, pineapple, chard, tomatoes, collard greens, raspberries, spinach, green beans, fennel, cranberries, asparagus, watermelon and winter squash.

7.4.2 Vitamin E

Vitamin E is a lipid-soluble vitamin found in cell membranes and circulating lipoproteins. It protects against oxidative damage by reacting directly with a variety of oxygen radicals. Its antioxidant capacity is strenthened by vitamin C-mediated regeneration [32]. Vitamin E is thought to play a role in preventing atherosclerosis [33]. This is corroborated by observations that animals deficient in vitamin E show higher isoprostane (marker of lipid peroxidation and oxidative stress) formation [29]. Moreover, vitamin E supplementation has been shown to inhibit isoprostane formation in both humans and animal models [34]. The major form of vitamin E in humans is α-tocopherol. Interactions between α-tocopherol and β-carotene are not as obvious as those reported with vitamin C, but α-tocopherol and β-carotene have been shown to exert a cooperative effect. This is best illustrated by their residing in different positions in the lipophilic compartment where they both scavenge free radicals [31].

Excellent sources of vitamin E include spinach, turnip greens and chard. Very good sources of vitamin E include mustard greens, cayenne pepper, sunflower seeds, almonds, bell peppers and asparagus. Good sources of vitamin E include collard greens, kale, tomatoes, cranberries, broccoli, Brussels sprouts, papaya, raspberries and carrots.

7.4.3 Carotenoids

Carotenoids are lipid-soluble antioxidants. Plasma levels of carotenoids are negatively correlated with isoprostane levels [28] and are inversely associated with inflammation, atherosclerosis, cardiovascular disease, sarcopenia and mortality [35]. They correlate positively with physical performance [36]. Carotenoid supplementation has been reported to improve antioxidant status and reduce lipid peroxidation [34]. The best known and most studied carotenoid is β-carotene, capable of rapidly quenching singlet oxygen [37]. β-carotene, α-carotene, β-cryptoxanthin, lycopene and lutein/zeaxanthin have all been associated with inflammation. Low-serum β-carotene levels were recently shown to be associated with an increased risk of mortality [35].

Orange-colored fruits and vegetables, including carrots, apricots, mangoes, squash, papaya and sweet potatoes contain significant amounts of beta-carotene, alpha-carotene, and beta-cryptoxanthin. Green vegetables, especially spinach, kale and collard greens, also contain beta-carotene. Other sources of carotenoids are salmon, shellfish, milk and eggs.

Vitamin C, vitamin E and carotenoids have been shown to act in synergy to prevent lipid peroxidation [31]. Higher serum antioxidant levels are associated with greater strength and improved physical performance [36], suggesting that oxidative damage may play an important role in the onset of disabling processes.

7.4.4 Vitamins B

The efficacy of antioxidation is complemented by the B vitamin group to a non-negligible extent. The complementarity of B-group vitamins' action is due to the roles played by enzymatic cofactors in the glutathione cycle, homocystein metabolism and cellular oxidation-reduction reactions [15]. Indeed, the flavin coenzymes—flavin mononucleotide (FMN) and flavin adenine dinucleotide (FAD)—are derivatives of vitamin B2 (riboflavin). They play an important role in both the respiratory cycle and energy production. FMN and FAD are electron transporters and oxidoreduction coenzymes. In red blood cells, FAD-dependent glutathione reductase is responsible for regenerating gluthathione, which is oxidised when glutathione peroxidase neutralises hydrogen peroxide. FAD, through its capacity to reoxidise NADPH, H+, stimulates erythrocyte glutathione reductase activity.

Thus, vitamin B2 should figure as an antioxidant vitamin, as it is a necessary cofactor involved in the glutathione cycle and for glutathione reductase activity. Other micronutrients such as polyphenols may also have significant antioxidant activity, possibly greater than that of vitamin E [38].

Finally, allyl sulphides, the sulphur compounds found in garlic, possess antioxidant properties by increasing the activity of superoxide dismutases (SOD), catalase, glutathione peroxidase and glutathione in cells [39].

Sources of vitamin B2 include crimini mushrooms, and calf liver, spinach summer squash, asparagus, chard, shiitake mushrooms, green beans, mustard greens, broccoli, collard greens, venison, turnip greens, eggs, yoghurt and cow's milk. Good sources of vitamin B include spinach, flaxseeds, shiitake mushrooms, salmon, chicken breast, asparagus (B1, B3), garlic, tuna, cauliflower and mustard greens (B6). Sources of vitamin B12 are limited to animal foods, including snapper, calf's liver, venison, shrimp, scallops and salmon.

In summary, antioxidants play important roles in many cellular and biochemical processes. However, the balance between oxidant and reducing forces is subtle. Trace elements with antioxidant properties such as selenium may become strongly pro-oxidant both *in vivo* and *in vitro*, if not present in appropriate properties. This is also the case with vitamins A, C and E, which may become pro-oxidant in some conditions [27]. For example, vitamin E becomes a pro-oxidant in isolated lipoprotein suspensions (e.g. parenteral nutrition solutions used in a clinical setting). The pro-oxidant effects of selenium have been investigated on cultured vascular cells exposed to parenteral nutrition solutions containing selenium in various forms and quantities. As part of preventing these potential deleterious effects of antioxidants, a study suggested that vitamin C could play an important role in preventing the pro-oxidant effect of Vitamin E in LDL oxidation [40].

To date no studies are available concerning possible vitamin deficit in masters athletes. However, masters athletes may present a greater risk of vitamin deficiencies due to age-related changes in the ability to absorb and metabolise vitamins and the detrimental effect of chronic diseases in older individuals.

7.5 ANTIOXIDANTS AND EXERCISE: ROLE OF VITAMIN SUPPLEMENTATION

7.5.1 Antioxidants and Acute Exercise

Long-duration physical exercise such as that undertaken by masters endurance athletes appears to alter the enzymatic and non-enzymatic defence systems [41]. Studies have reported a significant reduction in the erythrocyte superoxide dismutase concentration after exercise [41]. However, this reduction does not appear to depend on the duration of exercise. Indeed, reduced SOD was observed both after 30 seconds of supramaximal Wingate-type anaerobic exercise [42] and after a marathon [41]. In addition, the effect of training on SOD concentrations has been described in a few studies [43,44]. These report a greater resting SOD activity in trained subjects compared to non-trained subjects.

A reduction in circulating GSHPx concentrations after exercise was shown by several studies [42]. Reduced glutathione is one of the main elements involved in detoxifying the ROS formed during oxidative metabolism. So it is not unexpected to see a decrease in availability of this compound following exercise [45]. However, another study showed that 90 minutes of exercise at 60% of VO_{2max} had no effect on the reduced/oxidised glutathione ratio compared to resting values [46]. Thus, the reduced/oxidised glutathione ratio appears to vary with the duration of exercise and its intensity. For example, 30 minutes of pedalling at an intensity below the aerobic threshold does not induce oxidative stress, while an intensity above the anaerobic threshold tends to trigger indicators of this type of stress [17].

Reports pertaining to variations in vitamin concentrations during exercise are contradictory. Some reports indicate a reduction in α-tocopherol (vitamin E) after exercise suggesting that lipid peroxidation induced by participation in a 50-km ultra-marathon is associated with decreased vitamin E levels in athletes [47,48]. Other studies report an increase in vitamin E after dynamic exercise [49]. Yet another study suggests that plasma α-tocopherol levels appear unchanged immediately and 120 hours after a semi-marathon [50]. All these studies involve different types of exercise, sampling times, level of training of subjects and changes in plasma volumes, which could explain the different vitamin E responses to exercise.

For vitamin C, an increase in plasma ascorbic acid (vitamin C) from 52.7 to 67.0 mmol/L immediately after a 21-km running race was reported [51]. However, 24 hours after the race, the vitamin C concentration had dropped by 20% compared to the pre-race concentrations. The level remained low 48 hours later. The immediate post-exercise increase in vitamin C correlates with an increase in cortisol levels. Gleeson et al. suggest that the increase in ascorbic acid could be the result of concomitant cortisol release [51]. Duthie et al. [50] also describe an increase in vitamin C concentrations 5 minutes after a semi-marathon, but in this study levels had returned to baseline at 48 hours post-exercise. The changes in ascorbic acid observed at 5 minutes by Duthie et al. may be due to a 6% reduction in total plasma volume [50].

Plasma ß-carotene concentrations were also affected after a marathon [52]. The reduced availability of ß-carotene and other carotenoids after exercise appears to confirm their role in protecting the body against oxidative damage [41]. In older individuals, considerable evidence is available to support the suggestion that ageing skeletal muscle may be more susceptible to eccentric-exercise-induced injury than young skeletal muscle [53]. This intrinsic damage seen in older subjects may also be due to the accumulation of oxidised forms of proteins. With advancing age, rates of skeletal muscle lipid peroxidation (as well as antioxidant enzyme activities) have been shown to increase [54]. The accumulation of oxidised proteins in muscle may indicate that with age the increase in the rate of lipid peroxidation is greater than the increase in the activities of antioxidant enzymes.

7.5.2 Antioxidants and Chronic Exercise

Studies involving sprint activity [55] or endurance training [56] revealed no variations in muscle SOD activity. In contrast, other studies indicated a slight increase in SOD activity (40% to 60% above baseline), mainly in type IIb muscle fibres following training in animal models [57]. Many factors could explain these divergent results. For example, the different SOD isoenzymes, non-identical analysis methods and the intensity and duration of training. In addition, SOD and catalase levels may be altered in individuals who train intensively compared to moderately trained subjects [58].

Most studies in rats indicate identical catalase (CAT) activity, or reduced activity, after aerobic-type training. Although less data is available for humans, Miyazaki et al. [59] and Marsh et al. [60] confirm the observations from animal studies. They also note that there is no modification to catalase activity after completion of a training program. In contrast, catalase activity is increased increased in rats after 5 to 12 weeks of aerobic training and this increase appears to depend on the duration of training [61]. In humans, endurance training improves glutathione status as it does in animals [62]. An increase in GSH over the first 20 weeks of training, with stable high levels over the following 20 weeks has been reported in endurance runners population [62].

The antioxidant status of experienced runners between 20 and 40 years old (80–147 miles/week), moderately trained runners (16–43 miles/week) and sedentary subjects was examined in another study [63]. These authors report that the highest antioxidant capacities are detected in experienced runners. This population of runners have a higher catalase activity, as well as higher GSH and vitamin E levels. In corroboration of this positive effect of training on antioxidant levels, a mountain training session appears to increase plasma concentrations of vitamin C and E in professional cyclists [64]. Thus, chronic training appears to cause the antioxidant defence mechanisms to adapt, allowing an increase in the capacity to resist free radical damage. This adaptation does not involve large modifications to expression of antioxidant enzymes. Despite adapation, the resistance capacity is not optimal, and the massive production of free radicals during and after exercise can lead to extensive oxidation of biological macromolecules [13].

7.5.3 Antioxidants and Ageing

With ageing, increased production of free radicals may be related to changes to the enzymatic defence mechanisms and increasing mitochondrial dysfunction [65]. Several studies suggest that the majority of antioxidants are present in lower quantities as the body ages [66]. Various protective enzymes, including superoxide dismutase, catalase and glutathione peroxide in the liver and kidney, but not in the heart and brain, were also shown to decrease with age [67].

SOD and how it is affected by ageing has been reviewed [68]. In addition, a range of publications showed an age-related reduction in catalase and glutathione peroxide activity, both in mononuclear cells and plasma or erythrocyte platelets [69]. A study of American women showed a significant increase in oxidative stress in healthy women over 50 years of age compared to younger women [70]. Similarly, in healthy men over 60 years, the reduced glutathione pool is observed to be reduced, and a drop in erythrocyte antioxidant defences in the form of Cu, Zn-SOD and glutathione peroxidase are also reported [71]. However, despite this apparent consensus, the results described in the literature show that the relationship between antioxidant enzymes and ageing is not simple to establish.

7.6 VITAMIN SUPPLEMENTATION AND AGEING

Antioxidant status decreases in older subjects. Therefore the role of antioxidant micronutrients for this population appears essential. An optimal vitamin status helps fight the damaging effects of free radicals, and thus helps prevent accelerated cellular ageing [72]. In older healthy subjects who are independent and living at home, the prevalence of micronutrient deficiencies is comparable to that reported for younger subjects [73].

The benefits of a diet rich in fruit and vegetables are well known. These benefits have been attributed to their high levels of antioxidants and micronutrients (vitamins C, E, selenium, zinc, ß-carotene) and other microconstituants such as flavonoids and sulphides [74]. Various studies indicate that individuals who eat few fruit and vegetables and/or present low blood antioxidant levels are at a higher risk of developing diseases such as cancer, degenerative diseases and cardiovascular disease [75]. In addition, deficiencies in antioxidant vitamins have been associated with an increased cardiovascular risk and a higher incidence of cancer [76]. Finally, several studies suggest that a moderate selenium deficiency is associated with a significant drop in immune-competence [77]. Diseases involving oxidative stress are a human and financial burden, making them major public health issues. These diseases may be prevented or at least attenuated by increasing dietary intake of antioxidants.

All the results available in the literature highlight the need to optimise dietary intake of antioxidants. Beyond primary prevention, the antioxidant intake could also limit exercise-related oxidative stress and many related tissue injuries [12]. Furthermore in old exercisers, exercise greatly increases the production of oxygen radicals and the increased rates of lipid peroxidation resulting from oxygen radical production may cause skeletal damage. The consensus of the literature is that long- or short-term supplementation with vitamins has no ergogenic effect on exercise performance; however, the effects of these antioxidant vitamins may be subtle, and the positive health benefits of using vitamins may suggest an additive or synergistic effect when a vitamin is combined with regular exercise [5,78].

7.7 SUPPLEMENTATION AND EXERCISE IN MASTERS ATHLETES: PRACTICAL ASPECTS

7.7.1 Vitamin Supplementation, Fatigue and Recovery

Recovery following exercise can be split into the three following categories: (1) recovery immediately after exhausting exercise, (2) short-term recovery between repeats (e.g. between workloads) and (3) recovery between training sessions. The latter is particularly important as complete recovery between sessions is essential if performance is to progress. It also helps avoid excessive training or overtraining syndrome [79]. Fatigued subjects generally report muscle injuries, inflammation and a state of oxidative stress after intense physical exercise. When these effects are extensive they can temporarily exceed the body's defence capacities, limiting muscular recovery.

During training, several factors modify recovery capacity. On the one hand, acute fatigue after exercise or a training session is associated with peripheral phenomena and muscle injury lasting several days. These hinder full recovery leading to a progressive reduction in maximal voluntary force [79]. On the other hand, the central fatigue hypothesis suggests that the brain acts to protect the body by preventing excessive muscle injury. This protective mechanism could be the main influence on muscular performance, as measured during recovery [80]. Multiple strategies to improve or accelerate recovery during training have been described in the literature and include cryotherapy techniques, anti-inflammatory drugs and post-session massages [81].

Muscle injury may be linked to the formation of ROS (oxidative stress). Indeed, one hypothesis suggests that ROS are the main cause of injury to the muscle cells, rather than mechanical trauma. In this context, poor diet and ageing would further accentuate the muscle damage, contributing to increased fatigue and poor recovery [82,83].

This hypothesis has led to numerous investigations of the potential benefits of antioxidants and, more specifically, vitamin supplementation in preserving muscle function after acute exercise both in young [84] and older subjects [85]. An appropriate micronutritional intake could be beneficial through accelerating the return to hydromineral and antioxidant equilibrium necessary for muscular recovery. Many micronutritional supplements are currently available on the market. They are widely used by athletes to increase their antioxidant status.

The available data on the effects of vitamin supplementation on muscular recovery remain contradictory. For example, Goldfarb et al. showed that daily supplementation with vitamins E, C and mineral selenium for 14 days before and 2 days after eccentric exercise of the elbow flexors could help attenuate the increase in lipid peroxidation markers post-exercise in younger women aged 19–31 years [86]. More recently, Gauché et al. studied 24 well-trained runners aged 39.7 ± 1.7 years competing in a 65-km mountain running event [87]. They reported that the runners taking an antioxidant combination supplement (mainly consisting of vitamins E and C) for 21 days before and 2 days after the event recovered maximal strength of the thigh extensors more rapidly than athletes in a placebo group. Similarly, taking vitamin C alone before an effort has been shown to have protective effects against cellular damage induced by eccentric contractions [88]. Vitamin C, acting together with glutathione peroxidase, could protect cellular structures, such as the endoplasmic reticulum, against radical-induced membrane damage. Thus, taking an antioxidant complex could limit both lipid peroxidation and inflammation during and after exercise bouts [89].

More recently, Louis et al. studied the effect of an antioxidant complex on muscular fatigue in master endurance (cycling and running) athletes aged 66.1 ± 5.8 years [11]. The supplement was composed mainly of vitamins E and C, and was taken for 21 days before exercise [11]. The results of this study reveal an inverse correlation between fatigue and supplementation when investigating either cycling efficiency, during a 10-minute constant intensity cycling task (i.e. above the ventilatory threshold), or on muscular activity, recorded during dynamic and isometric exercises. During cycling exercises, fatigue induced a decrease in overall efficiency, with an increase in the VO_2 slow component and in agonistic muscular activity for both supplemented and placebo groups. However, these changes were significantly lower for the supplemented group. Moreover, despite a similar drop in maximal isometric voluntary torque after fatiguing exercise for both supplemented and placebo groups, the decrease in electromyographic frequency parameters (median frequency and mean power frequency) was significantly lower for the supplemented group. These results suggest a significant effect of vitamin and mineral supplementation on exercise tolerance in well-trained elderly subjects.

In a subsequent study Louis et al. studied the effect of this type of vitamin supplementation on recovery in masters athletes (50.8 ± 6.5 years) participating in a 3-week training program involving eccentric exercise [90]. Supplements were administered for 21 days before training, and throughout the 3-week training period. A positive effect of supplementation on inter-session recovery was observed, along with improvements in strength at the end of the training period. These results are comparable to those reported earlier by Hausswirth et al. who observed faster strength recovery after exhausting exercise when subjects receive supplements, with full recovery of maximal strength capacities 48 hours after exhausting exercises reported for the group receiving supplements and slower recovery in the placebo group [84].

While there have been contradictory finding on the effects of vitamin supplementation on exercise performance, recovery and ageing, recent studies on masters athletes suggest that supplementation combining several vitamins at the recommended doses over a period of 3 weeks improved recovery of performance levels, in particular after training involving eccentric exercises. However, these studies did not identify the mechanisms linking supplementation to an effect on muscle injury.

7.7.2 Vitamin Supplementation and Muscle Damage

Reports relating to the effect of vitamin supplementation, in particular with vitamin C, on muscle injury are contradictory. There is currently no convincing evidence that vitamin C or vitamin E taken individually protect against muscle damage [91]. Vitamin C is primarily found in the plasma and is not stored in the active tissue to any great extent. Therefore, raising plasma vitamin C levels to coincide with increased ROS production, such as during the inflammatory phase of muscle damage, could offer increased antioxidant protection at the time of peak ROS production.

The effects of an acute dose of ascorbic acid taken 2 hours before intermittent shuttle running for 90 minutes were investigated by using a placebo-controlled, crossover design in young subjects (22 ± 0.4 years) [92]. The results suggested that supplementation did not affect the moderate increases in serum CK, serum aspartate aminotransferase or delayed onset muscle soreness (DOMS). Subsequent studies also showed that vitamin C supplements taken for 3 days after intermittent shuttle running exercises had no effect on the increase in interleukin (IL)-6 response [93]. The same study found post-exercise supplementation with vitamin C did not affect any markers of muscle damage or lipid peroxidation. Similarly, Beaton et al. studied muscle damage in young healthy men who received either vitamin E or placebo for 30 days prior to eccentric contractions of the quadriceps [94]. They observed no effect of vitamin E on serum CK, torque loss or DOMS.

While supplemetation with either vitamin C or E alone does not appear to protect against DOMS, several other studies have examined the effects of combined supplements, usually containing vitamins C and E, and occasionally other antioxidants, on indices of oxidative stress and/or muscle damage reporting that an antioxidant complex could limit both lipid peroxidation and inflammation [91].

Earlier, Rokitski et al. showed that a complex with vitamin E (400 international units (IU) of vitamin E/kg) (15 mg per day of vitamin E corresponds to 22 IU) and vitamin C (200 mg) for 4 weeks in young trained subjects reduced the drop in creatine kinase levels after a marathon [52]. Furthermore, Viguie et al. reported that a mixture of antioxidants, containing 10 mg ß-carotene, 1000 mg vitamin C and 800 IU vitamin E taken over 8 weeks helps maintain glutathione levels, and attenuates the rise in CK observed after exercise on a treadmill at 65% of VO_{2max} [95]. Finally, Kaikkonen et al. observed that vitamin E (13.5 mg) and ubiquinone (90 mg) taken for 3 weeks have a minor effect on the CK response after a marathon [96].

Dietary supplementation in vitamins and micronutrients also appear to reduce the exercise-induce increase in markers of muscle injury. Jakeman and Maxwell studied 24 young physically active subjects and the effects of consuming vitamin E and vitamin C (400 mg each) for 21 days before and 7 days after eccentric exercise for 60 minutes [97]. They concluded that vitamin C has a protective effect against muscle injury induced by this type of exercise. According to Kanter et al. a supplement combining vitamins E and C and ß-carotene taken for 6 weeks reduces the resting and exercise levels of lipid peroxidation markers [98]. Similarly, Goldfarb et al. showed that supplementation with 400 IU of vitamin E, 1 g vitamin C and 90 mg selenium per day for 14 days before and 2 days after eccentric exercise of the elbow flexors reduced the rise in lipid peroxidation markers and stress proteins [86]. More recently, Mastaloudis et al. studied a group of 22 young runners during an ultra-marathon over 50 km and the effects of taking 1000 mg vitamin C and 300 mg vitamin E [99]. In these subjects, it appears that the treatment reduced lipid peroxidation. These investigators suggest that antioxidants such as vitamin E, C and selenium, when taken as combined supplements, appear to reduce lipid peroxidation.

Similarly Machefer et al. investigated the effect of a moderate mutivitamin and mineral supplementation containing mainly vitamin C (150.0 mg·day^{-1}), vitamin E (24.0 mg·day^{-1}) and β-carotene (4.8 mg·day^{-1}) prior to and during an extreme running competition—the Marathon des Sables—in 17 athletes (41.3 ± 2.6 yrs) [100]. The results suggested that the combination of multivitamin and mineral antioxidant complex prevented lipid peroxidation induced by repetition of exercises and may improve mobilisation and/or utilisation of antioxidant vitamins. However, according to both these studies, vitamin supplementation cannot prevent the considerable increase in inflammation markers induced by participation in an ultra-marathon.

In summary, the majority of studies have failed to demonstrate a protective effect of various individual supplementation strategies on markers of muscle damage. It is thus suggested that supplementing with vitamin C or vitamin E alone does not provide specific protection from the species of ROS formed during exercise. However, the combined effects of exogenous antioxidants may help protect the body against the potentially toxic effects of free radicals. Nevertheless, antioxidant intake should always remain within the recommended intake limits.

7.7.3 Vitamin Supplementation and Exercise: Negative Effects

While the combined effects of vitamin supplementation may have positive effects in athletes, recent research has found that long-term antioxidant supplementation at high doses, in particular with vitamin E, may increase mortality [101]. Based on the existing literature, there is no strong evidence for recommending antioxidant supplementation to athletes or other individuals habitually performing potentially damaging exercise. Given that antioxidants do not appear to help protect against muscle damage, and that vitamin E, in particular, may in fact be harmful, the casual use of large doses of antioxidants should be discouraged in healthy older adults and exercisers.

Masters athletes and older exercisers should note that antioxidant supplementation may not only fail to protect against muscle damage, but could in fact interfere with the cellular signalling functions of ROS [102]. A growing body of evidence exists describing the detrimental health effects of high doses of antioxidants taken as supplements. This is in contrast with studies showing the benefits of exercise training for performance. Indeed, although ROS are associated with harmful biological events, they are also essential to the development and optimal function of every cell.

Peternelj and Coombes recently reviewed the results of 23 studies and concluded that antioxidant supplementation interferes with training-induced adaptations [103]. The main findings of these studies are that loading the cell with high doses of antioxidants can blunt the positive effects of exercise training by interfering with important ROS-mediated physiological processes, such as vasodilation and insulin signalling. Therefore, ingesting antioxidant vitamins, rather than enhancing muscle performance, may actually slow the processes whereby individuals adapt to exercise through training.

7.8 CONCLUSION

Masters athletes need to match energy intake and expenditure to maintain optimal health and maximise sports performance. Intake of adequate calories and proportions of carbohydrate, fat and protein will sustain the energy requirements of training, recovery and competition. Masters endurance athletes in particular must include adequate vitamin (and mineral) intakes to maintain immune function.

Masters athletes who have a high energy intake should not require vitamin supplementation. However, given that both ageing and high-intensity exercise create oxidative stress, older athletes who are not taking adequate energy intakes or eating a healthy diet may compromise the health of their immune system. This cohort may benefit from vitamin supplementation based on the antioxidant vitamins A, C and E. Furthermore, recent studies in both young or masters athletes suggest that supplementation combining several vitamins at the recommended doses over a period of 3 weeks may improve recovery, in particular after training involving eccentric exercises. More research is required to examine the vitamin needs of masters athletes and older exercisers in general.

7.9 IMPLICATIONS FOR SPORTS MEDICINE PROFESSIONALS AND CLINICIANS

- Long-duration physical exercise appears to alter the enzymatic and non-enzymatic defence systems to oxidative stress.
- Physical training increases the capacity to resist free radical damage.
- An optimal vitamin status helps fight the damaging effects of free-radicals, and thus helps prevent accelerated cellular ageing.
- The combined effects of exogenous antioxidants such as vitamins can help protect the body against the potentially toxic effects of free radicals. Nevertheless, vitamin intake should always remain within the recommended limit.

7.10 IMPLICATIONS FOR MASTERS ATHLETES AND COACHES

- The available results on the effects of vitamin supplementation on muscular performance remain contradictory.
- Supplementing with vitamin C or vitamin E separately has no protective effect of on markers of muscle damage or recovery.
- Recent studies in both young or masters athletes show that supplementation combining several vitamins at the recommended doses over a period of 3 weeks improved recovery of performance levels, in particular after training involving eccentric exercises.
- Ingesting high doses of antioxidant vitamins can blunt the positive effects of exercise training especially on protein synthesis.
- To date there is no strong evidence for recommending vitamin supplementation to athletes or individuals of any age with an optimal vitamin status.

7.11 FUTURE RESEARCH DIRECTIONS

- Most of the previous studies on vitamin supplementation did not use a crossover design, thus it is possible that effects of vitamin supplementation are actually due to group differences.
- Few studies have been conducted examining the effects of vitamin supplementation in masters athletes. It is therefore difficult to raise pratical conclusions from sedentary elderly subjects on the benefits of vitamin supplementation in masters athletes.
- Randomised, controlled, crossover experiments on the effects of viatmin supplementation and/or antioxidants are needed, especially with well-trained endurance masters subjects.

REFERENCES

1. Bernard, T., Sultana, F., Lepers, R., Hausswirth, C. and Brisswalter, J., Age-related decline in olympic triathlon performance: Effect of locomotion mode, *Exp. Aging Res.* 36, 64–78, 2010.
2. Lepers, R. and Maffiuletti, N.A., Age and gender interactions in ultraendurance performance: Insight from the triathlon, *Med. Sci. Sports Exerc.* 43, 134–9, 2011.
3. Trappe, S., Marathon runners: How do they age? *Sports Med.* 37, 302–5, 2007.
4. Calder, P.C. and Kew, S., The immune system: A target for functional foods? *Brit. J. Nutr.* 88(Suppl 2), S165–77, 2002.
5. Brisswalter, J. and Louis, J., Vitamin supplementation benefits in masters athletes, *Sports Med.* 44(3), 311–8, 2014.
6. Burke, L.M. and Read, R.S., Diet patterns of elite Australian male triathletes, *Phys. Sportsmed.* 5, 140–55, 1987.

7. Nieman, D.C., Henson, D.A., McAnulty, S.R. et al., Vitamin E and immunity after the Kona Triathlon World Championship, *Med. Sci. Sports Exerc.* 36, 1328–35, 2004.
8. Knez, W.L. and Peake, J.M., The prevalence of vitamin supplementation in ultraendurance triathletes, *Int. J. Sport Nutr. Exerc. Metab.* 20, 507–14, 2010.
9. Wickens, A.P., Ageing and the free radical theory, *Respir. Physiol.* 128, 379–91, 2001.
10. Dunn-Lewis, C., Kraemer, W.J., Kupchak, B.R. et al., A multi-nutrient supplement reduced markers of inflammation and improved physical performance in active individuals of middle to older age: A randomized, double-blind, placebo-controlled study, *Nutr. J.* 7, 10:90, 2011.
11. Louis, J., Hausswirth, C., Bieuzen, F. and Brisswalter, J., Vitamin and mineral supplementation effect on muscular activity and cycling efficiency in masters athletes, *Appl. Physiol. Nutr. Metab.* 35(3), 251–60, 2010.
12. Mc Bride, C. and Kraemer, W.J., Effect of resistance exercise on free radical production. *Med. Sci. Sports Exerc.* 30, 67–72, 1998.
13. Leeuwenburgh, C. and Heinecke J.W., Oxidative stress and antioxidants in exercise. *Curr. Med. Chem.* 8, 829–38, 2001.
14. Boveris, A. and Cadenas, E., Mitochondrial production of superoxide anions and its relationship to the antimycin insensitive respiration, *FEBS Lett.* 54, 311–4, 1975.
15. Halliwell, B. and Gutteridge, J.M.C., *Free Radicals in Biology and Medicine*, Oxford University Press, New York, 1999.
16. Child, R.B., Wilkinson, D.M., Fallowfield, J.L. and Donnelly, A.E., Elevated serum antioxidant capacity and plasma malondialdehyde concentration in response to a simulated half-marathon run, *Med. Sci. Sports Exerc.* 30, 1603–7, 1998.
17. Sen, C.K., Oxidants and antioxidants in exercise, *J. Appl. Physiol.* 79, 675–86, 1995.
18. Rubin, B.B., Romaschin, A., Walker, P.M., Gute, D.C. and Korthuis, R.J., Mechanisms of postischemic injury in skeletal muscle: Intervention strategies, *J. Appl. Physiol.* 80, 369–87, 1996.
19. Granger, D.N. and Korthuis, R.J., Physiologic mechanisms of postischemic tissue injury, *Annu. Rev. Physiol.* 57, 311–32, 1995.
20. Souza, H.P., Laurindo, F.R., Ziegelstein, R.C., Berlowitz, C.O. and Zweier, J.L., Vascular NAD(P)H oxidase is distinct from the phagocytic enzyme and modulates vascular reactivity control, *Am. J. Physiol. Heart Circ. Physiol.* 280, H658–67, 2001.
21. Baggiolini, M., Chemokines and leukocyte traffic, *Nature* 392, 565–8, 1998.
22. Peacock, E.E., Inflammation and cellular response to injury, in *Wound Repair,* H.A.F. Dudley, ed., W.B. Saunders, Philadelphia, 1984, pp 1–14.
23. Sastre, J., Pallardó, F.V., García de la Asunción, J. and Viña, J., Mitochondria, oxidative stress and aging, *Free Radic. Res.* 32, 189–98, 2000.
24. Aoi, W. and Sakuma, K., Oxidative stress and skeletal muscle dysfunction with aging, *Curr. Aging Sci.* 4(2), 101–9, 2011.
25. Venkatraman, J.T. and Pendergast, D.R., Effect of dietary intake on immune function in athletes, *Sports Med.* 32, 323–37, 2002.
26. Fang, Y.Z., Yang, S. and Wu, G., Free radicals, antioxidants, and nutrition, *Nutrition* 18, 872–9, 2002.
27. Berger, M.M., Can oxidative damage be treated nutritionally? *Clin. Nutr.* 24, 172–83, 2005.
28. Block, G., Dietrich, M., Norkus, E.P. et al., Factors associated with oxidative stress in human populations, *Am. J. Epidemiol.* 156, 274–85, 2002.
29. Morrow, J.D. and Roberts, L.J., The isoprostanes: Unique bioactive products of lipid peroxidation, *Prog. Lipid Res.* 36, 1–21, 1997.
30. Fusco, D., Colloca, G., Lo Monaco, M.R. and Cesari, M., Effects of antioxidant supplementation on the aging process, *Clin. Interv. Aging.* 2, 377–87, 2007.
31. Niki, E., Noguchi, N., Tsuchihashi, H. and Gotoh, N., Interaction among vitamin C, vitamin E, and beta-carotene, *Am. J. Clin. Nutr.* 62, 1322S–1326S, 1995.
32. Maxwell, S.R., Prospects for the use of antioxidant therapies, *Drugs* 49, 345–61, 1995.
33. Steinberg, D. and Lewis A., Conner Memorial Lecture. Oxidative modification of LDL and atherogenesis, *Circulation* 95(4), 1062–71, 1997.
34. Upritchard, J.E., Schuurman, C.R., Wiersma, A. et al., Spread supplemented with moderate doses of vitamin E and carotenoids reduces lipid peroxidation in healthy, nonsmoking adults, *Am. J. Clin. Nutr.* 78, 985–92, 2003.
35. Hu, P., Reuben, D.B., Crimmins, E.M., Harris, T.B., Huang, M.H. and Seeman, T.E., The effects of serum beta-carotene concentration and burden of inflammation on all-cause mortality risk in high-functioning older persons: MacArthur studies of successful aging, *J. Gerontol. A Biol. Sci. Med. Sci.* 59, 849–54, 2004.

36. Cesari, M., Pahor, M., Bartali, B. et al., Antioxidants and physical performance in elderly persons: The Invecchiare in Chianti study, *Am. J. Clin. Nutr.* 79, 289–94, 2004.
37. Di Mascio, P., Murphy, M.E. and Sies, H., Antioxidant defense systems: The role of carotenoids, tocopherols, and thiols, *Am. J. Clin. Nutr.* 53, 194S–200S, 1991.
38. Mc Kay, M. and Blumberg, M., The role of tea in human health: An update, *J. Am. Col. Nutr.* 21, 1–13, 2002.
39. Borek, C., Antioxidant health effects of aged garlic extract, *J. Nutr.* 131, 1010S–1015S, 2001.
40. Nakamura, Y.K., Read, M.H., Elias, J.W. and Omaye, S.T., Oxidation of serum low-density lipoprotein (LDL) and antioxidant status in young and elderly humans, *Arch. Gerontol. Geriatr.* 42, 265–76, 2006.
41. Machefer, G., Groussard, C., Rannou-Bekono, F. et al., Extreme running competition decreases blood antioxidant defense capacity, *J. Am. Coll. Nutr.* 23, 358–64, 2004.
42. Groussard, C., Rannou-Bekono, F., Machefer, G. et al., Changes in blood lipid peroxidation markers and antioxidants after a single sprint anaerobic exercise, *Eur. J. Appl. Physiol.* 89, 14–20, 2003.
43. Lekhi, C., Gupta, P.H. and Singh, B., Influence of exercise on oxidant stress products in elite Indian cyclists, *Br. J. Sports Med.*, 41, 691–3, 2007.
44. Knez, W.L., Jenkins, D.G. and Coombes, J.S., Oxidative stress in half and full Ironman triathletes, *Med. Sci. Sports Exerc.* 39, 283–8, 2007.
45. Dringen, R., Metabolism and functions of glutathione in brain, *Prog. Neurobiol.* 62, 649–71, 2000.
46. Gohil, K., Viguie, C., Stanley, W.C., Brooks, G.A. and Packer, L., Blood glutathione oxidation during human exercise, *J. Appl. Physiol.* 64, 115–9, 1988.
47. Briviba, K., Watzl, B., Nickel, K. et al., A half-marathon and a marathon run induce oxidative DNA damage, reduce antioxidant capacity to protect DNA against damage and modify immune function in hobby runners, *Redox. Rep.* 10, 325–31, 2005.
48. Mastaloudis, A., Leonard, S.W. and Traber, M.G., Oxidative stress in athletes during extreme endurance exercise, *Free Rad. Biol. Med.* 31, 911–22, 2001.
49. Pincemail, J., Deby, C., Camus, G. et al., Tocopherol mobilization during intensive exercise, *Eur. J. Appl. Physiol.* 57, 189–91, 1988.
50. Duthie, G.G., Robertson, J.D., Maughan, R.J. and Morrice, P.C., Blood antioxidant status and erythrocyte lipid peroxidation following distance running, *Arch. Biochem. Biophys.* 282, 78–83, 1990.
51. Gleeson, M., Robertson, J.D. and Maughan, R.J., Influence of exercise on ascorbic acid status in man, *Clin. Sci.* 73, 501–5, 1987.
52. Rokitzki, L., Logemann, E., Sagredos, A.N., Murphy, M., Wetzel-Roth, W. and Keul, J., Lipid peroxidation and antioxidative vitamins under extreme endurance stress, *Acta. Physiol. Scand.* 151, 149–58, 1994.
53. Manfredi, T.G., Fielding, R.A., O'Reilly, K.P., Meredith, C.N., Lee, H.Y. and Evans, W.J., Plasma creatine kinase activity and exercise-induced muscle damage in older men, *Med. Sci. Sports Exerc.* 23, 1028–34, 1991.
54. Ji, L.L., Dillon, D. and Wu, E., Alteration of antioxidant enzymes with aging in rat skeletal muscle and liver, *Am. J. Physiol.* 258, R918–23, 1990.
55. Hellsten, Y., Apple, F.S. and Sjödin, B., Effect of sprint cycle training on activities of antioxidant enzymes in human skeletal muscle, *J. Appl. Physiol.* 81, 1484–7, 1996.
56. Tonkonogi, M., Walsh, B., Svensson, M. and Sahlin, K., Mitochondrial function and antioxidative defence in human muscle: Effects of endurance training and oxidative stress, *J. Physiol.* 528, 379–88, 2000.
57. Powers, S.K., Criswell, D., Lawler, J. et al., Influence of exercise and fiber type on oxidant enzyme activity in rat skeletal muscle, *Am. J.Physiol.* 266, R375–80, 1994.
58. Jenkins, R.R., Friedland, R. and Howald, H., The relationship of oxygen uptake to superoxide dismutase and catalase activity in human skeletal muscle, *Int. J. Sports Med.* 5, 11–4, 1984.
59. Miyazaki, H., Oh-ishi, S., Ookawara, T. et al., Strenuous endurance training in humans reduces oxidative stress following exhausting exercise, *Eur. J. Appl. Physiol.* 84, 1–6, 2001.
60. Marsh, S.A., Laursen, P.B. and Coombes, J.S., Effects of antioxidant supplementation and exercise training on erythrocyte antioxidant enzymes, *Int. J. Vitam. Nutr. Res.* 76, 324–31, 2006.
61. Powers, S.K. and Sen, C.K., Physiological antioxidants and exercise training, in *Handbook of Oxidants and Antioxidants in Exercise,* C.K. Sen, L. Packer and O. Hänninen, eds., Elsevier, Amsterdam, the Netherlands, 2000, pp. 221–241.
62. Evelo, C.T., Palmen, N.G., Artur, Y. and Janssen, G.M., Changes in blood glutathione concentrations, and in erythrocyte glutathione reductase and glutathione S-transferase activity after running training and after participation in contests, *Eur. J. Appl. Physiol.* 64, 354–8, 1992.

63. Robertson, J.D., Maughan, R.J., Duthie, G.G. and Morrice, P.C., Increased blood antioxidant systems of runners in response to training load, *Clin. Sci.* 80, 611–8, 1991.
64. Aguiló, A., Tauler, P., Pilar Guix, M., Villa, G., Córdova, A., Tur, J.A. and Pons A., Effect of exercise intensity and training on antioxidants and cholesterol profile in cyclists, *J. Nutr. Biochem.*14, 319–25, 2003.
65. Wei, Y.H., Lu, C.Y., Wei, C.Y., Ma, Y.S. and Lee, H.C., Oxidative stress in human aging and mitochondrial disease. Consequences of defective mitochondrial respiration and impaired anti-oxidant enzyme system, *Chin. J. Physiol.* 44, 1–11, 2001.
66. Pinzani, P., Petruzzi, E., Orlando, C. et al., Reduced serum antioxidant capacity in healthy centenarians, *Clin. Chem.* 43, 855–6, 1997.
67. Cand, F. and Verdetti, J., Superoxide dismutase, glutathione peroxidase, catalase, and lipid peroxidation in the major organs of the aging rats, *Free Radic. Biol. Med.* 7, 59–63, 1989.
68. Mc Cord, J.M., Superoxide dismutase in aging and disease: An overview, *Methods Enzymol.* 349, 331–42, 2002.
69. Guemouri, L., Artur, Y., Herbeth, B., Jeandel, C., Cuny, G. and Siest, G., Biological variability of superoxide dismutase, gluthathione peroxidase and catalase in blood, *Clin. Chem.* 37, 1932–7, 1991.
70. Trevisan, M., Browne, R., Ram, M. et al., Correlates of markers of oxidative status in the general population, *Am. J. Epidemiol.* 154, 348–56, 2001.
71. Cristol, J.P., Maggi, M.F., Bosc, J.Y. et al., Oxidative stress and chronic renal insufficiency: What can be a prophylactic approach? *C. R. Seances Soc. Biol. Fil.* 191(4), 603–16, 1991.
72. Harman, D., Role of anti-oxidant nutrient in aging, *Age* 18, 51–62, 1995.
73. Cruz, J.A., Moreiras-Varela, O., Van Staveren, W.A., Trichopoulou, A., and Roszkowski, W., Intake of vitamins and minerals, *Eur. J. Clin. Nutr.* 45, 121–38, 1991.
74. Hu, P., Plant-based food and prevention of cardiovascular diseases, *Am. J. Cln. Nutr.* 78, 544–52, 2003.
75. Rissanen, T.H., Voutilainen, S., Virtanen, J.K. et al., Low intake of fruit, berries, and vegetables is associated with excess mortality in men: The Kuopio Ischaemic Heart Diseases Risk Factor (KIHD) Study, *J. Nutr.* 133, 199–204, 2003.
76. Jacob, R.A. and Burri, B.J., Oxidative damage and defense, *Am. J. Clin. Nutr.* 63, 985S–90S, 1996.
77. James, J.S., Selenium: Important new review of health findings. *AIDS Treat. News*. 347, 3–4, 2000.
78. Evans, W.J., Vitamin E, vitamin C, and exercise, *Am. J. Clin. Nutr*. 72, 647S–52S, 2000.
79. Barnett, A., Using recovery modalities between training sessions in elite athletes: Does it help? *Sports Med.* 36, 781–96, 2006.
80. Lepers, R., Hausswirth, C., Maffiuletti, N., Brisswalter, J. and van Hoecke, J., Evidence of neuromuscular fatigue after prolonged cycling exercise, *Med. Sci. Sports Exerc.* 32, 1880–6, 2000.
81. Hausswirth, C., Louis, J., Bieuzen, F. et al., Effects of whole-body cryotherapy vs. far-infrared vs. passive modalities on recovery from exercise-induced muscle damage in highly-trained runners, *PLoS One* 6(12), e27749, 2011.
82. Davis, J.M., Alderson, N.L. and Welsh, R.S., Serotonin and central nervous system fatigue: Nutritional considerations, *Am. J. Clin. Nutr.* 72, 573S–8S, 2000.
83. Nielsen, P. and Nachtigall, D., Iron supplementation in athletes. Current recommendations, *Sports Med.* 26, 207–16, 1998.
84. Hausswirth, C., Caillaud, C., Lepers, R. and Brisswalter, J. Influence of a vitamin supplementation on locomotion gross efficiency after an ultra-trail race, *Sci. Sports*. 21(1), 8–12, 2006.
85. Gauche, E., Hausswirth, C., Bieuzen, F., Lepers, R., Rabita, J. and Brisswalter, J., Vitamin and mineral complex supplementation on maximal voluntary contraction decrease and biological markers following an eccentric exercise in elderly active people, *Sci. Sports*. 22, 201–9, 2007.
86. Goldfarb, A.H., Bloomer, R.J. and McKenzie, M.J., Combined antioxidant treatment effects on blood oxidative stress after eccentric exercise, *Med. Sci. Sports Exerc.* 37, 234–9, 2005.
87. Gauche, E., Lepers, R., Rabita, G. et al., Vitamin and mineral supplementation and neuromuscular recovery after a running race, *Med. Sci. Sports Exerc.* 38(12), 2110–7, 2006.
88. Maxwell, S.R., Jakeman, P., Thomason, H., Leguen, C. and Thorpe, G.H., Changes in plasma antioxidant status during eccentric exercise and the effect of vitamin supplementation, *Free Radic. Res. Commun.* 19, 191–202, 1993.
89. Powers, S.K. and Hamilton K., Antioxidants and exercise, *Clin. Sports Med.* 18, 525–36, 1999.
90. Louis, J., Hausswirth, C., Bieuzen, F. and Brisswalter, J., Influence of a vitamin supplementation on maximal muscular performance during a strength-training program in masters athletes, *Sci. Sports* 25, 253–9, 2011.

91. McGinley, C., Shafat, A. and Donnelly, A.E., Does antioxidant vitamin supplementation protect against muscle damage? *Sports Med.* 39(12), 1011–32, 2009.
92. Thompson, D., Williams, C., Kingsley, M. et al., Muscle soreness and damage parameters after prolonged intermittent shuttle-running following acute vitamin C supplementation, *Int. J. Sports Med.* 22, 68–75, 2001.
93. Thompson, D., Williams, C., Garcia-Roves, P., McGregor, S.J., McArdle, F. and Jackson, M.J., Post-exercise vitamin C supplementation and recovery from demanding exercise, *Eur. J. Appl. Physiol.* 89, 393–400, 2003.
94. Beaton, L.J., Allan, D.A., Tarnopolsky, M.A., Tiidus, P.M. and Phillips, S.M., Contraction- induced muscle damage is unaffected by vitamin E supplementation, *Med. Sci. Sports Exerc.* 34, 798–805, 2002.
95. Viguie, C.A., Frei, B., Shigenaga, M.K., Ames, B.N., Packer, L. and Brooks, G.A., Antioxidant supplementation affects indices of muscle trauma and oxidant stress in human blood during exercise, *Med. Sci. Sports Exerc.* 21, S16, 1989.
96. Kaikkonen, J., Kosonen, L., Nyyssönen, K. et al., Effects of combined coenzyme Q10 and d-alpha-tocopheryl; acetate supplementation on exercise-induced lipid peroxidation and muscular damage: A placebo-controlled double-blind study in marathon runners, *Free Rad. Res.* 29, 85–92, 1998.
97. Jakeman, P. and Maxwell, S., Effect of antioxidant vitamin supplementation on muscle function after eccentric exercise, *Eur. J. Appl. Physiol.* 67, 426–30, 1993.
98. Kanter, M.M., Nolte, L.A. and Holloszy, J.O., Effects of an antioxidant vitamin mixture on lipid peroxidation at rest and postexercise, *J. Appl. Physiol.* 74, 965–9, 1993.
99. Mastaloudis, A., Morrow, J.D., Hopkins, D.W., Devaraj, S. and Traber, M.G., Antioxidant supplementation prevents exercise-induced lipid peroxidation, but not inflammation, in ultramarathon runners, *Free Rad. Biol. Med.* 36, 1329–41, 2004.
100. Machefer, G., Groussard, C., Vincent, S. et al., Multivitamin-mineral supplementation prevents lipid peroxidation during 'the Marathon des Sables', *J. Am. Coll. Nutr.* 26, 111–20, 2007.
101. Soni, M.G., Thurmond, T.S., Miller, E.R., Spriggs, T., Bendich, A. and Omaye, S.T., Safety of vitamins and minerals: Controversies and perspective, *Toxicol. Sci.* 118, 348–55, 2010.
102. Jackson, M.J., Free radicals generated by contracting muscle: By-products of metabolism or key regulators of muscle function? *Free Radic. Biol. Med.* 44(2), 132–41, 2008.
103. Peternelj, T.T. and Coombes, J.S., Antioxidant supplementation during exercise training: Beneficial or detrimental?, *Sports Med.* 41, 1043–69, 2011.

8 Mineral Needs of Masters Athletes

Erica Hirsch, Mrinalini Sharma and Stella Lucia Volpe

CONTENTS

8.1 INTRODUCTION

In the past few decades there has been an increase in the number of older individuals participating in recreational and competitive sports. For example, the inaugural World Masters Games held in 1985 in Toronto, Canada had 8305 participants across 22 sports. The 2002 Melbourne, Australia World Masters Games hosted 24,886 participants across 26 sports [1]. It has also been reported that there was a greater increase in the participation of masters athletes who participated in the New York City Marathon compared to younger age groups [2].

The growth in the number of older individuals engaging in physical activity, whether recreational or competitive, can be attributed to several factors including health benefits, social benefits or a combination of both. Moreover, researchers have repeatedly demonstrated that a consistent involvement in physical activity reduces the risk of many chronic diseases [3,4]. Apart from the health reasons, factors such as prior success in sports and self-image also play an important role in motivating people to engage in physical activity during their later years of life [5].

Masters participants range widely in age, but are typically older than 30 years of age (certain masters sports competition may begin as early as 21 years of age), and may include highly conditioned, experienced competitive athletes who continue to compete after their formal athletic careers end. However, masters athletes also include 'walk-up' competitors with only sporadic training regimens, as well as those who resume competition after long periods of physical inactivity [1]. With increasing age, masters athletes competing in various sports decline linearly in performance until about 70 years of age, after which the rate of decline appears to accelerate [5–11]. Nonetheless, as the competition grows both nationally and internationally, competitive athletes of all ages continue to search for technical, physiological and biological advantages to gain a competitive edge in performance.

Nutrition is one aspect that can provide a completive edge to athletes, and is equally a part of the overall training program as the physical training itself. Athletes have become increasingly interested in the beneficial role that adequate overall nutrition can have on exercise performance. Though individuals are concerned about macronutrients (fat, carbohydrates and protein), micronutrients (vitamins and minerals) are also concerns for athletes of all ages. Vitamins and minerals are not only needed to maintain energy metabolism, but are also required to perform a wide variety of biochemical and physiological functions, like enzymatic activity and antioxidant defence; therefore, vitamins and minerals have the potential to influence physical performance [12–14].

Striegel et al. examined the use of nutritional supplements in masters athletes via questionnaire to 1560 participants of the World Masters Indoor Athletics Championships held in 2004 [11]. They found that 60.5% of all masters athletes who responded to their survey reported the actual use of nutritional supplements. The primary supplements used were vitamins (35.4%) and minerals (29.9%). Unlike elite young athletes who typically use nutritional supplements to improve athletic performance, masters athletes stated that they took supplements primarily for health reasons. In addition, more than half of the surveyed masters athletes obtained most of their nutritional supplement information from their physicians or pharmacies. Striegel et al. [11] observed that masters athletes who took nutritional supplement did not fit into a specific profile. In addition, because supplements may sometimes contain trace amounts of anabolic steroids, physicians and sports dieticians need to educate masters athletes to be cautious of taking supplements.

Nutrition, in general, has been well documented to influence athletic performance. Appropriate selection and timing of food, as well as fluid and supplement intakes, are considered essential for optimal health and exercise performance [15]. Apart from an increased need for adequate energy intakes, regular and intense training may also increase an athlete's requirement for vitamins and minerals. This may be as a result of decreased gastrointestinal absorption, increased losses via sweat, urine and/or faeces, increased degradation rates, increased need for tissue maintenance and repair, adaptation in the beginning stages of heavy training and/or acute training that may increase energy metabolism [13,15]. Marginal micronutrient deficiency may not have a great impact on sedentary individuals, but may adversely affect athletes [15,16].

Minerals are involved in many important physiological roles such as muscle contraction, normal heart rhythm, nerve impulse conduction, oxygen transport, oxidative phosphorylation, enzyme activation, bone health and acid-base balance of the blood, and many of these processes are accelerated during exercise [12]. Therefore, an adequate amount of minerals is required for optimal functioning in athletes of any age.

Mineral requirements for the older competitors are further complicated by changes associated with the ageing process (see Chapter 1). Low energy intakes, impaired nutrient absorption, chronic medical conditions and specific age-related factors influence mineral intake and requirements [16]. According to the joint statement from the American Dietetic Association (now called The Academy of Nutrition and Dietetics), Dietitians of Canada and the American College of Sports Medicine, athletes will not need vitamin and mineral supplements if adequate energy to maintain body weight is consumed from a variety of foods [16]. However, older athletes (with specific age-related health conditions) and athletes who restrict energy intake, use severe weight-loss practices, eliminate one or more food groups from their diet or consume high-carbohydrate diets with low micronutrient density, may require one or more supplements [15,16].

With the growing number of masters athletes participating in recreational and competitive sports, it is important to assess their nutritional needs. Minerals are not only necessary for a wide variety of biochemical and physiological processes, but they can also have a great impact on work capacity and performance. Mineral requirements can change with both exercise and advancing age. Therefore, it is important for masters athletes to ensure they are maintaining adequate mineral levels and understand how these minerals can impact their exercise performance. This chapter will focus on the following minerals: calcium, phosphorus, magnesium, iron, zinc and chromium. Mineral status within individuals, the importance of the minerals on optimal exercise performance and studies conducted on mineral supplementation will be discussed.

8.2 CALCIUM

8.2.1 Calcium Status within Individuals

Calcium is one of the most important minerals in the body, as well as the most abundant, accounting for 1.5% to 2% of the adult body weight. Approximately 99% of calcium is located in the teeth and bones, while the remaining 1% can be found in blood, muscle, nervous tissue and in intracellular and extracellular fluids [12]. While the skeleton has obvious structural roles, it also serves as a reservoir for calcium [17]. Calcium is required in various bodily functions including muscle contractions, nerve conduction, blood coagulation, hormone release, neurotransmitter release, glycogen metabolism, vision and cellular differentiation, proliferation and motility [12,17].

Homeostatic control processes such as absorption, excretion, secretion and storage in bone closely regulate the serum levels of calcium. Serum levels of calcium are maintained between 8.5 to 10.2 mg/dL (2.2 to 2.5 mmol/L) [12]. This tight regulation of calcium is achieved by the interaction of the three calcitropic hormones: parathyroid hormone (PTH), 1-25, dihydroxyvitamin D_3 (calcitriol) and calcitonin. When the serum calcium concentration falls below normal levels of 9 to 11 mg/dL, PTH release is stimulated. PTH stimulates (1) osteoclastic activity, resulting in bone resorption, or the release of calcium from the bones, (2) the increase of renal tubular reabsorption of calcium and (3) the activation of the most active form of vitamin D (calcitriol) that facilitates increased absorption of calcium in the small intestine, via increased production of calbindin, which requires vitamin D for its synthesis [12]. In contrast, when serum calcium levels are greater than 11 mg/dL, calcitonin causes increased calcium deposition in the bones by increasing osteoblastic activity, increasing calcium excretion in the urine and decreasing calcium absorption in the small intestine. Vitamin D plays a particularly important role in calcium homeostasis, because calcium cannot be absorbed in the gastrointestinal tract without the presence of vitamin D. As a result, vitamin D promotes growth and mineralisation of bones by maintaining calcium homeostasis.

Normal growth and development of the skeleton are dependent upon calcium. As part of skeletal growth and maturation, which typically continues until the early 20s, but can continue to the age of 30 years for some parts of the skeleton, calcium is accumulated in the skeleton at an average rate of 150 mg per day [17]. During maturity, homeostatic controls continue to keep calcium more or less at equilibrium. However, from about the age of 50 years for men and menopause in women, bone is lost from all skeletal sites with post-menopausal women particularly at risk for decreasing bone mineral density (BMD) because their oestrogen levels decrease significantly following menopause [18]. After 50 years of age for men, bone mass is lost at a rate of 0.4% per year; however, they generally do not have osteoporotic problems until their 80s. Women lose bone at a much greater rate than men. They lose 0.75% to 1% of their bone mass per year beginning in their early 30s. After menopause this rate can possibly triple, with many women losing 30% of their bone mass before their 70s [19]. As a result, bones become more brittle and fragile. This bone loss results in an increased risk and vulnerability to bone fracture. Consequently, there is a marked rise in fracture rate in both men and women in older age, but particularly in women. Maintaining weight-bearing exercise throughout life can prevent bone loss at such a dramatic rate.

8.2.2 Importance of Calcium on Optimal Exercise Performance

Strong bones are not only essential to maintaining health and skeletal integrity, but are integral to the success of athletes of any age. The skeletal structure provides the strength and rigidity necessary to train and compete in sports. Research indicates that age, gender and race are contributing factors in BMD [20]. While these factors are uncontrollable, they provide important information with respect to predispositions to fractures and other potentially serious bone conditions [20]. According to the National Osteoporosis Foundation; non-Hispanic white women are afflicted most often with a BMD condition, although women of other ethnicities are vulnerable as well. African American populations tend to have higher BMD than other races/ethnicities, including Asian and Hispanic in age- and gender-related studies [20–22]. This difference is significant because it is estimated that African American women have up to 50% lower incidence of hip fractures compared to their Caucasian counterparts [20].

Although increases in BMD have been recorded through the third decade of life, skeletal growth is nearly complete by 18 years of age in both males and females [20]. According to the National Institutes of Health Osteoporosis and Related Bone Diseases, the amount of peak bone mass achieved and the subsequent rate of bone loss are the determinants of BMD later in life [23]. Bones require a life-long calcium intake. It is of vital importance to maintain adequate calcium intake at all stages of life, from early in life for peak bone mass to be achieved, through later adulthood, for skeletal mass to be maintained and age-related bone loss minimised [17]. The importance of calcium is further underlined by the fact that most adults are consuming less than the required amounts of calcium and are at a greater risk for stress fractures and other medical conditions. Additionally, vitamin D deficiency has become a worldwide epidemic, with 50% of the global population at risk [24]. A deficiency in vitamin D will compromise the absorption of calcium.

Masters athletes are particularly vulnerable to calcium deficiency due to the natural decline in bone mass associated with advancing age and the demand they have for strong bones. Masters athletes should make a conscious effort in meeting their calcium requirements, because a deficiency could result in less than optimal athletic performance and overall health. It is imperative to maintain a balance between calcium intake through the diet and/or supplementation and calcium loss through the urine, faeces and sweat. As previously mentioned, calcitropic hormones homeostatically control serum calcium concentrations in the body. As the calcium status of athletes falls below a certain level, PTH stimulates bone resorption, leading to a lower BMD and increased risk of bone fractures.

Various researchers have repeatedly shown that athletes with stress fractures have lower calcium intakes and lower intakes of dairy products [25]. Furthermore, the incidence of hip fractures is lower in females and males who had higher lifetime calcium intakes (more than 800 mg/d), compared to those with low lifetime calcium intakes [25]. Additionally, it has been shown that exercise may increase calcium losses. Dressendorfer and colleagues [26] examined the effects of a 10-week intense endurance training in nine competitive male cyclists. They measured baseline and 24-h urinary calcium, magnesium, iron, zinc and copper levels in these male athletes. The supervised training was as follows: baseline period, volume phase (6 weeks of training at about 87% of maximal heart rate); interval phase (18 days of training at about 100% of maximal heart rate); and 10 days of unloading or tapering. The main training outcome for this study was a 20-km cycling time trial. While the participants' diets were not controlled, they maintained their normal body weight. Dressendorfer et al. [26] found that urinary calcium concentrations increased and serum calcium levels decreased below the clinical norm following the high-intensity interval phase. However, these changes were reversed following the tapering phase. Thus, it appears that calcium excretion may be increased with high-intensity training [26]. In addition, it has been reported that sweat calcium losses during exercise could be as high as 57 mg/h [12]. Calcium loss via sweat, however, varies with both exercise duration and temperature. Additionally, female athletes may be at the greatest risk for low BMD if energy intakes are low, dairy products are eliminated from the diet and a menstrual dysfunction is present [15].

Masters athletes, especially females, need to ensure that their diet is rich in calcium. Maintaining adequate calcium levels is not only essential to preventing bone loss, but is needed to ensure strong bones, which is integral to an athlete's success. Moreover, due to exercise-induced losses, it is important to replenish calcium that has been excreted.

8.2.3 Studies Conducted on Calcium Supplementation

Calcium requirements vary throughout an individual's life, with greater needs during childhood and adolescence, during pregnancy and lactation and later in life [17]. Owing to the importance of calcium in bone growth and repair and tissue maintenance, adequate intakes should be encouraged beginning in early childhood. Calcium can be obtained primarily through dairy products, as well as dark leafy green vegetables. Other sources include fatty fish, nuts and subtropical fruits [27].

Calcium supplementation can also help to maintain adequate calcium levels, but it should not be used in substitution of dietary intake. Rather, it should be used in conjunction with dietary sources. Additionally, calcium supplements should be taken with vitamin D, which will improve calcium absorption. The timing of calcium supplements is also important. For optimal absorption, two separate doses of 500 mg should be taken with 200 to 400 international units (IUs) of vitamin D_3. Calcium carbonate should be taken with meals, whereas calcium citrate can be taken at any time. Calcium citrate has been shown to be better absorbed and is not affected by low acidity in the stomach. If taken with food, they should not be taken with foods that reduce calcium absorption, such as oxalates and phytates (examples of foods high in oxalates and phytates include baked beans, kidney beans, raw green peppers and boiled potatoes).

Masters athletes should consume diets that contain adequate calcium, especially since low dietary calcium intake is associated with an increased risk of stress fractures. Additionally, with advancing age, a decrease in stomach acid production (achlorhydria) typically caused by a condition called atrophic gastritis commonly occurs (see Chapter 1 for other factors affecting nutritional status in older populations). This condition can make it more difficult to absorb essential nutrients, including calcium. In addition, as a person ages, the production of vitamin D in the skin from sun exposure is lower, resulting in less 25-hydroxyvitamin D circulating in the blood [28]. As a result, masters athletes need to increase their daily calcium and vitamin D intakes. The United States Recommended Dietary Allowance (RDA) for calcium for men and women 19 to 50 years of age, as well as for men 51 years and older, is 1000 mg/d, while women 51 years and older require 1200 mg/d [13]. Adequate intake of vitamin D for men and women 19 to 70 years of age is 600 IU/d. For men and women greater than 70 years of age, 800 IU/d of vitamin D is required [13].

Numerous researchers have examined the effectiveness of calcium supplementation on bone loss. These studies have revealed that the effectiveness of supplementation varies by skeletal site, menopausal age and with calcium intakes of the participants [29–31]. Calcium supplementation with higher doses of calcium than normally consumed in the diet offers some protection against age-related loss of bone in men and women, with the strongest effect seen in women with very low habitual calcium intakes (e.g. less than 400 mg/d) [31].

The timing of additional calcium supplementation following menopause also seems to be important. Researchers have shown that calcium supplementation for women during the first 5 years of menopause is not effective in hindering bone loss from trabecular regions of the skeleton, including those most vulnerable to osteoporotic fracture [32–34], but is effective in slowing cortical bone loss [33–36]. Post-menopausal women (more than 5 years since menopause onset) appear to be more responsive to supplemental calcium. Post-menopausal women who took calcium carbonate supplements (1500 mg/d) had reduced rates of bone loss and a lower risk of vertebral fractures [32]. Post-menopausal women who took a milk supplement (831 mg/d) for 1 year significantly increased the BMD at the proximal femur, but not at the lumbar or radial sites, whereas a walking program slightly increased lumbar BMD [37].

Calcium citrate malate supplementation appears to be better absorbed in post-menopausal women with low dietary intakes of calcium and is more effective in reducing bone loss than calcium carbonate [38,39]. Use of 500 mg of calcium citrate malate over 2 years in post-menopausal women reduced the loss of BMD of the lumbar vertebrae, proximal femur and radius [33]. Post-menopausal women who took a 1000-mg/d calcium supplement over 4 years significantly reduced the rate of total body BMD decline and experienced less fractures (hip, forearm and vertebral) than women in the placebo group [40].

Combined supplementation with calcium and vitamin D for 3 years significantly reduced non-vertebral fracture rates in both men and women (mean age, 71 years) [41]. However, only slight differences have been seen after calcium and vitamin D supplementation ceased. Older men and post-menopausal women (≥68 years of age) supplemented with both calcium (500 mg/d) and vitamin D (700 IU/d) for 3 years showed little difference in BMD of the spine and femoral neck than those receiving placebo 2 years after supplementation had ceased [38]. A modest benefit was observed in total BMD in men, but not in women [38].

While calcium supplementation can help maintain adequate calcium intake, precaution is advised because excessive calcium consumption may inhibit the absorption of other minerals such as zinc and iron. Diets high in calcium can result in a negative zinc balance with post-menopausal women especially affected. Increased calcium intake can also impact dietary iron absorption; consequently, anaemia and fatigue can result and negatively affect both physical activity and health status. The tolerable upper intake level (UL) for calcium is 2000 to 2500 mg/d for adults [13].

8.3 PHOSPHORUS

8.3.1 Phosphorus Status within Individuals

Phosphorus is the second most abundant inorganic element in the body, with the first being calcium. Approximately 85% of total body phosphorus is located in the skeleton, 1% in the blood and body fluids and the remaining 14% is associated with soft tissue such as muscle [12,42]. Phosphorus is typically combined with other inorganic elements or with organic compounds in the body [42]. Phosphorus has many functions in the body and is involved with several biologically important compounds. Phosphorus plays a vital role in bone mineralisation, energy transfer and storage (in the form of high energy phosphates), nucleic acid formation, cell membrane structure and acid-base balance [42]. In addition, phosphorus is fundamental to growth, maintenance and repair of all body tissues. In the body, most of the phosphorus is in the form of phosphate.

Phosphorus is widely distributed in foods [42]. Good sources of phosphorus include milk, milk products, eggs, meat, poultry and fish. Plant sources such as nuts, legumes, cereals and grains also contain phosphorus; however, animal products are better sources of available phosphorus compared with most plant foods [30,42]. Coffee, tea and soft drinks also contain small amounts of phosphorus. Because phosphorus is not usually found free, dietary phosphorus can be found in one of two forms: organic and inorganic. Organic phosphorus is bound to a variety of compounds such as proteins, sugars, and lipids. About 70% of dietary phosphorus is absorbed in its inorganic form [42]. While vitamin D enhances phosphorus absorption, phytates and excessive intakes of magnesium, calcium and aluminium inhibit phosphorous absorption [42].

The US RDA for phosphorous in males and females 11 to 24 years of age is 1200 mg/d [30]. The RDA for those 25 years of age and older is 800 mg/d [30]. Researchers have shown that both males' and females' average daily intakes are above the RDA, with adult males averaging 1500 mg/d and females averaging 1000 mg/d [12]. Because phosphorus is widely distributed in foods, it is unlikely that an individual would incur a deficiency. Most researchers have generally reported that the diets of athletes are adequate in phosphorus [12].

8.3.2 Importance of Phosphorus on Optimal Exercise Performance

Phosphorus is a key component to the development of skeletal tissue. In bone, phosphorus combines with calcium to form salts, called hydroxyapatite. PTH, calcitriol (1,25-dihydroxyvitamin D_3) and calcitonin influence phosphorus balance in the body and bone. Calcitonin decreases serum phosphorus concentrations by promoting the movement of phosphorus into the bone for mineralisation. In contrast, PTH and calcitriol stimulate resorption of phosphate from the bone, and as a result, serum phosphorus levels increase [42]. As a key component in bones, phosphorus plays a major role in both bone health and skeletal integrity. Strong bones are not only important in preventing bone fractures, but they are also integral to the masters athlete's sporting success since the skeletal structure provides the strength and rigidity necessary to train and compete in sports. Masters athletes may be at an increased risk for bone fractures. As part of the ageing process, bone mineral density declines. Therefore, masters athletes need to ensure they are consuming adequate amounts of phosphorus to maintain bone health. Failure to do so could have a detrimental effect on bone health and strength, and could ultimately lead to osteoporosis. Maintaining the calcium to phosphorus intake to a ratio of 2:1 or 1:1 is recommended to be optimal [13,30].

Phosphorus plays a major role in both energy storage and transport. High-energy phosphates, such as adenosine triphosphate (ATP), adenosine monophosphate (AMP) and creatine phosphate, are of vital importance in energy metabolism and athletic performance. ATP is the major fuel for the body and is used for a wide variety of biochemical and physiological processes. During exercise, muscles, as well as all of the other cells in the body, need a constant supply of ATP to perform work. In addition, creatine phosphate, synthesised in the muscle from ATP, provides energy to the muscles during high-intensity,short bouts of exercise [42].

Phosphorus also influences oxygen availability. Phosphorus is indirectly involved in oxygen delivery through the function of the phosphorus-containing molecule 2,3-diphosphoglycerate (2,3-DPG). In the red blood cells, 2,3-DPG influences oxygen release from haemoglobin [42]. Therefore, 2,3-DPG helps cells receive the oxygen they need. Decreased 2,3-DPG as a result of a phosphorus deficiency can diminish release of oxygen to tissues [42]. The molecule 2,3-DPG improves oxygen delivery to muscles during exercise, thus improving exercise capacity. A phosphorus deficiency could therefore greatly impact oxygen release and delivery to the muscle cells. This can have a substantial impact on overall health, as well as athletic performance. Masters athletes experience age-related declines in both their anaerobic and endurance capacity. A phosphorus deficiency could further hinder their exercise performance by compromising their aerobic capacity. Therefore, it is important for masters athletes to maintain adequate phosphorus intakes.

8.3.3 Studies Conducted on Phosphorus Supplementation

The concept of phosphate loading has been of interest to many athletes. Phosphate loading refers to the practice of ingesting a large quantity (4 g/d) of phosphate in the form of phosphate salts for several days before a competitive event [12]. The theoretical basis for using phosphate salts as an ergogenic (performance-enhancing) substance is based upon its metabolic functions. Phosphate salts (high-energy phosphates) play important roles in human metabolism and sport performance.

It is believed that phosphate loading may influence both aerobic and anaerobic energy systems and enhance performance [43].

In 1984, Cade et al. [44] conducted a study to examine the effects of phosphate loading. Ten young well-trained male distance runners were given 1 g of neutral-buffered sodium phosphate four times per day for 3 days prior to a maximal oxygen uptake test [44]. The phosphate loading resulted in an increase in both serum phosphorus and red blood cell 2,3-DPG concentrations. Additionally, the phosphate loading was associated with an increase in maximal oxygen uptake and a decrease in lactate concentration [44]. From these findings, the researchers hypothesised that the improvement of aerobic metabolism through phosphate loading was most likely caused by the increased formation of 2,3-DPG, which facilitates oxygen release from haemoglobin and delivery to the tissues. It is suggested that the increase of 2,3-DPG can displace more oxygen from haemoglobin which would increase oxygen delivery to tissues and thereby enhance performance [44]. Similar findings were observed in a study where the effects of phosphate loading was examined on six young trained male cyclists and triathletes. It was observed that phosphate loading attenuated anaerobic threshold, increased myocardial ejection fraction and fractional shortening, increased maximal oxidative capacity and enhanced endurance performance [45]. However, an increase in 2,3-DPG was not observed.

Others, however, have found no benefit on performance from ingesting a phosphate load. Duffy and Conlee [46] evaluated the effects of various dosage amounts of phosphate, as well as dosage duration prior to tests. In the first test, 1.24 g of phosphate salt was given 1 h before leg power isokinetic tests and high-intensity treadmill runs. In the second test, 3.73 g/d of the same formulation was ingested for 6 d prior to the same tests. Both acute and chronic phosphate loading had no effect on leg power tests or time to fatigue on treadmill runs in what age range, level of athlete and/or gender [46].

Thus the findings on phosphate loading effects appear equivocal. Some researchers support the ergogenic effects of phosphate salts on aerobic endurance, while others report no ergogenic effects. It is important to note that the studies that have been conducted differed in the type, amount and duration of phosphate ingested, the training level of the participants and the different exercise tests used [47]. The long-term effects of phosphate loading have not been studied. Because high levels of phosphorus can reduce serum calcium levels, studies are needed to examine the long-term effects of phosphate loading on bone mineral density, especially in masters athletes.

8.4 MAGNESIUM

8.4.1 Magnesium Status within Individuals

Magnesium functions in a wide range of biochemical and physiological processes. Magnesium is an essential mineral and cofactor for more than 300 enzymatic reactions [48]. Some of these activities include glycolysis, fat and protein metabolism, ATP hydrolysis, the second-messenger system, deoxyribonucleic acid (DNA) and ribonucleic acid (RNA) synthesis and cell growth and production. Moreover, magnesium plays a central role in the regulation of cell membrane stability and neuromuscular, cardiovascular, immune and hormonal functions [48,49]. Due to the wide variety of fundamental cellular activities, magnesium may be considered a potentially limiting element for human performance [48]. The body contains about 10 to 28 g of magnesium; about 60% of the body's magnesium is found in the bone, 26% in the muscle, 6% to 7% in other cells and about 1% in extracellular fluids [50].

Approximately 40% to 60% of magnesium is thought to be absorbed in adults with normal magnesium intake. As with most minerals, when magnesium intake exceeds the necessary recommended amount, absorption declines. Conversely, magnesium absorption becomes more efficient when magnesium status is poor and when magnesium intake is low [42]. Vitamin D and carbohydrates (lactose and fructose) enhance magnesium absorption, whereas phytates, fibre and excessive unabsorbed fatty acids inhibit magnesium absorption. Calcium and phosphorus also inhibit magnesium absorption, especially when magnesium intake is low and calcium and phosphorus intake are high [42].

The RDA for magnesium is 400 mg/d for males and 310 mg/d for females 19 to 30 years of age, and 420 mg/d for males and 320 mg/d for females 31 years of age and older [30]. Although magnesium deficiency is not widespread, magnesium intake has been reported to be suboptimal [49]. Suboptimal magnesium intake could be a result of consumption of highly refined and processed foods, as well as the use of fertilisers in farming that contain no magnesium.

A wide variety of foods and beverages contain magnesium. Beverages rich in magnesium include coffee, tea and cocoa. Good food sources of magnesium in food include nuts, legumes whole grain cereals, beans, peanut butter and green leafy vegetables [51]. Diets high in refined foods, meat and dairy products provide less magnesium than diets rich in vegetables and unrefined grains [12]. Substantial amounts of magnesium are lost during food processing and preparation techniques in many foods (e.g. wheat, flour, cereals, rice, vegetable and sugar) [49,51]. Often times, magnesium is lost during these processes and is not added back in as part of the enrichment process [49,51].

8.4.2 Importance of Magnesium on Optimal Exercise Performance

Magnesium plays a critical role in a wide variety of biochemical and physiological processes that are important to exercise performance [12]. Magnesium is involved in excitation coupling, serves as a modulator for numerous rate-limiting enzymes and is involved in muscle and nerve excitability by maintaining membrane electrical potentials [12,50]. In addition to being involved in glycolysis, fat and protein metabolism, magnesium is a modulator of oxygen transport and is involved in many oxidative-reduction and phosphorylation reactions [52]. Recent observations examining magnesium transporters within the mitochondria have shown that mitochondria contain high amounts of magnesium that, in addition to influencing mitochondrial enzymes, activate and stabilise cytochrome c oxidase, the enzyme that catalyses the final stage in aerobic respiration [52]. Therefore, magnesium plays a major role in oxygen transport and uptake and is of importance to endurance athletes of all ages.

Perhaps one of the most important roles magnesium plays is as a co-factor in ATP production and numerous ATP-dependent reactions. Thus, magnesium plays an essential role in energy metabolism and work capacity in athletes of all ages. Whether an athlete is engaging in an activity of low or high intensity, ATP must be constantly supplied to the muscles, as well as all the other cells in the body. As exercise becomes more strenuous, ATP turnover increases dramatically and needs to be synthesised quickly. The breakdown of ATP in muscles, as well as muscle and nerve excitability, result in muscle contractions that ultimately effect exercise performance. In addition, magnesium is thought to favourably influence adenine nucleotide degradation, which is believed to be a key contributory component in muscle fatigue [52].

Due to the many processes in which magnesium is involved, masters athletes should consume adequate amounts of the mineral. Based on self-reported dietary records, most athletic groups have a magnesium intake that is at or above the RDA [12]. The only athletes where magnesium intake may be compromised are those attempting to maintain low body weights, as is typical with wrestlers, martial artists, light-weight rowing crew members, jockeys, dancers, figure skaters and gymnasts. Because exercise increases urinary and sweat losses and alters blood magnesium levels, it is important for masters athletes, especially older endurance athletes living and training in hot and/or humid environments, to consume adequate magnesium in their diets.

Serum or plasma magnesium concentrations appear to be closely related to exercise intensity and duration. Short-term, high-intensity exercise has been shown to be associated with increased serum or plasma magnesium concentrations, whereas long-term endurance exercise has been shown to decrease concentrations [49]. While profuse sweating appears to account for a small loss of magnesium, most magnesium is lost in the urine. It has been reported that urinary magnesium excretion is increased after exercise, and the magnesium losses are significantly higher in athletes than untrained controls. Increased urinary excretion and alterations in blood magnesium levels can occur as a result of magnesium's redistribution during exercise. Magnesium may be released from one storage area to be used at an active site (e.g. exercising muscles) [49]. However, once magnesium is released from its stores, it is either used or excreted in the urine. Exercise-induced increases in urinary magnesium may also be due to metabolic acidosis, as well as increases in the hormones aldosterone and antidiuretic hormone (ADH). These hormones regulate magnesium handling by the kidneys and are increased in concentration during strenuous activity.

It is important that masters athletes meet the recommended intakes for magnesium since it plays a crucial role in many processes necessary for exercise. Exercise increases magnesium usage through increased muscle contraction, metabolic activity and sweat loss [52,53]. As a result, magnesium stores can become depleted, and if not replaced by the diet, can lead to a deficiency that may significantly hinder a masters athlete's work capacity and performance. Magnesium deficiency, and even marginal depletion, can impair oxygen delivery and thus the ability to undertake and complete sub-maximal exercise. As a result, endurance performance is reduced [52]. Furthermore, a deficiency can lead to injury, illness (due to magnesium's role in immune function), hypocalcaemia, reduced glucose breakdown, decreased bone remodelling and increased blood pressure through decreased enzyme efficiency and cellular instability [52].

Additionally, a magnesium deficiency can lead to muscle weakness, neuromuscular dysfunction and cramping or muscle spasms. Liu [53] reported a case study of a 24-year-old female tennis player who experienced severe carpopedal spasms following prolonged exercise. She was found to have low blood magnesium levels. The athlete was given 500 mg/d of magnesium gluconate to replace the magnesium loss. After several days of taking the supplement, her spasms ceased and her serum magnesium levels were normalised [53]. Severe muscle spasms and pain in the legs from strenuous exercise was also observed in another case study involving a 17-year-old male soldier [54]. The soldier had a low serum magnesium concentration and no other abnormalities. After examining his diet, it was evident that there was an inadequate intake of magnesium. Several days after being given intravenous infusions of magnesium sulphate, the male soldier had fewer muscle pains and the spasms had resolved [54].

In a larger study, Williamson et al. [55] evaluated serum magnesium and the incidence of muscle cramps in 109 trained cyclists before and after a 100-mile cycling race. Approximately 46% of the cyclists experienced muscle cramps. It was reported that serum magnesium levels declined pre- to post-race. The average decline for the cyclists who experienced muscle cramps was 0.12 mmol/L compared to 0.08 mmol/L for cyclists who did not experience muscle cramps. The muscle cramps and spasms experienced by these individuals were associated with a magnesium deficiency [55]. Magnesium plays an important role in neuromuscular function, nerve conduction, and muscular contraction; a deficiency can result in improper functioning and result in muscle spasms, cramps and convulsions.

Lukaski and Nielsen [56] evaluated the consequence of dietary magnesium restriction on biochemical measures markers and physiologic responses during sub-maximal exercise in 10 postmenopausal women (45 to 71 years of age). None of these women were receiving hormone replacement therapy. First, the participants consumed diets containing usual foods with the average magnesium content equal to 112 mg of magnesium per 2000 kilocalories (kcal) and were supplemented with 200 mg of magnesium/d for 35 days (control phase). Following the control phase, the women consumed a diet that consisted of 112 mg of magnesium/2000 kcal per day for 93 days (depletion phase). This was followed by 112 mg of magnesium/2000, supplemented with 200 mg magnesium/d for 49 d (repletion phase). Red blood cell magnesium concentration, magnesium retention and skeletal muscle magnesium concentration all significantly decreased when during the magnesium depletion phase. Peak oxygen uptake and peak heart rate significantly increased during standardised sub-maximal work during the depletion phase compared with the repletion phase. The researchers concluded that magnesium depletion results in increased energy needs and adversely impacts cardiovascular function in otherwise healthy women [56]. The results from this study emphasise the detrimental effects a diet deprived in magnesium can have on both exercise and overall health.

Masters athletes need to closely monitor their magnesium status because the normal ageing process can lead to inadequate magnesium levels. Ageing is often associated with magnesium inadequacy because total body magnesium and magnesium in the intracellular compartment tend to decrease with age [57]. Reduced magnesium intestinal absorption, reduced magnesium bone stores and excess urinary magnesium loss are also associated with ageing [57]. Perhaps the most prevalent cause of magnesium inadequacy in the older population is due to a poor dietary intake. Additionally, for health reasons, masters athletes may need to be on certain medications (e.g. diuretics, cancer medications, some antibiotics), which can inhibit magnesium absorption. Masters athletes need to maintain magnesium levels because a deficiency can weaken the immune system, increase blood pressure and decrease bone remodelling.

Older individuals are already more vulnerable to a weakened immune system, bone fractures and possibly higher blood pressure; though masters athletes, due to their fitness levels, tend to evade these problems, they are not impervious to them. Adequate levels of dietary magnesium are needed to protect against free radical damage, maintain adequate bone strength and keep blood pressure at normal levels. Masters athletes are also more vulnerable to reduced anaerobic and endurance work capacity as a result of the normal ageing process; however, not to the extent as their sedentary counterparts. A magnesium deficiency would only exacerbate the problem due to magnesium's role in a wide variety of processes that are important to exercise performance.

8.4.3 Studies Conducted on Magnesium Supplementation

A large number of biochemical and physiological processes that are important to exercise performance depend on magnesium. Although athletes generally have adequate magnesium intakes, except those trying to maintain low body weights, they can still experience exercise-induced magnesium losses that, if not replenished, can lead to a deficiency. Based on the belief that increased magnesium status may benefit performance, multiple researchers have investigated the effects of magnesium supplementation on exercise performance with the results appearing equivocal [58].

Magnesium supplementation has been shown to improve exercise performance in several studies. For example, Brilla and Haley examined the effects of dietary magnesium on strength in 26 untrained individuals 18 to 30 years of age [59]. This study consisted of a double-blind, 7-week strength training program, with 14 participants in the control group, and 12 participants supplemented with 8 mg/kg body weight/d of magnesium oxide (and the magnesium from the diet). Both groups performed the same strength training regimen three times per week over the 7-week study. Although both groups gained strength, the magnesium-supplemented group significantly increased absolute torque, relative torque adjusted for body weight and relative torque adjusted for lean body mass. The researchers suggested that magnesium's role may be at the ribosomal level in protein synthesis [59].

In a classic study from 1968, Ahlborg et al. conducted a study in which six healthy males, 21 to 25 years of age, received either 240 mg/d of magnesium asparate or a placebo for one day [60]. The men supplemented with magnesium had a 50% improvement in their endurance performance. Golf et al. found that male triathletes, 25 to 33 years of age, had a faster exercise performance time when supplemented with 413 mg/d of magnesium ororate for 4 weeks [61]. Brilla and Gunther reported a decrease in oxygen consumption and an increase in time to exhaustion on a treadmill run in 20 females and 12 males, 19 to 24 years of age, supplemented with 314 mg/d of magnesium oxide for 4 weeks [62].

Other researchers, however, have found no effects of magnesium supplementation on exercise performance. Terblanche et al. found no effect on performance during a marathon run when 16 males and four females, 25 to 49 years of age, were supplemented with 368 mg/d of magnesium asparate for 10 weeks [63]. Furthermore, no change in exercise performance was observed during cycling, treadmill run, and handcrank ergometer tests when 16 males and four females, 17 to 28 years of age, were supplemented with 500 mg/d of magnesium oxide for 3 weeks [64]. Additionally, Finstad et al. found no change in exercise performance or recovery during anaerobic and aerobic treadmill tests when 32 females, 18 to 32 years of age, were supplemented with 212 mg/d of magnesium oxide for 4 weeks [65].

The findings on magnesium supplementation's effect on exercise performance are conflicting. The equivocal results are likely due to several reasons including different magnesium supplements used, different doses used, varying length of supplementation duration, different types of exercise tests used and different types of athletes used. More research is required to evaluate if magnesium has a true ergogenic effect on athletic performance. In addition, there has been no research to date where magnesium supplementation in masters athletes has been examined. Regardless of the equivocal results in supplementation studies, magnesium plays a significant role in exercise performance and overall health [66], thus maintaining that an optimal magnesium intake via a healthy diet is important to masters athletes.

8.5 IRON

8.5.1 Iron Status within Individuals

Iron is often referred to as the metal of life. The human body contains approximately 2 to 4 g of iron [12]. Iron is found in the body in three main forms: storage iron (ferritin and hemosiderin), transport iron (transferrin) and oxygen transport iron (haemoglobin in the red blood cells and myoglobin in the muscle). The majority of iron, approximately 65%, is found in haemoglobin, with smaller quantities in the tissues as myoglobin, the cytochromes and iron-containing enzymes [12]. The remaining body iron is found in the blood or in storage [12,42]. Iron is stored as ferritin in the bone marrow, liver and spleen. Men have approximately 1000 mg of stored iron, whereas women only average 300 mg of stored iron [42]. The total amount of iron in a person is influenced by several factors including body weight, age, gender, pregnancy and state of growth [12,42].

An inverse relationship exists between the iron status of the individual and the amount of iron that is absorbed [67]. When iron stores become depleted, absorption of iron increases. On average, healthy adults absorb 10% to 15% of dietary iron. Dietary iron is found in one of two forms in foods: heme and non-heme. Heme iron is found in animal products (meat, fish, poultry), while non-heme iron is found in plant foods (fruits, vegetables, nuts, grains, tofu) and dairy products (milk, cheese, eggs) [12]. Heme iron is absorbed with much greater efficiency than non-heme iron, mainly because heme iron is not affected by gastrointestinal lumen factors. In addition, the absorption of heme is not affected by the diet composition, whereas non-heme absorption is [67,68]. Aside from heme iron being absorbed better than non-heme iron, other factors that affect iron absorption, including gastric acid (low pH), high demand for red blood cells (blood loss, high altitude, exercise training, pregnancy), low body stores of iron, meat protein factor (MPF), and ascorbic acid. In contrast, phytates and oxalates (which are high in many plant sources), polyphenols in tea and coffee, full body stores of iron, excess of other minerals (zinc, calcium, manganese), reduced gastric acid production (higher pH) and some antacids inhibit iron absorption [12,42]. The US RDA for women 19 to 50 years of age is 18 mg/d. The RDA for women 51 years of age and older is and 8 mg/d. The RDA for men 19 years of age and older is 8 mg/d. The tolerable upper intake level for iron for individuals 14 years of age and older is 45 mg/d [68].

8.5.2 Importance of Iron on Optimal Exercise Performance

Iron plays a critical role in the body because it is required for energy formation and the formation of oxygen-carrying proteins, haemoglobin and myoglobin, making it an essential nutrient for optimal oxygen delivery to the body's tissues [67,68]. Furthermore, iron plays a key role in the electron transport chain and oxidative phosphorylation, since mitochondrial enzymes and cytochromes are iron-containing proteins [67,68]. Iron is also important for the normal functioning of the nervous and immune systems. Therefore, insufficient iron stores may lead to a decline in health and athletic performance, especially in endurance athletes [67]. Despite iron's importance in metabolic processes and physical performance, iron depletion and deficiency are relatively common.

Iron deficiency is the most common nutritional deficiency in the world and is a major concern for approximately 15% of the world's population [42]. Furthermore, in the United States and Canada, approximately 6% to 25% of reproductive-age females and pregnant women are iron-deficient [42]. Iron depletion occurs in three stages: iron depletion, iron deficiency without anaemia and iron deficiency anaemia. Each biomarker altered in previous stages remains altered in the next stage. Iron depletion is marked by low serum ferritin levels (<20 ng/mL), but there is still stainable iron in the bone marrow, the site of red blood cell production. In stage 2 (iron deficiency without anaemia), there is an increase in total iron binding capacity (TIBC) (>400 mcg/dL), a decrease in serum iron levels (<60 mcg/dL), a decrease in transferring saturation (<30%) and an increase in erythrocyte protoporphyrin. Stage 3 (iron deficiency anaemia), is characterised by low haemoglobin concentrations (<14 g/dL in men and <11 g/dL in women), low hematocrit concentrations (<40% in men and <38% in women) and decreased mean corpuscular cell volume (<82 mm) [42,68].

In the United States, the incidence of iron deficiency anaemia among young athletes and non-athletes alike is only about 5% to 6%; however, the incidence of iron depletion is a relatively more common occurrence among athletes and has been reported to range between 30% and 50%, especially among female athletes, as well as male and female athletes who participate in endurance sports [12]. The high incidence of iron depletion among athletes is usually attributed to a diet poor in iron, as well as iron losses in sweat, gastrointestinal bleeding, haemolysis and haematuria [67–70]. Female athletes up to menopausal age are at a higher risk for iron deficiency since they often do not consume adequate amounts of dietary iron and have increased iron loss during menstruation. It is estimated that the average adult male has a total daily iron loss of 0.86 to 0.95 mg/d (0.5 mg through the gastrointestinal tract, 0.1 mg/d through the urinary tract and 0.24 to 0.33 mg/d from the skin). Women, on the other hand, tend to lose more with the estimated average daily iron loss of 1.4 mg/d (0.45 mg/d through the gastrointestinal tract, 0.1 mg/d through the urinary tract, 0.24 mg/d from the skin and 0.6 mg/d through the menses) [47]. Athletes of any age who are vegetarians or on a high-carbohydrate diet are also at an increased risk for iron deficiency anaemia, because these diets have poor iron availability due to the lack of (red) meat intake.

Iron is essential to athletic performance due to its role in oxygen transport [71]. Maintaining adequate iron levels in athletes of all ages is imperative since a deficiency can lead to muscle weakness, fatigue, impaired thermoregulation and impaired cognitive performance [12]. Furthermore, iron deficiency can have a detrimental impact on energy metabolism. When iron is deficient, the synthesis of haemoglobin is reduced; as a result of decreased haemoglobin, there is decreased oxygen transport, which ultimately reduces aerobic metabolism. Further, cytochrome production will also be decreased, leading to reduced ATP generation and energy metabolism. Finally, muscular aerobic enzymes are adversely affected due to the decreased oxygen-carrying capacity of myoglobin. Therefore, iron deficiency anaemia reduces the maximum oxygen uptake and aerobic efficiency, as well as the body's endurance capacity. Muscle function will be impaired and the capacity for prolonged exercise will be limited [12,69].

Masters athletes should pay particular attention to their iron intake since they are already vulnerable to age-related physiological changes that can hinder their athletic performance and work capacity. With increasing age, it appears that masters athletes competing in anaerobic events (e.g. high-intensity events such as sprinting or power lifting) decline linearly in performance until 70 years of age, after which the rate of decline appears to accelerate [1]. In both sedentary and well-trained older individuals, this decline in performance appears to be strongly associated to a decreased anaerobic work capacity [1]. Furthermore, age-related declines in endurance performance have been observed [72]. Endurance performance appears to be maintained until approximately 35 years of age. This is followed by modest decreases until 50 years of age, with a progressive decrease in performance; thereafter, with the greatest declines occurring after 70 years of age [72]. With iron deficiency anaemia, as a result of decreased intake of medications (see Chapter 13) that may decrease absorption, athletic performance may be further impaired. It is important to note that individuals who exercise prevent the degree of performance decline compared to their sedentary counterparts.

8.5.3 Studies Conducted on Iron Supplementation

Due to the fact that iron plays a major role in a number of metabolic reactions, the effects of iron depletion and deficiency can have a major impact on overall health, cognitive function and exercise performance [69]. With iron deficiency being so prevalent worldwide, even with the fortification of iron in foods supplementation may be necessary. Supplementation could also be beneficial to athletes of any age since they have greater iron losses during strenuous exercise, especially those participating in endurance exercise. Adequate iron levels are at the centre of an athlete's success due to its effect on aerobic metabolism, endurance capacity and thermoregulation.

The importance of iron in work performance has been demonstrated in a number of studies. Iron supplementation in athletes who are iron-deficient has been found to not only improve blood biochemical measures and iron status, but also increase work capacity by increasing oxygen uptake, reducing heart rate and decreasing lactate concentrations during exercise [16]. Edgerton and colleagues [73] studied 31 adult men and women 27 to 55 years of age. Iron supplementation in iron-deficient participants was found to decrease blood lactate concentrations and increase oxygen uptake during standardised testing compared to pre-treatment values [73]. After seven participants (1 male, 6 females) with low haemoglobin concentrations received a blood transfusion to correct anaemia, their work capacity was the same as that measured in the other participants with normal haemoglobin concentrations. These findings illustrate the importance of haemoglobin-associated iron to aerobic work performance [73]. Similar findings were observed in iron-deficient anaemic women, 22 to 65 years of age [74]. Iron supplementation not only improved iron status, but also increased work capacity and reduced heart rate and lactate concentration in this population [74].

Iron supplementation in iron-deficient, non-anaemic athletes has yielded equivocal results. Iron supplements have only been shown to enhance performance when iron deficiency anaemia exists. Iron supplementation in athletes with normal haemoglobin concentrations and iron status will not enhance performance. Although iron supplementation can increase serum ferritin concentrations in both anaemic and non-anaemic individuals, increases in ferritin levels unaccompanied by increases in haemoglobin concentration have not been shown to improve endurance performance [69,75].

Iron also plays an important role in thyroid hormone metabolism. Thus, a person with iron deficiency anaemia may have a lower resting metabolic rate (RMR) than his or her counterpart with normal iron levels [69]. Rosenzweig and Volpe [76] assessed two iron-deficient-anaemic female athletes, 18 (Athlete 1 [A1]) and 21 (Athlete 2 [A2]) years of age, were supplemented with 23 mg/d of elemental iron to assess its effects on iron, thyroid hormone status and RMR at 0, 8 and 16 weeks. Iron deficiency anaemia was clinically improved in both participants (haemoglobin: A1 = 11.0 to 13.0 to 12.6 g/dL and A2 = 11.5 to 13.9 to 12.6 g/dL, 0 to 8 to 16 weeks, respectively). Although serum ferritin levels improved in both participants (A1: 5.0 to 11.0 to 15.0 ng/dL and A2: 5.0 to 16.0 to 20.0 ng/dL; 0 to 8 to 16 weeks, respectively), 16 weeks of iron supplementation did not fully restore iron stores. RMR and total thyroxine increased in A1 but decreased in A2. Despite the fact that iron deficiency anaemia was corrected over a 16-week period, this did not directly affect RMR and thyroid hormone metabolism, likely due to the fact that this was a case study of only two female athletes. More studies of this nature need to be conducted in a larger sample size for more definitive results.

Iron supplementation is only effective when in iron depletion or iron deficiency anaemia. Iron supplementation is not useful as an ergogenic aid for athletes of any age, including masters athletes. Obtaining iron through iron-rich foods (e.g. red meat, poultry, dark leafy greens, dried fruit, legumes, artichokes) is the best method to maintain normal iron levels [68]. However, if iron depletion or iron deficiency anaemia is diagnosed, iron supplementation is warranted.

8.6 ZINC

8.6.1 Zinc Status within Individuals

Zinc is the second most prevalent trace mineral in the body and required for optimal athletic performance. Zinc is present in all organs, tissues and body fluids with the human body containing approximately 1.5 to 2.5 g of zinc. Approximately 60% of zinc in the body is found in the muscle, 29% in bone and about 1% in each of the following: gastrointestinal tract, skin, kidney, brain, lung and prostate [12,67].

Zinc is a metalloenzyme and is required for the structure and activity of more than 300 metabolic activities. Zinc's importance is reflected by its regulatory role on numerous functions and activities [48]. Zinc plays a role in growth, building and repair of muscle tissue, energy production, nucleic acid and protein synthesis, cellular differentiation and replication and glucose use and insulin secretion. Zinc is also required for many physiological systems such as immunity, reproduction, taste, wound healing, skeletal development, behaviour and gastrointestinal function [48]. Zinc homeostasis is maintained by changes in absorption and excretion. It is tightly regulated by the protein metallothionien which is located within the enterocytes, and sequesters zinc until it is needed, then releases it into the bloodstream [42].

Zinc is more bioavailable from animal foods compared to plant foods [68]. The best food sources of zinc include oysters and red meat [12]. Poultry, fish and other shellfish are other good sources [12]. The US RDA for zinc is 11 mg/d for men and 8 mg/d for women [68]; however, survey data indicate that a large number of North Americans have zinc intakes below the recommended levels [16]. Zinc absorption is enhanced by both vitamin D and dietary protein. Factors that inhibit zinc absorption include phytates, oxalates, fibre, high levels of iron and possibly calcium [68].

8.6.2 Importance of Zinc on Optimal Exercise Performance

Marginal zinc intake is more prevalent in women than men due to lower energy intake in women compared to men [10]. Furthermore, the nutritional habits of athletes during training and competition are quite different from the diet that is generally recommended to the majority of the population [77]. For instance, endurance athletes often adopt a diet high in carbohydrates and low in protein and fat. In addition, some athletes partake in voluntary food restriction when participating in activities in which body weight or physical appearance is a component of performance evaluation (e.g. wrestling, rowing, martial arts, figure skating and gymnastics) [10].

Decreases in serum zinc levels in some athletes may be attributed to a poor dietary intake as well as urinary and sweat losses. Older masters athletes are especially susceptible to zinc deficiencies as a result of lower energy intakes, impaired nutrient absorption, chronic medical conditions and increased physical activity levels that expose these individuals to the risk of developing a zinc deficiency. Physiologic functions required for optimal work performance are hampered by low zinc intakes. Low zinc intakes and low serum zinc concentrations have been linked to impaired muscle function, including reduced strength and increased propensity to fatigue [10], and decreased cardiorespiratory function and endurance [16]. Thus, low zinc status may lead to reduced physical function and hinder athletic performance [78].

Zinc is important to all athletes but especially to older athletes due to its ability to enhance tissue repair and immune function. Athletes are more prone to a weakened immune system due to the higher stress load that results from training. Low zinc status has been linked to lower plasma total protein thiol groups in masters athletes as a result of oxidative stress [28]. An optimum amount of zinc improves the immune function and helps to protect against oxidative stress; however, when zinc intakes are suboptimal, this antioxidant activity may be compromised.

Physical activity has been shown to effect zinc status with low plasma zinc levels having been reported in many athletes. The normal range for plasma zinc is 11.5 to 18.5 μmol/L [67,68]. Giolo et al. [79] assessed the zinc status of elite swimmers during different periods of their training. Eight elite male swimmers, 18 to 25 years of age, who had been swimming competitively for at least 5 years, were assessed over 14 weeks during the following intervals: before the basic and specific preparatory period (BSPP-baseline), at the end of the basic and specific preparatory period (post-BSPP) and at the end of the polishing (taper) period (PP). The researchers measured zinc concentrations in the plasma, erythrocyte, urine and saliva. The median plasma zinc concentrations were significantly below normal in all training periods: BSPP-baseline = 9 μmol/L; post-BSPP = 8.6 μmol/L; after PP μmol/L μmol/L). Below normal values were also observed in all other measures of zinc status, though salivary zinc levels did not correlate well with blood measures of zinc. Based on these results, elite swimmers may be at risk for a zinc deficiency, and should be monitored. Salivary zinc does not provide a good indicator of zinc status [79].

Similar findings of reduced circulating zinc concentrations and increased zinc loss via sweat have been reported in athletes by Anderson and colleagues [80]. Serum zinc values of nine runners, 23 to 46 years of age, were measured following a strenuous 6-mile run. The serum zinc values immediately following running did not differ from the pre-run values but decreased significantly within 2 hours of running. Two hours after running, urinary zinc concentration was elevated more than twofold compared to a non-run day [80]. Further, Anderson and colleagues observed that, on the day of the run, total urinary losses were more than 1.5-fold higher than those on the non-run day [80].

Zinc-dependent enzymes, most notably lactate dehydrogenase and carbonic anhydrase, play a critical role in exercise metabolism by regulating glycolysis and carbon dioxide removal [10]. Carbonic anhydrase may play a role in facilitating performance since it regulates the removal of carbon dioxide (a product of cellular aerobic energy production) from cells [78]. Carbonic anhydrase is found in red blood cells and helps red blood cells pick up carbon dioxide and releases it in the lungs to be exhaled. Zinc, however, needs to be bound to this enzyme for it to function. Preliminary data have indicated that the activity of carbonic anhydrase in red blood cells responds to dietary zinc [78]. Thus, a dietary zinc deficiency can be detrimental to respiratory function and could negatively impact cardiorespiratory, and thus, athletic performance.

In a double-blind, randomized crossover study, 14 men, 20 to 31 years of age, were fed low-zinc diets (3.8 mg/d) or zinc supplemented diets (18.7 mg/d) [78]. Low dietary zinc resulted in lower serum and erythrocyte zinc concentrations, lower zinc retention and lower total carbonic anhydrase activities in red blood cells. Peak oxygen uptake, carbon dioxide output and respiratory exchange ratio also decreased with the low-zinc diet. Furthermore, performance was impaired and physiologic function was altered during the sub-maximal exercise test due to a low zinc intake. These findings suggest that, as a result of low dietary zinc, there were significant reductions in zinc status, including red blood cell carbonic anhydrase activities, and impaired metabolic responses during exercise [78].

Masters athletes may already face age-related decreases in cardiorespiratory fitness in the absence of a zinc deficiency. It has been widely reported that, with ageing, there is a decrease in cardiovascular function [72]. Decreased aerobic capacity is attributed to decreases in maximal cardiac output, stroke volume and maximal heart rate [19].

To date, no one has utilised stable isotopes of zinc to assess the kinetics of zinc metabolism following an exhaustive exercise bout. Therefore, Volpe et al. [81] examined short-term changes in zinc kinetics using the stable isotope ^{70}Zn to identify the kinetics of zinc metabolism following an acute, strenuous bout of cycle ergometry exercise in sedentary men. They performed a cross-over design study in 12 healthy, sedentary young men, 25 to 35 years of age. ^{70}Zn was infused 10 min after an exhaustive exercise bout or at rest. Plasma zinc concentrations significantly decreased after exercise, with a mean nadir of 13.9% ± 4.1% observed at 70 min post-exercise. Based on their ^{70}Zn data, Volpe et al. [81] reported increases in the size of the rapidly exchangeable plasma zinc pool and the liver zinc pool, corresponding to a shift of plasma zinc into the interstitial fluid and liver after exercise, possibly reflecting the acute stress response of exhaustive exercise. This study demonstrated the changes in zinc during just one bout of exercise, which could result in decreased performance in those who exercise regularly and do not consume adequate amounts of zinc in their diets.

8.6.3 Studies Conducted on Zinc Supplementation

Suboptimal zinc intakes can lead to significant weight loss, low energy and reduced endurance performance. Wakimoto and Block [82] found that 75% of women 50 to 69 years of age and 90% of men over 70 years of age did not consume the RDA for zinc. Older athletes especially need to monitor their zinc consumption because they can suffer from decreased gastrointestinal absorption of zinc (see Chapter 1) and/or may be on medications for chronic illness (see Chapter 13) that may lead to zinc malaborption or urinary zinc loss. Many older athletes also supplement with calcium and iron, inhibitors of zinc absorption, leading to decreased bioavailability of zinc, and thus a possible greater risk of zinc deficiency.

In a double-blind, placebo-controlled, cross-over design study, Krotkiewski et al. [83] studied 16 middle-aged women who received a zinc supplement (30 mg/d) and a placebo for 14 days. Muscle strength and endurance were measured with an isokinetic, one-leg exercise at baseline and after 14 days. Compared to the placebo, zinc supplementation significantly increased dynamic isokinetic strength at 180°/s of angular velocity and isometric endurance [83]. Due to the fact that these muscle functions rely on recruitment of fast-twitch glycolytic muscle fibres, it was hypothesised that zinc supplementation enhanced the activity of lactate dehydrogenase, a zinc-dependent enzyme that converts lactate produced by the muscles back to pyruvate [48,83].

Van Loan and colleagues [84] also examined the effects of a very low zinc diet on muscular strength and endurance. Eight young males were placed on a zinc-restricted diet (≤0.05 mg/d) for 1 month. The zinc-restricted diet resulted in a significant decrease in plasma zinc concentrations to 24 mcg/dL. Isokinetic endurance of the shoulder flexors and extensors and knee extensors was significantly reduced by zinc depletion and was still substantially below baseline after 3 weeks of zinc repletion [84].

Zinc plays a significant role in the conversion of thyroxine (T_4) to the more active triiodothyronine (T_3). T_3 is involved with the body's overall metabolism, affecting health and exercise performance. Maxwell and Volpe [85] examined the effects of zinc supplementation on plasma zinc, serum ferritin, plasma T_3 and T_4, serum free T_3 and T_4 and thyroid-stimulating hormone (TSH) concentrations and RMR in two zinc-deficient, physically active college-age women (one was 19 years of age, the other was 25 years of age), who were supplemented with 26.4 mg/d of zinc gluconate for 4 months. They reported that zinc deficiency was corrected in both participants, while serum ferritin concentrations declined, categorising both participants as borderline iron-depleted. At 4 months, total T_3 concentrations increased in one participant, while all thyroid hormone concentrations increased in the other with RMR improved in both participants at 4 months. Because this was a case study, statistical analyses could not be performed. However, zinc supplementation seemed to be directly responsible for the increase in plasma zinc and decline in serum ferritin concentrations in both participants. Zinc supplementation seemed to result in the favourable effect on both total T_3 concentrations and RMR [85].

Although zinc supplementation may be effective after zinc repletion, high levels of zinc have been shown to decrease high-density lipoprotein cholesterol (HDL-C) concentrations as well as alter the status of other nutrients, such as magnesium [42,68]. Excess zinc intake can also negatively affect the absorption of iron and copper which can lead to anaemia and an impaired immune status [42]. Furthermore, large doses of zinc can significantly decrease calcium absorption, especially when zinc supplements are given with a low calcium intake [86]. Therefore, masters athletes must seek the advice of physicians or sports dieticians when starting supplementation to avoid health issues.

8.7 CHROMIUM

8.7.1 Chromium Status within Individuals

Chromium is an important but often overlooked mineral. The human body contains approximately 4 to 6 mg of chromium, which is primarily stored in the kidneys, liver, muscle, spleen, heart, pancreas and bone. The primary function of chromium is to potentiate the effects of insulin, a hormone critical to the metabolism and storage of carbohydrate, lipid and protein in the body [12,47]. Chromium is a cofactor with the protein chromodulin, which works with GLUT4 and insulin to help bring glucose into the cells.

Chromium exists in the trivalent form (Cr^{3+}) in foods. Good sources of chromium include meat, fish and poultry (especially organ meats) and whole grains. Other good sources of chromium include dark chocolate, cheese, select vegetables, fruits and spices as well as tea, beer and wine. Brewer's yeast is an especially significant source [12,42]. Food processing and refining decrease the chromium content in foods. Although the mode of absorption is not fully understood, it is known that about 0.4% to 2.5% of chromium intake is absorbed into the intestinal cells for use by the body [42,68]. Enhancers of chromium absorption include amino acids (phenylalanine, methionine and histidine) and ligands (picolinate). Vitamin C is also known to enhance chromium absorption. In contrast, antacids and phytates inhibit chromium absorption. There is no RDA for chromium; however, the Adequate Intake is to be 35 mcg/d for men and 25 mcg/d for women [68].

8.7.2 Importance of Chromium on Optimal Exercise Performance

Chromium is an essential mineral, yet 9 out of 10 people in the United States do not consume enough chromium due to processed foods and excessive chromium losses [87]. A diet high in processed foods and refined sugars and grains, which is typical for many in the Western world, could lead to low levels of chromium consumption with more than 90% of naturally occurring chromium in foods removed during the manufacturing processes used to produce these foods [87]. Moreover, high sugar intakes can increase urinary chromium loss. Chromium losses are also increased by stress, pregnancy, trauma, infection and exercise. Researchers hypothesise that diets containing high amounts of processed and refined foods, combined with the increased chromium loss in the urine caused by such a diet, can contribute to declining chromium levels in older adults [87].

Individuals at an increased risk for chromium deficiency include athletes, individuals with diabetes mellitus, pregnant women and the elderly [88,89]. Masters athletes are an especially vulnerable group, because exercise increases urinary chromium losses. Researchers have found that exercise substantially increases urinary chromium losses with double the amount of chromium lost in the urine on the day of exercise compared to a day of rest [88]. In response to exercise, chromium is mobilised from stores into the blood to be carried to target organs, such as the muscle, to enhance insulin function. However, once chromium is mobilised into the blood, it cannot be reabsorbed, and is ultimately excreted in the urine [47].

Masters athletes may be vulnerable to chromium deficiency because both the body's chromium reserves and tissue chromium levels decrease with age [90]. Diet, exercise, urinary losses and ageing can all lead to a chromium deficiency [90]. Chromium deficiency is characterised by decreased glycogen stores and elevated plasma glucose levels, increased serum insulin concentrations, increased serum total cholesterol levels and increased triacylglycerol concentrations [90]. A number of conditions, including fatigue, hypoglyacemia, heart disease and blurred vision are also known to result from chromium deficiency [84,91]. Impaired glucose tolerance and the incidence of diabetes mellitus, both of which are associated with chromium deficiency, become increasingly more common with age [90].

8.7.3 Studies Conducted on Chromium Supplementation

Chromium supplementation received attention in the mid-1990s based on the suggestion it may improve body composition by both increasing muscle mass and reducing body fat. However, researchers who used more accurate measures of body composition have not reported positive effects of chromium on muscle mass [89].

Chromium supplementation may have other health benefits, especially since insufficient dietary chromium has been linked to type 2 diabetes mellitus and cardiovascular disease. Chromium supplementation has been found to significantly improve glucose tolerance, insulin, insulin binding and low-density lipoprotein cholesterol (LDL-C) concentrations and HDL-C concentrations [89–91].

For athletes who are in weight-monitored sports, such as wrestling, martial arts, gymnastics and rowing, chromium's use as a possible weight-loss supplement is what gained it the most popularity. Volpe et al. [92] assessed the effects of chromium picolinate supplementation in 44 sedentary, overweight women (body mass indexes [BMIs] = 27 to 41 kg/m^2), who were 27 to 51 years of age. They conducted a double-blind, randomised, placebo-controlled study in moderately obese women on body weight, body composition and RMR. Volpe et al. [92] found that supplementation with 400 mcg/d of chromium picolinate did not result in changes in weight loss, body composition (evaluated by hydrostatic weighing) or RMR compared to women receiving an identical-looking placebo.

Volek et al. [93] more recently assessed the effects of 600 mcg/d of chromium picolinate in 16 overweight men (BMI = 31.1 ± 3.0 kg/m^2) who were randomly assigned to either the chromium group or the placebo group for 4 weeks. Volek et al. [93] reported no differences in glucose or insulin concentrations between the groups. They concluded that 4 weeks of chromium supplementation did not improve glycogen synthesis during recovery after high-intensity exercise followed by a high glycaemic index feeding.

Based on the aforementioned data, it does not appear that chromium has ergogenic effects on exercise performance or weight loss. Nonetheless, research on chromium's possible effect on type 2 diabetes mellitus may be more hopeful. Despite these results, it is still important that individuals of all ages consume whole foods and reduce the consumption of more processed foods to minimise deficiency of any nutrient.

8.8 CONCLUSIONS

This chapter presented the dietary needs and possible ergogenic effects of calcium, phosphorus, magnesium, iron, zinc and chromium with respect to masters athletes. Although some researchers reported positive effects of mineral supplementation, overall results appear equivocal, and most researchers have not reported positive effects of mineral supplementation on exercise performance. A methodical approach to the study of minerals and exercise performance in masters athletes is required. Masters athletes of differing age, gender and discipline (e.g. speed vs. endurance vs. team player) need to be studied. In addition, the same dose and type of mineral supplementation need to be evaluated over several different studies. Not until tightly controlled trials are performed can we definitively state the ergogenic effect (or no effect) of any mineral in athletes.

8.9 IMPLICATIONS FOR MASTERS ATHLETES AND COACHES

The results of the aforementioned research studies on the minerals reviewed in this chapter have been equivocal. Therefore, older athletes and coaches need to focus on consuming a varied diet, with less processed foods, to help enhance or maintain both their sports performance and health status. If a deficiency exists, supplementation would be warranted for that specific mineral. However, supplementation for the sake of supplementing is not warranted based on current evidence. If an older athlete chooses to supplement with a multi-vitamin/mineral supplement, it would be wise for that individual to choose a supplement that is well-balanced and does not exceed the national recommendations established for their country. In addition, if a person is taking any medication, they should consult with a physician to ensure there are no contraindications. There are many medication-nutrient interactions of which many people are unaware that are discussed in detail in Chapter 13.

8.10 IMPLICATIONS FOR SPORTS MEDICINE PROFESSIONALS AND CLINICIANS

Sports medicine professionals and clinicians need to be aware that an increasingly greater number of older individuals are not only exercising, but competing at high levels. These athletes need to be treated as the athletes they are, especially if they experience an injury. Nutrition needs to be a part of their training regime, and they should be referred to a registered dietician; in particular, one who specialises in sports nutrition and who is knowledgeable about the needs of athletes.

8.11 FUTURE RESEARCH DIRECTIONS

In general, more research in masters athletes is needed to better establish if they have greater mineral needs than non-athletes of similar age. A longitudinal approach needs to be established in masters athletes of similar age, gender and training. Furthermore, multiple studies need to be conducted using similar doses and duration. These studies will help establish if masters athletes require more minerals than the normal healthy person.

REFERENCES

1. Reaburn, P. and Dascombe, B., Anaerobic performance in masters athletes, *Eur. Rev. Aging Phys. Act.* 6, 39–53, 2009.
2. Jokl, P., Sethi, P.M. and Cooper, A.J., Master's performance in the New York City Marathon 1983–1999, *Br. J. Sports Med.* 38(4), 408–12, 2004.
3. Kujala, U.M., Sarna, S., Kaprio, J., Koskenvuo, M. and Karjalainen, J., Heart attacks and lower-limb function in master endurance athletes, *Med. Sci. Sports Exerc.* 31(7), 1041–6, 1999.
4. Maron, B.J., Arujo, C.G.S., Thompson, P.D. et al., Recommendations for preparticipation screening and the assessment of cardiovascular disease in masters athletes, *Circulation* 103(2), 327–34, 2001.
5. Trappe, S., Marathon runners. How do they age? *Sports Med.* 37(4–5), 302–5, 2007.
6. Tanaka, H. and Seals, D.R., Age and gender interactions in physiological functional capacity: Insight from swimming performance, *J. Appl. Physiol.* 82(3), 846–51, 1997.
7. Donato, A.J., Tench, K., Glueck, D.H., Seals, D.R., Eskurza, I. and Tanaka, H., Declines in physiological functional capacity with age: A longitudinal study in peak swimming, *J. Appl. Physiol.* 94(2), 764–9, 2002.
8. Evans, S.L., Davy, K.P., Stevenson, E.T. and Seals, D.R., Physiological determinants of 10-km performance in highly trained female runners of different ages, *J. Appl. Physiol.* 78(5), 1931–41, 1995.
9. Bird, S., Balmer, J., Olds, T. and Davidson, R.C.R., Differences between sexes and age-related changes in orienting speed, *J. Sports Sci.* 19(4), 243–52, 2001.
10. Lukaski, H.C., Magnesium, zinc and chromium nutriture and physical activity, *Am. J. Clin. Nutr.* 72(suppl), 585S–593S, 2000.
11. Striegel, H., Simon, P., Wurster, C., Neiss, A.M. and Ulrich, R., The use of nutritional supplements among masters athletes, *Int. J. Sports Med.* 27(3), 236–41, 2006.
12. Volpe, S.L. and Bland, E.G., Vitamins and minerals and exercise, in *Sports Nutrition: A Practice Manual for Professionals,* 5th Edition. C.A. Rosenbloom and E.J. Coleman, eds., The American Dietetic Association, Chicago, 2012, pp. 75–105.
13. Food and Nutrition Board of the Institute of Medicine, *Dietary Reference Intakes for Calcium and Vitamin D*, Food and Nutrition Board, National Academy Press, Washington, DC, 2011.

14. Maughan, R.J., Role of micronutrients in sport and physical activity, *Brit. Med. Bull.* 53(3), 683–90, 1995.
15. Williams, M.H., Dietary supplements and sports performance: Minerals, *J. Int. Soc. Sports Nutr.* 2(1), 43–9, 2005.
16. Rodriguez, N.R., DiMarco, N.M. and Langley, S., American College of Sports Medicine position stand. Nutrition and athletic performance. American Dietetic Association; Dietitians of Canada; American College of Sports Medicine, *Med. Sci. Sports Exerc.* 41(3), 709–31, 2009.
17. Cashman, K.D., Calcium intake, calcium bioavailability and bone health, *Brit. J. Nutr.* 87(Suppl 2), S169–77, 2002.
18. Riggs, B.L., The mechanisms of estrogen regulation on bone resorption, *J. Clin. Invest.* 106, 1203–4, 2000.
19. Maharam, L.G., Bauman, P.A., Kalman, D. and Sklonik, H., Masters athletes: Factors affecting performance, *Sports Med.* 28(4), 273–85, 1999.
20. Peer, K.S., Bone health in athletes: Factors and future considerations, *Orthop. Nurs.* 23(3), 24, 2004.
21. Kanis, J. A., *Textbook of Osteoporosis*, Blackwell Science, Oxford, England, 1996.
22. Wang, M.C., Aguirre, M., Bhudhikanok, G.S. et al., Bone mass and hip axis length in healthy Asian, black, Hispanic and white American youths, *J. Bone Min. Res.* 12, 1922–35, 1997.
23. National Institutes of Health, Osteoporosis and Related Bone Diseases, National Resource Center Peak bone mass, *NIH ORBD Newsletter*, 3(April), 1–2, 2001.
24. Vitamin D Council: Vitamin D Deficiency, http://www.vitamindcouncil.org/about-vitamin-d/, accessed 21 January 2014.
25. Myburgh, K.H., Hutchins, J., Fataar, A.B., Hough, S.F. and Noakes, T.D., Low bone density is an etiologic factor for stress fractures in athletes, *Ann. Intern. Med.* 113, 754–9, 1990.
26. Dressendorfer, R.H., Petersen, S.R., Moss Lovshin, S.E. and Keen, C.L., Mineral metabolism in male cyclists during high-intensity endurance training, *Int. J. Sport Nutr. Exer. Metab.* 12, 63–72, 2002.
27. Schaafsma, A., de Vries, P.J. and Saris, W.H.M., Delay of natural bone loss by higher intakes of specific minerals and vitamins, *Crit. Rev. Food Sci. Nutr.* 41(3), 225–49, 2001.
28. Rosenbloom, C. and Dunaway, A., Nutrition recommendations for masters athletes, *Clin. Sports Med.* 26, 91–100, 2007.
29. Kunstel, K., Calcium requirements for the athlete, *Curr. Sports Med. Rep.* 4(4), 203–6, 2005.
30. Food and Nutrition Board of the Institute of Medicine, *Dietary Reference Intakes for Calcium, Magnesium, Phosphorus, Vitamin D and Fluoride*, Food and Nutrition Board, National Academy Press, Washington, DC, 1997.
31. Theobald, H.E., Dietary calcium and health, *Nutr. Bull.* 30(3), 237–77, 2005.
32. Riis, B., Thomsen, K. and Christiansen, C., Does calcium supplementation prevent postmenopausal bone loss? A double-blind, controlled clinical study, *New Engl. J. Med.* 316, 173–7, 1987.
33. Dawson-Hughes, B., Dallai, G.E., Krall, E.A., Sandowski, L., Sahyoun, N. and Tannenbaum, S., A controlled trial of the effect of calcium supplementation on bone density in postmenopausal women, *New Engl. J. Med.* 323, 878–83, 1990.
34. Elders, P.J.M., Lips, P., Netelenbos, J.C. et al., Long-term effect of calcium supplementation on bone loss in perimenopausal women, *J. Bone Miner. Res.* 9, 938–70, 1994.
35. Polley, K.J., Nordin, B.E., Baghurst, P.A., Walker, C.J. and Chatterton, B.E., Effect of calcium supplementation on forearm bone mineral content in postmenopausal women: A prospective, sequential controlled trial, *J. Nutr.* 117(11), 1929–35, 1987.
36. Smith, E.L., Gilligan, C., Smith, P.E. and Sempos, C.T., Calcium supplementation and bone loss in middle-aged women, *Am. J. Clin. Nutr.* 50, 833–42, 1989.
37. Nelson, M.E., Fisher, E.C., Dilmanian, F.A., Dallal, G.E. and Evans, W.J., A 1-y walking program and increased dietary calcium in postmenopausal women: Effects on bone, *Am. J. Clin. Nutr.* 53, 1304–11, 1991.
38. Dawson-Hughes, B., Harris, S.S., Krall, E.A. and Dallal, G.E., Effect of withdrawal of calcium and vitamin D supplements on bone mass in elderly men and women, *Am. J. Clin. Nutr.* 72, 745–50, 2000.
39. Sacheck, J.M. and Roubenoff, R., Nutrition in the exercising elderly, *Clin. Sports Med.* 18(3), 565–84, 1999.
40. Reid, I.R., Ames, R.W., Evans, M.C., Gamble, G.D. and Sharpe, S.J., Long-term effects of calcium supplementation on bone loss and fractures in postmenopausal women: A randomized controlled trial, *Am. J. Med.* 98(4), 331–5, 1995.
41. Dawson-Hughes, B., Harris, S.S., Krall, E.A. and Dallal, G.E., Effect of calcium and vitamin D supplementation on bone density in men and women 65 years of age or older, *New Engl. J. Med.* 337, 670–6, 1997.

42. Gropper, S.S., Smith, J.L. and Groff, J.L., *Advanced Nutrition and Human Metabolism*. Wadsworth Publishing: Belmont, CA, 2009.
43. Czuba, M., Zajac, A., Poprzecki, S., Cholewa, J. and Woska, S., Effects of sodium phosphate loading on aerobic power and capacity in off road cyclists, *J. Sports Sci. Med.* 8, 591–9, 2009.
44. Cade, R., Conte, M., Zauner, C. et al., Effects of phosphate loading on 2,3-diphosphoglycerate and maximal oxygen uptake, *Med. Sci. Sports Exerc.* 16(3), 263–8, 1984.
45. Kreider, R.B., Miller, G.W., Schenck, D. et al., Effects of phosphate loading on metabolic and myocardial responses to maximal and endurance exercise, *Int. J. Sport Nutr.* 2(1), 20–47, 1992.
46. Duffy, D.J. and Conlee, R.K., Effects of phosphate loading on leg power and high intensity treadmill exercise, *Med. Sci. Sports Exerc.* 18, 674–7, 1986.
47. Haymes, E.M. and Clarkson, P.M. Minerals and trace minerals, in *Nutrition for Sport and Exercise*, J.R. Berning and S.N. Steen, eds., Jones and Bartlett Publishers, Sudbury, MA, 2006, pp. 77–99.
48. Lukaski, H.C., Vitamin and mineral status: Effects on physical performance, *Nutr.* 20, 632–44, 2004.
49. Bohl, C.H. and Volpe, S.L., Magnesium and exercise, *Crit. Rev. Food Sci. Nutr.* 42(6), 533–63, 2002.
50. Marier, J.R., Magnesium content of the food supply in the modern-day world, *Magnesium* 5, 1–8, 1986.
51. Carvil, P. and Cronin, J., Magnesium and implications on muscle function, *Strength Condition. J.* 32(1), 48–54, 2010.
52. Buchman, A.L., Keen, C., Commisso, J. et al., The effect of a marathon run on plasma and urine mineral and metal concentrations, *J. Am. Coll. Nutr.* 17, 124–7, 1998.
53. Liu, L., Hypomagnesaemia in a tennis player, *Phys. Sportsmed.* 11, 79–80, 1983.
54. Bilbey, D.L.J. and Prabhakaran, V.M., Muscle cramps and magnesium deficiency: Case reports, *Can. Fam. Physician* 42, 1348–51, 1996.
55. Williamson, S.L., Johnson, R.W., Hudkins, P.G. and Strate, S.M., Exertional cramps: A perspective study of biochemical and anthropometric variable in bicycle riders, *Cycling Sci.* 15, 20, 1993.
56. Lukaski, H.C. and Nielsen, F.H., Dietary magnesium depletion affects metabolic responses during submaximal exercise in postmenopausal women, *J. Nutr.* 132(5), 930–5, 2002.
57. Barbagallo, M., Belvedere, M. and Dominguez, L.J., Magnesium homeostasis and aging, *Magnes. Res.* 22(4), 235–46, 2009.
58. Volpe, S.L., Magnesium, in *Present Knowledge in Nutrition*, 10th Edition, J.W. Erdman, I. Macdonald and S. Zeisel, eds., ILSI Press, Washington, DC, 2012, pp. 743–66.
59. Brilla, L.R. and Haley, T.F., Effect of magnesium supplementation on strength training in humans, *J. Am. Coll. Nutr.* 11(3), 326–9, 1992.
60. Ahlborg, B., Ekelund, L.G. and Nilsson, C.G., Effect of potassium-magnesium-asparate on the capacity for prolonged exercise in man, *Acta Physiol. Scand.* 74, 238–45, 1968.
61. Golf, S.W., Bender, S. and Gruttner, J., On the significance of magnesium in extreme physical stress, *Cardiovasc. Drug Ther.* 12, 197–202, 1998.
62. Brilla, L.R. and Gunther, K.B., Effect of magnesium supplementation on exercise time to exhaustion, *Med. Exerc. Nutr. Health* 4, 230–3, 1995.
63. Terblanche, S., Noakes, T.D., Dennis, S.C., Marais, D. and Eckert, M., Failure of magnesium supplementation to influence marathon running performance or recovery in magnesium-replete subjects, *Int. J. Sports Nutr.* 2, 154–64, 1992.
64. Weller, E., Bachert, P., Hans-Michael, M., Friedmann, B., Bartsch, P. and Mairbaurl, H., Lack of effect of oral Mg-supplementation on Mg in serum, blood cells and calf muscle, *Med. Sci. Sports Exer.* 30, 1584–91, 1998.
65. Finstad, E.W., Newhouse, I.J., Lukaski, H.C., McAuliffe, J.E. and Stewart, C.R., The effect of magnesium supplementation on exercise performance, *Med. Sci. Sports Exer.* 33, 493–8, 2001.
66. Volpe, S.L., Magnesium in disease prevention and overall health, *Adv. Nutr.* 4(3), 378S–383S, 2013.
67. Haymes, E.M. and DeRuisseau, K.C., Trace minerals, in *Nutrition and the Strength Athlete*, C. Jackson, ed., CRC Press, Boca Raton, FL, 2000, pp. 97–113.
68. Food and Nutrition, Board of the Institute of Medicine, *Dietary Reference Intakes for Vitamin A, Vitamin K, Arsenic, Boron, Chromium, Copper, Iodine, Iron, Manganese, Molybdenum, Nickel, Silicon, Vanadium and Zinc*, Food and Nutrition Board, National Academy Press, Washington, DC, 1997.
69. Rosenzweig, P.H. and Volpe, S.L., Iron, thermoregulation and metabolic rate, *Crit. Rev. Food Sci. Nutr.* 39(2), 131–48, 1999.
70. Peeling, P., Dawson, B., Goodman, C., Landers, G. and Trinder, D., Athletic induced iron deficiency: New insights into the role of inflammation, cytokines and hormones, *Eur. J. Appl. Physiol.* 103, 381–91, 2008.
71. Volpe, S.L., Calcium, zinc, iron and exercise in women, *Top. Clin. Nutr.* 14(3), 43–52, 1999.

72. Reaburn, P. and Dascombe, B., Endurance performance in masters athletes, *Eur. Rev. Aging Phys. Act.* 5, 31–42, 2008.
73. Edgerton, V.R., Ohira, Y., Hettiarachchi, J., Senewiratne, B., Gardner, G.W. and Barnard, R.J., Elevation of hemoglobin and work tolerance in iron-deficient subjects, *J. Nutr. Sci. Vitaminol.* 27(2), 77–86, 1981.
74. Gardner, G.W., Edgerton, V.R., Senewiratne, B., Barnard, R.J. and Ohira, Y., Physical work capacity and metabolic stress in subjects with iron deficiency anemia, *Am. J. Clin. Nutr.* 30(6), 910–7, 1977.
75. Brittenham, G.M., New advances in iron metabolism, iron deficiency and iron overload, *Curr. Opin. Hematol.* 1, 101–6, 1994.
76. Harris Rosenzweig, P. and Volpe, S.L., Effect of iron supplementation on thyroid hormone levels and resting metabolic rate in two college female athletes: A case study, *Int. J. Sport Nutr. Exerc. Metab.* 10(4), 434–43, 2000.
77. Micheletti, A., Rossi, R. and Rufini, S., Zinc status in athletes: Relation to diet and exercise. *Sports Med.* 31(8), 577–82, 2001.
78. Lukaski, H.C., Low dietary zinc decreases erythrocyte carbonic anhydrase activities and impairs cardiorespiratory function in men during exercise, *Am. J. Clin. Nutr.* 81, 1045–51, 2005.
79. Giolo De Carvalho, F., Rosa, F.T., Marques Miguel Suen, V., Freitas, E.C., Padovan, G.J. and Marchini, J.S., Evidence of zinc deficiency in competitive swimmers, *Nutrition* 28(11–12), 1127–31, 2012.
80. Anderson, R.A., Polansky, M.M. and Bryden, N.A., Acute effects on chromium, copper, zinc and selected clinical variables in urine and serum of male runners, *Biol. Trace Element Res.* 6(4), 327–36, 1984.
81. Volpe, S.L., Lowe, N.M., Woodhouse, L.R. and King, J.C., Effect of maximal exercise on the short-term zinc kinetics of zinc metabolism in sedentary males, *Brit. J. Sports Med.* 41(3), 156–61, 2007.
82. Wakimoto, P. and Block, G., Dietary intake, dietary patterns and changes with age: An epidemiological perspective, *J. Gerontol.* 56A(II), 65–80, 2001.
83. Krotkiewski, M., Gudmundsson, P., Backstrom, P. and Mandroukas, K., Zinc and muscle strength and endurance, *Acta Physiol. Scand.* 116(3), 309–11, 1982.
84. Van Loan, M.D., Sutherland, B., Lowe, N.M., Turnlund, J.R. and King, J.C., The effects of zinc depletion on peak force and total work of knee and shoulder extensor and flexor muscles, *Int. J. Sport Nutr.* 9(2), 125–35, 1999.
85. Maxwell, C. and Volpe, S.L., Effect of zinc supplementation on thyroid hormone function: A case study of two college females, *Ann. Nutr. Metab.* 51(2), 188–94, 2007.
86. Spencer, H., Rubino, N., Kramer, L., Norris, C. and Osis, D., Effect of zinc supplements on the intestinal absorption of calcium, *J. Am. Coll. Nutr.* 6(1), 47–51, 1987.
87. Dolby, V., Chromium at the energy crossroads, *Better Nutr.* 60(5), 32, 1998.
88. Anderson, R.A., Polansky, M.M., Bryden, N.A., Roginski, E.E., Patterson, K.Y. and Reamer, D.C., Effect of exercise (running) on serum glucose, insulin, glucagon and chromium excretion, *Diabetes* 31(3), 212–6, 1982.
89. Kobla, H.V. and Volpe, S.L., Chromium, exercise and body composition, *Crit. Rev. Food Sci. Nutr.* 40(4), 291–308, 2000.
90. Bemden, M.G., Bemden, D.A. and Hartman, M.J., Chromium, in *Sports Nutrition: Vitamins and Trace Elements*, 2nd Edition, I. Wolinsky and J.A. Driskell, eds., CRC Press, Boca Raton, FL, 2005, pp. 267–74.
91. Anderson, R.A., Chromium metabolism and its role in disease processes in man, *Clin. Physiol. Biochem.* 4(1), 31–41, 1986.
92. Volpe, S.L., Huang, H.-W., Larpadisorn, K. and Lesser, I.I., Effect of chromium supplementation on body composition, resting metabolic rate and selected biochemical parameters in moderately obese women following an exercise program, *J. Am. Coll. Nutr.* 20(4), 293–306, 2001.
93. Volek, J.S., Silvestre, R., Kirwan, J.P. et al., Effects of chromium supplementation on glycogen synthesis after high-intensity exercise, *Med. Sci. Sports Exerc.* 38(12), 2102–9, 2006.

9 Fluid, Electrolytes and Hydration Needs of Masters Athletes

Kathryn Jackson

CONTENTS

9.1 INTRODUCTION

Hydration is an often overlooked nutritional factor that can influence exercise performance, particularly endurance exercise in the heat. It is commonly considered that a loss of only 2%–3% body water (BW) due to dehydration leads to exercise performance decrements [1], although any amount of dehydration can impair temperature regulation mechanisms in the body [2]. The effects of dehydration on thermoregulation can cause detrimental health outcomes, including impaired cognitive and cardiovascular functions and associated heat illness [3]. The effects of dehydration are not limited to masters athletes, but age-related fluid changes such as intra-cellular water loss compared to extra-cellular fluid losses during body water loss pose increased health and performance risks among older athletes [4,5].

Although endurance training and competition usually have a greater impact on fluid loss than sprint events [6], participation in competitions such as the many Masters Games competitions worldwide may involve more than one competitive event within a day. This scenario may increase the risk of dehydration if appropriate pre-event hydration and post-event rehydration are not attended to. Furthermore, the risk of dehydration in colder environments also must not be overlooked, as colder air is less saturated with water than warmer air, particularly at higher altitudes [2]. Expired air from the warmer respiratory system is more saturated than the inhaled air, increasing the risk of dehydration if strenuous exercise takes place without appropriate hydration strategies.

This chapter will focus on pre-, during- and post-exercise hydration needs of athletes, with particular emphasis on the unique requirements of masters athletes over the age of 35 years. Minor adjustments to standard hydration strategies are all that is needed among older athletes to ensure peak performance is not affected by dehydration or indeed by hyperhydration.

9.2 WATER AS AN ESSENTIAL NUTRIENT

Water is an essential nutrient as it is the basis of many biochemical and physiological functions in the human body. Water is also a carrier for waste disposal and an integral part of cell, tissue and organ structure. During exercise, water facilitates rapid delivery of nutrients and oxygen to working muscles and faster waste removal, while the role of water in thermoregulation is paramount. As the body core temperature increases with intensity and duration of exercise, extracellular water in the blood plasma compartment is partially diverted through blood vessels in the skin for radiant heat loss and evaporative cooling through sweat production. Loss of body water through sweat loss increases the electrolyte concentration (osmolality) in plasma [7]. For this reason it is counterproductive for dehydrated athletes to ingest salt tablets, with the further increase in plasma sodium concentration exacerbating the already hyperosmotic plasma. With as little as a 2%–3% loss of body weight as water, plasma electrolyte imbalances directly affect brain function [1,8]. Typical symptoms of these electrolyte imbalances include confusion, impaired muscle function and slowed reaction times [9]. Any of these symptoms can markedly impair exercise performance in athletes of any age.

The detection of body water loss and plasma electrolyte disturbances by brain cells triggers thirst, and in some cases 'sodium hunger' [10]. To restore water and electrolyte balance, reabsorptive actions in the kidney tubules are mediated by various hormones, including renin, antidiuretic hormone (ADH), and aldosterone [11]. Post-exercise plasma concentrations of these water- and salt-retaining hormones have been found to be lower among older athletes compared to their younger counterparts, particularly during post-exercise rehydration [12]. This may explain the blunted thirst reflex observed among older athletes [13], with the associated risk of incomplete rehydration following exercise. Without complete rehydration, older athletes are at risk of health complications such as increased blood pressure and cardiac strain and increased toxicity of medications [9], as well as performance decrements if further exercise is undertaken the same day or even the following day.

9.3 INFLUENCE OF AGE ON BODY WATER, THIRST AND FLUID INTAKE

Maintenance of water balance is less finely tuned among older adults [14], while renal function is also affected by ageing [15]. There is also a decreased ability to concentrate urine when fluid intake is suboptimal [16], leading to increased urine output [17] and subsequent blunting of the thirst sensation [13]. In addition, the decline in lean body mass with age can lead to a decrease in body water content which can be up to 4 litres loss in men and 6 litres loss in women by 80 years of age [16,18].

Any or each of these age-related water balance factors may increase the risk of dehydration, particularly during exercise and particularly in hot, humid environments. However, research among masters endurance runners [12] showed that age had no effect on fluid loss, which is supported by observations that osmoreceptor signalling in the kidneys is unaffected by increasing age [9]. Indeed endurance and resistance training among older adults may assist with maintenance of total body water, with associated improvements in cardiovascular and thermoregulatory function [4,19]. Further investigation of fluid balance in older athletes is clearly required.

Nonetheless, it is generally accepted that there is a decreased sweat output and delayed sweat response with age which increases the risk of increased core temperature during exercise [20]. Accompanied by attenuated vasodilatation of blood vessels [13] and decreased capillary density in skeletal muscle [21] in older adults, convective and evaporative heat loss due to decreased blood flow at the skin surface can be severely reduced during exercise among masters athletes. There follows an increased risk of hyperthermia in this older athlete population, even in the absence of dehydration.

9.4 DEHYDRATION

Dehydration describes a physiological state of low body water and is more correctly termed as hypohydration [2]. For the purposes of this chapter, the term dehydration will be used to describe a state of low body water.

Loss of body water as sweat during exercise is a physiological response to overheating of the core body temperature. Conduction of body water via the blood supply to the skin surface leads to whole body evaporative cooling. Indeed, much of the body water used for evaporative cooling is provided by the plasma compartment of blood (extra-cellular water) [8]. As the plasma volume is redirected to sweat production, more water is sourced from other body compartments to maintain a plasma volume that supports appropriate electrolyte concentrations [11]. However, both exercise and cognitive performance decrements are associated with overheating of the core body temperature due to an insufficient water intake to maintain evaporative cooling [8]. Various terms have been used to describe this pathological increase in core body temperature, including 'heat stroke' and 'heat exhaustion'. However, a succinct description of 'heat illness' encompasses various descriptions of the effects of elevated body core temperature, often due to dehydration [22].

The volume of water intake required to maintain hydration status is not clearly understood. Recommendations have been based on retrospective data in which water intake was compared with urine osmolality in healthy adults [1], while recommendations for sport and exercise suggest ingestion of approximately 1 L to 1.2 L/h for every hour of exercise, based upon the mean gastric emptying rate in well-hydrated adults and sweat rates, determined from energy expenditure and latent heat of evaporation calculations [9]. Rehydration strategies supported by the International Olympic Committee (IOC) suggest the post-exercise volume of fluid intake should be equivalent to weight lost during exercise (e.g. 0.5 kg weight loss ≅ 0.5 L fluid required) [23]. The fluid intake recommendation for exercise is in addition to a daily recommended baseline of approximately 1.4 L to replace obligatory water loss in urine, sweat, faeces and respiratory losses [24]. These fluid intake recommendations have recently been challenged by Tim Noakes who stated that these guidelines can lead to over-drinking and hyponatraemia (dilution of plasma electrolyte concentrations) with its attendant health risks [22]. This may be of particular relevance to older athletes if the attenuated sweat production with age [20] is accompanied by fluid intakes in excess of the amount of body water lost as sweat.

9.5 HYPONATRAEMIA AND WATER INTOXICATION

Hyponatraemia is defined as a serum sodium concentration less than 135 mmol/L in adults [25] and is usually a serum electrolyte dilution effect caused by excess water intake. Masters athletes are as vulnerable as all athletes to health and exercise performance decrements associated with hyperhydration (over-hydration), which usually manifests as hyponatraemia [26].

The risk of hyponatraemia is greater among endurance athletes than non-endurance athletes due to the prolonged duration of exercise and associated fluid intake. This risk is enhanced among older athletes who consume more water than is lost through sweat and urine output, due to the decrease in sweat output with age [20], and among those who hyperhydrate with water in low-sweat exercise conditions such as short duration exercise in cool, dry conditions. In addition, masters athletes are likely to take longer to complete endurance events such as a marathon compared to their younger counterparts [27], with the potential for further hyperhydration due to longer exercise duration and diligent water intake, but slower exercise pace and attendant lower sweat losses than faster or younger athletes. Similarly, non-endurance athletes in the older age group may be at risk if water or low-sodium beverage intakes (e.g. fruit juice, cordial or soft drinks) are higher than their fluid losses, when they diligently consume these fluids in exercise situations where there is a low risk of excessive fluid loss. Such an imbalance between water intake and output can lead to water intoxication, whereby the concentration of sodium in the bloodstream is diluted [26]. Conversely, hyponatraemic dehydration is rare, in which excessive sweat loss leads to large losses of plasma sodium, and yet this is the physiological state that is most commonly publicised in the media by various sports beverage manufacturers. There is some variability between individuals in the extent of electrolyte losses in sweat [2], but for most masters athletes the risk of excessive electrolyte loss is relatively low.

Water intoxication is a phenomenon which involves replacement of fluid losses without attention to sodium replacement. This scenario is more likely among endurance athletes participating in ultra-endurance events (see Chapter 15) such as Ironman triathlon competitions, particularly in hot and humid conditions in which the combination of prolonged exercise (>4 hours continuous exercise), heat and humidity contribute to excessive sodium and body water losses [28]. Typically hydration status is attended to with water intake, but electrolyte (particularly sodium) losses are not adequately replaced, leading to dilution of plasma sodium concentrations [22].

9.6 THE ROLE OF ELECTROLYTES IN HYDRATION

Electrolytes (mainly sodium and potassium) in dedicated sports beverages have a very specific role in maintaining hydration during exercise and assisting with rehydration following exercise. Unlike the popular media message that electrolytes added to sports drinks 'put back what the sweat takes out', loss of these micronutrients in sweat is not usually sufficient to require their specific replacement. Only in situations in which large volumes of sweat are produced, such as extreme endurance events performed in hot and humid environments, are the sodium and potassium losses sufficient to require their replacement. These electrolyte losses can be exacerbated by hypotonic fluid replacement beverages that lack electrolytes, such as plain water, cordial or soft drinks, leading to a dilution effect in blood plasma.

In most exercise circumstances, electrolytes are conserved in the body as the water component is lost as sweat [29], and the sweat becomes more dilute. As a result, sodium and potassium concentrations increase in blood plasma, until body water balance is restored through beverage intakes and renal adjustment. It is therefore counter-productive to consume salt tablets during exercise, as this will simply add to the already concentrated 'salt' in blood plasma, which may lead to transient increases in blood pressure in older vulnerable athletes. In addition, it is not known if the renal adjustment to restore body water balance after exercise is as effective in older athletes, as plasma concentrations of the electrolyte- and water-retaining hormones (aldosterone and ADH) are lower among older adults [12].

Sports drinks provide low concentrations of electrolytes (sodium and potassium) to assist with the rate of fluid uptake by the body. Sodium in particular assists with more rapid water absorption compared to water alone, as sodium is actively transported across the small intestine wall [30], dragging water with it. Absorption of plain water or low-sodium beverages across the intestine wall occurs by passive diffusion against a concentration gradient, which is slower than its assisted passage in the presence of sodium [31]. Post-exercise rehydration may also be more effectively achieved with commercial sports drinks, as the small amounts of electrolytes in these beverages will slightly increase their plasma concentrations, driving the thirst reflex [11]. This will lead to greater fluid intakes to restore electrolyte concentrations to within the normal range, ensuring more complete rehydration following exercise.

The risk of incomplete rehydration occurs when plain water or low sodium beverages are consumed and the plasma electrolyte concentrations are diluted. In this situation the thirst reflex is likely to be satisfied before rehydration is completed. However in masters athletes, for whom the thirst sensation may be blunted [13], there is an increased risk of incomplete rehydration if the hydration fluid is also low in sodium, as the thirst sensation is no longer a reliable indicator of complete rehydration. Further research is required in this area of rehydration for masters athletes, particularly with sports drinks compared to plain water and low-sodium beverages.

Sodium concentrations in appropriate sports drinks vary between 10–30 mmol per litre of fluid [32]. These relatively low electrolyte concentrations are sufficient to replace any small sodium losses during usual exercise, even endurance exercise, while assisting with water absorption and maintenance of the thirst reflex. Further electrolyte replacement is easily achieved with post-exercise food intake, although sweat and urine electrolyte losses are likely to be relatively low under normal exercise or cool or thermoneutral conditions.

Over recent years, recommendations for higher-sodium sports beverages have been introduced to satisfy the needs of extreme endurance athletes [33], such as Ironman triathlons, for whom large sweat losses may lead to plasma electrolyte losses and hyponatraemic dehydration. However, it must be stressed that this is an extreme exercise situation that is not usually encountered by masters athletes nor indeed most endurance athletes. Individual hydration and electrolyte replacement strategies should be attended to among masters athletes who compete in these events.

9.7 ELECTROLYTES AND MUSCLE CRAMPS

The addition of potassium, sodium and/or magnesium to sports beverages and various sports supplements is often promoted by commercial interests to prevent exercise-associated muscle cramps (EAMCs). These promotions are based mainly on older evidence [34] that described heat cramps due to hyponatraemia and water intoxication, which are often confused with EAMC. The aetiologies of heat cramps and EAMC are distinctly different, with the latter less well understood but thought to be associated with altered neuromuscular function [35,36]. Various dietary risk factors for EAMC have been suggested, including electrolyte imbalances and dehydration [37]. For the prevention and treatment of EAMC, there is currently no definitive scientific evidence to support the addition of extra sodium, potassium, magnesium or any other electrolytes to the diet by specific food selection or supplementation, as there is no evidence to suggest a causative relationship between loss of electrolytes in sweat and EAMC [35,36,38] in most athletes, except those who compete in prolonged exercise in hot, humid environments where there is a greater risk of hyponatraemia. However, there are observed exceptions such as those athletes who show excessive sodium losses in sweat in non-extreme exercise conditions and experience concomitant muscle cramps [39]. In these less common circumstances, sodium replacement has been an effective treatment for EAMC [37], although some evidence still suggests a role for dehydration in the development of EAMC [39,40]. Masters athletes may be more at risk of EAMC than their younger counterparts, as muscle cramps in general are more likely to occur and more frequently among the older population [41].

Hypomagnesaemia (magnesium deficiency) may also be associated with muscle cramps [41] but this deficiency is not caused by the very small magnesium losses in sweat during exercise. Generally magnesium deficiency is only seen among those with poor nutrition or specific medical conditions and is not due to dehydration and prolonged exercise.

9.8 THE EFFECTS OF CAFFEINE AND ALCOHOL ON HYDRATION STATUS

9.8.1 CAFFEINE

Caffeine (1,3,7-trimethylxanthine) is a central and peripheral nervous system stimulant [42] consumed daily throughout the world in beverages and foods. Typical caffeine concentrations in common beverages and foods are shown in Table 9.1 [43].

Since caffeine was removed from the World Anti-Doping Agency (WADA) banned substances list in 2004, use of caffeine among athletes as an ergogenic aid has increased [44]. Removal of caffeine from the WADA list was due mainly to the large variability in habitual caffeine-containing dietary and beverage intakes and the inter-individual variability in the urinary detection test (previously banned urinary threshold of 12 μg/mL). Therefore urinary concentrations of caffeine and its metabolites could not accurately indicate supplement intakes.

TABLE 9.1
Caffeine Content of Some Common Caffeine-Containing Beverages and Foods

Beverage or Food	Caffeine (mg/serve)	Serve Size
Coffee from ground beans	253	Long black (250 mL)
Coffee from ground beans	146	Espresso/short black (75 mL)
Instant coffee	175	1 teaspoon (5 g) powder/granules
Regular Tea brewed from leaves or tea bags	46	Black tea, standard mug (240 mL)
Coca Cola™	38	375-ml can
Diet Coke™	48	375-ml can
Coke Zero™	34	375-ml can
Iced coffee, fat reduced	90	600-ml carton
Red Bull™ energy drink	80	250-ml can
Powerade Energy Edge™ sports drink	108	450-ml bottle
Glaceau Vitamin Water Energy™	75	500-ml bottle
Milk chocolate, plain	50	250-g block
Dark chocolate, plain	148	250-g block

Source: Food Standards Australia New Zealand. *NUTTAB 2010 Online Searchable Database*. Canberra: Commonwealth of Australia, 2011. Available at http://www.foodstandards.gov.au/science/monitoringnutrients/nutrientables/nuttab/Pages/default.aspx, accessed 6 February 2014.

Historically, caffeine has been regarded as a diuretic which may promote dehydration, particularly if consumed in a sporting context [45]. It was thought that caffeine induces fluid and electrolyte losses through increased urine output, exacerbating fluid losses from increased sweat production, particularly among endurance athletes in the heat. However, much of this evidence comes from studies with laboratory rodents fed high doses of caffeine [46], the results of which cannot be translated directly to humans. More recent research has shown that caffeine consumed prior to exercise in doses equivalent to usual dietary intakes (~300 mg; two short black coffees) does not increase the risk of dehydration or heat illness [37,47]. Higher doses of caffeine (6 mg/kg body weight) (~420 mg for a 70-kg adult; 1 long black coffee + 600-mL bottle Diet Coke™ + 250-mL can of Red Bull™) prior to exercise, even in hot environments, also has no adverse effects on hydration status or thermoregulation [48] despite a slight increase in urine output at doses above 300 mg [37,49]. Even long-term caffeine intake (e.g. habitual coffee drinkers) does not lead to dehydration or heat illness during exercise [48].

Although the risk of dehydration among older athletes is enhanced with age [21], older habitual consumers of caffeine beverages should not be concerned about fluid and electrolyte losses during exercise. Nonetheless it would be prudent to adhere to appropriate hydration practices, as endurance exercise in the heat is more likely to lead to dehydration and heat illness than pre-exercise caffeine intake.

9.8.2 Alcohol

The effects of alcohol intake on hydration status are usually considered in a post-exercise context. Celebratory drinks or enjoying an alcoholic beverage of choice after arduous exercise need not be banned, but some simple rehydration steps should be followed prior to alcohol consumption. These steps include adequate hydration with water or commercial sports drinks prior to commencement of exercise, maintenance of sufficient fluid intake during exercise, and adequate rehydration with water or sports drinks immediately after completion of exercise. Complete post-exercise rehydration should be accomplished before alcoholic beverages are consumed.

TABLE 9.2
Typical Ethanol Concentrations (G/100 mL) in Common Alcoholic Beverages

Beverage	Ethanol Concentration Range (%)
Wine (red, white, sparkling)	8–14
Port (fortified wine)	14.2
Beer (ale, bitter, draught, lager, stout)	3.3–5.7
Beer (low alcohol, <1% alcohol w/v)	0.7
Beer (reduced alcohol or light beer)	2.1
Beer (carbohydrate modified)	3.6
Spirits (distilled)	35–60
Cider (fermented from apples)	3.7–3.9
Liqueurs	12.4–14.2
Sake	14–16

Source: Food Standards Australia New Zealand. *NUTTAB 2010 Online Searchable Database*. Canberra: Commonwealth of Australia, 2011. Available at http://www.foodstandards.gov.au/science/monitoring nutrients/nutrientables/nuttab/Pages/default.aspx, accessed 6 February 2014.

Alcohol (ethanol; ethyl alcohol) exerts a dehydrating effect through inhibition of antidiuretic hormone (ADH). The result is increased urine production, with 1 g of alcohol purportedly leading to 10 mL excess urine production, but only if the alcoholic beverage has an ethanol concentration greater than 4% [50]. Typical ethanol concentrations of alcoholic beverages are shown in Table 9.2 [43]. Post-exercise alcohol consumption can exacerbate dehydration that had already occurred during exercise, which may lead to inadequate rehydration before exercise on the following day and poor competition or training performance, as well as cardiovascular risks due to poor thermoregulation. It is unlikely that complete rehydration can be achieved prior to exercise if athletes arrive at competition or training in a state of dehydration, as gastric emptying is delayed, leading to slowed delivery of fluid for body functions and increased exercise-related nausea [51].

Dehydration can also limit post-exercise muscle glycogen replenishment. The most likely mechanism is replacement of post-exercise dietary carbohydrate intake with alcohol [52], although studies with laboratory rats suggest that ethanol may mitigate in impaired post-exercise glucose uptake and glycogen synthesis by skeletal muscle, particularly following high-intensity exercise [53]. Alcohol-mediated decreases in insulin secretion were not evident in the cited human and rodent studies, suggesting that impaired glycogen repletion is not due to the suppression of insulin secretion that can accompany alcohol-induced hypoglycaemia [54].

In summary, while habitual intakes of caffeine-containing foods and beverages among older athletes may not lead directly to dehydration, the post-exercise effects of alcohol- and exercise-induced dehydration may lead to incomplete recovery, particularly as the thirst drive is possibly diminished in older athletes. There is the risk of inadequate muscle glycogen availability for the next day's training or competition and exacerbation of pre-existing dehydration from the previous day's exercise. Not only will fatigue occur more quickly in these circumstances, but the likelihood of further dehydration, and the attendant heat illness, increased heart rate and elevated blood pressure, could pose serious health risks to older athletes, particularly those who may have co-morbidities such as hypertension or heart disease.

9.9 CONCLUSION

There are very few contraindications to exercise in older adults, and any increased risk of dehydration with exercise in this population is easily prevented with simple and practical hydration strategies. However, as water balance is less finely controlled among older athletes, hydration should be conscientiously addressed by masters athletes and older exercisers prior to, during and post-exercise. Blunting of the thirst sensation among older athletes is of particular relevance, as the more recent recommendation for complete hydration suggests that athletes should consume fluids according to thirst [22]. Reliance upon quenching of thirst for complete hydration, particularly during and after endurance or multiple one-day events, may put masters athletes at risk of dehydration. Nonetheless, attention to pre-hydration strategies and maintaining regular fluid intakes during exercise should enable masters athletes to avoid the health risks and performance decrements associated with dehydration.

The choice of fluids is of utmost importance in all athletes but of particular importance to masters athletes. Among all athletes there is a risk of hyponatraemia from water intoxication if water is the sole beverage of choice, particularly during and post-exercise. Masters athletes who rightly are diligent about fluid intake with exercise should embrace the use of appropriate commercial sports drinks. The small amounts of added electrolytes in these beverages assist with maintenance of the thirst reflex, which is of added importance among older athletes for whom thirst may be an unreliable indicator of the volume of fluid required for complete rehydration. In addition, the carbohydrate content of commercial sports drinks can supplement both intra-muscular and liver glycogen stores during exercise and provide substrate for glycogen replacement post-exercise, while concomitantly attending to hydration needs.

Caffeinated beverages need not be avoided by masters athletes unless acute intakes of caffeine are greater than 300 mg. Evidence suggests that caffeine *per se* does not produce a diuretic effect sufficient to lead to dehydration with exercise in the older athlete population, even among habitual caffeine consumers. If large (>300 mg) acute doses of caffeine are used as an ergogenic aid, appropriate attention to other fluid intakes would be prudent in order to prevent dehydration in older athletes in whom renal water retention may be compromised by age. Conversely, post-exercise alcohol consumption can exacerbate exercise-induced dehydration, although appropriate post-exercise rehydration strategies prior to alcohol consumption can allow masters athletes to still celebrate their competition success and enjoy post-event socialising.

Readers interested in more in-depth discussion and reviews of the area of hydration, ageing and sports performance are encouraged to read a number of reviews [55–57].

9.10 IMPLICATIONS FOR SPORTS MEDICINE PROFESSIONALS AND CLINICIANS

The following implications are suggested for sports medicine professionals and clinicians working with older exercisers and masters athletes:

- Monitor hydration status, particularly post-exercise.
  - Measure changes in pre- versus post-exercise body weight, using the same operator and same weighing scales.
  - Weigh the athlete in competition (or training) clothes, without shoes.
  - Wring out clothes before post-exercise weigh-in to avoid inclusion of sweat loss absorbed by clothes in weight measurements.
  - Ensure athlete has voided as much urine as possible before the weigh-in, to account for water lost in the production of urine.
  - Measure fluid intake during exercise to add to the pre-exercise body weight measurement.
- Replace pre- versus post-exercise weight differential with equivalent fluid volume.
  - For every gram of weight loss, consume 1 mL of appropriate fluid (water or commercial sports drink only); 0.5 kg weight loss $\cong$ 500 mL (0.5 L) fluid replacement required.
  - Perceived symptoms of dehydration may be hyperthermia without significant dehydration, and weight-matched fluid replacement may be counter-productive (see Noakes [22] for clinical rationale).

- If athlete collapse occurs, do not assume this is due to dehydration. Other possible causes may include
  - Water intoxication. Check the type and volume of fluid consumed by the athlete pre-, during- and post-exercise.
  - Post-exercise hypotension.
  - Other cardiac-related malfunctions.

9.11 IMPLICATIONS FOR MASTERS ATHLETES AND COACHES

The following implications are suggested for masters athletes and coaches of masters athletes:

- Monitor hydration status according to the suggestions in Section 9.10.
- Dehydration can also be monitored by examination of urine colour.
  - Pale yellow urine indicates the athlete is well-hydrated.
  - Dark yellow urine suggests dehydration, but ingestion of medications containing yellow dye will also colour the urine.
- Rehearse type and volume of fluid intake for a competition event in similar environmental and race conditions to that expected on competition day. This allows for any untoward hydration-related outcomes to be corrected before competition day.
- Practise with *ad libitum* (voluntary) fluid intake, so that personalised fluid requirements can be established and then adopted for competition day.
  - This approach may maximise an individual athlete's exercised performance rather than following rigid one-size-fits-all fluid intake guidelines.
  - Check pre- versus post-exercise weight difference to determine an approximate estimate of post-exercise hydration status and required volume of fluid intake during exercise when competition day arrives.
- An alternative to *ad libitum* fluid intake is to follow current fluid intake recommendations of 250 mL fluid (water or sports drink) every 15 to 20 minutes during exercise.
- Have your own (labelled) drink bottles with your preferred fluid placed at drink stations for endurance events. Practise consuming fluids at similar distance-placed drink stations, to determine the appropriate volume required to meet an individual athlete's hydration (and energy) needs.
- Do not introduce unfamiliar fluids on competition day, as there is a risk that unfamiliar fluids may cause gastro-intestinal discomfort, vomiting and/or diarrhoea.
  - Train and compete with water and commercial sports drink only.
  - Beverages with added protein, fat or high (>10% w/v) carbohydrate concentrations can slow gastric emptying rate, causing gastro-intestinal discomfort and/or exacerbate exercise-induced dehydration.
- Temperature of beverages has minimal effect on rate of delivery of fluid into the bloodstream.
  - Chilled beverages may be more palatable, leading to a larger volume of intake, and may also be less likely to cause gastrointestinal discomfort compared to warm beverages.
  - Flavour of the beverage is also important to palatability and therefore to the volume of fluid consumed.

9.12 FUTURE RESEARCH DIRECTIONS

- The evidence about water loss during exercise for masters athletes is equivocal. While some evidence suggests renal water-retaining hormones (renin, ADH and aldosterone) are lower following exercise in older athletes, leading to greater urinary water loss, others state that age has no effect on fluid loss as renal osmoreceptor signalling is unaffected by age. More research is needed to address this area.

- There needs to be clarification of the effect of ageing on renal function during exercise, to ascertain the effects of age on renal hormone functions and their relationship to osmoreceptor function in water balance in this population. Currently these two mechanisms have only been investigated separately.
- The mechanism of blunted thirst sensation among older athletes requires further investigation, to determine whether this physiological phenomenon is directly related to decreased renal hormone function or other mechanisms, including decreased sweat output, particularly as the evidence for increased urinary water loss among older athletes is equivocal.
- Further investigation is required to determine whether the recommendation for *ad libitum* fluid intake during exercise is appropriate for older athletes.
- If the thirst sensation is blunted in these athletes, there is a theoretical risk that *ad libitum* fluid intake may be insufficient to achieve full rehydration status, particularly during and post-exercise.

REFERENCES

1. Popkin, B.M., D'Anci, K.E. and Rosenberg, I.H., Water, hydration and health, *Nutr. Rev.* 68, 439–58, 2010.
2. McArdle, W.D., Katch, F.I. and Katch, V.L., *Sports and Exercise Nutrition*, Lippincott, Williams & Wilkins, Baltimore, 2009.
3. Rodriguez, N.R., DiMarco, N.M. and Langley, S., Nutrition and athletic performance. Joint position statement: American College of Sports Medicine, American Dietetic Association, Dietitians of Canada, *Med. Sci. Sports Exerc.* 41, 709–31, 2009.
4. Pickering, G., Hydration et exercise physique chez la personne âgée, *Sci. Sport* 13, 5–9, 1998.
5. Ritz, P., Salle, A. and Berrut, G., Body water variations in the elderly, *Nutr. Clin. Metabol.* 18, 205–11, 2004.
6. Jeukendrup, A.E., Nutrition for endurance sports: Marathon, triathlon and road cycling, *J. Sports Sci.* 29(Suppl 1), S91–9, 2011.
7. Jéquier, E. and Constant, F., Water as an essential nutrient: The physiological basis of hydration, *Eur. J. Clin. Nutr.* 64, 115–23, 2010.
8. Thornton, S.N., Thirst and dehydration: Physiology and consequences of dysfunction, *Physiol. Behav.* 100, 15–21, 2010.
9. Sawka, M.N., Burke, L.M., Eichner, E.R., Maughan, R.J., Montain, S.J. and Stachenfeld, N.S., Exercise and fluid replacement. American College of Sports Medicine position stand, *Med. Sci. Sports Exerc.* 39, 377–90, 2007.
10. Borer, K.T., *Exercise Endocrinology*, Human Kinetics, Champaign, IL, 2003.
11. Louden, J.D., Regulation of fluid and electrolyte balance, *Anaesth. Intens. Care Med.* 13, 302–8, 2012.
12. Galbo, H., Influence of aging and exercise on endocrine function, *Int. J. Sport Nutr. Exerc. Metab.* 11, S49–57, 2001.
13. Reilly, T. and Waterhouse, J., Circadian aspects of body temperature regulation in exercise, *J. Thermal. Biol.* 34, 161–70, 2009.
14. Ritz, P., Body water spaces and cellular hydration during healthy aging, *Ann. NY Acad. Sci.* 904, 474–83, 2000.
15. Bennett, J.A., Dehydration: Hazards and benefits, *Geriatr. Nurs.* 21, 84–8, 2000.
16. Steen, B., Body water in the elderly—a review, *J. Nutr. Health Aging.* 1, 142–5, 1997.
17. Maharam, L.G., Bauman, P.A., Kalman, D., Skolnik, H. and Perle, S.M., Masters athletes: Factors affecting performance, *Sports Med.* 28, 273–85, 1999.
18. Gille, D., Overview of the physiological changes and optimal diet in the golden age generation over 50, *Eur. Rev. Aging Phys. Act.* 7, 27–36, 2010.
19. Best, S., Caillaud, C. and Thompson, M., The effect of ageing and fitness on thermoregulatory response to high-intensity exercise, *Scand. J. Med. Sci. Sports.* 22, e29–37, 2012.
20. Campbell, W.W. and Geik, R.A., Nutritional considerations for the older athlete, *Nutr.* 20, 603–8, 2004.
21. Tarnopolsky, M., Nutritional consideration in the aging athlete, *Clin. J. Sports Med.* 18, 531–8, 2008.
22. Noakes, T.D., A modern classification of the exercise-related heat illness, *J. Sci. Med. Sport.* 11, 33–9, 2008.

23. Maughan, R.J., Burke, L.M. and Coyle, E.F., eds., *Food, Nutrition and Sports Performance II. The International Olympic Committee Consensus on Sports Nutrition*, Routledge, London, 2004.
24. Stipanuk, M.H. and Caudell, M.A., eds., *Biochemical, Physiological and Molecular Aspects of Human Nutrition*, Elsevier Saunders, St. Louis, MO, 2013.
25. Chorley, J., Cianca, J. and Divine, J., Risk factors for exercise-associated hyponatraemia in non-elite marathon runners, *Clin. J. Sport Med.* 17, 471–7, 2007.
26. Noakes, T.D., Changes in body mass alone explain almost all of the variance in the serum sodium concentrations during prolonged exercise. Has commercial influence impeded scientific endeavor? *Br. J. Sports Med.* 45, 475–7, 2011.
27. Tanaka, H. and Seals, D.R., Endurance exercise performance in masters athletes: Age-associated changes and underlying physiological mechanisms, *J. Physiol.* 586, 55–63, 2008.
28. Noakes, T.D. and Speedy, D.B., Case proven: Exercise associated hyponatraemia is due to overdrinking, *Br. J. Sports Med.* 40, 567–72, 2006.
29. Valtin, H., 'Drink at least 8 glasses of water a day'. Really? Is there scientific evidence for '8 × 8'? *Am. J. Physiol.* 283, R993–1004, 2002.
30. Katch, V.L., McArdle, W.D. and Katch, F.I., *Essentials of Exercise Physiology*, Lippincott, Williams & Wilkins, Baltimore, 2011.
31. Shi, X. and Passe, D.H., Water and solute absorption from carbohydrate-electrolyte solutions in the human proximal small intestine: A review and statistical analysis, *Int. J. Sport Nutr. Exerc. Metab.* 20, 427–42, 2010.
32. Burke, L. and Deakin, V., eds., *Clinical Sports Nutrition*, McGraw-Hill, Sydney, 2010.
33. Valentine, V., The importance of salt in the athlete's diet, *Curr. Sports Med. Rep.* 6, 237–40, 2007.
34. McGee, S.R., Muscle cramps, *Arch. Intern. Med.* 150, 511–18, 1990.
35. Schwellnus, M.P., Drew, N. and Collins, M., Muscle cramping in athletes—risk factors, clinical assessment and management, *Clin. Sports Med.* 27, 183–94, 2008.
36. Minetto, M.A., Holobar, A., Botter, A. and Farina, D., Origin and development of muscle cramps, *Exerc. Sport Sci.* 41, 3–10, 2013.
37. Ganio, M.S., Casa, D.J., Armstrong, L.E. and Maresh, C.M., Evidence-based approach to lingering hydration questions, *Clin. Sports Med.* 26, 1–16, 2007.
38. Sulzer, N.U., Schwellnus, M.P. and Noakes, T.D., Serum electrolytes in Ironman triathletes with exercise-associated muscle cramping, *Med. Sci. Sports Exerc.* 37, 1081–5, 2005.
39. Schwellnus, M.P., Cause of exercise associated muscle cramps (EAMC)—altered neuromuscular control, dehydration or electrolyte depletion? *Br. J. Sports Med.* 43, 401–8, 2009.
40. Casa, D.J., Exercise in the heat. I. Fundamentals of thermal physiology, performance implications and dehydration, *J. Athl. Train.* 34, 246–52, 1999.
41. Gaby, A.R., Nutritional interventions for muscle cramps, *Integr. Med.* 6, 20–3, 2007.
42. Higgins, J.P., Tuttle, T.D. and Higgins, C.L., Energy beverages: Content and safety, *Mayo Clin. Proc.* 85, 1033–41, 2010.
43. Food Standards Australia New Zealand. *NUTTAB 2010 Online Searchable Database*. Canberra: Commonwealth of Australia, 2011, http://www.foodstandards.gov.au/science/monitoringnutrients/nutrientables/nuttab/Pages/default.aspx, accessed 6 February 2014.
44. Del Coso, J., Munoz, G., Murloz-Guerra, J. and Cela, C., Prevalence of caffeine use in elite athletes following its removal from the World Anti-Doping Agency list of banned substances, *Appl. Physiol. Nutr. Metab.* 36, 555–61, 2011.
45. Greer, F., Commentary. Myth buster: Caffeine does not exhibit a diuretic effect during exercise performance, *Indian J. Med. Res.* 132, 11–3, 2010.
46. Ruxton, C.H.S., The impact of caffeine on mood, cognitive function, performance and hydration: A review of benefits and risks, *Nutr. Bull* 33, 15–25, 2008.
47. Armstrong, L.E., Casa, D.J., Maresh, C.M. and Ganio, M.S., Caffeine, fluid-electrolyte balance, temperature regulation and exercise-heat tolerance, *Exerc. Sport Sci. Rev.* 35, 135–40, 2007.
48. Lopez, R.M. and Casa, D.J., The influence of nutritional ergogenic aids on exercise heat tolerance and hydration status, *Curr. Sports Med. Rep.* 8, 192–9, 2009.
49. Maughan, R.J. and Griffin, J., Caffeine ingestion and fluid balance: A review, *J. Hum. Nutr. Dietet.* 16, 411–20, 2003.
50. Vella, L.D. and Cameron-Smith, D., Alcohol, athletic performance and recovery, *Nutrients* 2, 781–9, 2010.
51. Van Nieuwenhoven, M.A., Vriens, B.E., Brummer, R.J. and Brouns, E., Effect of dehydration on gastrointestinal function at rest and during exercise in humans, *Eur. J. Appl. Physiol.* 83, 578–584, 2000.

52. Burke, L.M., Collier, G.R., Broad, E.M. et al., Effect of alcohol intake on muscle glycogen storage after prolonged exercise, *J. Appl. Physiol.* 95, 983–90, 2003.
53. Peters, T.J., Nikolovski, S., Raja, G.H., Palmer, N. and Fournier, P.A., Ethanol acutely impairs glycogen repletion in skeletal muscle following high intensity short duration exercise in the rat, *Addict Biol.* 1, 289–95, 1996.
54. Marks, V., Alcohol and carbohydrate metabolism, *Clin. Endocrinol. Metab.* 7, 333–49, 1978.
55. Hooper, L., Bunn, D., Jimoh, F.O. and Fairweather–Tait, S.J., Water-loss dehydration and aging, *Mech. Ageing Dev.* doi: 10.1016/j.mad.2013.11.009 (Epub ahead of print).
56. Garth, A.K. and Burke, L.M., What do athletes drink during competitive sporting activities? *Sports Med.* 43(7), 539–64, 2013.
57. Goulet, E.D., Dehydration and endurance performance in competitive athletes, *Nutr. Rev.* 70(Suppl 2), S132–6, 2012.

10 Supplement Use in Masters Athletes

Ben Desbrow, Greg Shaw and Gary Slater

CONTENTS

10.1 INTRODUCTION

Organised sport and regular physical activity provides many benefits to older individuals including health benefits, social interaction, and the maintenance of self-identity and self-esteem [1]. While community-based guidelines and general nutrient reference values (NRVs) are suitable for addressing the nutritional needs associated with both sport and physical activity, some masters athletes are involved in sport at a level of commitment that creates unique nutritional requirements.

Implementing strategies to achieve these special nutritional needs can enhance the effectiveness of both training and competition performances. Many commercial companies have exploited the link between food and sports performance as a strategy by which to market supplements as a way of achieving outcomes of interest to athletes, including direct performance enhancement, facilitating recovery, promoting fat loss or building muscle mass and strength. In addition, many dietary supplements are also promoted for the enhancement of general health, the avoidance of chronic disease and the treatment of medical conditions, making the supplement market a difficult area to charter for the masters athlete and older exerciser.

This chapter aims to initially define dietary supplements, describe the supplement practices of masters athletes, explore issues of inadvertent doping associated with supplement use, and finally provide dietary supplement recommendations for older exercisers and masters athletes.

10.2 DEFINING A DIETARY SUPPLEMENT

'Dietary supplement' is a broad term with numerous definitions in the literature and in practice. Unlike science that needs a definition to guide research and investigation, athlete practices are not guided by a single and overarching definition of this term. Masters athletes may not be aware that a product they are consuming for the purpose of enhancing health or athletic performance is classified as a dietary supplement. It is important in the context of this chapter to discuss how dietary supplements are classified or defined to ensure masters athletes are aware of the range of products available while recognising key differences between products. There are numerous influencers that can impact a working definition of dietary supplements including the regulatory frameworks for foods and therapeutic agents in different countries, the form of products and the proposed mechanisms of action.

10.2.1 The Regulation of Dietary Supplements

In most countries or regions there is a governing body (or bodies) that regulate the manufacture and marketing of foods and therapeutic agents. Such organisations provide a working definition of a dietary supplement within their jurisdiction. For example, in the United States a dietary supplement is defined by the Dietary Supplement Health and Education Act of 1994 (DSHEA) as 'a product (other than tobacco) intended to supplement the diet that bears or contains one or more of the following dietary ingredients: a vitamin; a mineral; a herb or other botanical; an amino acid; a dietary substance for use by man to supplement the diet by increasing the total dietary intake; or a concentrate, metabolite, constituent, extract, or combination of any ingredient described previously' [2]. Within Europe a dietary supplement is defined as 'foodstuffs the purpose of which is to supplement the normal diet and which are concentrated sources of nutrients (meaning vitamins and minerals) or other substances with a nutritional or physiological effect, alone or in combination, marketed in dose form, namely forms such as capsules, pastilles, tablets, pills and other similar forms, sachets of powder, ampoules of liquids, drop dispensing bottles, and other similar forms of liquids and powders designed to be taken in measured small unit quantities' [3]. These food supplements are unable to claim the ability to cure or treat a disease but may make the claim to affect a physiological function. For example a food supplement cannot claim to cure heart disease but may make the claim to reduce cholesterol.

Within Australia, products commonly defined as dietary supplements in the United States or Europe fall into two different categories regulated by two different bodies. Formulated sports foods are regulated by the Food Standard Australia and New Zealand (FSANZ) and are defined as *foods or mixtures of foods specifically formulated to assist sports people in achieving specific nutritional or performance goals* [4]. Alternatively, dietary supplements are regulated by the Therapeutic Goods Administration (TGA) and are not as clearly defined as in other countries. Broadly, a dietary supplement is considered a therapeutic good and a therapeutic good is defined as being taken for the purpose of

a. Preventing, diagnosing, curing or alleviating a disease, ailment, defect or injury in persons
b. Influencing, inhibiting or modifying a physiological process in persons
c. Testing the susceptibility of persons to a disease or ailment
d. Influencing, controlling or preventing conception in persons
e. Testing for pregnancy in persons
f. The replacement or modification of parts of the anatomy in persons [5]

Therefore, the definition of a dietary supplement in Australia is regulated based on the proposed purpose of the product not the specified ingredients or components. Masters athletes need to be aware of what constitutes a dietary supplement in various jurisdictions around the world as increased international competition (e.g. World Masters Games, Pan Pacific Masters Games) and the availability of dietary supplements over the internet has resulted in older athletes potentially being exposed to products and ingredients not approved for sale in their country. Of course, the importation of ingredients/products that are considered supplements in one country may be prohibited by customs laws in another, with individuals subjected to the consequences of any breached laws.

10.2.2 The Form Supplements Take

Dietary supplements can be presented in a number of forms including solid foods, drinks, small-volume liquids, powders, capsules and tablets. They are commonly administered via two distinct routes: oral or infusion, with the latter route including intramuscular and intravascular administration. While it can be argued that intravascular and intramuscular injection of nutrients should be classified as a medical procedure carrying risks rather than a nutritional intervention, it is noted that athletes report self-administration of injectable dietary nutrients as a way of supplementing dietary sources [6]. Dietary supplements that require infusion should only be considered by a medical procedures. Dietary supplements that require this route of administration may be considered by a medical professional to correct a nutritional deficiency diagnosed against an established requirement. It is important to recognise that a range of products, including peptides and pro-hormones, have been promoted or popularised as dietary supplements which are in fact pharmaceutical agents and even though they are available freely from sources that sell dietary supplements they should not be considered as such [7]. Masters athletes thinking of using these products for anti-ageing reasons should first seek the advice of a trained medical professional, specifically one familiar with the World Anti-Doping Agency (WADA) code [8].

10.2.3 Dietary Supplements Mode of Action

An early definition of sports supplements divided products into nutritional supplements and ergogenic aids based on the intended rationale for their use or mode of action [9]. Ergogenic aids have been defined as products claiming to 'provide a direct enhancement of sports performance by mechanisms other than meeting the goals of everyday nutrition' [9]. These mechanisms might include effects on the central nervous system, or by supplying metabolites or co-factors that are important in metabolism. The classification of nutritional supplements included formulated sports foods which were defined as specialised products in a food form with a composition, size or presentation intended to 'provide a convenient and practical means of meeting a known nutrient requirement to optimise daily training or competition performance' [10]. Examples of such products include liquid meal supplements, sports drinks, sports gels and sports bars [10]. It is the purposeful formulation of these foods from specific ingredients that classify them as dietary supplements, warranting their inclusion in investigations of supplementation practices of both young and older athletes. Indeed, they have been shown to contribute substantially to the nutrient intake of younger athletes [11]. Micronutrient supplements used to prevent or treat a known nutritional deficiency (i.e. iron, vitamin D and multivitamin supplements) are another example of nutritional supplements.

While the classification of products as nutritional supplements or ergogenic aids may have provided some logical definitions in the past, two recent and significant changes have blurred these previously distinct supplement categories. Firstly, the supplement industry now produces large numbers of multi-ingredient sports foods which contain ergogenic ingredients in addition to traditional nutrient components. Food and beverage items which fall within this group could be referred to as 'functional sports foods' and include examples such as sports drinks containing added caffeine and sports bars containing creatine. Secondly, scientific knowledge regarding nutritional factors affecting performance has increased, necessitating a broader scope for performance-enhancing supplements. For instance a probiotic (specific bacteria ingested for the purpose of optimising gut microflora) may be considered ergogenic by reducing the incidence, severity and duration of upper respiratory tract infections [12,13], thereby allowing the athlete to achieve uninterrupted training without illness.

10.3 PROGRAMS TO GUIDE SAFE PRACTICE

More recently, to incorporate all the above considerations and provide athletes with clear direction for supplement use, programs based on the strength of the evidence of the efficacy of a product have

TABLE 10.1
Australian Institute of Sport (AIS) Sport Supplement Program Categorisations

Category	Supplements Included
Group A: Supported for use in specific situations in sport and provided to AIS athletes for evidence-based uses	Sports drinks, gels and confectionery Liquid meals and whey protein Sports bar Calcium supplement Iron supplement Probiotics Multivitamin/mineral Vitamin D Electrolyte replacement Caffeine Creatine Bicarbonate
Group B: Deserving of further research and considered for provision to AIS athletes under a research protocol	B-alanine Beetroot juice/nitrate Anti-oxidants C and E Carnitine HMB Fish oils Quercetin Probiotics for immune support Other polyphenols as anti-oxidants and anti-inflammatories
Group C: No meaningful proof of beneficial effects and not provided to AIS athletes	Ribose Coenzyme Q10 Vitamins outside A use Ginseng Other herbals (Cordyceps, Rhodiola Rosea) Glucosamine Chromium picolinate Oxygenated waters MCT oils ZMA Inosine Pyruvate Others—if you can't find it anywhere, it probably deserves to be here
Group D: Banned or at high risk of contamination and should not be used by AIS athletes	Stimulants: • Ephedrine • Strychnine • Sibutramine geranium oil and associated compounds (e.g. methylhexanamine) • Bitter orange and associated compounds (e.g. octopamine and synephrine) • Other herbal stimulants Pro-hormones and hormone boosters: • DHEA • Androstenedione • 19-norandrostenione/ol • Other pro-hormones • Tribulus terrestris and other testosterone boosters Glycerol Colostrum

Source: Australian Institute of Sport: AIS Supplement Group Classification System. Available at http://www.ausport.gov.au/ais/nutrition/supplements/classification_test, accessed 5 March 2014.

emerged. One such example is the Australian Institute of Sport (AIS) Sports Supplement Framework. It provides the expertise and resources developed during the implementation of the AIS Sports Supplement Program (2000–13), allowing Australian sporting organisations and agencies to develop their own sports supplement programs and guidelines [14]. Within this program, evidence of supplement efficacy is considered by a panel of experts using a mix of subjective and objective criteria. Once evaluated, a dietary supplement is then allocated into one of four groups (A, B, C and D). This categorisation is based on the level of scientific evidence available for performance enhancement and the relative risk of a dietary supplement containing (potentially through inadvertent contamination) a banned substance (see Table 10.1). The most visible component of the program is an education program available to all via the AIS website [14]. The education program tries to influence the supplement practices of athletes of all ages by empowering them to make informed decisions with background information on the specific dietary supplement, safety guidelines and also evidence-based supplement protocols [14].

In summary, what defines a dietary supplement is broad, confusing and is changing rapidly. It is therefore the responsibility of masters athletes, their coaches, sports scientists and masters sport administrators to ensure programs are in place to help guide and educate older athletes on what is effective and safe use of dietary supplements.

10.4 SUPPLEMENTATION PRACTICES OF MASTERS ATHLETES

Dietary supplementation has become a mainstream practice driving a lucrative industry. In the United States alone the sports nutrition and weight loss sector of the supplement industry was estimated at US$22.7 billion [15], representing a 10% compound growth rate over 13 years to 2010 [15]. The increase in monetary spending on dietary supplements follows a comparative increase in the prevalence of use of dietary supplements in the general population of the United States. Between 2003 and 2006, 44% of males and 54% of females reported using dietary supplements [16]. This is an increase from the 35% and 43% in males and females, respectively [16], who reported using dietary supplements between 1988–1994 [17]. Within Australia, recent evidence from consecutive national nutrition surveys indicates that supplement use also continues to rise. In 2011–12, 33% of females (up from 27% in 1995) and 24% (up from 15% in 1995) of males reported consuming a dietary supplement on the day prior to interview [18].

In the United States, upwards of 60% of the elderly population report use of dietary supplements on a daily basis, with health-conscious and physically active individuals also more likely to take supplements [19]. This may, in part, reflect the successful marketing of athletes portrayed as high supplement users with the employment of athletes as brand ambassadors by supplement companies providing anecdotal testimonials or paid scripted promotions [20]. In addition, athletes are portrayed in marketing campaigns as having higher or different nutritional requirements which need to be met via the use of dietary supplements.

Contrary to this perception, dietary supplement research undertaken before 1994 showed usage rates in athletes that were only modestly higher than the general public [17,21]. For example, a review of 51 studies involving 10,274 participants found a mean prevalence of dietary supplement use by younger athletes of 46% [21]. This is compared to values of 40% within the general population at a similar time point [17]. Furthermore, in a direct comparison to a group of control subjects, Sundgot-Borgen and colleagues found that younger athletes reported higher supplement usage (53%) compared to controls (42%) [22].

Dietary supplement use in athletic populations appears to have increased over the last 15 years, mimicking general population trends. Large-scale studies completed within the last 5 years have reported mean usage rates by athletes of between 66% and 93% [23,24]. Although there is ample information on the supplement practices of junior, college, sub-elite and elite athletes, little information is available on the prevalence of supplement use in the masters athlete community.

In one of the most comprehensive studies examining supplement use in masters athletes, 60% of track and field athletes competing at the 2004 World Masters Indoor Athletics Championships reported using some form of dietary supplement [25]. This level of dietary supplement consumption is similar to those of other world-class track and field athletes [24]. These masters athletes primarily used vitamin and mineral supplements for health-related reasons although many still consumed supplements to enhance sports performance. The athletes sourced supplements from pharmacies, supermarkets, the Internet and drug stores [25]. Interestingly, just over half of the masters athletes using supplements reported getting them through the health care system in their country [25]. Masters athletes report physicians as preferred sources of supplement information, a group not known for expert nutrition knowledge [26]. This is despite the fact that individuals are also unlikely to self-disclose their supplementation practices to physicians [27], thus leaving the masters athlete at risk of inappropriate product selection and ingestion protocols as well as increasing their risk of committing a doping offence through the inadvertent ingestion of products contaminated with doping substances [28].

Although the prevalence of dietary supplement use in athletes is of interest, the safety and efficacy of dietary supplement use is of greatest concern. That is, to ensure that any misguided use of dietary supplementation (e.g. 'polypharmacy') does not lead to negative health implications, especially in older athletes who may be at increased risk of chronic disease. In most countries individuals would argue that the regulatory bodies responsible for supplement industry legislation should ensure that any negative health outcomes associated with supplement use are addressed as a priority. However, with the globalisation of the supplementation industry and the increased incidence of individuals frequently consuming multi-ingredient supplements, negative health consequence reports from supplement ingestion are on the rise [29,30].

For those masters athletes on prescription drugs, co-ingesting popular herbal or complementary medicines such as St John's wort, ginko, ginseng, kava, ginger and echinacea may also have significant clinical consequences [31]. Despite this, such herbal preparations are rarely considered in assessments of supplementation practices or disclosed during interaction with health care providers [27,32]. The prevalence of this polysupplementation is high amongst older adults, with upwards of one-third being at risk of interaction between their medications, herbs or nutritional supplements [33]. A detailed discussion of medication and nutrient interactions issues in masters athletes is presented in Chapter 13.

10.5 RATIONALE FOR SUPPLEMENT USE

Athletes take supplements for two primary reasons: the enhancement of health and/or the enhancement of athletic performance [25]. Broadly speaking, masters athletes are no different to other athletic groups in this regard. However, as individuals mature, the emphasis of health versus performance considerations may change and an awareness of the possible reasons why masters athletes take supplements is an important consideration when consulting older athletes or interpreting their supplement intake patterns.

Health-related supplements can take many forms and are often target-marketed toward the prevention or management of a health challenge. A supplement may proclaim broad effects relating to the prevention of 'at-risk' disease(s) (e.g. B group vitamins—folic acid, vitamin B-6 and vitamin B-12 for heart health—or antioxidants—beta-carotene, lycopene, vitamins C, E, and/or A for cancer prevention). These supplements may be consumed by otherwise healthy individuals where behaviour is influenced by a concern regarding prevalent health conditions or due to genetic susceptibility considerations as indicated by a family history.

For older athletes with established or perceived health challenges, dietary supplements also promote their capacity to assist in condition management by 'curing' or 'alleviating' a disease, ailment or injury (e.g. glucosamine to support the structure and function of joints in those suffering from osteoarthritis or magnesium to avoid excessive magnesium losses associated with hyperglycaemia in diabetes mellitus). Given ageing is directly associated with many disease processes [34], increasing age may create a strong trigger for health-related dietary supplementation in older athletes.

Masters athletes may also take dietary supplements to directly influence competition performance, or to indirectly alter performance with supplements designed to affect training and adaptation, enhance recovery or to alter body composition. Whilst very few masters athletes self-report the purposeful use of illicit drugs and doping substances [25], it is not rare for nutritional supplements to be contaminated with trace amounts of anabolic androgenic steroids or pro-hormones [35]. Athletes of any age who take supplements are therefore at risk of committing an inadvertent anti-doping rule violation. In addition, athletes of all ages should be aware that no differentiation is made between the inappropriate use of prohibited supplements for performance or health enhancement regardless of competition level or age grouping. For example, if a 55-year-old cyclist decides (without specific medical clearance) to start taking a coenzyme Q10 supplement for their 'heart condition' and that supplement is inadvertently contaminated with a prohibited pro-hormone, the use of this prohibited substances is viewed equally in terms of doping code violations. This is in accordance with the WADA strict liability principle, where any athlete is ultimately responsible for any substance found in their body, regardless of how it got there or why it was taken [8].

10.6 RECOMMENDATIONS

It is beyond the scope of this chapter to systematically discuss the full spectrum of dietary supplements that have evidence for ergogenic effects. Furthermore, the range of supplements promoted in the marketplace, plus the emerging evidence for their scientific support (or lack thereof) is in a constant state of flux, making it difficult to provide specific guidelines. Moreover, specific recommendations for supplement use amongst masters athletes should take into consideration several issues, which can vary markedly from one athlete to another.

The provision of appropriate recommendations on supplement use to masters athletes should involve consideration of the same issues as those for younger athletes. These include

- Specific motivation for participating in regular physical activity and sport. For example, to decrease all-cause mortality and increase physiological function to facilitate maintenance or improvement in activities of daily living versus competing in senior or masters-level events focused on enhancing sports performance.
- Current dietary intake, including both macro- and micronutrients with an associated consideration of daily energy requirements, plus fluid intake.
- Underlying medical conditions and associated prescribed pharmacotherapies, and where appropriate, herbal or complementary therapies, which may impact on nutrient needs directly or indirectly via drug-nutrient, herbal-nutrient or drug-herbal interactions (see Chapter 13).
- Training load and competition schedule.
- Other nutrition-related objectives such as changes of body composition.
- Financial constraints.
- Previous experiences including identification if an individual is a responder or not (i.e. perceived effect or documented via detailed monitoring).

Given the above, it is impractical to provide detailed recommendations for supplement prescription amongst masters athletes. The contemporary supplement categorisation scheme developed by the AIS and other bodies is an excellent platform from which to explore evidence-based supplement strategies for masters athletes. However, the unique physiological and metabolic characteristics of masters athletes relative to their younger counterparts will need to be taken into consideration.

Three examples are provided relating to sports drinks, high biological value (HBV) protein and osteoarthritis

- The reduced thirst response [36] and delayed gastric emptying [37] associated with ageing, at least in ageing non-athletes, may make the use of palatable, sodium-containing beverages like sports drinks particularly valuable.

- The anabolic resistance to food intake proposed to occur amongst older individuals may be overcome with ingestion of HBV proteins such as whey protein (see Chapter 6) which are a very energy-efficient method of stimulating muscle protein synthesis [38], especially when used to fortify existing foods so as other nutrient needs are addressed simultaneously.
- The increasing incidence of osteoarthritis amongst masters athletes may demand greater consideration of nutritional factors such as the use of omega-3 polyunsaturated fatty acids amongst this population relative to their younger counterparts to assist in the management of this debilitating condition [39].

In conclusion, while the process of considering the supplement needs of masters athletes is the same as that of younger athletes, the actual prescription of products, if any, may contrast markedly depending on the individual athlete, their dietary intake, health status and nutrition-related goals.

10.7 CONCLUSIONS

What defines a dietary supplement is broad and can vary throughout various jurisdictions around the world, creating a confusing and ever-changing landscape for the masters athlete. This is exacerbated by an industry which now produces large numbers of multi-ingredient products with numerous health and/or performance claims. In an effort to empower athletes of all ages to make informed decisions about supplements, a number of classification schemes have been established such as that developed by the AIS. This contemporary approach categorises supplements based on the level of scientific evidence for performance enhancement as well as the risk to health and inadvertent doping. Such programs should help guide and educate masters athletes on what is effective and safe use of dietary supplements. It is therefore the responsibility of masters athletes, coaches, sports scientists and masters sport administrators to ensure these programs are supported and advocated to their athletes.

Similar to their younger peers, masters athletes are regular users of dietary supplements. While the motivation for supplement use may be broader amongst masters athletes compared to their younger peers, masters athletes remain avid consumers of sports and other supplements. Direct ergogenic effects (see Chapter 11) remain a motivation for masters athletes but they are also motivated to enhance or maintain health status (see Chapters 12 and 13). This potentially opens up a broader range of supplements masters athletes may be interested in, including herbal or complementary therapy products.

A number of factors need to be taken into consideration when exploring supplementation issues with masters athletes. These include the unique physiological and metabolic adaptations that occur with ageing, including underlying medical conditions, plus the specific motivation for exercise and/or dietary interventions, current training loads and competition schedule, specific dietary needs, prior experiences and other related issues such as finances available. Current guidance on dietary supplements for masters athletes is primarily based on scientific evidence from the broader younger athletic population. Given the unique physiological adaptations that occur with ageing, there is a clear need to investigate the performance and risk potential of specific supplements across a range of sporting environments in masters athletes.

10.8 IMPLICATIONS FOR SPORTS MEDICINE PROFESSIONALS AND CLINICIANS

With more than one in two masters athletes reporting the use of a dietary supplement primarily for health reasons [25], it is that essential health care professionals working within the sports environment have an understanding of this high-profile component of sports nutrition practice. While masters athletes report medical professionals as important sources of dietary supplement information [25], many of these professionals do not feel confident or comfortable in offering advice regarding supplement use [26]. Without guidance, the masters athlete may be at risk of adverse outcomes from their supplementation protocols, including financial and health implications, or contravening drugs in sport regulations. Given this, sports medicine professionals should consider referral to suitably trained performance nutrition experts such as sports dieticians.

Masters athletes are a unique sub-group of the sporting population because they have the potential for medical issues related to ageing and a concurrent involvement in athletic pursuits. Medical professionals need to regularly investigate in detail the supplement practices of their masters athletes, recognising that this population rarely voluntarily discloses such information [40]. Information should be sought on the range of products ingested, including the specific protocols that address frequency of ingestion and individual doses across the full spectrum of supplements, including herbal preparations, plus health- and sport-outcome-focused products. This enables the sports medicine professional to make an informed judgement in regards to the potential achievement of desired outcomes and associated cost versus benefit assessment of the product, but also to the risk of adverse drug-nutrient interactions (see Chapter 13) and doping risk. Medical practitioners should focus on patients who report the use of multiple supplements as recent evidence suggests that this intake in combination with medications could lead to greater frequency of adverse events such as headaches, heart problems, chest and abdominal pain, rashes and nausea [40].

The case study below of a masters athlete highlights some of the potential issues medical professionals and clinicians need to be concerned with.

Dave is a 55-year-old track cyclist competing at the World Masters Games in 2 months' time. He has been on hypertension medication for over 5 years. Recently in preparation for the games he has been training hard for the individual pursuit event, trying to increase both his power and speed. He was told by a fellow athlete that he needed to be more explosive in training and competition and he should think about using something like a pre-workout supplement. Dave is told these supplements are purported to help give you a 'kick' and may be really beneficial to his training and competition performance. The fellow athlete that suggested the pre-workout supplement attends the same medical practice as Dave and is always diligent at checking out supplements for doping purposes. Dave thinks it must therefore be all right to take the supplement but decides to check out the ingredient list of this supplement online, just in case. The ingredient list is full of ingredients he doesn't recognise, grouped under a 'proprietary blend'. He decides to look up the ingredient list on his WADA iPhone application and there is nothing that the code says is banned. He decides to take the dietary supplement.

After a few sessions of taking the supplement he feels very anxious and 'unwell' at training. On a subsequent visit to the doctor Dave only reports symptoms and fails to report the use of his pre-workout supplement. Based on Dave's reported symptoms, Dave's doctor feels he is training too hard and should reduce his load slightly prior to the games to freshen up. When he reduces his training load he stops his high-intensity efforts and therefore the use of the pre-workout supplement. Dave's symptoms disappear and he heads to the masters games feeling confident.

At the World Masters Games Dave decides due to the nature of the event and the fact that he may not be there again he should double the 10-g serve of his pre-workout supplement and consumes it an hour prior to his event. After his warm-up Dave feels awful and has to see the event doctor for support who identifies that Dave has tachycardia yet is hypotensive and strongly recommends he doesn't race. Dave decides to pull out of the race and is left wondering what went wrong. Upon closer inspection of the pre-workout supplement the race doctor identifies two key ingredient categories that could have caused issues with Dave's body: first, the stimulant caffeine, and second, nitrate precursors. Within the proprietary blend there is an ingredient section called 'Performance blend'. Listed in this section are the ingredients methylxanthine, guarana and kola nut. These are all sources of caffeine and after further investigation it is revealed that the supplement contains a total of 300 mg of caffeine. Doubling the dose provided 600 mg of caffeine to Dave (who only partakes in coffee after road training rides). At 70 kg this amount of caffeine equates to 8 $mg \cdot kg^{-1}$ body mass. Doses in this range have previously been reported to result in a range of side effects, including tachycardia, palpitations, insomnia, tremor, headache, abdominal pain, nausea, vomiting and diarrhoea [41].

Within the proprietary blend there was an ingredient section called 'NO Releasers'. Listed in this section were L-arginine, beetroot concentrate and rhubarb concentrate. Beetroot and rhubarb are both significant sources of dietary nitrate. Moderate dietary nitrate sources have been shown to reduce blood pressure after consumption [42]. L-arginine has only been shown at high doses to cause side effects such as hypotension [43] but may have exacerbated Dave's situation.

As an alternative approach, recognising Dave was a competitive masters athlete, his doctor should have investigated Dave's supplementation practices in more detail, exploring all of the products he consumed and their protocol of ingestion. Dave could then have passed on the ingredient list of the supplements he was taking. This would have allowed his doctor the ability to search an online dietary supplement database (e.g. http://www.nlm.nih.gov/medlineplus/druginformation.html) looking for potential supplement medication interactions especially in relation to his blood pressure prescription. Given this, Dave would not have had to deviate from his training program in the weeks leading up to the World Masters Games and could have competed knowing he'd done everything in training to perform at his best.

10.9 IMPLICATIONS FOR MASTERS ATHLETES AND COACHES

With athletes and coaches working closely together to optimise performance it is not uncommon for masters athletes to use coaches for advice on dietary supplements [25]. It is becoming more common for both masters and age group athletes to be tested for doping control purposes at major competitions and events. It is therefore important that athletes and their coaches stay well informed about the risk associated with dietary supplements and potential inadvertent doping outcomes. The case study below illustrates an interaction between a coach and masters athlete that ends badly.

Michelle is a masters swimmer competing at an international level. Michelle used to compete at a competitive level as a younger swimmer in the early 1980s. Back then dietary multi-vitamin supplementation was all she ever took. This new era of dietary supplements has her totally confused and bewildered. As a masters swimmer she is struggling to maintain an ideal performance body composition. Her training is going well and she is on track to potentially break the world masters record for the 100-m freestyle.

In a discussion with her coach one day she outlines her goals for the coming months and identifies her problem losing fat mass and achieving the body composition she wants. She is seeing someone to help her with nutrition but she finds it difficult to stick to the program outlined and often strays. Her coach sympathises with her and suggests a dietary supplement he is taking called 'Super Duper Slimmer'. He exclaims he has lost 10 kg of fat and never feels hungry and never craves the bad things. Michelle goes to the local health food store where the sales representative agrees with her coach on the effectiveness of the fat-loss supplement. The salesperson also states that the supplement is all natural and a quick skim of the label revels that all the ingredients are either plant names Michelle is familiar with or roots or extract of roots. Michelle decides to take the supplement and all of a sudden feels she has lots of energy, is losing fat mass and is never hungry. A month later Michelle is at the National Masters Swimming titles and wins the 100-m freestyle in World Record time. Michelle hops out of the pool and is greeted by a doping control officer who informs her she has a test to ensure her record is ratified. Without thinking she has anything to worry about Michelle complies and continues to enjoy her win. A month later a letter comes in the mail from the National Masters Swimming Association informing Michelle she has failed an in-competition doping test for a substance called 'octopamine', a WADA in-competition banned stimulant. Michelle had never heard of this and definitely knew she didn't knowingly ingest it. An Internet search takes her to a supplement website talking about octopamine and the fact that it can be found in a plant called bitter orange. This is where Michelle felt a sinking feeling; she remembered reading it on the supplement label she was taking. Michelle had to accept the ban and served a 2-year ban for doping.

Although octopamine is present in small amounts in bitter orange it is not considered the main natural source of octopamine. However, some supplement companies around the world are currently being accused of adulterating supplements by adding synthetic forms of stimulants at levels not available in natural ingredients. Michelle unfortunately consumed a supplement that was adulterated with artificially elevated levels of octopamine. Coaches need to be aware that certain categories of dietary supplements like those that claim to enhance fat loss usually contain a stimulant to increase metabolic rates. These categories of supplements increase the risk of consuming a banned substance and should be avoided by athletes subject to doping control.

Given the current sporting environment, masters athletes and their coaches need to have a global understanding of the sport and health supplement environment. A particular issue of importance to athletes who compete under anti-doping codes involves the inadvertent ingestion of prohibited substances that can be present in supplements, either as stated ingredients or undeclared components and contaminants. This can lead to an unintentional violation of the anti-doping code, often referred to as an inadvertent doping outcome, with major consequences to the athlete's reputation and ability to participate in competition. Given the complexity of issues associated with supplement use, masters athletes should be directed to professionals with expertise in the prescription of health and sports supplements, such as sports dieticians. Their expertise can help direct the use of protocols to derive the optimal benefits from supplements that are scientifically supported while minimising the potential for negative effects to health and performance.

10.10 FUTURE RESEARCH DIRECTIONS

Very little is known about the supplementation practices of the masters athlete. Research is warranted to explore this issue across a range of sports and athletic abilities, especially given the increasingly competitive nature of masters events. However, rather than just explore the prevalence of supplementation, greater insight will be obtained by taking a holistic approach to the issue, sourcing information on dosage protocols, motives and rationale for ingestion, significant sources of supplement information and provision, as well as other pertinent information such as nutrition knowledge and associated dietary intake of macro- and micronutrients.

Given the unique physiological and metabolic adaptations that may be evident amongst masters athletes, controlled investigations exploring the potential value of specific supplements are warranted. A logical starting point for this may be exploration of supplements within the A and B category of supplements within the AIS supplementation program; that is, products with known or promising value amongst adult athletic populations. With an ever-increasing calendar of masters sporting competitions, opportunities to explore this unique population will continue to emerge. Major multi-sport games such as the World Masters Games would be an excellent avenue for exploring these issues across a range of sporting disciplines.

Readers interested in examining the issues surrounding supplement use in athletes are directed to a number of detailed reviews [44–47].

REFERENCES

1. Galloway, M.T. and Jokl, P., Aging successfully: The importance of physical activity in maintaining health and function, *J. Am. Acad. Orthop. Surg.* 8(1), 37–44, 2000.
2. Food and Drug Administration, Dietary Supplement Health and Education Act of 1994, http://www.fda.gov/RegulatoryInformation/Legislation/FederalFoodDrugandCosmeticActFDCAct/SignificantAmendmentstotheFDCAct/ucm148003.htm, accessed 23 January 2014.

3. European Parliament and Council, Directive 2002/46/EC of the European Parliament and of the Council of 10 June 2002 on the approximation of the laws of the member states relating to food supplements, http://eur-lex.europa.eu/LexUriServ/LexUriServ.do?uri=CELEX:32002L0046:en:NOT, accessed 23 January 2014.
4. Food Standard Australia and New Zealand, Standard 2.9.4 Formulated Supplemental Sports Foods, http://www.comlaw.gov.au/Details/F2011C00549, accessed 26 January 2014.
5. Therapuetic Goods Administration, Therapuetic Goods Act 1989, http://www.comlaw.gov.au/Details/C2012C00355, accessed 23 January 2014.
6. Corrigan, B. and Kazlauskas, R., Medication use in athletes selected for doping control at the Sydney Olympics (2000), *Clin. J. Sport Med.* 13(1), 33–40, 2003.
7. Australian Crime Commission 2013, Organised crime and drugs in sport, new generation performance and image enhancing drugs and organised criminal involvement in their use in professional sport, Canberra: Australian Crime Commission, AC Commission, p. 47, http://www.crimecommission.gov.au/publications/other/organised-crime-drugs-sport, accessed 23 January 2014.
8. World Anti-Doping Agency, World Anti-Doping Code, http://www.wada-ama.org/en/world-anti-doping-program/sports-and-anti-doping-organizations/the-code/, accessed 23 January 2014.
9. Burke, L. and Deakin, V., *Clinical Sports Nutrition*, McGraw-Hill, Sydney, Australia, 2010.
10. Burke, L., Broad, E., Cox, G. et al., Supplements and sports foods, in *Clinical Sports Nutrition*, 4th Ed., L. Burke and V. Deakin, eds., McGraw-Hill, Sydney, Australia, 2010, pp. 419–500.
11. Lun, V., Erdman, K.A. and Reimer, R.A., Evaluation of nutritional intake in Canadian high-performance athletes, *Clin. J. Sport Med.* 19(5), 405–11, 2009.
12. West, N.P., Pyne, D.B., Cripps, A.W. et al., Lactobacillus fermentum (PCC®) supplementation and gastrointestinal and respiratory-tract illness symptoms: A randomised control trial in athletes, *Nutr. J.* 10, 30, 2011.
13. Gleeson, M., Bishop, N.C., Oliveira, M. and Tauler, P., Daily probiotic's (lactobacillus casei shirota) reduction of infection incidence in athletes, *Int. J. Sport Nutr. Exerc. Metab.* 21(1), 55–64, 2011.
14. Australian Institute of Sport, Supplements, http://www.ausport.gov.au/ais/nutrition/supplements, accessed 23 January 2014.
15. Nutrition Business Journal, Sports nutrition returns to form with big sales and investor interest, *Nutr. Bus. J.* XVI(2), 1, 2011.
16. Bailey, R.L., Gahche, J.J., Lentino, C.V. et al., Dietary supplement use in the United States, 2003–2006, *J. Nutr.* 141(2), 261–266, 2011.
17. Ervin, R.B., Wright, J.D. and Kennedy-Stephenson, J., Use of dietary supplements in the United States, 1988–94, *Vital Health Stat. 11.* (244), i–iii, 1–14, 1999.
18. Australian Bureau of Statistics, Australian Health Survey: Nutrition First Results—Foods and Nutrients, 2011–12. Access online http://www.abs.gov.au/ausstats/abs@nsf/Lookup/by%20Subject/4364.0.55.007~2011-12~Main%20Features~Supplements~400, 2014.
19. Houston, D.K., Johnson, M.A., Daniel, T.D. and Poon, L.W., Health and dietary characteristics of supplement users in an elderly population, *Int. J. Vitam. Nutr. Res.* 67(3), 183–91, 1997.
20. Burke, L. and Cox, G., eds., *The Complete Guide to Food for Sports Performance*, Allen and Unwin, Sydney, Australia 2010.
21. Sobal, J. and Marquart, L.F., Vitamin/mineral supplement use among athletes: A review of the literature, *Int. J. Sport Nutr.* 4(4), 320–34, 1994.
22. Sundgot-Borgen, J., Berglund, B. and Torstveit, M.K., Nutritional supplements in Norwegian elite athletes—impact of international ranking and advisors, *Scand. J. Med. Sci. Sports* 13(2), 138–44, 2003.
23. de Silva, A., Samarasinghe, Y., Senanayake, D. and Lanerolle, P., Dietary supplement intake in national-level Sri Lankan athletes, *Int. J. Sport Nutr. Exerc. Metab.* 20(1), 15–20, 2010.
24. Tscholl, P., Alonso, J.M., Dolle, G., Junge, A. and Dvorak, J., The use of drugs and nutritional supplements in top-level track and field athletes, *Am. J. Sports Med.* 38(1), 133–40, 2010.
25. Striegel, H., Simon, P., Wurster, C., Niess, A.M. and Ulrich, R., The use of nutritional supplements among master athletes, *Int. J. Sports Med.* 27(3), 236–41, 2006.
26. Vetter, M.L., Herring, S.J., Sood, M., Shah, N.R. and Kalet, A.L., What do resident physicians know about nutrition? An evaluation of attitudes, self-perceived proficiency and knowledge, *J. Am. Coll. Nutr.* 27(2), 287–98, 2008.
27. Mehta, D.H., Gardiner, P.M., Phillips, R.S. and McCarthy, E.P., Herbal and dietary supplement disclosure to health care providers by individuals with chronic conditions, *J. Altern. Complement. Med.* 14(10), 1263–9, 2008.

28. Geyer, H., Parr, M.K., Mareck, U., Reinhart, U., Schrader, Y. and Schanzer, W., Analysis of non-hormonal nutritional supplements for anabolic-androgenic steroids—results of an international study, *Int. J. Sports Med.* 25(2), 124–9, 2004.
29. Prosser, J.M., Majlesi, N., Chan, G.M., Olsen, D., Hoffman, R.S. and Nelson, L.S., Adverse effects associated with arginine alpha-ketoglutarate containing supplements, *Hum. Exp. Toxicol.* 28(5), 259–62, 2009.
30. FitzSimmons, C.R. and Kidner, N., Caffeine toxicity in a bodybuilder, *J. Accid. Emerg. Med.* 15(3), 196–7, 1998.
31. Izzo, A.A. and Ernst, E., Interactions between herbal medicines and prescribed drugs: An updated systematic review, *Drugs* 69(13), 1777–98, 2009.
32. Canter, P.H. and Ernst, E., Herbal supplement use by persons aged over 50 years in Britain: Frequently used herbs, concomitant use of herbs, nutritional supplements and prescription drugs, rate of informing doctors and potential for negative interactions, *Drugs Aging* 21(9), 597–605, 2004.
33. Loya, A.M., Gonzalez-Stuart, A. and Rivera, J.O., Prevalence of polypharmacy, polyherbacy, nutritional supplement use and potential product interactions among older adults living on the United States-Mexico border: A descriptive, questionnaire-based study, *Drugs Aging* 26(5), 423–36, 2009.
34. Australian Institute of Health and Welfare, Australia's Health 2012, http://www.aihw.gov.au/publication-detail/?id=10737422172, accessed 23 January 2014.
35. Geyer, H., Parr, M., Koehler, K., Mareck, U., Schanzer, W. and Thevis, M., Nutritional supplements cross-contaminated and faked with doping substances, *J. Mass Spectrom.* 43, 892–902, 2008.
36. Ainslie, P.N., Campbell, I.T., Frayn, K.N. et al., Energy balance, metabolism, hydration, and performance during strenuous hill walking: The effect of age, *J. Appl. Physiol.* 93(2), 714–23, 2002.
37. Bhutto, A. and Morley, J.E., The clinical significance of gastrointestinal changes with aging, *Curr. Opin. Clin. Nutr. Metab. Care.* 11(5), 651–60, 2008.
38. Pennings, B., Groen, B., de Lange, A. et al., Amino acid absorption and subsequent muscle protein accretion following graded intakes of whey protein in elderly men, *Am. J. Physiol. Endocrinol. Metab.* 302(8), E992–9, 2012.
39. Lopez, H.L., Nutritional interventions to prevent and treat osteoarthritis. Part i: Focus on fatty acids and macronutrients, *PM. R.* 4(5 Suppl), S145–54, 2012.
40. Timbo, B.B., Ross, M.P., McCarthy, P.V. and Lin, C.T., Dietary supplements in a national survey: Prevalence of use and reports of adverse events, *J. Am. Diet. Assoc.* 106(12), 1966–74, 2006.
41. Higdon, J.V. and Frei, B., Coffee and health: A review of recent human research, *Crit. Rev. Food Sci. Nutr.* 46(2), 101–23, 2006.
42. Kenjale, A.A., Ham, K.L., Stabler, T. et al., Dietary nitrate supplementation enhances exercise performance in peripheral arterial disease, *J. Appl. Physiol.* 110(6), 1582–91, 2011.
43. Alvares, T.S., Meirelles, C.M., Bhambhani, Y.N., Paschoalin, V.M. and Gomes, P.S., L-arginine as a potential ergogenic aid in healthy subjects, *Sports Med.* 41(3), 233–48, 2011.
44. Morenete-Sanchez, J. and Zabala, M., Doping in sport: A review of elite athletes' attitudes, beliefs, and knowledge, *Sports Med.* 43(6), 395–411, 2013.
45. Liddle, D.G. and Connor, D.J., Nutritional supplements and ergogenic aids, *Prim. Care* 40(2), 487–505, 2013.
46. Koncic, M.Z. and Tomczyk, M., New insights into dietary supplements used in sport: Active substances, pharmocological and side effects, *Curr. Drug Targets* 14(9), 1079–92, 2013.
47. Bishop, D., Dietary supplements and team-sport performance, *Sports Med.* 40(2), 995–1017, 2010.

11 Ergogenic Aids for Masters Athletes

Vincent J. Dalbo, Michael D. Roberts and Aaron T. Scanlan

CONTENTS

11.1 INTRODUCTION

The field of sports nutrition has become increasingly popular, but much of the information presented to the general public is in the form of marketing hype rather than scientific evidence. As a result, information is often presented in a manner to convince potential consumers that supplements provide performance gains that are not physiologically possible. Therefore, medical and allied health professionals, coaches and consumers such as masters athletes must be aware of products/ingredients that are present within supposed ergogenic aids in order to make informed decisions before purchasing products that are unlikely to provide a performance benefit.

The first aim of this chapter is to increase the reader's awareness about ergogenic aids/supplements in order to help medical and allied health professionals, coaches and consumers identify products/substances that may promote health. More importantly given the scope of this book, a secondary aim of the chapter is to increase sport performance in masters athletes. In order to be completely open with the reader, the authors of this chapter each consume supplements daily and have published peer-reviewed papers on the safety [1–3] and efficacy of ergogenic aids to potentially extend life [4], aid fat metabolism [3,5,6], promote weight loss [3,7], increase skeletal muscle hypertrophy [8,9] and enhance sport performance [2,10,11].

11.2 SELECTING THE CORRECT SUPPLEMENTS

Potential consumers are overloaded with choices when attempting to purchase an ergogenic aid from a health food or online store and it may be getting to the point where consumers may have too many options. There are very few ingredients that have been found to consistently enhance athletic performance or promote physiological adaptations that over long durations may be able to enhance athletic performance. Given that supplements can be viewed as an investment in one's own personal health, analogies can be drawn. As a result consumers should consider the following suggestions prior to purchasing a supplement:

1. Only purchase/consume products that you fully understand. For instance, do not consume creatine because it has been shown to enhance skeletal muscle strength [4,12–14] unless you understand the mechanisms in which creatine exerts its effects. Understanding the physiological mechanisms by which the supplement exerts its effects will enable you to have a realistic expectation of the results you can expect from the supplement and allow you to tailor your training program to enable you to get the best performance benefit while consuming the supplement.
2. Be wary of overcomplicated blends contained within ergogenic aids (proprietary blends). If a supplement contains a proprietary blend, a red flag should be raised as you do not know how much of the ingredients included in the proprietary blend are in the product. Hence, if you don't understand each of the active ingredients, know how much of an ingredient is in the product, or if the product is overly complicated, then you should think twice before purchasing or consuming it.
3. Renowned investor Warren Buffet has stated that most investors should only make 20 investment decisions in their lifetime [15], which is another principle that can apply to the consumption of ergogenic aids. With ergogenic aids, less is often more; only purchase and consume raw products or ergogenic aids that contain substances in known quantities that have been scientifically shown to be effective in enhancing performance.

11.2.1 Unwrapping the Secret of Proprietary Blends

A major event regarding nutritional supplements came into effect in the United States on October 25, 1994, termed The Dietary Supplement Health and Education Act (DSHEA). According to DSHEA the labels of dietary supplements must list the names and amounts of dietary ingredients contained in a serving, with a serving being defined as the recommended amount of the supplement to be consumed on one occasion. However, when dietary ingredients in a supplement are considered to be a proprietary blend, only the total amount of the blend needs to be listed in order of predominance by weight [16]. It is generally advised to avoid supplements containing proprietary blends because the consumer is unaware of the specific amount of product contained in the blend. For example, a company could market a supplement containing a 305-mg propriety blend of caffeine, rice powder, creatine, beta-alanine (β-alanine) and leucine. In this instance, the product could contain 250 mg of caffeine, 50 mg of rice powder, 3 mg of creatine, 1 mg of β-alanine and 1 mg of leucine. The reality is that the supplement will most likely give the user the psychological impression that it is effective because caffeine has the ability to enhance mood [17], cognitive abilities [18], feelings of alertness [19], improve reaction time [20] and aerobic performance [21]. Conversely, the creatine, β-alanine and leucine would be consumed in too low a dose to stimulate an ergogenic effect. As a result, the consumer would likely be paying for a very expensive caffeine supplement.

It is well established that training and nutritional requirements vary greatly for competitive aerobic and anaerobic athletes. However, there is great overlap in regard to nutritional supplements that may enhance exercise performance for aerobic and anaerobic athletes, particularly for masters athletes. Therefore, the following sections will discuss commonly consumed ergogenic aids that may promote the athletic performance of masters athletes.

11.3 ERGOGENIC AIDS TO BUILD/MAINTAIN SKELETAL MUSCLE MASS

Ageing is marked by a significant decrease in skeletal muscle mass and strength starting as early as the third decade of life [22–24]. The loss of skeletal muscle mass and strength is a concern for aerobic and anaerobic athletes as skeletal muscle function is vital for optimising performance in each type of activity. As a result, masters athletes, particularly those ≥55 years of age, should strive to at least maintain their current level of skeletal muscle functionality. Fortunately, cost-effective ergogenic aids are available that have the potential to help masters athletes maintain skeletal muscle function.

11.3.1 Protein Supplementation

Adequate protein consumption is not only important for the masters athlete, but the population as a whole. Unfortunately, Campbell et al. reported that 15%–38% of men and 27%–41% of women consume less than the Recommended Daily Allowance (RDA) of 0.8 g/kg/day of protein [25]. In this regard, it is becoming established that the RDA of protein is insufficient to protect older adults from sarcopenic muscle loss [26,27]. At this point you may be asking how this information relates to the masters athlete. Simply stated, if you are an athlete and you are consuming ≤0.8 g/kg/day of protein you are likely not consuming enough protein to maintain your skeletal muscle mass, and even more likely, you are not optimising your physiological potential.

The next logical question one may ask is 'How much protein should I be consuming?' Unfortunately, this is a difficult question to answer; however, Dr. Marc Tarnopolsky, the author of Chapter 6 of this book, recently provided protein recommendations for aerobic and anaerobic athletes (Figures 11.1 and 11.2).

As can be seen in Figure 11.1, protein requirements are increased for athletes engaging in aerobic exercise. The increased protein requirements are the result of amino acid oxidation that occurs during endurance exercise [28]. Thus, protein requirements range from 0.8 to 1.0 g/kg/day in sedentary and recreational endurance active adults (males and females), 1.1–1.2 g/kg/day for moderate-intensity endurance athletes and 1.4–1.6 g/kg/day for elite endurance athletes [29]. As can be seen

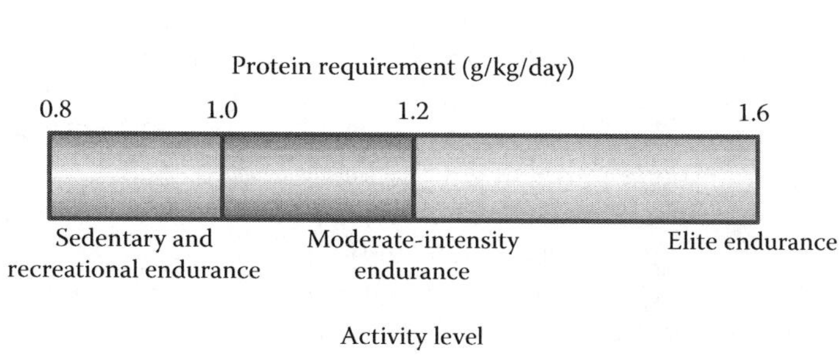

FIGURE 11.1 Continuum of protein requirements for aerobic athletes. (Based on recommendations by Tarnopolsky, M.A., Protein and amino acid needs for training and bulking up, in *Clinical Sports Nutrition*, L. Burke and V. Deakin, eds., McGraw-Hill Medical, New York, 2010.)

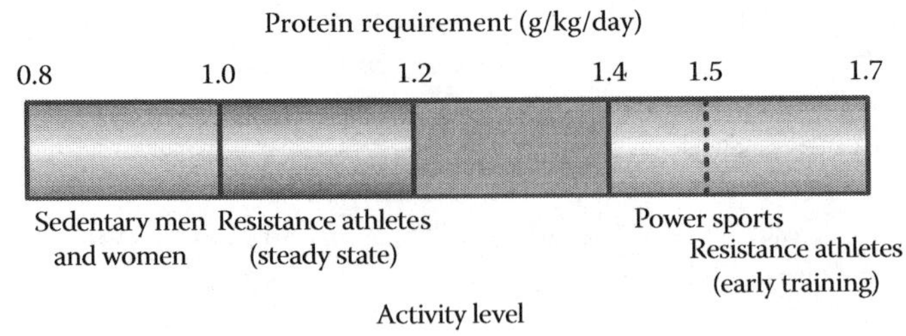

FIGURE 11.2 Continuum of protein requirements for anaerobic athletes. (Based on recommendations by Tarnopolsky, M.A., Protein and amino acid needs for training and bulking up, in *Clinical Sports Nutrition*, L. Burke and V. Deakin, eds., McGraw-Hill Medical, New York, 2010.)

in Figure 11.2, protein requirements are also increased in anaerobic athletes given that more amino acids are required for the maintenance of a higher amount of skeletal muscle mass [29].

As a result, protein requirements range from 1.1–1.2 g/kg/day for resistance-trained athletes who have reached steady state performance and 1.5–1.7 g/kg/day for resistance-trained athletes early in the training cycle [29]. The increased protein consumption for athletes in early stages of training is the result of accelerated myofibrillar protein accretion that occurs within the first several months following the initiation of a resistance training program [29].

In line with these recommendations, athletes engaging in sports that require strength and endurance components such as mixed martial arts, football and rugby should consume 1.5–1.7 g/kg/day of protein due to amino acid oxidation that is likely to occur during practice and competition [29]. The lower-level protein requirements presented for aerobic and anaerobic athletes may be suitable for female athletes as leucine oxidation has been found to be lower in females compared to males at rest and following a 38-day exercise program [30]. It is important to note the protein requirements may need to be increased for masters athletes [31], particularly for older adults (≥55 years), as research has found 1.0–1.3 g/kg/day of protein may be necessary to maintain nitrogen balance and counteract decreased protein synthesis efficiency, impaired insulin sensitivity and reduced energy intake, all common characteristics of older adults [32,33]. For more detailed discussion on the protein needs of masters athletes, see Chapter 6.

11.3.1.1 Protein Timing

We have all heard the statement 'It is all about timing'. In the case of protein consumption, this statement holds particularly true. Much is known about the amount of protein and amino acids that should be consumed per meal and the timing of protein surrounding exercise, with much less known about the timing of protein throughout the course of the day. Based on the current literature, it is advisable for masters athletes to consume between 25–30 g of protein per meal, which should contain approximately 10 g of essential amino acids [27]. The lower limit of the protein recommendation of 25 g is based on research which found that older adults need to consume approximately 10–15 g of essential amino acids to stimulate muscle protein synthesis [27]. While the upper limit recommendation of 30 g is derived from a research study which found a similar anabolic response to occur from 30 and 90 g of protein consumption in younger and older adults [34], additional protein that is consumed over the recommended dose (~30 g per serving) is likely to be oxidised for energy [35]. Whether this occurs in masters athletes remains to be investigated.

Now that we know the amount of protein to consume per meal, the next question becomes, what is the ideal time to consume protein in relation to exercise bouts? It would be advisable for masters athletes to consume protein prior to, during and following a training bout [36]. The importance of protein consumption surrounding exercise is highlighted in an investigation by Hulmi et al. who reported the consumption of 15 g of whey protein isolate immediately prior to and following a twice-weekly resistance training program to significantly increase acute (1 and 48 h post-exercise) and chronic (following 21 weeks of training) intramuscular signalling pathways that are known to aid in building skeletal muscle mass. In addition, the researchers reported body mass and leg muscle thickness to be significantly increased in participants consuming whey protein 10 and 20 weeks following the initiation of the investigation [37]. This work is consistent with the findings of others who have reported muscle protein synthesis to be increased with the immediate consumption of protein following a bout of resistance exercise [38,39].

Although research examining the timing of protein surrounding resistance exercise has yielded equivocal results in regard to meaningful physiological adaptations (i.e. increased muscle strength), [40], there appears to be an optimal period for the uptake of amino acids and glucose into skeletal muscle [41,42]. The optimal time period has yet to be clearly defined, but appears to occur when muscle protein synthesis is elevated in response to exercise [40]. In this regard, muscle protein synthesis is increased 48 hours following exercise [43], and protein consumption at any point within 48 hours following a bout of exercise should produce a synergistic effect on rates of muscle protein synthesis and thus promote protein accretion [44]. However, consuming protein closely surrounding exercise has been reported to have a more beneficial effect on skeletal muscle hypertrophy than the consumption of protein at various points throughout the day [37,45]. In fact, protein timing may be more important for older athletes due to a variety of physiological adaptations that occur with ageing [44].

Based on recommendations from Phillips et al. it advisable for masters athletes to consume between 25–30 g of protein 30–45 minutes prior to and through the duration of exercise and another 25–30 g of protein within 1 hour following exercise, particularly for older (≥55 years) athletes, to ensure amino acid availability for muscle protein repair/anabolism following a bout of exercise [44].

Protein consumption is important surrounding exercise but another essential issue is protein timing throughout the remainder of the day. Research suggests the optimal dose of protein is 25–30 g per bolus, which should contain approximately 10 g of essential amino acids [27]. However, research examining protein timing throughout the course of the day is limited [40]. One investigation reported the consumption of ~10 g of essential amino acids every 2–5 hours would be sufficient for maintaining positive net protein balance in skeletal muscle [46]. However, another investigation reported the consumption of one protein-rich meal (80% of daily protein requirement) per day surrounded by two low-protein-rich meals to provide better responses in terms of lean body mass and protein balance than the consumption of five protein-rich meals consumed every 4 hours throughout the day [47]. Nonetheless, each of these investigations was conducted in non-athletic populations and the primary purpose was to determine optimal feeding strategies to maintain muscle in older adults [46,47].

As a result, it may be advisable for masters athletes to strive to consume a protein-rich meal every 3–5 hours throughout the course of the day to ensure sufficient amino acid availability required for skeletal muscle development following a training bout. Regarding exercise, it is advisable the protein be a fast-acting protein such as whey or skim milk found in dairy products or supplements [40]. Throughout the course of the day, a combination of slower- (i.e. casein) and faster-acting protein may be advisable. Prior to sleep, a slower-acting protein will be the best option [40,48]. More research is needed on both protein timing and quantities in masters athletes.

11.3.1.2 Protein Type

Recently, Phillips et al. conducted an analysis of nine investigations (241 participants) that examined the effects protein supplementation on changes in lean body mass. Of the investigations examined, three reported on the effects of milk (n = 42), eight on the effects of whey protein (n = 91), three on isolated soy protein (n = 51) and seven on the effects of carbohydrate (n = 67). The average duration for each investigation was 11.2 weeks (range: 8–16 weeks). The mean improvement in lean mass among all studies was 1.9 ± 0.5 kg, whey protein: 2.9 ± 1.6 kg, milk: 2.7 ± 1.3 kg, soy protein: 1.4 ± 0.6 kg and carbohydrate: 0.9 ± 0.6 kg. Hence, this report demonstrates that it is advantageous for masters athletes to consume protein following a training bout. Moreover, these data suggest that whey protein was more effective than soy protein for promoting skeletal muscle hypertrophy [44].

11.3.1.3 Conclusions

- Masters athletes consuming the RDA of 0.8 g/kg/day of protein are not consuming enough protein to optimise performance
- Protein consumption surrounding an exercise bout can help maintain skeletal muscle function in older adults
- A fast-acting protein source such as milk or whey protein should be consumed prior to, preferably during, and within 1 hour following an exercise bout

11.3.2 Leucine

The branch-chain amino acid leucine is arguably one of the most important supplements for any athlete. Cell culture and animal studies have reported leucine to stimulate both muscle protein synthesis [49,50] and mammalian target of rapamycin (mTOR) signalling [51]. In other words, leucine is able to activate signalling cascades that regulate muscle protein synthesis and build skeletal muscle [52]. As can be seen in Figure 11.3, leucine also has a stimulatory effect on insulin [53]. This is important, particularly for older athletes, as skeletal muscle accretion is determined by muscle protein synthesis—muscle protein breakdown [44].

In younger healthy individuals, muscle protein breakdown has been found to occur at relatively negligible levels, but in older adults muscle protein breakdown can have a significant influence on the development of skeletal muscle mass [44]. While insulin is limited in its capacity as an anabolic agent, it is highly effective at limiting skeletal muscle breakdown [44,54,55]. As a result, leucine may be even more important for older athletes (≥55 years) compared to younger athletes (≤35 years).

11.3.2.1 Leucine Supplementation

Leucine is effective at increasing muscle protein synthesis [40], but the amount of leucine required to yield significant performance improvements has yet to be fully elucidated. For example, 6.7 g of essential amino acids containing 1.7 g of leucine has been reported to significantly increase muscle protein synthesis rates in younger (29.7 ± 2.3 years) but not older adults (66.6 ± 2.3 years). However, when the amount of leucine in the 6.7 g of essential amino acids was increased to 2.8 g the older adults also experienced a significant increase in muscle protein synthesis rates [56]. In this regard, a later study examined the effects of the daily consumption of 7.5 g/day of leucine consumed in 2.5-g boluses with each meal for a period of 12 weeks in older adults (71.0 ± 16.0 years). However, leucine had no effect on lean mass, fat mass, percent body fat, leg volume or leg cross-sectional area [57]. It must be noted the protein consumption of the adults in this investigation was 0.99 ± 0.06 g/kg/day

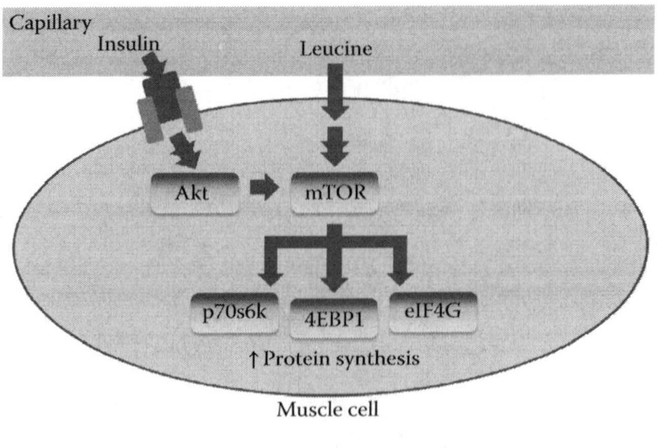

FIGURE 11.3 Influence of leucine on mTOR pathway activity.

which may have provided enough protein/leucine to optimise muscle protein synthesis given the participant's level of physical activity.

Koopman et al. examined the effect of a carbohydrate (25 g of glucose), carbohydrate and protein (25 g of glucose and 33.3 g of whey protein) and a carbohydrate, protein and leucine (25 g of glucose, 33.3 g of whey protein and 16.6 g of leucine) beverage on plasma insulin response and rates of whole-body protein breakdown, synthesis, oxidation and net protein balance following a bout of resistance exercise [53]. Leucine was found to provide a significant benefit as the carbohydrate, protein, leucine beverage had the greatest effect on plasma insulin response and net protein balance, as well as reduced protein breakdown and oxidation and increased protein synthesis compared to the carbohydrate beverage alone [53]. A plausible theory to explain the equivocal results regarding the ability of leucine to elicit meaningful physiological adaptations could be that when consuming high doses of protein, leucine intake may already be sufficient to activate the proteins regulating muscle protein synthesis [44] and as a result supplementing with leucine provides no additional benefit.

11.3.2.2 Leucine Dosing Suggestions

Leucine appears to be a viable supplement for masters athletes, but as yet it is difficult to quantify a suggested dose based on limited available research. As a result, the best recommendations that can be made based on the existing literature are to supplement 5 g of leucine with meals, particularly for those masters athletes who are on a vegetarian/vegan diet, are ≥55 years of age or are consuming a meal with less than 25–30 g of protein. Since leucine is also able to enhance the insulin response [53] and stimulate muscle protein synthesis [49,50], it is most likely advisable to place ~5 g of leucine in training beverages.

11.3.2.3 Conclusions

- Leucine is effective at enhancing muscle protein synthesis
- Research examining the ability of leucine supplementation to produce meaningful physiological adaptations following supplementation has yielded equivocal results
- Leucine supplementation may provide the best benefits for those on a vegetarian/vegan diet, those ≥55 years of age and those who tend to consume less than 25–30 g of protein per meal

11.3.3 Creatine

Creatine is one of the most popular ergogenic aids with sales exceeding $400 million in 2004 [58]. As a result of the popularity of creatine, much work has been conducted on the safety and efficacy of creatine supplementation [1,4,12]. Creatine has been proposed to enhance performance through a variety of mechanisms including cell swelling which may serve to reduce whole-body proteolysis and amino acid oxidation [59], positively influence the expression of myogenic transcription factors [60,61], increase satellite cell mitotic activity [62,63] and allow for increased exercise volume by positively influencing the energy producing capacity of the phosphocreatine energy system [12,64]. A visual schematic of the influence of creatine supplementation on skeletal muscle and high-energy phosphates can be seen in Figure 11.4.

Given the available literature, creatine is highly recommended for masters athletes involved in strength and power sports [4,12]. Creatine is also highly recommended for all older athletes (≥55 years) because of its potential ability to slow the rate of muscle loss with age and improve muscle function in older adults [4,65].

For older endurance athletes, the use of creatine supplementation is not as straightforward. The majority of literature on the topic does not support the use of creatine supplementation for performance enhancement during endurance events [66,67]; however, creatine has not been found to hinder endurance performance [67]. As a result, it could be suggested that if your event relies primarily on aerobic metabolism it is not necessary to consume creatine; however, if your event is of long

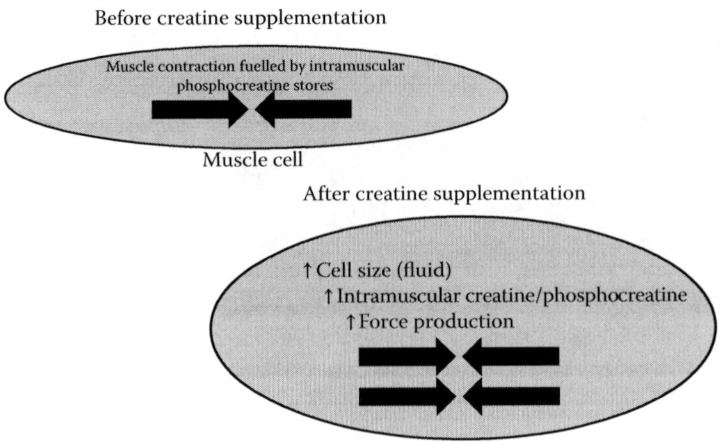

FIGURE 11.4 Effects of creatine supplementation on skeletal muscle.

duration (≥2 hours) or you are exercising for extended periods in hot and/or humid environments, creatine supplementation may be able to reduce the risk for heat injury through its ability to increase water retention within muscle cells [1]. In this regard, numerous investigations have reported creatine supplementation to increase total body water while others have reported decreased heart rate and reduced body temperature following prolonged exercise at a given intensity in hot and humid environments [1,68,69]. Consequently, any masters athlete competing for extended durations (e.g. marathon, triathlon), particularly in hot and/or humid conditions, should consider the use of creatine to help preserve body water and modulate body temperature [1]. Given the ability of creatine to help preserve skeletal muscle function with age, it is advisable that any older person, including masters athletes (≥55 years) consume a creatine supplement [4]. If necessary, to enhance performance, masters athletes should be able to eliminate all excess intramuscular stores of creatine from skeletal muscle in approximately 6 weeks following cessation of use [70].

11.3.3.1 Dosing Suggestions

The most common dosing strategy for creatine is the consumption of a loading phase (20 g/day consumed in four 5-g doses) which lasts for 3 to 5 days, followed by a maintenance phase of 5 g/day. The loading phase is proposed to reduce the amount of time necessary to saturate skeletal muscle with creatine and phosphocreatine. However, creatine supplementation can be effective without the loading phase but it will take a longer duration of time for skeletal muscle to become saturated with creatine and phosphocreatine [71,72]. Therefore, dosing is in the hands of the user. However, it is recommended that the loading phase should not exceed 20 g/day, because excess creatine will simply be eliminated in urine. While 5 g/day of creatine is sufficient for maintaining intramuscular total creatine and phosphocreatine levels once saturated, the 5 g/day of creatine is also sufficient to increase intramuscular levels of creatine and phosphocreatine until the muscle becomes saturated. It should also be noted that research clearly demonstrates that 5 g/day is sufficient for performance enhancement and increases in performance are not linear with dose, meaning consuming 10 g/day will not elicit a better performance outcome than consuming 5 g/day.

11.3.3.2 Conclusions

- Creatine may be the most cost-effective supplement for masters strength and power athletes
- Creatine is effective for all older athletes (≥55 years) because of its ability to help preserve skeletal muscle function with age
- Creatine may reduce the risk of heat injury in endurance athletes of all ages while exercising in hot and/or humid conditions

11.4 OTHER SUPPLEMENTS OF INTEREST

Particularly for older masters athletes (≥55 years), a primary concern is maintaining skeletal muscle function with age. However, there are a few other supplements that may help enhance sports performance including β-alanine and caffeine.

11.4.1 β-Alanine

β-alanine is a non-essential amino acid that can potentially indirectly enhance performance of extremely high intensity (110% of VO_2 peak), short duration (1–5 minutes) bouts of exercise [73,74]. β-alanine may enhance performance by increasing intramuscular levels of another amino acid, carnosine [75]. It is well established that acidosis can increase fatigue during exercise and therefore increasing the body's buffering capacity may improve high-intensity, short-duration exercise performance [76,77]. The importance of carnosine has been previously described by Tallon et al., who reported carnosine concentrations in body builders of 40 mmol/kg dry mass [78] compared to the average human of 16 mmol/kg dry mass [79]. Tallon et al. estimated carnosine to account for 20% of total buffering capacity in body builders compared to 10% in the typical population [78]. In theory, if an athlete of any age increases the amount of carnosine present in skeletal muscle, they can enhance their ability to buffer acidic concentrations during high-intensity exercise and thus delay fatigue.

Intramuscular carnosine concentrations may be able to be enhanced by two mechanisms—training and/or supplementation [73]. Since this chapter is focused on ergogenic aids, we will focus on discussing supplementation. Carnosine is synthesised in muscle and other tissues from β-alanine and L-histidine by carnosine synthetase. Carnosine synthetase has a higher binding affinity for L-histidine than β-alanine, and L-histidine is found in higher concentrations in the human body than β-alanine. As a result, β-alanine is the rate-limiting enzyme in the production of carnosine [73]. In this regard, Harris et al. examined the effects of a 4-week β-alanine supplementation protocol on skeletal muscle carnosine concentrations [80]. Participants in the low-dose group consumed 3.2 g/day of β-alanine each week, while participants in the high-dose group consumed 4.0 g/day during week one, increasing to 6.4 g/day during week four. Skeletal muscle carnosine concentrations increased in the low-dose group by 7.80 ± 0.36 mmol/kg dry mass, while the high dose resulted in an increase of 11.04 ± 2.68 mmol/kg dry mass, which is consistent with findings from a later study [74].

11.4.1.1 Does β-Alanine Enhance Performance?

In theory, β-alanine should be able to enhance short-duration, high-intensity bouts of exercise but athletes should not be overly excited about β-alanine yet, as research regarding the efficacy of β-alanine has been equivocal [73,81]. In this regard, research provides some evidence that β-alanine may be able increase anaerobic threshold [73] and potentially performance involving high-intensity exercise [79]. However, other investigations have found β-alanine to have no effect on fatigue rates during line drills in college football players [82] or 400-msprint running times [75]. Results from the available literature would suggest that physiologically, β-alanine has the ability to enhance exercise performance but studies examining the efficacy of β-alanine on athletic performance have not found these physiological changes to result in meaningful performance adaptations. Given the relatively expensive cost and limited support for its efficacy to enhance performance, the recreational athlete may find better value for their money with supplements other than β-alanine. However, there may be a place for the use of β-alanine in elite athletes where minimal performance improvements can translate into success. However, more research needs to be conducted in this area, particularly in relation to masters athletes.

11.4.1.2 Dosing

A common side effect of β-alanine supplementation is paresthesia which is a sensation of tingling, burning, prickling or numbness to a person's skin with no apparent long-term physical effects.

An early investigation reported 10 mg/kg or approximately 800 mg of β-alanine to be the maximal single dose that could be consumed without experiencing significant symptoms of paresthesia [80]. Moreover, β-alanine concentrations peaked 30–40 minutes following consumption and returned to baseline 3 hours following consumption [80]. As a result, an individual supplementing with β-alanine could consume multiple doses throughout the day in 3-hour intervals. In this regard, the consumption of 6.4 g/day of β-alanine consumed in eight doses of 800 mg appears more effective at enhancing skeletal muscle carnosine levels than the consumption of 3.2 g/day of β-alanine consumed in four doses of 800 mg [80]. Finally, controlled release capsules have been developed allowing for the single dose consumption of 1600 mg without the presentation of paresthesia, allowing users to consume fewer daily doses of β-alanine [75,83]. As a result, masters athletes wishing to experiment with β-alanine should aim to consume 6.4 g/day, which can be accomplished with eight doses of 800 mg of β-alanine, or with four doses of 1600 mg with controlled release β-alanine capsules.

11.4.1.3 Conclusions

- Research supporting the efficacy of β-alanine supplementation has been equivocal; currently β-alanine is not recommended for the recreational athlete
- β-alanine supplementation may be most applicable to competitive masters athletes engaging in high-intensity, short-duration bouts of exercise likely to induce high intracellular acidosis

11.4.2 Caffeine

Caffeine is the most commonly consumed pharmacological agent in the world [84]. As a result, much research has been conducted on the physiological and performance effects of caffeine [85,86]. Research suggests caffeine has the ability to provide ergogenic benefits to both sleep-deprived [87] and endurance athletes [88].

Caffeine has been proposed to have several positive physiological effects. However, the only positive effect that can be achieved within the physiological concentration range of caffeine consumption is through the inhibition of adenosine receptors [89,90]. Caffeine non-selectively blocks adenosine receptors, thus serving as a competitive inhibitor of adenosine [91,92], which acts as a modulator of central nervous system neurotransmission [93]. Some of the potential ergogenic effects of caffeine include bronchial dilation [91], the relaxation of bronchial smooth muscle [91], an increase in respiratory rate [91], an increase in calcium release from the sarcoplasmic reticulum which may increase contractile force during submaximal exercise intensities [94], a reduction in pain perception [95], increased alertness [96] and improvements in ratings of perceived exertion [97].

Research strongly supports the use of caffeine for endurance athletes competing in cycling [98], rowing [99] and jogging [88], as well as sleep-deprived athletes such as those competing in events lasting for extended durations such as ultra-endurance marathons and adventure races [87]. For example, an early investigation found caffeinated coffee (330 mg of caffeine) to increase exercise time to exhaustion at 80% of VO_{2max} on a cycler ergometer [98]. To the contrary, the majority of research does not support the use of caffeine for muscle strength and force output [100,101].

It is also important to note the source of caffeine is important as caffeine obtained in the form of tea or coffee is likely to function in a manner different than caffeine alone. For instance, Graham et al. had participants run at 85% of VO_{2max} until voluntary exhaustion under five conditions: placebo in water, decaffeinated coffee, regular coffee, decaffeinated coffee supplemented with caffeine, and caffeine in water. In each caffeine trial the caffeine dose was 4.45 mg/kg of body mass and the volume of liquid was 7.15 mg/kg. Each drink was consumed 1 hour prior to exercise. Of interest was the finding that during each caffeine condition, epinephrine levels were significantly increased, but endurance was only increased in the caffeine in water trial. The researchers have speculated that caffeine alone may be superior to obtaining caffeine in the form of drinks such as tea and coffee because tea and coffee contain numerous compounds that may counteract some of the effects of caffeine [88]. Thus, recommendations for caffeine dosing are made on the assumption that caffeine is consumed in the form of a supplement such as NoDoz.

11.4.2.1 Dosing

Effective dosing strategies include the consumption of 3–6 mg/kg of body mass consumed 1 hour prior to exercise [102] or 1–2 mg/kg of body mass consumed during exercise [103]. Plasma concentrations of caffeine peak 30–90 minutes following consumption [102] and caffeine has a half-life of 4–6 hours, and as a result circulating levels of caffeine remain near peak levels for approximately 3–4 hours [90].

Possible concerns around dosing could include caffeine habituation and dehydration. However, neither of these issues inhibits the ergogenic effects of caffeine. Specifically, no relationship has been reported between caffeine habits and degree of performance response in 1500-meter runners [104] or muscle force development [94]. In regard to dehydration, numerous studies have reported no effect of caffeine on sweat rates, plasma volume, electrolytes or core temperature [90,105,106]. While caffeine is a mild diuretic as it increases the secretion of rennin (an enzyme that helps mediate extracellular volume), this occurs over a period of several hours [107], and this effect appears to be overridden with the initiation of exercise [105].

11.4.2.2 Conclusions

- Caffeine can enhance endurance performance by acting as a competitive inhibitor of adenosine
- Caffeine is a potentially ergogenic supplement for endurance athletes
- Caffeine supplementation should not increase risk for heat injury

Readers interested in learning more about other ergogenic aids and their effect on athletes and older individuals are directed to a number of previously published reviews [108–111].

11.5 IMPLICATIONS FOR SPORTS MEDICINE PROFESSIONALS, CLINICIANS, MASTERS ATHLETES AND COACHES

Athletes, coaches, clinicians and sports medicine professionals should have a thorough understanding of commonly utilised supplements, including their ergogenic effects, possible dangers and potential uses for enhancing performance.

- A large proportion of older adults do not consume enough protein per day. Increasing protein consumption can help optimise performance, particularly in older (≥55 years) masters athletes.
- Creatine is likely the most cost-effective performance-enhancing supplement on the market.
- Creatine may function to reduce the risk of heat injury.
- β-alanine is a popular supplement but research has not reported β-alanine to consistently enhance athletic performance.
- Caffeine is a widely used sport supplement that has consistently been found to enhance athletic performance in a variety of tasks. It should be noted that caffeine consumed in tea/coffee/soft drinks is likely not able to produce the same ergogenic effects as caffeine alone taken as a supplement.
- Before consuming any supplement, ensure the following:
    - The product is safe. Just because a product is sold over-the-counter does not necessarily mean the product is safe, so make decisions based on research evidence rather than marketing hype.

- The product has consistently been found to elicit the performance benefits you are seeking to attain such as an increase in strength or aerobic capacity.
- The proper dosing strategy, such as how much of the supplement to consume per day.
- Be aware of any potential adverse effects.

11.6 FUTURE RESEARCH DIRECTIONS

This chapter has focused on supplements for the masters athlete. The majority of research to date has been conducted on the use of supplements in college-aged and young adults (18–35 years) and can be applied, without too many assumptions or concerns, to healthy older populations. However, limited work has examined the effects of supplements in older adults (≥55 years), where the ability exists for supplements to not only enhance performance but also improve quality of life. Specific studies of interest are the following:

- Effect of protein intake on skeletal muscle mass in older (≥55 years) adults.
- Effect of creatine supplementation on recovery from an acute exercise bout (aerobic or anaerobic) in older adults (≥55 years).
- Effects of long-term (52-week) creatine supplementation and resistance exercise on skeletal muscle mass and strength in older adults (≥55 years).
- With time, novel supplements of interest will be developed and studies will be required to determine the safety and efficacy of use. An area of interest appears to be myostatin blocking agents.

REFERENCES

1. Dalbo, V.J., Roberts, M.D., Stout, J.R. and Kerksick, C.M., Putting to rest the myth of creatine supplementation leading to muscle cramps and dehydration, *Br. J. Sports Med.* 42(7), 567–73, 2008.
2. Dalbo, V.J., Roberts, M.D., Hassell, S.E., Moon, J.R. and Kerksick, C.M., Effects of a mineral antioxidant complex on clinical safety, body water, lactate response, and aerobic performance in response to exhaustive exercise, *Int. J. Sport Nutr. Exerc. Metab.* 20(5), 381–92, 2010.
3. Roberts, M.D., Dalbo, V.J., Hassell, S.E., Stout, J.R. and Kerksick, C.M., Efficacy and safety of a popular thermogenic drink after 28 days of ingestion, *J. Int. Soc. Sports Nutr.* 5, 19, 2008.
4. Dalbo, V.J., Roberts, M.D., Lockwood, C.M., Tucker, P.S., Kreider, R.B. and Kerksick, C.M., The effects of age on skeletal muscle and the phosphocreatine energy system: Can creatine supplementation help older adults, *Dyn. Med.* 8, 6, 2009.
5. Dalbo, V.J., Roberts, M.D., Stout, J.R. and Kerksick, C.M., Effect of gender on the metabolic impact of a commercially available thermogenic drink, *J. Strength Cond. Res.* 24(6), 1633–42, 2010.
6. Dalbo, V.J., Roberts, M.D., Stout, J.R. and Kerksick, C.M., Acute effects of ingesting a commercial thermogenic drink on changes in energy expenditure and markers of lipolysis, *J. Int. Soc. Sports Nutr.* 5, 6, 2008.
7. Poole, C.N., Roberts, M.D., Dalbo, V.J. et al., The combined effects of exercise and ingestion of a meal replacement in conjunction with a weight loss supplement on body composition and fitness parameters in college-aged men and women, *J. Strength Cond. Res.* 25(1), 51–60, 2011.
8. Roberts, M.D., Dalbo, V.J., Hassell, S.E., Brown, R. and Kerksick, C.M., Effects of preexercise feeding on markers of satellite cell activation, *Med. Sci. Sports Exerc.* 42(10), 1861–9, 2010.
9. Dalbo, V.J., Roberts, M.D., Hassell, S. and Kerksick, C.M., Effects of pre-exercise feeding on serum hormone concentrations and biomarkers of myostatin and ubiquitin proteasome pathway activity, *Eur. J. Nutr.* 52(2), 477–87, 2012.
10. Lockwood, C.M., Moon, J.R., Tobkin, S.E. et al., Minimal nutrition intervention with high-protein/low-carbohydrate and low-fat, nutrient-dense food supplement improves body composition and exercise benefits in overweight adults: A randomized controlled trial, *Nutr. Metab. (Lond)* 5, 11, 2008.
11. Roberts, M.D., Lockwood, C., Dalbo, V.J., Volek, J. and Kerksick, C.M., Ingestion of a high-molecular-weight hydrothermally modified waxy maize starch alters metabolic responses to prolonged exercise in trained cyclists, *Nutrition* 27(6), 659–65, 2011.

12. Rawson, E.S. and Volek, J.S., Effects of creatine supplementation and resistance training on muscle strength and weightlifting performance, *J. Strength Cond. Res.* 17(4), 822–31, 2003.
13. Volek, J.S., Duncan, N.D., Mazzetti, S.A. et al., Performance and muscle fiber adaptations to creatine supplementation and heavy resistance training, *Med. Sci. Sports Exerc.* 31(8), 1147–56, 1999.
14. Law, Y.L., Ong, W.S., GillianYap, T.L., Lim, S.C. and Von Chia, E., Effects of two and five days of creatine loading on muscular strength and anaerobic power in trained athletes, *J. Strength Cond. Res.* 23(3), 906–14, 2009.
15. Miles, R.P., *101 Reasons to Own the World's Greatest Investment: Warren Buffett's Berkshire Hathaway*, John Wiley & Sons, Inc., New York, 2001.
16. United States Food and Drug Administration, *Guidance for Industry: Statement of Identity, Nutrition Labeling and Ingredient Labeling of Dietary Supplements; Small Entity Compliance Guide*, United States Food and Drug Administration, Silver Spring, MD, 1999.
17. Childs, E. and de Wit, H., Enhanced mood and psychomotor performance by a caffeine-containing energy capsule in fatigued individuals, *Exp. Clin. Psychopharmacol.* 16(1), 13–21, 2008.
18. Haskell, C.F., Kennedy, D.O., Wesnes, K.A. and Scholey, A.B., Cognitive and mood improvements of caffeine in habitual consumers and habitual non-consumers of caffeine, *Psychopharmacology (Berl).* 179(4), 813–25, 2005.
19. Wesensten, N.J., Killgore, W.D. and Balkin, T.J., Performance and alertness effects of caffeine, dextroamphetamine, and modafinil during sleep deprivation, *J. Sleep. Res.* 14(3), 255–66, 2005.
20. Jacobson, B.H. and Edgley, B.M., Effects of caffeine on simple reaction time and movement time, *Aviat. Space Environ. Med.* 58(12), 1153–6, 1987.
21. Kovacs, E.M., Stegen, J. and Brouns, F., Effect of caffeinated drinks on substrate metabolism, caffeine excretion, and performance, *J. Appl. Physiol.* 85(2), 709–15, 1998.
22. Young, A., Stokes, M. and Crowe, M., The size and strength of the quadriceps muscles of old and young men, *Clin. Physiol.* 5(2), 145–54, 1985.
23. Young, A., Stokes, M. and Crowe, M., Size and strength of the quadriceps muscles of old and young women, *Eur. J. Clin. Invest.* 14(4), 282–7, 1984.
24. Lindle, R.S., Metter, E.J., Lynch, N.A. et al., Age and gender comparisons of muscle strength in 654 women and men aged 20–93 yr, *J. Appl. Physiol.* 83(5), 1581–7, 1997.
25. Campbell, W.W., Trappe, T.A., Wolfe, R.R. and Evans, W.J., The recommended dietary allowance for protein may not be adequate for older people to maintain skeletal muscle, *J. Gerontol. A Biol. Sci. Med. Sci.* 56(6), M373–80, 2001.
26. Wolfe, R.R. and Miller, S.L., The recommended dietary allowance of protein: A misunderstood concept, *JAMA* 299(24), 2891–3, 2008.
27. Paddon-Jones, D. and Rasmussen, B.B., Dietary protein recommendations and the prevention of sarcopenia, *Curr. Opin. Clin. Nutr. Metab. Care* 12(1), 86–90, 2009.
28. Wagenmakers, A.J., Muscle amino acid metabolism at rest and during exercise: Role in human physiology and metabolism, *Exerc. Sport Sci. Rev.* 26, 287–314, 1998.
29. Tarnopolsky, M.A., Protein and amino acid needs for training and bulking up, in *Clinical Sports Nutrition*, L. Burke and V. Deakin, eds., McGraw-Hill Medical, New York, 2010.
30. McKenzie, S., Phillips, S.M., Carter, S.L., Lowther, S., Gibala, M.J. and Tarnopolsky, M.A., Endurance exercise training attenuates leucine oxidation and BCOAD activation during exercise in humans, *Am. J. Physiol. Endocrinol. Metab.* 278(4), E580–7, 2000.
31. Dalbo, V.J., Stout, J.R. and Kerksick, C.M., Nutrient timing considerations for the military, aged, metabolically-challenged populations, and children, in *Nutrient Timing: Metabolic Optimization for Health, Performance, and Recovery*, C.M. Kerksick, ed., CRC Press, Boca Raton, FL, 2012.
32. Paddon-Jones, D., Short, K.R., Campbell, W.W., Volpi, E. and Wolfe, R.R., Role of dietary protein in the sarcopenia of aging, *Am. J. Clin. Nutr.* 87(5), 1562S–66S, 2008.
33. Morais, J.A., Chevalier, S. and Gougeon, R., Protein turnover and requirements in the healthy and frail elderly, *J. Nutr. Health Aging* 10(4), 272–83, 2006.
34. Symons, T.B., Schutzler, S.E., Cocke, T.L., Chinkes, D.L., Wolfe, R.R. and Paddon-Jones, D., Aging does not impair the anabolic response to a protein-rich meal, *Am. J. Clin. Nutr.* 86(2), 451–6, 2007.
35. Tarnopolsky, M.A., Atkinson, S.A., MacDougall, J.D., Chesley, A., Phillips, S. and Schwarcz, H.P., Evaluation of protein requirements for trained strength athletes, *J. Appl. Physiol.* 73(5), 1986–95, 1992.
36. Ivy, J. and Portman, R., *Nutrient Timing: The Future of Sports Nutrition*, Basic Health Publications, Inc., Laguna Beach, CA, 2004.

37. Hulmi, J.J., Tannerstedt, J., Selanne, H., Kainulainen, H., Kovanen, V. and Mero, A.A., Resistance exercise with whey protein ingestion affects mTOR signaling pathway and myostatin in men, *J. Appl. Physiol.* 106(5), 1720–9, 2009.
38. Tipton, K.D., Elliott, T.A., Cree, M.G., Aarsland, A.A., Sanford, A.P. and Wolfe, R.R., Stimulation of net muscle protein synthesis by whey protein ingestion before and after exercise, *Am. J. Physiol. Endocrinol. Metab.* 292(1), E71–6, 2007.
39. Wilkinson, S.B., Tarnopolsky, M.A., Macdonald, M.J., Macdonald, J.R., Armstrong, D. and Phillips, S.M., Consumption of fluid skim milk promotes greater muscle protein accretion after resistance exercise than does consumption of an isonitrogenous and isoenergetic soy-protein beverage, *Am. J. Clin. Nutr.* 85(4), 1031–40, 2007.
40. Hulmi, J.J., Lockwood, C.M. and Stout, J.R., Effect of protein/essential amino acids and resistance training on skeletal muscle hypertrophy: A case for whey protein, *Nutr. Metab (Lond.)* 7, 51, 2010.
41. Tipton, K.D., Rasmussen, B.B., Miller, S.L. et al., Timing of amino acid-carbohydrate ingestion alters anabolic response of muscle to resistance exercise, *Am. J. Physiol. Endocrinol. Metab.* 281(2), E197–206, 2001.
42. Levenhagen, D.K., Gresham, J.D., Carlson, M.G., Maron, D.J., Borel, M.J. and Flakoll, P.J., Postexercise nutrient intake timing in humans is critical to recovery of leg glucose and protein homeostasis, *Am. J. Physiol. Endocrinol. Metab.* 280(6), E982–93, 2001.
43. Phillips, S.M., Tipton, K.D., Aarsland, A., Wolf, S.E. and Wolfe, R.R., Mixed muscle protein synthesis and breakdown after resistance exercise in humans, *Am. J. Physiol.* 273(1 Pt 1), E99–107, 1997.
44. Phillips, S.M., Tang, J.E. and Moore, D.R., The role of milk- and soy-based protein in support of muscle protein synthesis and muscle protein accretion in young and elderly persons, *J. Am. Coll. Nutr.* 28(4), 343–54, 2009.
45. Esmarck, B., Andersen, J.L., Olsen, S., Richter, E.A., Mizuno, M. and Kjaer, M., Timing of postexercise protein intake is important for muscle hypertrophy with resistance training in elderly humans, *J. Physiol.* 535(Pt 1), 301–11, 2001.
46. Cuthbertson, D., Smith, K., Babraj, J. et al., Anabolic signaling deficits underlie amino acid resistance of wasting, aging muscle, *FASEB J.* 19(3), 422–4, 2005.
47. Arnal, M.A., Mosoni, L., Boirie, Y. et al., Protein pulse feeding improves protein retention in elderly women, *Am. J. Clin. Nutr.* 69(6), 1202–8, 1999.
48. Boirie, Y., Dangin, M., Gachon, P., Vasson, M.P., Maubois, J.L. and Beaufrere, B., Slow and fast dietary proteins differently modulate postprandial protein accretion, *Proc. Natl. Acad. Sci. U.S.A.* 94(26), 14930–5, 1997.
49. Kimball, S.R. and Jefferson, L.S., New functions for amino acids: Effects on gene transcription and translation, *Am. J. Clin. Nutr.* 83(2), 500S–7S, 2006.
50. Anthony, J.C., Yoshizawa, F., Anthony, T.G., Vary, T.C., Jefferson, L.S. and Kimball, S.R., Leucine stimulates translation initiation in skeletal muscle of postabsorptive rats via a rapamycin-sensitive pathway, *J. Nutr.* 130(10), 2413–9, 2000.
51. Atherton, P.J., Smith, K., Etheridge, T., Rankin, D. and Rennie, M.J., Distinct anabolic signalling responses to amino acids in C2C12 skeletal muscle cells, *Amino Acids* 38(5), 1533–9, 2010.
52. Kimball, S.R. and Jefferson, L.S., Signaling pathways and molecular mechanisms through which branched-chain amino acids mediate translational control of protein synthesis, *J. Nutr.* 136(1 Suppl), 227S–31S, 2006.
53. Koopman, R., Wagenmakers, A.J., Manders, R.J. et al., Combined ingestion of protein and free leucine with carbohydrate increases postexercise muscle protein synthesis in vivo in male subjects, *Am. J. Physiol. Endocrinol. Metab.* 288(4), E645–53, 2005.
54. Fujita, S., Rasmussen, B.B., Cadenas, J.G., Grady, J.J. and Volpi, E., Effect of insulin on human skeletal muscle protein synthesis is modulated by insulin-induced changes in muscle blood flow and amino acid availability, *Am. J. Physiol. Endocrinol. Metab.* 291(4), E745–54, 2006.
55. Chow, L.S., Albright, R.C., Bigelow, M.L., Toffolo, G., Cobelli, C. and Nair, K.S., Mechanism of insulin's anabolic effect on muscle: Measurements of muscle protein synthesis and breakdown using aminoacyl-tRNA and other surrogate measures, *Am. J. Physiol. Endocrinol. Metab.* 291(4), E729–36, 2006.
56. Katsanos, C.S., Kobayashi, H., Sheffield-Moore, M., Aarsland, A. and Wolfe, R.R., A high proportion of leucine is required for optimal stimulation of the rate of muscle protein synthesis by essential amino acids in the elderly, *Am. J. Physiol. Endocrinol. Metab.* 291(2), E381–7, 2006.
57. Verhoeven, S., Vanschoonbeek, K., Verdijk, L.B. et al., Long-term leucine supplementation does not increase muscle mass or strength in healthy elderly men, *Am. J. Clin. Nutr.* 89(5), 1468–75, 2009.

58. Grande, B. and Graves, S., Creatine supplementation: Forms, function, and effects, *Strength Cond. J.* 27, 62–8, 2005.
59. Berneis, K., Ninnis, R., Haussinger, D. and Keller, U., Effects of hyper- and hypoosmolality on whole body protein and glucose kinetics in humans, *Am. J. Physiol.* 276(1 Pt 1), E188–95, 1999.
60. Hespel, P., Op't Eijnde, B., Van Leemputte, M. et al., Oral creatine supplementation facilitates the rehabilitation of disuse atrophy and alters the expression of muscle myogenic factors in humans, *J. Physiol.* 536(Pt 2), 625–33, 2001.
61. Young, R.B. and Denome, R.M., Effect of creatine on contents of myosin heavy chain and myosin-heavy-chain mRNA in steady-state chicken muscle-cell cultures, *Biochem. J.* 218(3), 871–6, 1984.
62. Dangott, B., Schultz, E. and Mozdziak, P.E., Dietary creatine monohydrate supplementation increases satellite cell mitotic activity during compensatory hypertrophy, *Int. J. Sports Med.* 21(1), 13–6, 2000.
63. Olsen, S., Aagaard, P., Kadi, F. et al., Creatine supplementation augments the increase in satellite cell and myonuclei number in human skeletal muscle induced by strength training, *J. Physiol.* 573(Pt 2), 525–34, 2006.
64. Casey, A., Constantin-Teodosiu, D., Howell, S., Hultman, E. and Greenhaff, P.L., Creatine ingestion favorably affects performance and muscle metabolism during maximal exercise in humans, *Am. J. Physiol.* 271(1 Pt 1), E31–7, 1996.
65. Gotshalk, L.A., Volek, J.S., Staron, R.S., Denegar, C.R., Hagerman, F.C. and Kraemer, W.J., Creatine supplementation improves muscular performance in older men, *Med. Sci. Sports Exerc.* 34(3), 537–43, 2002.
66. van Loon, L.J., Oosterlaar, A.M., Hartgens, F., Hesselink, M.K., Snow, R.J. and Wagenmakers, A.J., Effects of creatine loading and prolonged creatine supplementation on body composition, fuel selection, sprint and endurance performance in humans, *Clin. Sci. (Lond.)* 104(2), 153–62, 2003.
67. Engelhardt, M., Neumann, G., Berbalk, A. and Reuter, I., Creatine supplementation in endurance sports, *Med. Sci. Sports Exerc.* 30(7), 1123–9, 1998.
68. Kilduff, L.P., Georgiades, E., James, N. et al., The effects of creatine supplementation on cardiovascular, metabolic, and thermoregulatory responses during exercise in the heat in endurance-trained humans, *Int. J. Sport Nutr. Exerc. Metab.* 14(4), 443–60, 2004.
69. Easton, C., Turner, S. and Pitsiladis, Y.P., Creatine and glycerol hyperhydration in trained subjects before exercise in the heat, *Int. J. Sport Nutr. Exerc. Metab.* 17(1), 70–91, 2007.
70. Greenhaff, P.L., Creatine and its application as an ergogenic aid, *Int. J. Sport Nutr.* (5 Suppl), S100–10, 1995.
71. Gotshalk, L.A., Kraemer, W.J., Mendonca, M.A. et al., Creatine supplementation improves muscular performance in older women, *Eur. J. Appl. Physiol.* 102(2), 223–31, 2008.
72. Brose, A., Parise, G. and Tarnopolsky, M.A., Creatine supplementation enhances isometric strength and body composition improvements following strength exercise training in older adults, *J. Gerontol. A Biol. Sci. Med. Sci.* 58(1), 11–9, 2003.
73. Artioli, G.G., Gualano, B., Smith, A., Stout, J. and Lancha, A.H., Jr., Role of beta-alanine supplementation on muscle carnosine and exercise performance, *Med. Sci. Sports Exerc.* 42(6), 1162–73, 2010.
74. Hill, C.A., Harris, R.C., Kim, H.J. et al., Influence of beta-alanine supplementation on skeletal muscle carnosine concentrations and high intensity cycling capacity, *Amino Acids* 32(2), 225–33, 2007.
75. Derave, W., Ozdemir, M.S., Harris, R.C. et al., Beta-alanine supplementation augments muscle carnosine content and attenuates fatigue during repeated isokinetic contraction bouts in trained sprinters, *J. Appl. Physiol.* 103(5), 1736–43, 2007.
76. Bishop, D., Edge, J., Davis, C. and Goodman, C., Induced metabolic alkalosis affects muscle metabolism and repeated-sprint ability, *Med. Sci. Sports Exerc.* 36(5), 807–13, 2004.
77. Bouissou, P., Defer, G., Guezennec, C.Y., Estrade, P.Y. and Serrurier, B., Metabolic and blood catecholamine responses to exercise during alkalosis, *Med. Sci. Sports Exerc.* 20(3), 228–32, 1988.
78. Tallon, M.J., Harris, R.C., Boobis, L.H., Fallowfield, J.L. and Wise, J.A., The carnosine content of vastus lateralis is elevated in resistance-trained bodybuilders, *J. Strength Cond. Res.* 19(4), 725–9, 2005.
79. Harris, R.C., Marlin, D.J., Dunnett, M., Snow, D.H. and Hultman, E., Muscle buffering capacity and dipeptide content in the thoroughbred horse, greyhound dog and man, *Comp. Biochem. Physiol. A Comp. Physiol.* 97(2), 249–51, 1990.
80. Harris, R.C., Tallon, M.J., Dunnett, M. et al., The absorption of orally supplied beta-alanine and its effect on muscle carnosine synthesis in human vastus lateralis, *Amino Acids* 30(3), 279–89, 2006.
81. Sale, C., Saunders, B. and Harris, R.C., Effect of beta-alanine supplementation on muscle carnosine concentrations and exercise performance, *Amino Acids* 39(2), 321–33, 2010.

82. Hoffman, J.R., Ratamess, N.A., Faigenbaum, A.D. et al., Short-duration beta-alanine supplementation increases training volume and reduces subjective feelings of fatigue in college football players, *Nutr. Res.* 28(1), 31–5, 2008.
83. Hoffman, J., Ratamess, N.A., Ross, R. et al., Beta-alanine and the hormonal response to exercise, *Int. J. Sports Med.* 29(12), 952–8, 2008.
84. Keisler, B.D. and Armsey, T.D., 2nd, Caffeine as an ergogenic aid, *Curr. Sports Med. Rep.* 5(4), 215–9, 2006.
85. Burke, L.M., Caffeine and sports performance, *Appl. Physiol. Nutr. Metab.* 33(6), 1319–34, 2008.
86. Ganio, M.S., Klau, J.F., Casa, D.J., Armstrong, L.E. and Maresh, C.M., Effect of caffeine on sport-specific endurance performance: A systematic review, *J. Strength Cond. Res.* 23(1), 315–24, 2009.
87. McLellan, T.M., Bell, D.G. and Kamimori, G.H., Caffeine improves physical performance during 24 h of active wakefulness, *Aviat. Space Environ. Med.* 75(8), 666–72, 2004.
88. Graham, T.E., Hibbert, E. and Sathasivam, P., Metabolic and exercise endurance effects of coffee and caffeine ingestion, *J. Appl. Physiol.* 85(3), 883–9, 1998.
89. Davis, J.M., Zhao, Z., Stock, H.S., Mehl, K.A., Buggy, J. and Hand, G.A., Central nervous system effects of caffeine and adenosine on fatigue, *Am. J. Physiol. Regul. Integr. Comp. Physiol.* 284(2), R399–404, 2003.
90. Graham, T.E., Caffeine and exercise: Metabolism, endurance and performance, *Sports Med.* 31(11), 785–807, 2001.
91. Chou, T., Wake up and smell the coffee. Caffeine, coffee, and the medical consequences, *West. J. Med.* 157(5), 544–53, 1992.
92. Bell, D.G., McLellan, T.M. and Sabiston, C.M., Effect of ingesting caffeine and ephedrine on 10-km run performance, *Med. Sci. Sports Exerc.* 34(2), 344–9, 2002.
93. Cauli, O. and Morelli, M., Caffeine and the dopaminergic system, *Behav. Pharmacol.* 16(2), 63–77, 2005.
94. Tarnopolsky, M. and Cupido, C., Caffeine potentiates low frequency skeletal muscle force in habitual and nonhabitual caffeine consumers, *J. Appl. Physiol.* 89(5), 1719–24, 2000.
95. Motl, R.W., O'Connor, P.J. and Dishman, R.K., Effect of caffeine on perceptions of leg muscle pain during moderate intensity cycling exercise, *J. Pain* 4(6), 316–21, 2003.
96. Zwyghuizen-Doorenbos, A., Roehrs, T.A., Lipschutz, L., Timms, V. and Roth, T., Effects of caffeine on alertness, *Psychopharmacology (Berl.)* 100(1), 36–9, 1990.
97. Doherty, M. and Smith, P.M., Effects of caffeine ingestion on rating of perceived exertion during and after exercise: A meta-analysis, *Scand. J. Med. Sci. Sports* 15(2), 69–78, 2005.
98. Costill, D.L., Dalsky, G.P. and Fink, W.J., Effects of caffeine ingestion on metabolism and exercise performance, *Med. Sci. Sports* 10(3), 155–8, 1978.
99. Bruce, C.R., Anderson, M.E., Fraser, S.F. et al., Enhancement of 2000-m rowing performance after caffeine ingestion, *Med. Sci. Sports Exerc.* 32(11), 1958–63, 2000.
100. Astorino, T.A., Rohmann, R.L. and Firth, K., Effect of caffeine ingestion on one-repetition maximum muscular strength, *Eur. J. Appl. Physiol.* 102(2), 127–32, 2008.
101. Greer, F., Morales, J. and Coles, M., Wingate performance and surface EMG frequency variables are not affected by caffeine ingestion, *Appl. Physiol. Nutr. Metab.* 31(5), 597–603, 2006.
102. Tarnopolsky, M.A., Caffeine and creatine use in sport, *Ann. Nutr. Metab.* 57 (Suppl 2), 1–8, 2010.
103. Cox, G.R., Desbrow, B., Montgomery, P.G. et al., Effect of different protocols of caffeine intake on metabolism and endurance performance, *J. Appl. Physiol.* 93(3), 990–9, 2002.
104. Wiles, J.D., Bird, S.R., Hopkins, J. and Riley, M., Effect of caffeinated coffee on running speed, respiratory factors, blood lactate and perceived exertion during 1500-m treadmill running, *Br. J. Sports Med.* 26(2), 116–20, 1992.
105. Wemple, R.D., Lamb, D.R. and McKeever, K.H., Caffeine vs caffeine-free sports drinks: Effects on urine production at rest and during prolonged exercise, *Int. J. Sports Med.* 18(1), 40–6, 1997.
106. Wells, C.L., Schrader, T.A., Stern, J.R. and Krahenbuhl, G.S., Physiological responses to a 20-mile run under three fluid replacement treatments, *Med. Sci. Sports Exerc.* 17(3), 364–9, 1985.
107. Robertson, D., Frolich, J.C., Carr, R.K. et al., Effects of caffeine on plasma renin activity, catecholamines and blood pressure, *N. Engl. J. Med.* 298(4), 181–6, 1978.
108. Liddle, D.G. and Connor, D.J., Nutritional supplements and ergogenic aids, *Prim. Care* 40(2), 487–505, 2013.
109. Schubert, M.M. and Astorino, T.A., A systematic review of the efficacy of ergogenic aids for improving running performance, *J. Strength Cond. Res.* 27(6), 1699–707, 2013.
110. Cherniak, E.P., Ergogenic dietary aids for the elderly, *Nutrition* 28(3), 225–9, 2012.
111. Moon, A., Heywood, L., Rutherford, S. and Cobbold, C., Creatine supplementation: Can it improve quality of life in the elderly without associated resistance training? *Curr. Aging Sci.* 6(3), 251–7, 2013.

12 Nutrients, Health and Chronic Disease in Masters Athletes

Janelle A. Gifford, Helen T. O'Connor, Alexandra L. Honey and Ian D. Caterson

CONTENTS

12.1 INTRODUCTION

Masters athletes are a heterogeneous group, comprised of adults who have been active all their lives through to those just embarking on new exercise regimes, perhaps as a way of treating an existing chronic disease. They provide a model for studying the health benefits of adoption and sustained engagement in physical activity during middle to older age [1]. Unfortunately there is limited research conducted on masters athletes and studies available are often methodologically flawed. However, available evidence would suggest that masters athletes have better general health, a lower prevalence of lifestyle diseases and decreased all-cause mortality by virtue of their engagement in physical activity [2,3]. Adults who have healthy lifestyles (healthy diet and physical activity) whether lifelong, adopted during middle age, or adopted as healthy older adults may have lower rates of these diseases and decreased all-cause mortality when compared to those who do not [1,4–7].

Along with nutrition interventions, physical activity is a frequently recommended therapy for the prevention and management of many chronic conditions including obesity, type 2 diabetes, cardiovascular disease (CVD), stroke, dyslipidaemias, hypertension, osteoarthritis (OA), osteoporosis, neurological and cognitive disorders and cancer [8]. This chapter will examine the available evidence describing the prevalence of lifestyle diseases in masters athletes and the benefits or potential risks of exercise training in this group. Finally, nutritional interventions to prevent or treat chronic lifestyle diseases in masters athletes that are also consistent with optimising athletic performance will be outlined.

12.2 CHRONIC CONDITIONS AND NUTRIENT RECOMMENDATIONS FOR PREVENTION AND TREATMENT

12.2.1 Metabolic Conditions: Obesity/Type 2 Diabetes

12.2.1.1 Definition, Presentation and Prevalence

Metabolic conditions encompass a number of disorders including obesity, type 2 diabetes, hyperlipidaemia and hypertension [9]. Whilst they are related, this section discusses obesity and type 2 diabetes; hyperlipidaemia and hypertension are discussed in a subsequent section in relation to CVD. Obesity, or excess adiposity, is most commonly assessed using the body mass index (BMI). The World Health Organization (WHO) define obesity as a BMI over 30 kg/m^2 (see Table 12.1). Waist circumference is an alternative measure for obesity, and a strong predictor for increased cardiovascular risk [9]. A measure of >102 cm in men and >88 cm in women is considered obese [10]. It is generally useful as a population indicator of appropriateness of weight for height and at a population level a BMI > 30 kg/m^2 is strongly associated with increased morbidity and mortality. It is also acknowledged that some populations have different body proportions and so interpretation of BMI may vary across populations. For example, the cut-off at which risk of disease increases may be lower for Asian populations [11]. It is also well known that BMI is not a reliable indicator of excess adiposity in active individuals with higher muscularity (e.g. in football, heavy weight rowing, weightlifting, throwing disciplines in athletics).

Obesity is a known risk factor for type 2 diabetes [12], a metabolic disorder characterised by chronic hyperglycaemia resulting from defects in either insulin secretion or insulin action or both. Type 2 diabetes is due to insulin resistance and a relative deficiency in insulin secretion and results in disturbances of carbohydrate, fat and protein metabolism [9]. Diabetes can be detected in patients who present with symptoms of hyperglycaemia such as increased thirst, increased urination, fatigue and infections along a spectrum to those with severe hyperglycaemic states. It may also be detected via routine screening of glucose levels or an oral glucose tolerance test. Table 12.2 [13] shows diagnostic criteria used by WHO.

Metabolic conditions can present independently, but may also occur concurrently, fulfilling the criteria for metabolic syndrome. Metabolic syndrome is defined by International Diabetes Federation

TABLE 12.1
The International Classification of Adult Underweight, Overweight and Obesity according to BMI

	BMI (kg/m^2)	
Classification	**Principal Cut-Off Points**	**Additional Cut-Off Points**
Underweight	<18.50	<18.50
Severe thinness	<16.00	<16.00
Moderate thinness	16.00–16.99	16.00–16.99
Mild thinness	17.00–18.49	17.00–18.49
Normal range	18.50–24.99	18.50–22.99
		23.00–24.99
Overweight	≥25.00	≥25.00
Pre-obese	25.00–29.99	25.00–27.49
		27.50–29.99
Obese	≥30.00	≥30.00
Obese class I	30.00–34.99	30.00–32.49
		32.50–34.99
Obese class II	35.00–39.99	35.00–37.49
		37.50–39.99
Obese class III	≥40.00	≥40.00

Source: Adapted from World Health Organization, Global database on body mass index. Available at http://apps.who.int/bmi/index.jsp?introPage=intro_3.html, accessed December 12, 2013.
Note: Additional cut-off points may be used in different population groups.

TABLE 12.2
World Health Organization Diagnostic Criteria for Diabetes and Intermediate Hyperglycaemia

	Fasting Plasma Glucose		**2-Hour Plasma Glucose**[a]
Diabetes	≥7.0 mmol/L (126 mg/dL)	OR	≥11.0 mmol/L (200 mg/dL)
Impaired glucose tolerance (IGT)	≥11.0 mmol/L (126 mg/dL)	AND	≥7.8 mmol/L (140 mg/dL) and <11.1 mmol/L (200 mg/dL)
Impaired fasting glucose (IFG)	6.1–6.9 mmol/L (110–125 mg/dL)	AND[b]	<7.8 mmol/L (140 mg/dL)

Source: World Health Organization and International Diabetes Federation, Definition and diagnosis of diabetes mellitus and intermediate hyperglycemia: report of a WHO/IDF consultation, World Health Organization, Geneva, 2006.
[a] Venous plasma glucose 2 hours after ingestion of 75-g oral glucose load. If 2-hour plasma glucose is not measured, status is uncertain as diabetes or IGT cannot be excluded.
[b] If measured.

criteria [14] as those with central obesity (waist circumference ≥94 cm for Caucasian men and ≥80 cm for Caucasian women), plus any two of the following criteria:

- Raised triglyceride level: >1.7 mmol/L (150 mg/dL)
- Reduced high-density lipoprotein cholesterol (HDL-C): <1.03 mmol/L (40 mg/dL) in males and <1.29 mmol/L (50 mg/dL) in females, or specific treatment for this lipid abnormality
- Raised blood pressure: SBP ≥ 130 mm Hg or DBP ≥ 85 mmHg, or treatment of previously diagnosed hypertension
- Raised fasting plasma glucose ≥ 5.6 mmol/L (100 mg/dL), or previously diagnosed type 2 diabetes

Those individuals with metabolic syndrome are at a greater risk of CVD than those with one risk factor alone.

The prevalence of obesity, type 2 diabetes and metabolic syndrome is rising in both the developed and developing world [15,16] and also increases with advancing age [17]. Analysis in 2010 by the International Association for the Study of Obesity and the International Obesity Taskforce estimates that worldwide, approximately 1.0 billion adults are currently overweight (BMI 25–29.9 kg/m^2) and a further 475 million are obese [18]. When Asian-specific cut-off points for the definition of obesity (body mass index >28 kg/m^2) are taken into account for the relevant countries, the number of adults considered obese globally is over 600 million [18]. It is estimated that there were around 366 million cases of diabetes worldwide in 2011 [19], with at least 85%–90% of these being type 2 diabetes. There are few data on prevalence of obesity, glucose intolerance and type 2 diabetes in masters athletes, but since physical activity is known to reduce body weight and improve whole-body insulin sensitivity, rates for these conditions should be lower amongst long-term athletes, and glycaemic control better amongst those who have taken up or maintained physical activity in later years.

The largest study examining BMI in masters athletes was conducted at the World Masters Games (WMG) held in Australia in 2009 [16]. In terms of participant numbers, the WMG is the largest international sporting competition worldwide and in 2009 attracted 28,089 competitors across 95 countries and 28 sports [16]. This study compared self-reported BMI in over 6000 WMG participants who responded to an online survey (male ~52%; female ~48%; mean age ~52 yr) to an Australian population sample where data was collected in over 12,000 participants as part of a National Health Survey (2007–2008) [20]. Linear and Loess regression was performed to describe the relationship between BMI and age in both samples. In comparison to the general Australian population sample where BMI increased with age, this trend was reversed in the WMG athletes [16].

Previously, Kettunen and others reported no cases of type 2 diabetes amongst 102 track and field participants in the 1985 World Veterans Games athletes at a 16-year follow-up compared to 9% of 777 controls [2]. This relationship may be discipline-specific, with a previous study of over 2000 subjects showing a relative risk (RR) of 0.24 and 0.52 for endurance and mixed-sport masters athletes, while power-sport masters athletes were found to have a similar risk (RR 1.21) as control subjects [21]. In younger athletes, lower insulin resistance has been reported amongst rowers and short-distance track athletes, whilst higher insulin resistance was found amongst archers and field-throwing athletes compared to control subjects [22].

Thus it appears that masters athletes, particularly those involved with endurance activities, have a lower risk of obesity and glucose intolerance/insulin resistance.

12.2.1.2 Medical Risks with Physical Activity

There is growing evidence that regular exercise prevents metabolic disease and should be part of treatment regimes to manage metabolic conditions [8]. Regular exercise is associated with improved glycaemic control, improved insulin sensitivity, preferential use of fat during less intense exercise and improved metabolism of post-meal lipids [8,23].

The major risk of physical activity in those with metabolic conditions largely relates to the increased risk of CVD amongst these individuals. For example, athletes with diabetes are 2–4 times more likely than unaffected individuals to develop early CVD and possibly death [24]. Overall, the benefits of exercise far outweigh the risks but there are some potential adverse effects amongst those with metabolic conditions who begin competing at a higher level. Sudden, intense exercise in previously sedentary individuals, or those who haven't trained for many years, can result in myocardial ischaemia, or infarction, and death [25]. In obese patients, other potential issues include an increased risk of soft tissue injury and joint damage.

Type 2 diabetes has a number of complications, both microvascular and macrovascular, that could potentially impact on an older athlete's performance. For example, the presence of peripheral neuropathy and foot deformities may increase the risk of foot ulceration, particularly if footwear is ill-fitting [26]. Control of blood sugars in diabetes is also an important consideration when endeavouring to compete at a high level, particularly in those who require insulin. People with well-controlled diabetes requiring insulin generally have reduced treatment requirements with exercise, and this increases the risk of hypoglycaemia. In contrast, people with poorly controlled diabetes may get a paradoxical elevation in blood glucose during exercise, increasing the risk of severe hyperglycaemic states [27,28].

12.2.1.3 Screening Recommendations

The screening recommendations for masters athletes with metabolic conditions largely relates to screening for CVD (see Section 12.2.2). Masters athletes with diabetes should be screened for both microvascular and macrovascular complications, with the aim to prevent any adverse outcomes. As part of routine care, all athletes with diabetes should have a BMI, blood pressure and foot check every 6 months, along with an annual assessment of lipids, HbA_{1c} and microalbuminuria, and two yearly ophthalmology reviews [29]. Additionally, a screening stress electrocardiogram (ECG) in men with diabetes who have no symptoms of CVD has been shown to have prognostic value [24].

Readers are referred to further screening guidelines for more detail [30–32].

12.2.1.4 Medications and Nutrient Interactions

Pharmacological management of metabolic conditions may result in an increased risk of adverse side effects in athletes. HMG CoA reductase inhibitors, used in the treatment of hypercholesterolaemia, can produce a statin-induced myopathy [33]. In athletes of any age who are training, symptoms may be mistaken for muscle pains resulting from training. Medication for diabetes can lead to multiple issues during exercise. Insulin requirements change with exercise depending on glucose control, so regular monitoring of blood sugar is required in masters athletes with type 2 diabetes [28]. Endurance athletes taking Metformin are theoretically at an increased risk of lactic acidosis, although evidence to support this is lacking. Nutritional supplements used by some athletes should be taken cautiously; for example, creatine may interact with Metformin, increasing the risk of renal impairment and lactic acidosis [34]. For more details on medication-nutrient interactions, see Chapter 13.

12.2.1.5 Nutrition Recommendations in Prevention and Treatment

To promote weight or fat loss, an energy deficit is required between intake and expenditure. Masters athletes may approach this by increasing energy expenditure via additional training but care must be taken to ensure that this does not result in overtraining or injury [35]. A modest reduction in daily energy intake while maintaining or slightly increasing energy expenditure is usually the most effective way to achieve an energy deficit. The relative balance between intake and expenditure is best determined at an individual level; however, mild to modest energy deficits of 10%–20% from that required for weight maintenance are generally recommended [8]. Manipulation or periodising energy intake over different phases of the training cycle is often required to achieve this.

The macronutrient (carbohydrate, fat, protein) distribution of the dietary energy consumed to optimise weight/fat loss and compliance to the energy deficit remains controversial in the obesity literature despite extensive investigation of this aspect of weight management [35]. In athletic individuals of any age, the macronutrient distribution also needs to support and optimise training adaptations and recovery in addition to assisting with loss of weight, specifically fat rather than lean mass. Masters athletes engaged in prolonged endurance events (e.g. triathlon, marathon running) will have a greater requirement for carbohydrate than those athletes involved in strength-based events (e.g. shot put, weightlifting) [36]. Despite this, there is increasing recent support in the obesity literature for macronutrient distributions which favour higher protein (~25% of energy) and moderate (~50%–55%) carbohydrate intake with total fat less than 30% of energy for both weight loss and weight loss maintenance [37]. Unfortunately, prescription of protein and carbohydrate intake based on energy distribution rather than intake as g/kg/d is known to be less useful for athletes, particularly those at the higher and lower extremes of energy requirement [38]. Effective macronutrient prescription in masters athletes seeking weight or fat loss therefore requires an individual approach which balances the requirements of training against the benefits of a higher protein, moderate carbohydrate intake which appears to assist with fat loss, improved satiety and retention of lean mass [35]. For more details on energy requirements for masters athletes, see Chapter 3.

The potential benefit of low glycaemic index (GI) carbohydrates for weight management should also be considered in masters athletes as these are also linked with improved satiety (feelings of fullness) and better maintenance of lost weight [37]. As higher GI carbohydrates are associated with faster recovery of glycogen stores, it may be that the GI is also periodised with greater emphasis on higher GI carbohydrates when rapid recovery of glycogen or maintenance of blood glucose during prolonged training or competition is required (see Chapter 4). Greater incorporation of low GI carbohydrates would also be recommended in masters athletes with glucose intolerance or type 2 diabetes (see below).

There are a number of other dietary aspects which may also assist with weight management in masters athletes but detailed coverage is beyond the scope of this chapter. Briefly, dietary prescription should consider the benefit of a higher dietary fibre intake and also a reduction in the energy density of meals and snacks [39]. Masters athletes and coaches should especially be careful of using sports foods which are low in fibre and energy dense yet often less satiating than regular foods [35]. Higher intake of dairy calcium may also be beneficial for fat loss when energy intake is restricted [40,41]. Masters athletes may be drawn to a wide range of diets or supplements promoted to reduce weight or fat for which there is little evidence of efficacy. These diets may not provide adequate nutrients for health [35] and to optimise training and there is a risk with supplements of a positive drug test (see Chapter 10). Commercial weight loss programs may also be appealing. Although some of these provide sound guidance, the dietary prescriptions are based on sedentary through to moderately active individuals and not athletes [36]. Professional guidance from a sports dietician/nutritionist will assist masters athletes with achieving and monitoring weight and fat loss while maintaining health, lean mass and optimising training/competition outcomes.

In general, the dietary pattern for treatment and prevention of type 2 diabetes is similar to that recommended for good health for most individuals. However, there is some overlap in specific dietary recommendations for the prevention and treatment of type 2 diabetes, weight management and management of CVD, since weight reduction of 5%–10% of weight delays or reduces the risk of type 2 diabetes development, and improves glycaemic control and risk of diabetes complications such as CVD [42,43]. Readers are directed to recommendations on weight management and CVD to supplement their reading on type 2 diabetes. Specific nutrients and strategies that may be of benefit in prevention and management of type 2 diabetes for masters athletes are described below.

Carbohydrate intake may need to be more carefully managed for athletes of any age with type 2 diabetes. It is usually useful to aim for consistency in carbohydrate intake at meals and snacks throughout the day to minimise fluctuations in blood glucose levels. Carbohydrate is often recommended for fuelling intake before, during and after exercise, especially if exercise is prolonged [38,44,45]. The recommendations for carbohydrate intake for athletes without type 2 diabetes prior to exercise should generally be observed with medication adjusted if necessary. For masters athletes on insulin or an insulin secretagogue (a medication that promotes insulin secretion) whose blood glucose is <5.6 mmol/L (100 mg/dL) prior to beginning exercise, extra carbohydrate is recommended [46]. People with type 2 diabetes with blood glucose <5.6 mmol/L (100 mg/dL) prior to exercise who are treated with diet, metformin, glucosidase inhibitors and/or thiazolidinediones without insulin/insulin secretagogues generally do not need supplementary carbohydrate [46].

During exercise, glucose uptake and utilisation by muscle is increased, plasma insulin decreases and hepatic glucose production increases [47]. Muscle glycogen stores are utilised, and circulating glucose and free fatty acids are increasingly utilised as the duration of exercise increases [48]. Blood glucose levels will fall if no food is consumed after 60–90 minutes of moderate–high-intensity exercise [47]. Muscle glycogen stores will be depleted and need replenishing for subsequent exercise.

These processes occur both in the absence of and in the presence of type 2 diabetes [47]. Thus, recommendations with regard to amounts and timing of carbohydrate intake around exercise are generally the same for masters athletes without diabetes for fuel provision and recovery (see Chapter 4 for a detailed discussion on the carbohydrate needs of masters athletes before, during and after exercise).

A low glycaemic load as part of a Mediterranean diet pattern has been found to reduce the incidence of type 2 diabetes [49]. Moreover, systematic reviews demonstrate that low GI carbohydrate foods may assist with weight management [50] and improve glycaemic control [51]. However, there are many factors that influence the GI factor of meals including particle size, type of starch (proportion of amylose to amylopectin), presence of fat and protein, acidity and processing [52]. Thus, the ability to apply the GI concept practically has been questioned [53]. Around exercise, low GI carbohydrate choices prior to an activity may be beneficial where access to fuel sources during an exercise session is limited [38]. While high GI choices appear to promote more rapid glycogen recovery, the effect on subsequent performance is not consistent and needs further investigation [44]. Additionally, carbohydrate foods with a range of nutrients may be important in recovery processes apart from refuelling, such as repair and immune system function [44]. Thus, GI is among several factors to be considered in determining optimal carbohydrate sources for masters athletes.

Carbohydrate from whole grain cereals, fruit, vegetables and dairy are important for all masters athletes and is equally important in the prevention and management of type 2 diabetes. It is recommended that Australian and New Zealand men and women consume 38 and 28 g dietary fibre per day, respectively, as suggested targets for chronic disease prevention [54]. There is good evidence that type 2 diabetes risk is reduced with the consumption of non-starch polysaccharides (NSP) [55], the main component of dietary fibre [56]. Foods rich in NSP include whole grain cereals, fruit and vegetables [55] and may also be important in weight management, induce higher satiation and smooth glycaemic responses following meals [53]. The NSP β-glucan, found in oats and barley, may slow glucose absorption [57] and reduce insulin response [58], thus assisting in the management of blood glucose control as well as increase satiety and reduce energy intake in meals subsequent to intake [58]. Dairy foods are another source of healthy carbohydrate for masters athletes with evidence suggesting an association with dairy (milk, yoghurt and cheese) with reduced risk of developing type 2 diabetes [53] (see Section 12.2.2 and Section 12.5 for more on suggested dairy intake).

Replacing saturated fats (saturated fatty acids [SFAs]) and trans fats with monounsaturated fats (monounsaturated fatty acids [MUFAs]) or polyunsaturated fats (polyunsaturated fatty acids [PUFAs]) may reduce the risk of developing diabetes and improve insulin sensitivity as well as reduce the risk of coronary heart disease (CHD) [59,60]. Since people with diabetes are at higher risk of CVD, specific dietary recommendations for prevention and treatment of CVD, including modification of fat type, are included in the next section. These should be observed for masters athletes at risk of or having had a diagnosis of type 2 diabetes.

Lastly, there is increasing evidence that the consumption of coffee is associated with a reduced risk of type 2 diabetes [61,62]. The recent systematic review to underpin the Australian Dietary Guidelines found a probable association with the consumption of four cups of coffee per day with reduced risk of type 2 diabetes [63]. Whilst the mechanisms are unclear, it is possible there is a thermoregulatory effect of caffeine that favourably influences glucose metabolism [64], that the magnesium in coffee may beneficially affect glucose control [65] and insulin sensitivity [66,67] or that specific phenolic compounds (e.g. chlorogenic acid) may produce beneficial metabolic effects [68]. It is evident that different types of coffee consumption (e.g. instant, brewed, filtered, decaffeinated) are practiced across populations [63] and serve size in studies may vary widely [61]. The reduced risk of type 2 diabetes observed in the systematic review by van Dam and colleagues was most likely to be associated with drip-filtered coffee [61]. Although findings are positive in relation to glucose metabolism and type 2 diabetes risk, caution is needed in recommendations on coffee intake since it may have also have some negative health effects [69]. For example, diterpenes in unfiltered coffee may contribute to raised cholesterol and therefore increase the risk of CVD [70].

In conclusion, lifestyle intervention (diet and physical activity) can potentially reduce the risk of the development of type 2 diabetes by up to 58% [71,72]. Nutritious carbohydrate foods that are low GI and high in fibre, as well as unsaturated fats and low fat dairy are usually a good choice for masters athletes in regular training and are consistent with prevention and management of type 2 diabetes.

12.2.2 Cardiovascular Disease

12.2.2.1 Definition, Presentation and Prevalence

CVD encompasses four main categories, all of which often co-exist due to similar pathogenesis in the affected blood vessels. These include coronary artery disease (CAD) (including angina, myocardial infarction, cardiac failure, arrhythmias or sudden cardiac death), cerebrovascular disease (stroke or transient ischaemic attacks), peripheral vascular disease and aortic atherosclerosis (abdominal and thoracic aneurysms) [9]. The risk of developing CVD increases with age [8], with a strong family history and male gender comprising other non-modifiable risk factors. The main risk factors for the development of CVD are potentially modifiable, and these include hypertension, hyperlipidaemia, smoking, inactivity, obesity, diabetes mellitus and depression [71].

CVDs are by far the leading cause of death globally [72]. The prevalence of CVD increases with age; in Australia, 13% of 35–44-year-olds and 23% of 45–54-year-olds report long-term conditions; however, this increases to 63% for those 75 years and older [73]. Although more women than men (20% compared to 16%) report having CVD, the proportion of males and females reporting heart, stroke and vascular diseases is similar [73]. Masters athletes with a mean age of ~46 years who continue to exercise may have a lower risk for CVD (including total cholesterol, low-density lipoprotein [LDL] cholesterol, HDL cholesterol, triglycerides and blood pressure) compared to those who do not continue to exercise, sedentary control subjects [74] and non-athletes of the same age [74–76].

12.2.2.2 Medical Risks with Physical Activity

Regular physical activity is well known to be beneficial in reducing the risk of CVD [25,30,71]. Regular exercise may reduce the risk of myocardial infarction and other coronary events through improvements in blood pressure, lipid profile, adiposity and insulin sensitivity [25,71].

CVD is much more prevalent amongst masters athletes when compared to their younger counterparts [77], and as such, the incidence of atherosclerotic-related complications during or post-physical activity is increased [25,78]. Overall, however, masters athletes are generally a lower CVD risk group than their matched sedentary contemporaries [31]. Despite the obvious benefits of moderate-intensity physical exercise on the cardiovascular profile of older people, competitive and more vigorous exercise may increase the risk of adverse cardiac events, in both asymptomatic athletes and those with known cardiovascular disease [24,25]. The mechanisms responsible may be related to spasm of the coronary arteries, increased heart rate and blood pressure causing increased arterial shear, or increased platelet aggregation secondary to raised circulating catecholamines [24]. The physiological alterations that occur during exercise and immediately post-exercise can increase the risk of both myocardial ischaemia and arrhythmias [24].

Atherosclerotic CVD is responsible for the majority of cardiac morbidity and death associated with physical exercise [24]. Other cardiac conditions, however, may increase the risk of syncope or sudden cardiac death including cardiomyopathy and hypertrophic or dilated and arrhythmias/conduction abnormalities including atrial fibrillation, sick sinus syndrome, ventricular tachycardia or fibrillation [30].

Ageing results in a decline in aerobic cardiovascular function, with reduced maximal heart rate, stroke volume, blood pressure and overall cardiac output [8]. If the oxygen demand of the heart is exceeded during exercise, ischaemia will result, increasing the risk of adverse cardiovascular outcomes [25]. Sports are generally classified according to their myocardial oxygen requirement, and this can be applied to masters athletes in an attempt to categorise the potential risk associated with their sport [25]. Higher-intensity exercise is usually limited to those at low risk for CVD, and is not advisable for those with documented CVD [30]. It is also thought that the emotional impact of high-intensity competitive sports for masters athletes may result in the masking of angina, increasing the risk of myocardial infarction [30]. Currently, the American Heart Association recommends general restrictions on high-intensity competitive sports in those with any of the conditions below [30]:

- Impaired left ventricular systolic function under resting conditions (ejection fraction <50%)
- Evidence of exercise-induced myocardial ischaemia, including angina, positive ECG or positive imaging findings with exercise testing
- Evidence of exercise-induced frequent or complex supraventricular or ventricular arrhythmias, including non-sustained ventricular tachycardia or exercise-induced systolic hypotension

12.2.2.3 Screening Recommendations

The aim of screening is to reduce the risk of coronary events by identifying athletes with asymptomatic CVD and to determine the appropriate level of exercise intensity an athlete with known CVD can resume [23,25,28,30].

All screening should involve history, examination and appropriate investigations. During the screening process modifiable risk factors such as hypertension, hyperlipidaemia, obesity and diabetes mellitus should be identified and addressed. Prior to the commencement of vigorous exercise, attempts should be made to normalise blood pressure, lipids and body weight through lifestyle modifications and/or pharmacological management. Participation in masters sport should particularly be restricted until blood pressure is controlled for those doing highly static sports such as weight lifting [30]. Smokers should be advised to cease smoking.

Screening investigations largely involve ECG and exercise stress ECG, with or without an echocardiogram, depending on individual medical and personal history. A screening ECG has previously been recommended for all masters athletes [24,25,30], although its diagnostic value for detecting ischaemic heart disease is limited in asymptomatic athletes. It may provide unexpected results, such as an old infarction, arrhythmia or inherited cardiac conditions, so may be performed as part of a physicians assessment [30], particularly for older patients with coronary risk factors who are engaged in leisure sport activity [79]. The diagnosis of hypertrophic cardiomyopathy, long QT or Wolff-Parkinson-White syndrome is likely to be more common in younger athletes, but may also be present [30].

A symptom-limited exercise stress test is recommended for all moderate- to high-risk athletes, which includes men >45 years and women >55 years with one or more cardiovascular risk factor (hypertension, hyperlipidaemia, diabetes mellitus or strong family history). They should continue with prescribed medication whilst competing and/or training. Such an exercise ECG has good sensitivity and specificity in these athletes (with high pre-test probability) but has poor predictive accuracy in low-risk athletes. In asymptomatic athletes, the sensitivity and specificity of exercise testing is lower for women than men, so testing is controversial.

12.2.2.4 Medications and Nutrient Interactions

Medications commonly used in the management of cardiovascular disease and its risk factors include beta blockers, digoxin, HMG-CoA reductase inhibitors, angiotensin-converting enzyme (ACE) inhibitors and warfarin. Prior to competition each athlete should confirm that their medication is not prohibited during competition. This can be done through the World Anti-Doping Agency or via the Australian Sports Drug Medical Advisory Committee. While the issues related to medication use in masters athletes are discussed in detail in the next chapter, Table 12.3 below lists medications commonly used and potential side effects that may impact on performance in masters athletes managing cardiovascular disease.

TABLE 12.3
Common Medications Used for Cardiovascular Disease and Side Effects

Medication	Clinical Use	Side Effects and Potential Effects on Masters Athletes
Beta blockers (e.g. Metoprolol, Atenolol)	Hypertension, cardiac failure or post myocardial infarction	May cause hypotension and reduce maximum heart rate achievable; prohibited in sports such as darts or billiards [80]
Digoxin	Cardiac failure and arrhythmias	Reduced effect during high-intensity exercise, increasing the risk of arrhythmia
HMG CoA reductase inhibitors	Hyperlipidaemia, post-myocardial infarction and post-CVA	Increased risk of myositis, and symptoms may be masked in high-intensity exercise
Nitrates	Angina in ischaemic heart disease	May lead to excessive vasodilation when in hot climates, resulting in syncope
Warfarin	CVA prevention in atrial fibrillation and post-mechanical valve replacement	Increased risk of uncontrolled bleeding and bruising, particularly in contact sports; influenced by dietary intake of vitamin K rich foods, so athletes need to maintain a balanced diet

12.2.2.5 Nutrition Recommendations in Prevention and Treatment

Obesity and increased waist circumference are major risk factors for CHD and are associated with other CVD risk factors including dyslipidaemia, hypertension, insulin resistance and type 2 diabetes [81]. Modest body weight reduction of 5%–10% can improve the cardiovascular risk profile in overweight or obese individuals [42,43]. Overweight masters athletes with increased central (abdominal) adiposity and CVD should refer to the previous section on strategies to reduce body fat.

Alternatively, it has been postulated that functional hypothalamic amenorrhea, characterised by hypoeostrogenaemia and associated with low-energy availability/energy deficiency, may impact on cardiovascular health and particularly endothelial function [82,83]. Energy availability is the amount of energy intake remaining after exercise energy expenditure is subtracted with energy balance estimated to be around 188 kJ/kg of fat-free mass per day in healthy young adults, while energy availability below 125 kJ/kg fat-free mass per day suppresses reproductive function [84,85]. There is some evidence to suggest that women who have experienced previous oestrogen deficiency or menstrual cycle irregularity may be at increased risk for CVD [86,87]. Endothelial dysfunction itself has been associated with menstrual dysfunction in 18–36-year-old athletes [88,89] and is considered an early marker for the development of atherosclerosis [90]. It seems prudent for masters athletes who have experienced pre-menopausal amenorrhea or who have previously engaged in sports where dietary restriction or low body weight was encouraged to be screened for CVD. Premenopausal masters athletes should maintain optimal energy availability for reproductive function.

Dietary quality also has a crucial role in CVD prevention and treatment across a wide range of foods and nutrients. Fat intake and effect of different fat types are possibly the most discussed of these dietary factors in relation to CVD. SFA in particular is often targeted to reduce cholesterol levels and thereby influence CVD risk. In fact, individual types of SFAs have both negative and positive effects on plasma lipid level [91,92], but may negatively influence other factors that affect CVD risk such as vascular function and blood pressure [91]. The recent Food and Agriculture Organization of the United Nations (FAO) report on fats, fatty acids and human nutrition concluded that overall there is convincing evidence that reducing SFA intake and replacing it with PUFA or MUFA reduces the risk of CHD [60]. There is also convincing evidence that trans fats from partially hydrogenated vegetable oils increase CHD risk factors and events [60]. While food sources of fat are usually a mixture of fat types, SFA is predominantly found in animal foods (e.g. fatty meats, chicken skin) and processed baked goods, trans fats may be found naturally in some animal foods and in hydrogenated fats, while unsaturated fats are generally found in plant foods and fish. From the latter, long-chain PUFAs from the omega-3 and omega-6 families of PUFAs are of particular interest.

Dietary sources of PUFAs from foods such as oily fish (e.g. salmon, tuna, sardines and mackerel), nuts and seeds (e.g. walnuts, pecans, hazelnuts, pine nuts, sunflower seeds and linseed/flaxseed), margarines, and vegetable oils have cardio-protective effects, potentially mediated through physiological processes via cell membranes and gene expression, although the exact mechanisms are still to be elucidated [93]. Anti-inflammatory and anti-coagulant activity may also provide cardiovascular benefit [53]. Evidence suggests that consumption of oily fish appears to be particularly beneficial in protection against CVD because of its very-long-chain polyunsaturated omega-3 fatty acids, especially eicosapentaenoic acid (EPA) and docosahexaenoic acid (DHA). Those with a higher fish intake have a lower risk of death from CHD [94–96] and stroke [97,98]. Data from large systematic reviews demonstrate that consumption of 250 mg/day of EPA + DHA (one to two servings of oily fish/week) may reduce the risk of CHD death by up to 36% [99,100].

In normal ageing, vascular walls thicken and may lose their elasticity, resulting in hypertension and reduction in maximal workload under stress [101]. However, studies indicate that fish oil may favourably influence cardiovascular function in conjunction with exercise. In overweight individuals with mild high blood pressure, high cholesterol or high triglycerides, DHA-rich fish oil supplementation (~1.9 g EPA + DHA) significantly reduced triglycerides and improved HDL cholesterol, arterial vasodilation, heart rate and heart rate variability, while exercise improved arterial compliance [102,103]. Elite young Australian Rules Football players consuming the same DHA-rich fish oil supplements during pre-season also significantly lowered triglycerides and heart rate during sub-maximal exercise, whilst attenuating a rise in diastolic blood pressure compared to sunflower oil supplementation [104]. In well-trained young male cyclists, fish oil supplementation (3.2 g EPA + DHA) may lower heart rate during incremental workloads to exhaustion, as well as steady state exercise, whilst decreasing whole body oxygen consumption [105]. In these latter studies, improvements in performance were either not detected or not measured. However, there was improvement in CV function and/or risk factors without performance decrement which may be a useful outcome for masters athletes.

Plant-based diets also have a protective effect on CVD, especially amongst older adults [106]. WHO stated that 31% of deaths from ischemic heart disease and 11% of deaths from stroke worldwide were caused by diets poor in fruit and vegetables [107]. Scientific evidence that vegetables (including legumes and beans) are protective against cardiovascular disease has strengthened, with probable evidence that each additional daily serving of vegetables reduces the risk of CHD and stroke, with higher intakes indicating even stronger protection [53]. Fruit is also protective, with 7% increase in protective effect with each additional serving per day [53].

Components of plant foods that provide benefit are numerous. The constituents of fruits and vegetables that are postulated to provide benefit include vitamins C and E and phytochemicals which may reduce inflammation and oxidation of cholesterol [108–110], potassium and magnesium which may lower blood pressure [54] and soluble fibre [111] and isoflavones [112] which may lower cholesterol. Nitrate, of which vegetables (e.g. green leafy vegetables and beetroot) are a major source [113], has been shown to have vascular benefits including blood pressure reduction [114–116], improvement in endothelial function [114], inhibition or attenuation of platelet aggregation [114], as well as improve exercise performance in subjects up to 38 years old where age was specified [115,117–121], Additionally, there is good evidence that consumption of 1–3 servings of whole grain cereals, especially oats and barley, is associated with reduced risk of CVD [53] with clinical trials showing reduction in total and LDL levels [63].

Nuts provide a useful source of PUFAs as well as other nutrients thought to be protective in cardiovascular disease [122]. An association between the consumption of 65–110 g nuts per day and lowered cholesterol has been suggested [53], possibly due to phytosterols which reduce cholesterol [122], the displacement of saturated fat with unsaturated fat in the diet [53] or potential anti-inflammatory/anti-atherogenic properties [123]. Polyphenols in tea such as catechins may assist in the reduction of hypertension and atherosclerosis, and beneficially influence endothelial function [124] and consumption of green and black tea may be protective against stroke [53]. Tea may therefore be both protective against CVD as well as being a useful source of daily hydration [125].

The recent release of the Australian Dietary Guidelines saw an increase in the number of servings of dairy recommended for men over 70 to 3-1/2 and women over the age of 50 to four per day [53], or the equivalent of 1 l of low-fat milk per day. This is an important change given the evidence to support the benefits of low-fat dairy in CVD reduction, the provision of carbohydrate and high-biological-value protein for athletes for fuelling and muscle growth and repair, and the reduction in recommended amounts from the "classic" carbohydrates group (breads and cereals groups). Consumption of dairy foods is associated with reduced risk of ischemic heart disease, myocardial infarction, stroke and hypertension [53]. Unfortunately, calcium absorption across the small intestine may be reduced with ageing [126]. However, there are some strategies that athletes can utilise to maximise calcium absorption (see Section 12.5).

The prevalence of hypertension increases with increasing age [127], and more so in postmenopausal women than in similar-aged men [128]. Similarly, de Matos and colleagues recently reported a prevalence of 7% and 13% amongst Finnish male and female athletes, respectively, with the majority of these being over 35 years old [77]. However, reduction of blood pressure in middle age significantly reduces lifetime risk for CVD [129]. In a cohort of 61,858 males and females followed for an average of 14 years from age 55 years, Allen and colleagues found that those who were able to maintain normal or decrease to normal blood pressure during middle age reduced their lifetime risk of CVD to 35%–40% (men) and 22%–25% (women) from an estimated lifetime risk of 52.5% and 39.9%, respectively [129].

There is convincing evidence that reduction of sodium intake of 1.8 g/day reduces blood pressure in both normotensive and hypertensive adults [53], and some evidence that reduction of sodium intake of 1 g/day reduces the risk of cardiovascular events [53]. Additionally, sensitivity of blood pressure to dietary sodium may increase with age [130], meaning that increases in dietary sodium in an older population may be more likely to increase blood pressure. However, exercise lowers the risk of hypertension [32]. Moreover, previous research has shown that 6 months of aerobic activity in older subjects can reduce sensitivity to dietary sodium [131].

Although athletes are often advised to acutely increase sodium intake to assist with hydration levels for exercise, it may be prudent to observe the general recommendation of less than 2300 mg sodium/day or 1600 mg sodium/day for disease prevention [54] and in higher-risk older adults. Masters athletes travelling to exercise at altitude may need to take particular care, since high altitude is known to increase blood pressure and potentially exacerbate pre-existing hypertension [132]. Alternatively, while a recent study suggests that thermoregulation in older endurance-trained males is no different than in younger counterparts [133], normal physiological responses to ageing may result in a greater susceptibility to hypohydration and heat stress in older athletes compared to younger athletes [134]. While the risks of hypertension and hyponatraemia should generally be considered because older individuals have a slower water and sodium excretion [135], standard commercial sports drinks may be the superior choice for masters athletes undertaking prolonged training or competition in high heat or humidity areas where there is risk of heat stress. Voluntary fluid intake is superior and restores plasma volume faster with carbohydrate-electrolyte beverage compared to water for older adults exercising in the heat [136]. The fluid, electrolyte and hydration needs of masters athletes is discussed in detail in Chapter 9.

While specific nutrients are often highlighted in disease prevention, certain dietary patterns are known to be protective against CVD and provide a framework athletes can modify for athletic performance. Dietary patterns low in foods like fruits, vegetables and cereals (among others) have been associated with a higher risk for CHD and mortality in middle-aged men [137] and with middle-aged women consuming a diet rich in vegetables, fruit, legumes, fish, poultry and whole grains having been reported to experience a 28% lower risk of CVD [138]. Among known preventive patterns are the Mediterranean diet [139,140], Dietary Approaches to Stop Hypertension (DASH) diet

[141–144] and plant-based diets [140,145]. These diets are characterised by olive oil, bread, high fruit and vegetable intake, fish and moderate amounts of dairy foods and wine (Mediterranean) [139]; low-sodium, high fruit and vegetable intake, low- or non-fat dairy and whole grains (DASH) [144] and high intake of plant-based foods (not necessarily devoid of meat).

12.2.3 Musculoskeletal Conditions

12.2.3.1 Definition, Presentation and Prevalence

Musculoskeletal conditions encompass any disorder involving bones, joints and periarticular structures such as muscles, cartilage, tendons and ligaments [9]. Masters athletes are susceptible to similar musculoskeletal injuries as are their younger counterparts [146], but there are a number of conditions, in particular OA, osteoporosis and tendon ruptures, that are of increased importance [32].

OA is characterised by loss of articular hyaline cartilage, with new bone proliferation and remodelling of the joint surface [9,146]. This is likely to be the most common cause of pain and functional limitation [8], particularly in the knees, hips and shoulders. The risk of arthritis increases with age [8,32,147]. There is insufficient evidence to suggest participation in exercise *per se* causes OA [148–150]. However, development of OA in masters athletes may relate to exercise intensity [151], type of sport [32,152] and previous injury or trauma to the affected joint. Moderate exercise appears to result in a reduction in pain and improved physical functioning in knee OA [153].

Osteoporosis is a condition of reduced bone mineral density (BMD), causing micro-architectural deterioration of bone tissue, increasing the risk of fracture, particularly in the spine, hip and wrist [9,154]. The World Health Organization reports that OA affects 9.6% of men and 18% of women over 60 years old [155], whilst osteoporosis affects around 5% and 2.4% of women and men around 50 years old, and 50% and 20% of women and men aged 85 [156]. Prevalence across groups of masters athletes may vary. Knee OA is reported to occur in around 3% of shooters, through 14%–20% of runners and 31% of weight lifters in current and former older-age athletes [152]. Osteoathritic changes in the dominant shoulder of tennis players has also been reported in 33% of compared to 11% for control subjects [157].

Similarly, more active older individuals often have higher whole-body or site-specific BMD [158–161] and former elite athletes may have higher BMD [161,162] and lower risk of osteoporotic fracture [163,164] than control subjects. However, changes in BMD with age may vary according to sport (impact or weight-bearing) and previous menstrual dysfunction [165,166]. Older runners may have higher lumbar spine BMD than cyclists [167] and swimmers [159], while swimmers may have higher arm BMD than runners [161]. Exclusive participation in non-weight-bearing sports like cycling may lead to greater BMD decline [168–169]. Nichols et al. recently reported that a significantly greater percentage of male masters cyclists compared to non-athletes (mean age ~51) met criteria for osteopaenia or osteoporosis at baseline (84.2% vs. 50.0%) and at 7-year follow-up (89.5% compared to 61.1%) and concluded that a higher risk of fracture with cycling falls warranted attention [170]. However, road cycling may confer greater risk than other types of cycling such as mountain biking or if cycling is combined with other sporting activity [171]. Csermesly and colleagues recently found that incidence (42.1% compared to 30.4%) and severity (average BMD of the lumbar spine 71.6 ± 3.9, compared to 84.8 ± 7.8) of osteoporosis was significantly higher in perimenopausal women who had experienced secondary amenorrhoea (cycle length > 3 months) during adolescence compared to those with eumennorrhoea [166]. Of 180 recently surveyed Australian exercising women (18–40 years), 45% did not think that amenorrhea affected bone health, and a significantly greater proportion (22%) of women in lean-build sports (running/athletics, triathlon, swimming, cycling, dancing, rowing) compared to those in non-lean-build sports (3.2%) reported that they would take no action if they experienced amenorrhea [168]. Masters athletes who have been engaged in sports in their younger years where dietary restriction, low body weight or with an aesthetic nature (e.g. jockeys, dancers and gymnasts) may be at greater risk of low BMD through previous insufficiency of nutrients or low energy availability [169].

12.2.3.2 Medical Risks with Physical Activity

Physical activity has many health benefits, and these largely outweigh the risks [8,30,172]. The effects on the musculoskeletal system can, however, be conflicting. Whilst it is thought that weight-bearing exercise improves bone density [8], peak bone mass is reached during late adolescence and early adulthood [154], so the effect of weight-bearing exercise on bone density in adulthood is less defined [8]. Osteopaenia or osteoporosis in athletes participating in non-weight-bearing sports such as cycling, makes them at a high risk of fracture when involved in collisions as seen in competitive cycling [173].

The risk of masters athletes developing OA or tendon/ligament damage depends on multiple factors including age, prior joint injuries or deformities, the type of sport (weight-bearing, high torsional load vs. low impact such as swimming or cycling) and the intensity of the exercise [147]. Tendon and ligament tensile strength declines with age [32], resulting in an increased risk of Achilles tendon ruptures, rotator cuff tears and tendinopathy such as at the lateral elbow (tennis elbow) [32].

12.2.3.3 Screening Recommendations

The most important screening method in masters athletes is a thorough medical and exercise history, screening for symptoms and signs of OA, prior injuries and for the risk factors for osteoporosis. Mass screening of the general population for osteoporosis [154] or OA is not recommended. Osteoporotic risk factors such as a prior fracture, malabsorption history, family history, smoking or long-term corticosteroid use should prompt further investigation. Vitamin D levels should also be checked, as this is important for improved bone mineralisation [174]. Screening imaging in OA is not usually necessary, as x-ray findings often do not correlate with physical findings [172].

12.2.3.4 Medications and Nutrient Interactions

Symptoms control is the mainstay of treatment for OA, and there should be confirmation that analgesics prescribed are not prohibited in sport. Long-term bisphosphonate use (for the treatment of osteoporosis) may be associated with a small increased risk of atypical (mid-shaft) femoral fractures [175], which may be increased in contact/high intensity masters sports such as rugby union and soccer.

12.2.3.5 Nutrition Recommendations in Prevention and Treatment

Nutritional recommendations for musculoskeletal conditions will focus on OA and osteoporosis. Obesity is the main preventable risk factor for large joint OA [176], and dietary approaches for the management of OA principally focus on reduction of load on weight-bearing joints. Messier and colleagues have demonstrated a four-fold reduction in knee joint forces (per step taken) per kilogram reduction in body weight after diet and exercise intervention in overweight sedentary individuals [177]. While participants in this study lost a mean of 2.6% body weight, a recent meta-analysis shows that >5.1% body weight loss at a rate of 0.24% reduction per week may be required to achieve significant improvement in disability due to knee OA in obese patients [178]. Recent studies suggest that it is fat mass (vs. body weight *per se*) that is associated with higher risk of knee OA, whilst muscle mass may be protective potentially due to an associated increase in cartilage volume or muscular absorption of force around the joint [179,180]. Thus, an overweight masters athlete with OA of the knee, and potentially the hip, should aim to reduce body fat while maintaining lean muscle mass (see Section 12.2.1). Masters athletes aiming to reduce risk of developing OA should maintain muscle mass and normal body weight.

Nutritional supplements may often be recommended to athletes of any age to alleviate the effects of OA. So-called antioxidants (e.g. vitamins A, C, E and selenium) do not generally show benefit in treatment of OA [181–185]. Evidence for the efficacy of fish oils and omega-3 supplementation in OA is also currently lacking [185] although they may be beneficial for joint inflammation as seen in rheumatoid arthritis [186]. Recommendations of supplemental glucosamine, a natural component of articular cartilage [187], may be made to masters athletes with OA to relieve pain. Studies suggest a potential role of glucosamine for normalisation of cartilage metabolism or anti-inflammatory function [188,189]. However, a recent Cochrane review of studies including nearly 5000 subjects concluded that although glucosamine was as safe as placebo, a beneficial effect on pain and function was not consistent across brands of glucosamine [187]. Chondroitin sulphate is another supplement that may be recommended, and while it has not shown consistent effect alone, in combination with glucosamine it may provide pain relief for those with moderate–severe OA pain [190,191]. Masters athletes are advised to seek advice from a sports physician and relevant anti-doping authorities before considering supplements for management of OA.

Reduction in bone mass (BM) and BMD may begin as early as 35–40 years in normal ageing [192], increasing the risk of bone fracture. The skeleton is made up of cortical (dense) bone (80%) and trabecular (spongy) bone (20%) with a reduction in the former influenced by calcium deprivation and the latter by falling sex steroids [192,193]. The reduction of oestrogen at menopause for women can be particularly devastating. At menopause, urinary calcium losses increase and calcium absorption may decrease, resulting in a 0.5%–1.0% reduction in BMD per year post-menopause [194]. Women can potentially lose one third of their cortical and half of their trabecular bone from youth to old age, while men may lose 50%–70% that of females [192,193]. Low BM in the elderly may be due to excessive losses, inadequate peak BM (PBM; achieved around 18–20 years old in females and 18–23 years in males) [195] or a combination of these [192].

Dietary intake of calcium is critical for bone health and is inadequate across many age groups, including adolescent girls [196] (when calcium accretion increases [194]), and in middle- and older-aged men and women [197] when risk of bone injury increases. There are few data on the dietary intake of masters athletes. Beshgetoor et al. compared female masters runners and cyclists (mean age 50.4 years) taking supplements compared with those who did not [198]. They found that calcium intakes were 791 ± 174 mg without supplementation, which is well below recommended daily intakes for 31–50-year-old females (1000 mg/day) and over 50 year olds (1200–1300 mg) [54,199]. Hawkins et al. found a similar level of calcium intake with mean intake increasing over time to an adequate level in some middle–older-age female runners after calcium supplementation (age at baseline of the 4.8-year study period ranged from 46.3 ± 0.8 years for pre-menopausal women to 60.0 ± 10.4 years for post-menopausal women not on oestrogen therapy) [200]. Whilst the latter study found a maintenance of BMD in runners over 5 years regardless of hormone replacement therapy or menstrual status [200], studies overall seem to show inconsistent effect of calcium intake over peri-menopausal and early post-menopausal years since the primary reason for reduced BM at this time is diminishing hormone levels [201]. Calcium intake above recommended doses do not appear to achieve extra benefit [202] and requirements do not appear to be elevated due to physical activity [203]. There is some suggestion that calcium supplementation may increase risk of cardiovascular disease in older women [204], but this finding is not consistent [204,205].

Vitamin D is also critical to bone health as it is essential for both calcium absorption and bone remodelling [202]. Reduction in Vitamin D synthesis in the skin with ageing and poor sunlight exposure can both contribute to poor bone health [192]. With recent attention on potential links of poor vitamin D status with a range of chronic diseases, statistics are emerging indicating vitamin D deficiencies across most age groups [206]. Indeed, vitamin D recommendations in the United States have recently been revised upwards, with other countries potentially to follow suit. The US recommended daily allowance for 31–50-year-olds (600 international units [IU], 15 μg) is now triple Australia and New Zealand's Adequate Intake of 200 IU (5 μg) and is 200 IU (5 μg) higher for each of the older age groups above 50 with 800 IU (20 μg) being the requirement for those above 70 in the United States [54,199,205]. The dietary intake of middle-aged Australian men and women is likely to be inadequate even against the lower recommendations, with mid-tertile intake at around 3.5 ± 1.0 μg/day [197]. There are few studies reporting on the vitamin D status of athletes [206] and masters athletes, or on intake in this group. However, Beshgetoor et al. reported vitamin D intake in female masters athletes met dietary requirements for vitamin D [198], which would not be adequate against newer recommendations, even in their supplemented group.

Thus, to maximise bone health, it appears prudent to for masters athletes to consume adequate energy and aim for recommended calcium levels via intake of calcium-rich foods like dairy (e.g. milk, cheese, yoghurt), calcium-fortified soy products and salmon with bones. If supplementation is taken, calcium from combined diet and supplement should not exceed nutrient reference values [204], and may be best taken in a divided dose (e.g. one-third morning, two-thirds evening) to optimise the effect by suppressing the nocturnal increase in bone resorption [207]. Masters athletes are encouraged to consume vitamin D from dietary sources such as fatty fish (e.g. North Sea salmon, herring, mackerel), fortified milk and spreads, liver, eggs and ultraviolet (UV)-exposed mushrooms. However, it is unlikely that adequate serum levels of vitamin D will be obtained in the diet. Prudent exposure to sunlight and adequate energy intake is also recommended for the older athlete.

12.2.4 Neurological Function

12.2.4.1 Definition, Presentation and Prevalence

Neurological conditions encompass any disorder of the brain, spinal cord and peripheral nerves. The aetiology of each disorder varies greatly, as does the presentation. Presentation may include numbness in the distribution of one nerve, movement disorders, seizures, hemiparesis (weakness on one side of the body) and stroke. Other issues with neurological conditions include cognitive impairment and depression.

Unfortunately there are little data on the prevalence of various neurological conditions in masters athletes. As some conditions are limiting or even prohibitive for physical activity, it is likely that the prevalence is lower in masters athletes than in the general population. However, there are some conditions including spinal cord injury, spina bifida and intellectual disability where there is a long history of sports participation through disabled sport programs and the Paralympic Games.

In those with neurological conditions where regular physical activity is possible, there is evidence that this is generally health-protective although there are some specific risks. There is also accumulating evidence that regular physical activity is beneficial for cognition and that physical activity through the lifespan may improve cognitive function and also delay the onset, progression or severity of diseases such as dementia and Alzheimer's [208]. As this chapter has outlined, exercise improves metabolic and cardiovascular health but in addition it is known to induce positive changes in regional brain volume and brain-derived neurotrophic factor (BDNF) [208]. Animal studies also suggest aerobic exercise can result in brain neuro- and angiogenesis. While the existing evidence suggests these changes are beneficial to brain function, more research is required, particularly teasing out the types and dose of exercise that are most beneficial. Evidence of the benefits of exercise (both aerobic and resistance training) for the prevention and clinical management of depression and anxiety is well established but probably underutilised in clinical practice [209,210].

12.2.4.2 Medical Risks with Physical Activity

The overall benefits of exercise in athletes with neurological conditions are likely to outweigh the risks. There are few studies reviewing the risks associated with high-level competition, but in general, exercise within the limitations of the disability would be recommended.

Certain conditions such as multiple sclerosis, Parkinson's disease and stroke, may impair an athlete's functional ability and balance, increasing the risk of falls and injury. People with epilepsy are at increased risk of drowning [211], and of most injury types, when compared to the general population [212], so athletes should be aware of the risks associated with some competitive sports. Sensory impairment, particularly involving the lower limbs, may be associated with a higher risk of foot ulceration. Sports requiring good balance, such as cycling, may be associated with an increased risk of injury from falls.

12.2.4.3 Screening Recommendations

Diagnosis would be dependent on symptoms and screening would not be recommended. Prior to commencing exercise, the functional ability of the masters athlete should be assessed by medical and/or allied health professionals with experience with athletes and appropriate aids prescribed as recommended.

12.2.4.4 Medications and Nutrient Interactions

The spectrum of neurological disease is very broad, as is its treatment. For Parkinson's disease, levodopa can result in marked motor fluctuations after about 5 years of treatment. These include 'freezing' or dyskinesias [33], which could increase the risk of injury and falling. Antiepileptic medication can have side effects including ataxia [33], affecting balance and ability to participate in sport. Chapter 13 discusses in depth the medications and nutrient interactions in masters athletes.

12.2.4.5 Nutrition Recommendations in Prevention and Treatment

Dietary therapy for masters athletes with neurological disorders depends on the specific condition and is strongly linked to symptom management. Both total body weight and lean mass loss are relatively common to a number of neurological conditions and may result from increased energy expenditure (associated with tremors in Parkinson's disease) through to difficulty in shopping, cooking or self feeding, chewing and swallowing. Typically by this stage most individuals would no longer be participating in competitive sport. Ongoing assessment of the individual masters athlete is paramount and involves the input of a speech therapist to assess chewing and swallowing capacity and an occupational therapist to assess competency with shopping, cooking and feeding. Dietetic input with menus of suitable food textures, supplemental foods or beverages and monitoring of intake and body weight is essential.

12.2.5 Cancer

12.2.5.1 Definition, Presentation and Prevalence

Cancer is the abnormal growth of cells, proliferating in an uncontrolled manner. There are many different types, affecting solid organs, skin or blood/bone marrow, and the presentation varies according to the organs involved [9]. Although cancer prevalence data in masters athletes is lacking, the scientific evidence supporting physical activity as a means of cancer prevention is strong or convincing for particular cancers including colon, colorectal and breast; probable for prostate and possible for lung and endometrial cancers [213]. A recent study of 2448 elite male athletes and 1712 referents followed up via the Finnish Cancer Registry for cancer incidence during 1986–2010 found that former athletes had less incidence of cancer, although smoking was also less frequent amongst this cohort [214]. Unfortunately, the best types and dose of exercise for cancer prevention still require further study. However, by virtue of sustained physical activity and lower prevalence of obesity which is linked to a number of cancers, masters athletes are likely at a reduced risk of cancers. In the case of some cancers including colorectal, breast and prostate cancer, a dose-response relationship has been reported with risk decreasing as activity levels increase [213].

12.2.5.2 Medical Risks with Physical Activity

There is growing evidence of the benefit of exercise in both the prevention of cancer and during the recovery phase in cancer patients [213]. Cancer and its treatment modalities such as chemotherapy, radiotherapy or surgery, can cause a broad range of adverse effects in both the short and long term. These may include fatigue, nausea, loss of body weight, shortness of breath, pain, impaired immunity and paraesthesiae (sensation of tingling, burning, pricking or numbness of the skin) [215]. As such, masters athletes wishing to return to competition should do so within the limits of their physical ability. The stage, type of cancer and type of treatment will all affect individual masters athletes differently.

There are certain circumstances in which exercise may increase the risk of adverse effects in cancer patients. Chemotherapy (and haematological malignancies) can often result in reduced levels of white cells, platelets and haemoglobin. During periods of reduced immunity, athletes should avoid public facilities and swimming where the risks of infection are increased [213]. High-impact and contact sports should also be avoided when platelet counts are very low, due to an increased risk of bleeding. These sports should also be avoided in those with known primary bone cancer or metastases, as fracture risk may be increased [213]. A low haemoglobin may reduce the athletes exercise tolerance and ability to compete at a high level. Finally, in patients with peripheral neuropathy or ataxia (lack of muscle coordination) secondary to cancer therapy, competing in sports requiring balance may increase their risk of injury [213].

12.2.5.3 Screening Recommendations

Masters athletes endeavouring to return to training after (or during) treatment for cancer should be aware of the potential adverse effects outlined above. General screening for low blood counts should be performed, but due to the diversity and specificity of treatments available, a generalised screening approach is not available. The medical team should be consulted for any specific individual screening recommendations related to the specific treatment modality [215].

12.2.5.4 Medications and Nutrient Interactions

Cancer treatment is an ever-growing field, and treatments are customised to both the type of cancer and the patient [215]. The treating medical team should be consulted on any possible interactions. Chapter 13 discusses in depth the medications and nutrient interactions in masters athletes.

12.2.5.5 Nutrition Recommendations in Prevention and Treatment

Nutritional therapy is best targeted to the individual and in particular is often focussed on promoting recovery from cancer treatment. The cancer itself and treatment therapies may alter appetite and/or induce nausea. Maintaining bodyweight, lean mass and an adequate and balanced diet is a key nutritional goal when undergoing treatment. Supplemental nutrition often in the form of higher-energy/-protein beverages may be needed to support intake when appetite or intake is poor. Conversely, in some individuals where overweight or obesity is evident then gradual weight loss may be warranted.

A large body of research exists on diet and cancer with the view to inform guidelines on and anti-cancer diet. It is estimated that 30%–40% of all cancers can be prevented by diet and lifestyle [216]. While a comprehensive review of the dietary factors associated with cancer risk is beyond the scope of this chapter, numerous reviews have previously been published [216–218]. A number of dietary factors appear to be protective including cruciferous vegetables (e.g. broccoli, cauliflower, Brussels sprouts), the nutrients selenium, vitamin B12, vitamin D, anti-oxidants (e.g. vitamin C found in many citrus fruits and a wide variety of vegetables, and vitamin E found in some nuts, wheat germ and sunflower oils), and carotenoids (sources include red and orange fruits and vegetables), lycopene (e.g. tomato, watermelon, pink guava), lutein (e.g. spinach, broccoli) and cryptoxanthin (e.g. oranges, watermelon).

Nutritional risk factors for cancer appear to be diets low in fibre, higher in red and processed meat, an imbalance between omega-3 and 6 fatty acid intake and excessive alcohol consumption [216–219].

12.3 CONCLUSION

Masters athletes provide a unique model for examining the health benefits of good nutrition and physical activity during middle to older age [1]. Unfortunately there is limited research conducted on this cohort and the available literature examining chronic disease in masters athletes is predominantly cross sectional with participant numbers small. There is also a significant publication bias to masters athletes participating in endurance events such as running or cycling with limited data on other sports. Masters athletes are almost always compared to age-matched sedentary controls rather than recreationally active individuals so the benefits of competitive athletic training as opposed to recreational exercise are unable to be delineated.

Despite this, in most cases we have presented evidence to indicate superior health in this group in relation to major chronic disease. Masters athletes who follow nutrition guidelines presented here for prevention of chronic disease are likely to enjoy a reduced risk of these diseases and increased longevity.

Readers interested in increasing their knowledge in this area are encouraged to look at a number of published reviews [220–224].

12.4 IMPLICATIONS FOR SPORTS MEDICINE PROFESSIONALS AND CLINICIANS

- Prior to commencing (or recommencing) training masters athletes should be screened for cardiovascular disease and other medical conditions.
- Blood pressure should be controlled by lifestyle changes and pharmacotherapy prior to commencing training.
- For those with diabetes, exercise may lower blood sugar and therefore oral hypoglycaemic or insulin therapy may need to be altered.
- Exacerbation of osteoarthritis pain may occur when commencing training and athletes should be aware of this and the potential for tendon and soft tissue injury.

12.5 IMPLICATIONS FOR MASTERS ATHLETES AND COACHES

- Lower energy requirements of older individuals mean that a food planning for fuelling and performance should be carefully mapped to include high-nutrient-dense foods for chronic disease prevention. For example, carbohydrate-containing foods like dairy and high fibre vegetables (legumes) and fruits, and whole grain cereals can supply both fuel for aerobic exercise and protective benefits against chronic disease.
- It makes good sense to ensure consumption of low-fat dairy with heart and bone protective qualities for older adults as well as being a great source of carbohydrate and protein for fuelling. Calcium absorption is affected by enhancers (e.g. vitamin D_3 and carbohydrates such as lactose) and inhibitors (e.g. oxalic acid in spinach and phytic acid in high-phytate bran cereal), as well as calcium load with absorption inversely related to the amount of calcium consumed at one time [225]. It is important that masters athletes are aware of known enhancers and inhibitors, and do spread the servings of food containing calcium over the course of the day.
- While food sources of calcium have similar effects as supplements on bone health, they have not been associated with cardiovascular effects [226]. Since there is some suggestion that calcium supplementation may increase risk of cardiovascular disease in older women [207], it is advisable to consume up to (but not exceed) calcium requirements from food sources where possible.
- Inclusion of fish and/or fish oil supplements may improve CVD risk factors and function without performance decrements in masters athletes. The National Heart Foundation of Australia recommends 500 mg/day of fish oil for all Australians or 1000 mg/day for those with documented CHD from three to five 150-g servings of oily fish per week, fish oils and fish oil capsules and foods and drinks enriched in omega-3 [228].

- Oily fish can provide both protein and omega-3 fats for cardiovascular health. Most white fish consumed in Australia has only limited amounts of omega-3 oils [229], with the best sources including salmon, tuna, sardines and mackerel.
- Population guidelines for Australians and New Zealanders recommend that SFA and trans fats together should equate to no more than 10% of total energy intake to reduce risk of chronic disease [54], while the Heart Foundation recommends SFA be reduced to <7% and trans fats <1% of total energy intake [227]. Athletes should trim fat off meat, avoid fatty meats, remove skin from chicken, avoid processed baked and fried goods, and read food labels to ensure saturated fat intake is low. SFA should be replaced with MUFA and PUFA foods from foods like oily fish, nuts, oils and spreads.
- Aim for 2300 mg sodium/day or 1600 mg sodium/day for disease prevention and higher-risk older adults such as those with existing CVD or hypertension. Sports drinks may be the best choice for masters athletes training and competing in hot/humid environments as they have greater potential for heat stress. Aim to determine and allocate any specific sodium requirements for exercise and spread the balance of suggested requirements in the remainder of daily intake. Accommodating sodium requirements for exercise may require a lower sodium intake for non-exercise-related food and beverage intake.
- Providing dietary advice to masters athletes may be more complex due to the need to incorporate dietary strategies for the treatment of disease (e.g. CVD, type 2 diabetes) with optimal sports nutrition practice. A sports dietician who is skilled in both sports and clinical practice has the required training to provide such expert advice.

12.6 FUTURE RESEARCH DIRECTIONS

- Assessment of typical daily diets, knowledge, attitudes and beliefs in relationship to chronic disease in masters athletes across various sport groups (e.g. team sports, endurance, speed and power). Although epidemiological evidence supports a link of longevity with particular dietary patterns [230], it would be useful to understand how to adapt these for athletic performance in the masters cohort.
- Qualitative research in dietary patterns, challenges and attitudes towards diet for chronic disease prevention in masters athletes compared to their younger counterparts would be helpful to understand how practitioners can support this cohort in healthy ageing as well as performance.
- Specific research on the potential benefits of fish/fish oil consumption on the health and performance of masters athletes with and without CVD risk factors is warranted.
- How/whether sodium recommendations for hypertensive masters athletes should be adjusted.
- Assessment of the impact of low-energy availability in peri-menopause is warranted especially for female athletes in sports with high risk of falls/contact related fracture.

REFERENCES

1. Rosenbloom, C. and Bahns, M., What can we learn about diet and physical activity from masters athletes, *Nutr. Today* 40(6), 267–72, 2005.
2. Kettunen, J.A., Kujala, U.M., Kaprio, J. and Sarna, S., Health of master track and field athletes—A 16-year follow-up study, *Clin. J. Sport Med.* 16(2), 142–8, 2006.
3. Grimsmo, J., Maehlum, S., Moelstad, P. and Arnesen, H., Mortality and cardiovascular morbidity among long-term endurance male cross country skiers followed for 28–30 years, *Scand. J. Med. Sci. Sports* 21(6), E351–8, 2011.
4. King, D.E., Mainous, A.G., 3rd, and Geesey, M.E., Turning back the clock: Adopting a healthy lifestyle in middle age, *Am. J. Med.* 120(7), 598–603, 2007.

5. Booth, F.W., Laye, M.J. and Roberts, M.D., Lifetime sedentary living accelerates some aspects of secondary aging, *J. Appl. Physiol.* 111(5), 1497–504, 2011.
6. Hamer, M., Lavoie, K.L. and Bacon, S.L., Taking up physical activity in later life and healthy ageing: The English longitudinal study of ageing, *Br. J. Sports Med.* 48(3), 239–43, 2013.
7. Chomistek, A.K., Cook, N.R., Flint, A.J. and Rimm, E.B., Vigorous-intensity leisure-time physical activity and risk of major chronic disease in men, *Med. Sci. Sports Exerc.* 44(10), 1898–905, 2012.
8. Chodzko-Zajko, W.J., Proctor, D.N., Fiatarone Singh, M.A. et al., American College of Sports Medicine position stand. Exercise and physical activity for older adults, *Med. Sci. Sports Exerc.* 41(7), 1510–30, 2009.
9. Haslett, C., Chilvers, E.R., Boon, N.A., Colledge, N.R. and Hunter, J.A.A., *Davidson's Principles and Practice of Medicine*, 19th Ed., Churchill Livingstone, New York, 2002.
10. National Health and Medical Research Council, Clinical practice guidelines for the management of overweight and obesity in adults, Commonwealth of Australia, Canberra, Australia, 2003.
11. WHO Expert Consultation, Appropriate body-mass index for Asian populations and its implications for policy and intervention strategies, *Lancet* 363(9403), 157–63, 2004.
12. Kyrou, I., Haukeland, J.W., Bhala, N. and Kumar, S., Metabolic syndrome, diabetes and non-alcoholic steatohepatitis, in *Clinical Obesity*, 3rd Ed., P. Kopelman, I.D. Caterson and W. Dietz, eds., Blackwell Publishing, Oxford, England, 2010.
13. World Health Organization and International Diabetes Federation, Definition and diagnosis of diabetes mellitus and intermediate hyperglycemia: Report of a WHO/IDF consultation, World Health Organization, Geneva, 2006.
14. Tonkin, A., Barter, P., Best, J. et al., National Heart Foundation of Australia and the Cardiac Society of Australia and New Zealand: Position statement on lipid management—2005, *Heart Lung Circ.* 14(4), 275–91, 2005.
15. World Health Organization, Global database on body mass index, http://apps.who.int/bmi/index.jsp?-introPage=intro_3.html, accessed 12/12/13.
16. Walsh, J., Climstein, M., Heazlewood, I.T. et al., The Loess regression relationship between age and BMI for both Sydney World Masters Games athletes and the Australian national population, *Int. J. Biol. Med. Sci.* 1(1), 33–6, 2011.
17. Wang, Y. and Beydoun, M.A., The obesity epidemic in the United States—Gender, age, socioeconomic, racial/ethnic, and geographic characteristics: A systematic review and meta-regression analysis, *Epidemiol. Rev.* 29, 6–28, 2007.
18. International Obesity Taskforce, Obesity the global epidemic, http://www.iaso.org/iotf/obesity/obesitytheglobalepidemic/, accessed 12/12/13.
19. Whiting, D.R., Guariguata, L., Weil, C. and Shaw, J., IDF Diabetes Atlas: Global estimates of the prevalence of diabetes for 2011 and 2030, *Diabetes Res. Clin. Pract.* 94(3), 311–21, 2011.
20. Australian Bureau of Statistics, National Health Survey: Summary of Results 2007–2008 (reissue) (4364.0), http://www.abs.gov.au/ausstats/abs@.nsf/mf/4364.0/, accessed 13/12/13.
21. Kujala, U.M., Kaprio, J., Taimela, S. and Sarna, S., Prevalence of diabetes, hypertension, and ischemic-heart-disease in former elite athletes, *Metabolism* 43(10), 1255–60, 1994.
22. Chen, Y.L., Huang, C.Y., Lee, S.D. et al., Discipline-specific insulin sensitivity in athletes, *Nutrition* 25(11–12), 1137–42, 2009.
23. Ryan, A.S., Exercise in aging: Its important role in mortality, obesity and insulin resistance, *Aging Health* 6(5), 551–63, 2010.
24. Freeman, J., Froelicher, V. and Ashley, E., The ageing athlete: Screening prior to vigorous exertion in asymptomatic adults without known cardiovascular disease, *Br. J. Sports Med.* 43(9), 696–701, 2009.
25. Whiteson, J.H., Bartels, M.N., Kim, H. and Alba, A.S., Coronary artery disease in masters-level athletes, *Arch. Phys. Med. Rehabil.* 87(3), S79–81, 2006.
26. Baker IDI Heart and Diabetes Institute, The George Institute for Global Health, and Adelaide Health Technology Assessment (The University of Adelaide), National evidence-based guideline on prevention, identification and management of foot complications in diabetes (part of the guidelines on management of type 2 diabetes) 2011, National Health and Medical Research Council, Melbourne, Australia, 2011.
27. Berger, M., Berchtold, P., Cuppers, H.J. et al., Metabolic and hormonal effects of muscular exercise in juvenile type diabetics, *Diabetologia* 13(4), 355–65, 1977.
28. Shugart, C., Jackson, J. and Fields, K.B., Diabetes in sport, *Sports Health* 2(1), 29–38, 2010.
29. The Royal Australian College of General Practitioners and Diabetes Australia, *General Practice Management of Type 2 Diabetes—2014–15*, The Royal Australian College of General Practitioners, Melbourne, Australia, 2014.

30. Maron, B.J., Araujo, C.G.S., Thompson, P.D. et al., Recommendations for preparticipation screening and the assessment of cardiovascular disease in masters athletes—An advisory for healthcare professionals from the working groups of the World Heart Federation, the International Federation of Sports Medicine, and the American Heart Association Committee on Exercise, Cardiac Rehabilitation, and Prevention, *Circulation* 103(2), 327–34, 2001.
31. Pigozzi, F., Spataro, A., Alabiso, A. et al., Role of exercise stress test in master athletes, *Br. J. Sports Med.* 39(8), 527–31, 2005.
32. American Academy of Family Physicians, American Academy of Orthopaedic Surgeons, American College of Sports Medicine et al., Selected issues for the master athlete and the team physician: A consensus statement, *Med. Sci. Sports Exerc.* 42(4), 820–33, 2010.
33. Rossi, S., *Australian Medicines Handbook 2011*, Australian Medicines Handbook Pty Ltd, Adelaide, 2011.
34. Saidi, H. and Mani, M., Severe metabolic acidosis secondary to coadministration of creatine and metformin, a case report, *Am. J. Emerg. Med.* 28(3), 388.e5–.e6, 2010.
35. O'Connor, H. and Caterson, I., Weight loss and the athlete, in *Clinical Sports Nutrition*, L. Burke and V. Deakin, Eds., McGraw-Hill Australia Pty Ltd, North Ryde, Australia, 2010, pp. 116–48.
36. O'Connor, H. and Slater, G., Losing, gaining and making weight for athletes, in *Sport and Exercise Nutrition*, S. Lanham-New, S. Stear, M. Sherriffs, and A. Collins, eds., Wiley-Blackwell, West Sussex, United Kingdom, 2011, pp. 210–32.
37. Larsen, T.M., Dalskov, S.M., van Baak, M. et al., Diets with high or low protein content and glycemic index for weight-loss maintenance, *N. Engl. J. Med.* 363(22), 2102–13, 2010.
38. Burke, L., Preparation for competition, in *Clinical Sports Nutrition*, L. Burke and V. Deakin, eds., McGraw-Hill Australia Pty Ltd, North Ryde, Australia, 2010, pp. 304–29.
39. Rolls, B.J., The role of energy density in the overconsumption of fat, *J. Nutr.* 130(2), 268S–71S, 2000.
40. Abargouei, A.S., Janghorbani, M., Salehi-Marzijarani, M. and Esmaillzadeh, A., Effect of dairy consumption on weight and body composition in adults: A systematic review and meta-analysis of randomized controlled clinical trials, *Int. J. Obes.* 36(12), 1485–93, 2012.
41. Dougkas, A., Reynolds, C.K., Givens, I.D., Elwood, P.C. and Minihane, A.M., Associations between dairy consumption and body weight: A review of the evidence and underlying mechanisms, *Nutr. Res. Rev.* 24(1), 72–95, 2011.
42. Wing, R.R., Lang, W., Wadden, T.A. et al., Benefits of modest weight loss in improving cardiovascular risk factors in overweight and obese individuals with type 2 diabetes, *Diabetes Care* 34(7), 1481–6, 2011.
43. Vidal, J., Updated review on the benefits of weight loss, *Int. J. Obes.* 26, S25–8, 2002.
44. Burke, L., Nutrition for recovery after training and competition, in *Clinical Sports Nutrition*, L. Burke and V. Deakin, eds., McGraw-Hill Australia Pty Ltd, North Ryde, Australia, 2010, pp. 358–92.
45. Maughan, R., Fluid and carbohydrate intake during exercise, in *Clinical Sports Nutrition*, L. Burke and V. Deakin, eds., McGraw-Hill Australia Pty Ltd, North Ryde, Australia, 2010, pp. 330–57.
46. Sigal, R.J., Kenny, G.P., Wasserman, D.H., Castaneda-Sceppa, C. and White, R.D., Physical activity/exercise and type 2 diabetes—A consensus statement from the American Diabetes Association, *Diabetes Care* 29(6), 1433–8, 2006.
47. Deakin, V., Wilson, D. and Cooper, G., Special needs: The athlete with diabetes, in *Clinical Sports Nutrition*, L. Burke and V. Deakin, eds., McGraw-Hill Australia Pty Ltd, North Ryde, Australia, 2010, pp. 578–601.
48. Sigal, R.J., Kenny, G.P., Wasserman, D.H. and Castaneda-Sceppa, C., Physical activity/exercise and type 2 diabetes, *Diabetes Care* 27(10), 2518–39, 2004.
49. Rossi, M., Turati, F., Lagiou, P. et al., Mediterranean diet and glycaemic load in relation to incidence of type 2 diabetes: Results from the Greek cohort of the population-based European Prospective Investigation into Cancer and Nutrition (EPIC), *Diabetologia* 56(11), 2405–13, 2013.
50. Thomas, D.E., Elliott, E.J. and Baur, L., Low glycaemic index or low glycaemic load diets for overweight and obesity, *Cochrane Database Syst. Rev.* Jul 18(3), 2007.
51. Thomas, D. and Elliott, E.J., Low glycaemic index, or low glycaemic load, diets for diabetes mellitus, *Cochrane Database Syst. Rev.* Jan 21(1), 2009.
52. Pi-Sunyer, F.X., Glycemic index and disease, *Am. J. Clin. Nutr.* 76(1), 290S–8S, 2002.
53. National Health and Medical Research Council, Australian Dietary Guidelines, Commonwealth of Australia, Canberra, Australia, 2013.
54. Department of Health and Ageing, National Health and Medical Research Council, and Health, Ministry of Health, Nutrient Reference Values for Australia and New Zealand: Executive Summary, Commonwealth of Australia, Canberra, Australia, 2006.

55. World Health Organization and Food and Agriculture Organisation of the United Nations, Joint WHO/FAO Expert Consultation on Diet, Nutrition and the Prevention of Chronic Diseases, http://www.who.int/dietphysicalactivity/publications/trs916/download/en/index.html, accessed 13/12/13.
56. Englyst, K.N., Liu, S. and Englyst, H.N., Nutritional characterization and measurement of dietary carbohydrates, *Eur. J. Clin. Nutr.* 61(Suppl 1), S19–39, 2007.
57. Kerckhoffs, D., Brouns, F., Hornstra, G. and Mensink, R.P., Effects on the human serum lipoprotein profile of beta-glucan, soy protein and isoflavones, plant sterols and stanols, garlic and tocotrienols, *J. Nutr.* 132(9), 2494–505, 2002.
58. Beck, E.J., Tosh, S.M., Batterham, M.J., Tapsell, L.C. and Huang, X.F., Oat beta-glucan increases postprandial cholecystokinin levels, decreases insulin response and extends subjective satiety in overweight subjects, *Mol. Nutr. Food Res.* 53(10), 1343–51, 2009.
59. Riserus, U., Willett, W.C. and Hu, F.B., Dietary fats and prevention of type 2 diabetes, *Prog. Lipid Res.* 48(1), 44–51, 2009.
60. Food and Agriculture Organization of the United Nations, Fats and fatty acids in human nutrition: Report of an expert consultation, Food and Agriculture Organisation of the United Nations, Geneva, 2010.
61. van Dam, R.M. and Hu, F.B., Coffee consumption and risk of type 2 diabetes—A systematic review, *JAMA* 294(1), 97–104, 2005.
62. Huxley, R., Lee, C.M.Y., Barzi, F. et al., Coffee, decaffeinated coffee, and tea consumption in relation to incident type 2 diabetes mellitus: A systematic review with meta-analysis, *Arch. Intern. Med.* 169(22), 2053–63, 2009.
63. National Health and Medical Research Council, A review of the evidence to address targeted questions to inform the revision of the Australian Dietary Guidelines, Commonwealth of Australia, Canberra, Ausralia, 2011.
64. Yoshioka, K., Kogure, A., Yoshida, T. and Yoshikawa, T., Coffee consumption and risk of type 2 diabetes mellitus, *Lancet* 361(9358), 703, 2003.
65. Song, Y., He, K., Levitan, E.B., Manson, J.E. and Liu, S., Effects of oral magnesium supplementation on glycaemic control in type 2 diabetes: A meta-analysis of randomized double-blind controlled trials, *Diabetic Med.* 23(10), 1050–6, 2006.
66. Guerrero-Romero, F., Tamez-Perez, H.E., Gonzalez-Gonzalez, G. et al., Oral magnesium supplementation improves insulin sensitivity in non-diabetic subjects with insulin resistance. A double-blind placebo-controlled randomized trial, *Diabetes Metab.* 30(3), 253–8, 2004.
67. Mooren, F.C., Kruger, K., Volker, K., Golf, S.W., Wadepuhl, M. and Kraus, A., Oral magnesium supplementation reduces insulin resistance in non-diabetic subjects—A double-blind, placebo-controlled, randomized trial, *Diabetes Obes. Metab.* 13(3), 281–4, 2011.
68. van Dijk, A.E., Olthof, M.R., Meeuse, J.C., Seebus, E., Heine, R.J. and van Dam, R.M., Acute effects of decaffeinated coffee and the major coffee components chlorogenic acid and trigonelline on glucose tolerance, *Diab. Care* 32(6), 1023–5, 2009.
69. Pimentel, G.D., Zemdegs, J.C.S., Theodoro, J.A. and Mota, J.F., Does long-term coffee intake reduce type 2 diabetes mellitus risk?, *Diabetol. Metab. Syndr.* 1(1), 2009.
70. Cornelis, M.C. and El-Sohemy, A., Coffee, caffeine, and coronary heart disease, *Curr. Opin. Clin. Nutr. Metab. Care* 10(6), 745–51, 2007.
71. Briffa, T., Maiorana, A., Allan, R. et al., National Heart Foundation of Australia physical activity recommendations for people with cardiovascular disease, National Heart Foundation of Australia, Sydney, Australia, 2006.
72. World Health Organization, The Global burden of disease: 2004 update, World Health Organization, Geneva, 2008.
73. Australian Bureau of Statistics, Cardiovascular Disease in Australia: A snapshot, 2004–05 (4821.0.55.001), http://www.abs.gov.au/ausstats/abs@.nsf/mf/4821.0.55.001, accessed 22/12/13.
74. Dey, S.K., Ghosh, C., Debray, P. and Chatterjee, M., Coronary artery disease risk factors and their association with physical activity in older athletes, *J. Cardiovasc. Risk* 9(6), 383–92, 2002.
75. Hernelahti, M., Kujala, U.M., Kaprio, J., Karjalainen, J. and Sarna, S., Hypertension in master endurance athletes, *J. Hypertens.* 16(11), 1573–7, 1998.
76. Kujala, U.M., Sarna, S., Kaprio, J., Koskenvuo, M. and Karjalainen, J., Heart attacks and lower-limb function in master endurance athletes, *Med. Sci. Sports Exerc.* 31(7), 1041–6, 1999.
77. De Matos, L., Caldeira, N.D.O., Perlingeiro, P.D., Dos Santos, I.L.G., Negrao, C.E. and Azevedo, L.F., Cardiovascular risk and clinical factors in athletes: 10 years of evaluation, *Med. Sci. Sports Exerc.* 43(6), 943–50, 2011.

78. Mathews, S.C., Narotsky, D.L., Bernholt, D.L. et al., Mortality among marathon runners in the United States, 2000–2009, *Am. J. Sports Med.* 40(7), 1495–500, 2012.
79. Corrado, D., Basso, C. and Thiene, G., Sudden cardiac death in athletes: What is the role of screening?, *Curr. Opin. Cardiol.* 27(1), 41–8, 2012.
80. World Anti-Doping Agency, The World Anti-Doping Code: The 2012 Prohibited List International Standard, http://www.wada-ama.org/Documents/World_Anti-Doping_Program/WADP-Prohibited-list/2012/WADA_Prohibited_List_2012_EN.pdf, accessed 5/12/13.
81. Mann, J. and Chisholm, A., Cardiovascular diseases, in *Essentials of Human Nutrition*, J. Mann and A.S. Truswell, eds., Oxford University Press, Oxford, United Kingdom, 2007, pp. 282–312.
82. O'Donnell, E., Goodman, J.M. and Harvey, P.J., Cardiovascular consequences of ovarian disruption: A focus on functional hypothalamic amenorrhea in physically active women, *J. Clin. Endocrinol. Metab.* 96(12), 3638–48, 2011.
83. Temme, K.E. and Hoch, A.Z., Recognition and rehabilitation of the female athlete triad/tetrad: A multidisciplinary approach, *Curr. Sport. Med. Rep.* 12(3), 190–9, 2013.
84. Loucks, A.B. and Thuma, J.R., Luteinizing hormone pulsatility is disrupted at a threshold of energy availability in regularly menstruating women, *J. Clin. Endocrinol. Metab.* 88(1), 297–311, 2003.
85. Loucks, A.B., Verdun, M. and Heath, E.M., Low energy availability, not stress of exercise, alters LH pulsatility in exercising women, *J. Appl. Physiol.* 84(1), 37–46, 1998.
86. Kaplan, J.R. and Manuck, S.B., Ovarian dysfunction and the premenopausal origins of coronary heart disease, *Menopause* 15(4), 768–76, 2008.
87. Solomon, C.G., Hu, F.B., Dunaif, A. et al., Menstrual cycle irregularity and risk for future cardiovascular disease, *J. Clin. Endocrinol. Metab.* 87(5), 2013–7, 2002.
88. Hoch, A.Z., Papanek, P., Szabo, A., Widlansky, M.E., Schimke, J.E. and Gutterman, D.D., Association between the female athlete triad and endothelial dysfunction in dancers, *Clin. J. Sport Med.* 21(2), 119–25, 2011.
89. Rickenlund, A., Eriksson, M.J., Schenck-Gustafsson, K. and Hirschberg, A.L., Amenorrhea in female athletes is associated with endothelial dysfunction and unfavorable lipid profile, *J. Clin. Endocrinol. Metab.* 90(3), 1354–9, 2005.
90. Davignon, J. and Ganz, P., Role of endothelial dysfunction in atherosclerosis, *Circulation* 109(23 Suppl 1), III27–32, 2004.
91. Iggman, D. and Riserus, U., Role of different dietary saturated fatty acids for cardiometabolic risk, *Clin. Lipidol.* 6(2), 209–23, 2011.
92. Astrup, A., Dyerberg, J., Elwood, P. et al., The role of reducing intakes of saturated fat in the prevention of cardiovascular disease: Where does the evidence stand in 2010?, *Am. J. Clin. Nutr.* 93(4), 684–8, 2011.
93. Jung, U.J., Torrejon, C., Tighe, A.P. and Deckelbaum, R.J., n–3 Fatty acids and cardiovascular disease: Mechanisms underlying beneficial effects, *Am. J. Clin. Nutr.* 87(6), 2003S–9S, 2008.
94. He, K., Song, Y., Daviglus, M.L. et al., Accumulated evidence on fish consumption and coronary heart disease mortality: A meta-analysis of cohort studies, *Circulation* 109(22), 2705–11, 2004.
95. Whelton, S.P., He, J., Whelton, P.K. and Muntner, P., Meta-analysis of observational studies on fish intake and coronary heart disease, *Am. J. Cardiol.* 93(9), 1119–23, 2004.
96. König, A., Bouzan, C., Cohen, J.T. et al., A quantitative analysis of fish consumption and coronary heart disease mortality, *Am. J. Prev. Med.* 29(4), 335–46, 2005.
97. He, K., Song, Y., Daviglus, M.L. et al., Fish consumption and incidence of stroke: A meta-analysis of cohort studies, *Stroke* 35(7), 1538–42, 2004.
98. Bouzan, C., Cohen, J.T., Connor, W.E. et al., A quantitative analysis of fish consumption and stroke risk, *Am. J. Prev. Med.* 29(4), 347–52, 2005.
99. Mozaffarian, D., Fish and n–3 fatty acids for the prevention of fatal coronary heart disease and sudden cardiac death, *Am. J. Clin. Nutr.* 87(6), 1991S–6S, 2008.
100. Musa-Veloso, K., Binns, M.A., Kocenas, A. et al., Impact of low v. moderate intakes of long-chain n-3 fatty acids on risk of coronary heart disease, *Br. J. Nutr.* 106(08), 1129–41, 2011.
101. Gille, D., Overview of the physiological changes and optimal diet in the golden age generation over 50, *Eur. Rev. Aging Phys. Act.* 7(1), 27–36, 2010.
102. Hill, A.M., Buckley, J.D., Murphy, K.J. and Howe, P.R., Combining fish-oil supplements with regular aerobic exercise improves body composition and cardiovascular disease risk factors, *Am. J. Clin. Nutr.* 85(5), 1267–74, 2007.
103. Ninio, D.M., Hill, A.M., Howe, P.R., Buckley, J.D. and Saint, D.A., Docosahexaenoic acid-rich fish oil improves heart rate variability and heart rate responses to exercise in overweight adults, *Br. J. Nutr.* 100(5), 1097–103, 2008.

104. Buckley, J.D., Burgess, S., Murphy, K.J. and Howe, P.R.C., DHA-rich fish oil lowers heart rate during submaximal exercise in elite Australian Rules footballers, *J. Sci. Med. Sport* 12(4), 503–7, 2009.
105. Peoples, G.E.P., McLennan, P.L.P., Howe, P.R.C.P. and Groeller, H.P., Fish oil reduces heart rate and oxygen consumption during exercise, *J. Cardiovasc. Pharmacol.* 52(6), 540–7, 2008.
106. Bamia, C., Trichopoulos, D., Ferrari, P. et al., Dietary patterns and survival of older Europeans: The EPIC-Elderly Study (European Prospective Investigation into Cancer and Nutrition), *Public Health Nutr.* 10(6), 590–8, 2007.
107. World Health Organization, The World Health Report 2002: Reducing risks, promoting healthy life, World Health Organization, Geneva, 2002.
108. Hamilton, C.A., Low-density lipoprotein and oxidised low-density lipoprotein: Their role in the development of atherosclerosis, *Pharmacol. Ther.* 74(1), 55–72, 1997.
109. Thompson, H.J., Heimendinger, J., Diker, A. et al., Dietary botanical diversity affects the reduction of oxidative biomarkers in women due to high vegetable and fruit intake, *J. Nutr.* 136(8), 2207–12, 2006.
110. Wannamethee, S.G., Lowe, G.D.O., Rumley, A., Bruckdorfer, K.R. and Whincup, P.H., Associations of vitamin C status, fruit and vegetable intakes, and markers of inflammation and hemostasis, *Am. J. Clin. Nutr.* 83(3), 567–74, 2006.
111. Theuwissen, E. and Mensink, R.P., Water-soluble dietary fibers and cardiovascular disease, *Physiol. Behav.* 94(2), 285–92, 2008.
112. Taku, K., Umegaki, K., Sato, Y., Taki, Y., Endoh, K. and Watanabe, S., Soy isoflavones lower serum total and LDL cholesterol in humans: A meta-analysis of 11 randomized controlled trials, *Am. J. Clin. Nutr.* 85(4), 1148–56, 2007.
113. Lidder, S. and Webb, A.J., Vascular effects of dietary nitrate (as found in green leafy vegetables and beetroot) via the nitrate-nitrite-nitric oxide pathway, *Br. J. Clin. Pharmacol.* 75(3), 677–96, 2013.
114. Webb, A.J., Patel, N., Loukogeorgakis, S. et al., Acute blood pressure lowering, vasoprotective, and antiplatelet properties of dietary nitrate via bioconversion to nitrite, *Hypertension* 51(3), 784–90, 2008.
115. Lansley, K.E., Winyard, P.G., Fulford, J. et al., Dietary nitrate supplementation reduces the O_2 cost of walking and running: A placebo-controlled study, *J. Appl. Physiol.* 110(3), 591–600, 2011.
116. Coles, L. and Clifton, P., Effect of beetroot juice on lowering blood pressure in free-living, disease-free adults: A randomized, placebo-controlled trial, *Nutr. J.* 11(1), 106, 2012.
117. Bailey, S.J., Winyard, P., Vanhatalo, A. et al., Dietary nitrate supplementation reduces the O_2 cost of low-intensity exercise and enhances tolerance to high-intensity exercise in humans, *J. Appl. Physiol.* 107(4), 1144–55, 2009.
118. Lansley, K.E., Winyard, P.G., Bailey, S.J. et al., Acute dietary nitrate supplementation improves cycling time trial performance, *Med. Sci. Sports Exerc.* 43(6), 1125–31, 2011.
119. Bailey, S.J., Fulford, J., Vanhatalo, A. et al., Dietary nitrate supplementation enhances muscle contractile efficiency during knee-extensor exercise in humans, *J. Appl. Physiol.* 109(1), 135–48, 2010.
120. Hoon, M.W., Johnson, N.A., Chapman, P.G. and Burke, L.M., The effect of nitrate supplementation on exercise performance in healthy individuals: A systematic review and meta-analysis, *Int. J. Sport Nutr. Exerc. Metab.* 23(5), 522–32, 2013.
121. Hoon, M.W., Jones, A.M., Johnson, N.A. et al., The effect of variable doses of inorganic nitrate-rich beetroot juice on simulated 2,000 m rowing performance in trained athletes, *Int. J. Sports. Physiol. Perform.* in press, 2014.
122. Segura, R., Javierre, C., Lizarraga, M.A. and Ros, E., Other relevant components of nuts: Phytosterols, folate and minerals, *Br. J. Nutr.* 96(Suppl 2), S36–44, 2006.
123. Ziemke, F. and Mantzoros, C.S., Adiponectin in insulin resistance: Lessons from translational research, *Am. J. Clin. Nutr.* 91(1), 258S–61S, 2010.
124. Curin, Y. and Andriantsitohaina, R., Polyphenols as potential therapeutical agents against cardiovascular diseases, *Pharmacol. Rep.* 57, 97–107, 2005.
125. Ruxton, C.H. and Hart, V.A., Black tea is not significantly different from water in the maintenance of normal hydration in human subjects: Results from a randomised controlled trial, *Br. J. Nutr.* 106(4), 588–95, 2011.
126. Cefalu, C.A., Theories and mechanisms of aging, *Clin. Geriatr. Med.* 27(4), 491–506, 2011.
127. Australian Bureau of Statistics, 2009–2010 Year Book Australia, 91 Ed., Commonwealth of Australia, Canberra, Australia, 2010.
128. Lawes, C.M.M., Vander Hoorn, S., Law, M.R., Elliott, P., MacMahon, S. and Rodgers, A., Blood pressure and the global burden of disease 2000. Part 1: Estimates of blood pressure levels, *J. Hypertens.* 24(3), 413–22, 2006.

129. Allen, N., Berry, J.D., Ning, H., Van Horn, L., Dyer, A. and Lloyd-Jones, D.M., Impact of blood pressure and blood pressure change during middle age on the remaining lifetime risk for cardiovascular disease: The cardiovascular lifetime risk pooling project, *Circulation* 125(1), 37–44, 2012.
130. Weinberger, M.H. and Fineberg, N.S., Sodium and volume sensitivity of blood-pressure—Age and pressure change over time, *Hypertension* 18(1), 67–71, 1991.
131. Dengel, D.R., Brown, M.D., Reynolds, T.H., Kuskowski, M.A. and Supiano, M.A., Effect of aerobic exercise training on blood pressure sensitivity to dietary sodium in older hypertensives, *J. Hum. Hypertens.* 20(5), 372–8, 2006.
132. Vearrier, D. and Greenberg, M.I., Occupational health of miners at altitude: Adverse health effects, toxic exposures, pre-placement screening, acclimatization, and worker surveillance, *Clin. Toxicol.* 49(7), 629–40, 2011.
133. Best, S., Caillaud, C. and Thompson, M., The effect of ageing and fitness on thermoregulatory response to high-intensity exercise, *Scand. J. Med. Sci. Sports* 22(4), E29–37, 2012.
134. Reaburn, P., Nutrition issues for the aging athlete, in *Clinical Sports Nutrition*, L. Burke and V. Deakin, eds., McGraw-Hill Australia Pty Ltd, North Ryde, Australia, 2010, pp. 547–77.
135. Sawka, M.N., Burke, L.M., Eichner, E.R., Maughan, R.J., Montain, S.J. and Stachenfeld, N.S., Exercise and fluid replacement, *Med. Sci. Sports Exerc.* 39(2), 377–90, 2007.
136. Baker, L.B., Munce, T.A. and Kenney, W.L., Sex differences in voluntary fluid intake by older adults during exercise, *Med. Sci. Sports Exerc.* 37(5), 789–96, 2005.
137. Meyer, J., Doring, A., Herder, C., Roden, M., Koenig, W. and Thorand, B., Dietary patterns, subclinical inflammation, incident coronary heart disease and mortality in middle-aged men from the MONICA/KORA Augsburg cohort study, *Eur. J. Clin. Nutr.* 65(7), 800–7, 2011.
138. Heidemann, C., Schulze, M.B., Franco, O.H., van Dam, R.M., Mantzoros, C.S. and Hu, F.B., Dietary patterns and risk of mortality from cardiovascular disease, cancer, and all causes in a prospective cohort of women, *Circulation* 118(3), 230–7, 2008.
139. Perez-Lopez, F.R., Chedraui, P., Haya, J. and Cuadros, J.L., Effects of the Mediterranean diet on longevity and age-related morbid conditions, *Maturitas* 64(2), 67–79, 2009.
140. Guallar-Castillon, P., Rodriguez-Artalejo, F., Tormo, M.J. et al., Major dietary patterns and risk of coronary heart disease in middle-aged persons from a Mediterranean country: The EPIC-Spain cohort study, *Nutr. Metab. Carbiovasc. Dis.* 22(3), 192–9, 2012.
141. Chen, S.T., Maruthur, N.M. and Appel, L.J., The effect of dietary patterns on estimated coronary heart disease risk: Results from the Dietary Approaches to Stop Hypertension (DASH) trial, *Circ. Cardiovasc. Qual. Outcomes* 3(5), 484–9, 2010.
142. Fung, T.T., Chiuve, S.E., McCullough, M.L., Rexrode, K.M., Logroscino, G. and Hu, F.B., Adherence to a DASH-Style diet and risk of coronary heart disease and stroke in women, *Arch. Intern. Med.* 168(7), 713–20, 2008.
143. Van Horn, L., McCoin, M., Kris-Etherton, P.M. et al., The evidence for dietary prevention and treatment of cardiovascular disease, *J. Am. Diet. Assoc.* 108(2), 287–331, 2008.
144. Sacks, F.M., Svetkey, L.P., Vollmer, W.M. et al., Effects on blood pressure of reduced dietary sodium and the Dietary Approaches to Stop Hypertension (DASH) diet. DASH-Sodium Collaborative Research Group, *N. Engl. J. Med.* 344(1), 3–10, 2001.
145. Brunner, E.J., Mosdøl, A., Witte, D.R. et al., Dietary patterns and 15-y risks of major coronary events, diabetes, and mortality, *Am. J. Clin. Nutr.* 87(5), 1414–21, 2008.
146. Browne, J.A., The mature athlete with hip arthritis, *Clin. Sports Med.* 30(2), 453–62, 2011.
147. Buckwalter, J.A. and Martin, J.A., Sports and osteoarthritis, *Curr. Opin. Rheumatol.* 16(5), 634–9, 2004.
148. Chakravarty, E.F., Hubert, H.B., Lingala, V.B., Zatarain, E. and Fries, J.F., Long distance running and knee osteoarthritis—A prospective study, *Am. J. Prev. Med.* 35(2), 133–8, 2008.
149. Urquhart, D.M., Tobing, J.F.L., Hanna, F.S. et al., What is the effect of physical activity on the knee joint? A systematic review, *Med. Sci. Sports Exerc.* 43(3), 432–42, 2011.
150. Willick, S.E. and Hansen, P.A., Running and osteoarthritis, *Clin. Sports Med.* 29(3), 417–28, 2010.
151. Michaelsson, K., Byberg, L., Ahlbom, A., Melhus, H. and Farahmand, B.Y., Risk of severe knee and hip osteoarthritis in relation to level of physical exercise: A prospective cohort study of long-distance skiers in Sweden, *PloS One* 6(3), 2011.
152. Takeda, H., Nakagawa, T., Nakamura, K. and Engebretsen, L., Prevention and management of knee osteoarthritis and knee cartilage injury in sports, *Br. J. Sports Med.* 45(4), 304–9, 2011.
153. Bosomworth, N.J., Exercise and knee osteoarthritis: Benefit or hazard?, *Can. Fam. Phys.* 55(9), 871–8, 2009.

154. Nordin, C., Prince, R. and Seeman, E., Consensus statement on the prevention and management of osteoporosis, *Med. J. Aust.* 167(5), 241, 1997.
155. Woolfe, A.D. and Pfleger, B., Burden of major musculoskeletal conditions, *Bull. World Health Organ.* 81(9), 646–56, 2003.
156. Kanis, J.A., Johnell, O., Oden, A., Jonsson, B., De Laet, C. and Dawson, A., Risk of hip fracture according to the World Health Organization criteria for osteopenia and osteoporosis, *Bone* 27(5), 585–90, 2000.
157. Maquirriain, J., Ghisi, J.P. and Amato, S., Is tennis a predisposing factor for degenerative shoulder disease?, A controlled study in former elite players, *Br. J. Sports Med.* 40(5), 447–50, 2006.
158. Chen, K.T. and Yang, R.S., Effects of exercise on lipid metabolism and musculoskeletal fitness in female athletes, *World J. Gastroenterol.* 10(1), 122–6, 2004.
159. Velez, N.F., Zhang, A., Stone, B., Perera, S., Miller, M. and Greenspan, S.L., The effect of moderate impact exercise on skeletal integrity in master athletes, *Osteoporosis Int.* 19(10), 1457–64, 2008.
160. Wiswell, R.A., Hawkins, S.A., Dreyer, H.C. and Jaque, S.V., Maintenance of BMD in older male runners is independent of changes in training volume or (V) over dot O(2)peak, *J. Gerontol. A Biol. Sci. Med. Sci.* 57(4), M203–8, 2002.
161. Andreoli, A., Celi, M., Volpe, S.L., Sorge, R. and Tarantino, U., Long-term effect of exercise on bone mineral density and body composition in post-menopausal ex-elite athletes: A retrospective study, *Eur. J. Clin. Nutr.* 66(1), 69–74, 2012.
162. Lynch, N.A., Ryan, A.S., Evans, J., Katzel, L.I. and Goldberg, A.P., Older elite football players have reduced cardiac and osteoporosis risk factors, *Med. Sci. Sports Exerc.* 39(7), 1124–30, 2007.
163. Kettunen, J.A., Impivaara, O., Kujala, U.M. et al., Hip fractures and femoral bone mineral density in male former elite athletes, *Bone* 46(2), 330–5, 2010.
164. Tveit, M., Rosengren, B.E., Nyquist, F., Nilsson, J.A. and Karlsson, M.K., Former male elite athletes have lower incidence of fragility fractures than expected, *Med. Sci. Sports Exerc.* 45(3), 405–10, 2013.
165. Gibson, J.H., Harries, M., Mitchell, A., Godfrey, R., Lunt, M. and Reeve, J., Determinants of bone density and prevalence of osteopenia among female runners in their second to seventh decades of age, *Bone* 26(6), 591–8, 2000.
166. Csermely, T., Halvax, L., Vizer, M. et al., Relationship between adolescent amenorrhea and climacteric osteoporosis, *Maturitas* 56(4), 368–74, 2007.
167. Beshgetoor, D., Nichols, J.F. and Rego, I., Effect of training mode and calcium intake on bone mineral density in female master cyclists, runners, and non-athletes, *Int. J. Sport Nutr.* 10(3), 290–301, 2000.
168. Miller, S.M., Kukuljan, S., Turner, A.I., van der Pligt, P. and Ducher, G., Energy deficiency, menstrual disturbances, and low bone mass: What do exercising Australian women know about the female athlete triad?, *Int. J. Sport Nutr. Exerc. Metab.* 22(2), 131–8, 2012.
169. American College of Sports Medicine, The female athlete triad, *Med. Sci. Sports Exerc.* 39(10), 1867–82, 2007.
170. Nichols, J.F. and Rauh, M.J., Longitudinal changes in bone mineral density in male master cyclists and nonathletes, *J. Strength Cond. Res.* 25(3), 727–34, 2011.
171. Olmedillas, H., Gonzalez-Aguero, A., Moreno, L.A., Casajus, J.A. and Vicente-Rodriguez, G., Cycling and bone health: A systematic review, *BMC Med.* 10, 2012.
172. Dieppe, P.A., Cushnaghan, J. and Shepstone, L., The Bristol 'OA500' Study: Progression of osteoarthritis (OA) over 3 years and the relationship between clinical and radiographic changes at the knee joint, *Osteoarthritis Cartilage* 5(2), 87–97, 1997.
173. Nichols, J.F., Palmer, J.E. and Levy, S.S., Low bone mineral density in highly trained male master cyclists, *Osteoporosis Int.* 14(8), 644–9, 2003.
174. Rosen, C.J., Vitamin D insufficiency, *N. Engl. J. Med.* 364(3), 248–54, 2011.
175. Schilcher, J., Michaelsson, K. and Aspenberg, P., Bisphosphonate use and atypical fractures of the femoral shaft, *N. Engl. J. Med.* 364(18), 1728–37, 2011.
176. Powell, A., Teichtahl, A.J., Wluka, A.E. and Cicuttini, F.M., Obesity: A preventable risk factor for large joint osteoarthritis which may act through biomechanical factors, *Br. J. Sports Med.* 39(1), 4–5, 2005.
177. Messier, S.P., Gutekunst, D.J., Davis, C. and DeVita, P., Weight loss reduces knee-joint loads in overweight and obese older adults with knee osteoarthritis, *Arthritis Rheum.* 52(7), 2026–32, 2005.
178. Christensen, R., Bartels, E.M., Astrup, A. and Bliddal, H., Effect of weight reduction in obese patients diagnosed with knee osteoarthritis: A systematic review and meta-analysis, *Ann. Rheum. Dis.* 66(4), 433–9, 2007.
179. Berry, P.A., Wluka, A.E., Davies-Tuck, M.L. et al., The relationship between body composition and structural changes at the knee, *Rheumatology* 49(12), 2362–9, 2010.

180. Sowers, M.F., Yosef, M., Jamadar, D., Jacobson, J., Karvonen-Gutierrez, C. and Jaffe, M., BMI vs. body composition and radiographically defined osteoarthritis of the knee in women: A 4-year follow-up study, *Osteoarthritis Cartilage* 16(3), 367–72, 2008.
181. Canter, P.H., Wider, B. and Ernst, E., The antioxidant vitamins A, C, E and selenium in the treatment of arthritis: A systematic review of randomized clinical trials, *Rheumatology* 46(8), 1223–33, 2007.
182. Peregoy, J. and Wilder, F.V., The effects of vitamin C supplementation on incident and progressive knee osteoarthritis: A longitudinal study, *Public Health Nutr.* 14(4), 709–15, 2011.
183. Wluka, A.E., Stuckey, S., Brand, C. and Cicuttini, F.M., Supplementary vitamin E does not affect the loss of cartilage volume in knee osteoarthritis: A 2 year double blind randomized placebo controlled study, *J. Rheumatol.* 29(12), 2585–91, 2002.
184. Brand, C., Snaddon, J., Bailey, M. and Cicuttini, F., Vitamin E is ineffective for symptomatic relief of knee osteoarthritis: A six month double blind, randomised, placebo controlled study, *Ann. Rheum. Dis.* 60(10), 946–9, 2001.
185. Rosenbaum, C.C., O'Mathuna, D.P., Chavez, M. and Shields, K., Antioxidants and antiinflammatory dietary supplements for osteoarthritis and rheumatoid arthritis, *Altern. Ther. Health Med.* 16(2), 32–40, 2010.
186. Cleland, L.G., James, M.J. and Proudman, S.M., Dietary fats and inflammation: The medicinal use of fish oil, *Nutr. Diet.* 66(1), 4–6, 2009.
187. Towheed, T.E., Maxwell, L., Anastassiades, T.P. et al., Glucosamine therapy for treating osteoarthritis, *Cochrane Database Syst. Rev.* Apr 18(2), 2005.
188. Igarashi, M., Sakamoto, K. and Nagaoka, I., Effect of glucosamine, a therapeutic agent for osteoarthritis, on osteoblastic cell differentiation, *Int. J. Mol. Med.* 28(3), 373–9, 2011.
189. Nagaoka, I., Igarashi, M., Hua, J., Ju, Y., Yomogida, S. and Sakamoto, K., Recent aspects of the anti-inflammatory actions of glucosamine, *Carbohydr. Polym.* 84(2), 825–30, 2011.
190. Bruyere, O. and Reginster, J.Y., Glucosamine and chondroitin sulfate as therapeutic agents for knee and hip osteoarthritis, *Drugs Aging* 24(7), 573–80, 2007.
191. Distler, J. and Anguelouch, A., Evidence-based practice: Review of clinical evidence on the efficacy of glucosamine and chondroitin in the treatment of osteoarthritis, *J. Am. Acad. Nurse Pract.* 18(10), 487–93, 2006.
192. Horwath, C. and van Staveren, W., Nutrition and ageing, in *Essentials of Human Nutrition*, J. Mann and A.S. Truswell, eds., Oxford University Press, Oxford, United Kingdom, 2007, pp. 502–14.
193. Goulding, A., Major minerals: Calcium and magnesium, in *Essentials of Human Nutrition*, J. Mann and A.S. Truswell, eds., Oxford University Press, Oxford, United Kingdom, 2007, pp. 112–24.
194. Food and Agriculture Organization of the United Nations and World Health Organization, FAO/WHO expert consultation on human vitamin and mineral requirements, Food and Agriculture Organization of the United Nations, Rome, Italy, 2001.
195. Boot, A.M., de Ridder, M.A.J., van der Sluis, I.M., van Slobbe, I., Krenning, E.P. and de Muinck Keizer-Schrama, S.M.P.F., Peak bone mineral density, lean body mass and fractures, *Bone* 46(2), 336–41, 2010.
196. Commonwealth Scientific Industrial Research Organisation Preventative Health National Research Flagship and University of South Australia, Australian National Children's Nutrition and Physical Activity, Department of Health and Ageing, Australian Food and Grocery Council, and Department of Agriculture Fisheries and Forestry, 2008.
197. Bonthuis, M., Hughes, M.C.B., Ibiebele, T.I., Green, A.C. and van der Pols, J.C., Dairy consumption and patterns of mortality of Australian adults, *Eur. J. Clin. Nutr.* 64(6), 569–77, 2010.
198. Beshgetoor, D. and Nichols, J.F., Dietary intake and supplement use in female master cyclists and runners, *Int. J. Sport Nutr. Exerc. Metab.* 13(2), 166–72, 2003.
199. Institute of Medicine, Dietary Reference Intakes for Calcium and Vitamin D, Institute of Medicine, Washington, DC, 2011.
200. Hawkins, S.A., Schroeder, E.T., Dreyer, H.C., Underwood, S. and Wiswell, R.A., Five-year maintenance of bone mineral density in women master runners, *Med. Sci. Sports Exerc.* 35(1), 137–44, 2003.
201. Kerr, D., Khan, K. and Bennell, K., Bone, exercise and nutrition, in *Clinical Sports Nutrition*, 4th Ed., L. Burke and V. Deakin, eds., McGraw-Hill Australia Pty Ltd, North Ryde, Australia, 2010, pp. 200–21.
202. Sanders, K.M., Nowson, C.A., Kotowicz, M.A., Briffa, K., Devine, A. and Reid, I.R., Calcium and bone health: Position statement for the Australian and New Zealand Bone and Mineral Society, Osteoporosis Australia and the Endocrine Society of Australia, *Med. J. Aust.* 190(6), 316–20, 2009.
203. Institute of Medicine and Food and Nutrition Board, Dietary Reference Intakes for Calcium, Phosphorus, Magnesium, Vitamin D and Fluoride 1997, National Academy Press, Washington, DC, 1997.
204. Reid, I.R. and Bolland, M.J., Calcium supplementation and vascular disease, *Climacteric* 11(4), 280–6, 2008.

205. Lewis, J.R., Calver, J., Zhu, K., Flicker, L. and Prince, R.L., Calcium supplementation and the risks of atherosclerotic vascular disease in older women: Results of a 5-year RCT and a 4.5-year follow-up, *J. Bone Miner. Res.* 26(1), 35–41, 2011.
206. Willis, K.S., Peterson, N.J. and Larson-Meyer, D.E., Should we be concerned about the vitamin D status of athletes?, *Int. J. Sport Nutr. Exerc. Metab.* 18(2), 204–24, 2008.
207. Scopacasa, F., Need, A.G., Horowitz, M., Wishart, J.M., Morris, H.A. and Nordin, B.E.C., Effects of dose and timing of calcium supplementation on bone resorption in-early menopausal women, *Horm. Metab. Res.* 34(1), 44–7, 2002.
208. Voss, M.W., Nagamatsu, L.S., Liu-Ambrose, T. and Kramer, A.F., Exercise, brain, and cognition across the life span, *J. Appl. Physiol.* 111(5), 1505–13, 2011.
209. Rodriguez, N.R., DiMarco, N.M., Langley, S. et al., Nutrition and athletic performance, *Med. Sci. Sports Exerc.* 41(3), 709–31, 2009.
210. Daley, A., Exercise and depression: A review of reviews, *J. Clin. Psychol. Med. Settings* 15(2), 140–7, 2008.
211. Bell, G.S., Gaitatzis, A., Bell, C.L., Johnson, A.L. and Sander, J.W., Drowning in people with epilepsy—How great is the risk?, *Neurology* 71(8), 578–82, 2008.
212. Kwon, C.S., Liu, M.F., Quan, H.D. et al., The incidence of injuries in persons with and without epilepsy—A population-based study, *Epilepsia* 51(11), 2247–53, 2010.
213. Hayes, S.C., Spence, R.R., Galvao, D.A. and Newton, R.U., Australian Association for Exercise and Sport Science position stand: Optimising cancer outcomes through exercise, *J. Sci. Med. Sport* 12(4), 428–34, 2009.
214. Sormunen, J., Bäckmand, H.M., Sarna, S. et al., Lifetime physical activity and cancer incidence—A cohort study of male former elite athletes in Finland, *J. Sci. Med. Sport*, in press.
215. Schmitz, K.H., Courneya, K.S., Matthews, C. et al., American College of Sports Medicine Roundtable on Exercise Guidelines for Cancer Survivors, *Med. Sci. Sports Exerc.* 42(7), 1409–26, 2010.
216. Donaldson, M.S., Nutrition and cancer: A review of the evidence for an anti-cancer diet, *Nutr. J.* 3, 19, 2004.
217. Robien, K., Demark-Wahnefried, W. and Rock, C.L., Evidence-based nutrition guidelines for cancer survivors: Current guidelines, knowledge gaps, and future research directions, *J. Am. Diet. Assoc.* 111(3), 368–75, 2011.
218. Romaguera, D., Vergnaud, A.C., Peeters, P.H. et al., Is concordance with World Cancer Research Fund/American Institute for Cancer Research guidelines for cancer prevention related to subsequent risk of cancer? Results from the EPIC study, *Am. J. Clin. Nutr.* 96(1), 150–63, 2012.
219. World Cancer Research Fund and American Institute for Cancer Research, Food, nutrition, and the prevention of cancer: A global perspective. American Institute for Cancer Research/World Cancer Research Fund, American Institute for Cancer Research, 1997, World Cancer Research Fund & American Institute for Cancer Research, 1997.
220. Fardet, A. and Boirie, Y., Associations between diet-related diseases and impaired physiological mechanisms: A holistic approach based on meta-analyses to identify targets for preventive nutrition, *Nutr. Rev.* 71(10), 643–56, 2013.
221. Cameron, K.A., Healthy aging: Programs that make a difference—Part 1, *Consult. Pharm.* 27(4), 239–53, 2012.
222. Cameron, K.A., Healthy aging: Programs for self-management of chronic disease second of a 2-part series, *Consult. Pharm.* 27(5), 330–5, 2012.
223. Smith, S.M., Soubhi, H., Fortin, M., Hudon, C. and O'Dowd, T., Managing patients with multimorbidity: Systematic review of interventions in primary care and community settings, *BMJ*, 345, e5205, 2012.
224. González-Vallinas, M., González-Castejón, M., Rodríguez-Casado, A. and Ramírez de Molina, A., Dietary phytochemicals in cancer prevention and therapy: A complementary approach with promising perspectives, *Nutr. Rev.* 71(9), 585–99, 2013.
225. Heaney, R.P., Weaver, C.M. and Lee Fitzsimmons, M., Influence of calcium load on absorption fraction, *J. Bone Miner. Res.* 5(11), 1135–8, 1990.
226. Reid, I.R., Bolland, M.J., Avenell, A. and Grey, A., Cardiovascular effects of calcium supplementation, *Osteoporosis Int.* 22(6), 1649–58, 2011.
227. National Heart Foundation of Australia, Position Statement: Dietary fats and dietary sterols for cardiovascular health, National Heart Foundation of Australia, 2009.
228. National Heart Foundation of Australia, Position Statement: Fish, fish oils, n-3 polyunsaturated fatty acids and cardiovascular health, National Heart Foundation of Australia, 2008.
229. Soltan, S. and Gibson, R.A., Levels of omega 3 fatty acids in Australian seafood, *Asia Pac. J. Clin. Nutr.* 17(3), 385–90, 2008.
230. Ziegler, C.C. and Sidani, M.A., Diets for successful aging, *Clin. Geriatr. Med.* 27(4), 577–89, 2011.

13 Drug and Nutrient Interactions in Masters Athletes

Kathleen M. Knights and Arduino A. Mangoni

CONTENTS

13.1 INTRODUCTION

> Show me a drug with no side effects and I'll show you a drug with no actions.
>
> **Sir Derrick Dunlop**
> *1902–1980*

Herodicus, a sports physician from the fifth century BC, combined his knowledge of sports physiology and medicine advocating that physical health was a balance between a strict diet, regular training and physical activity [1]. The benefit of a simple balanced diet and regular exercise appears to have been lost prior to the Christian era. Galen (131 AD–201 AD), a Greek physician famed for his role as a surgeon to the gladiators of Pergamos is also, like Herodicus, considered a father of sports medicine [2].

In contrast to current accepted practices in the twenty-first century, Galen actively advocated the use of medications to enhance competitive performance which at that time was blood-thirsty gladiatorial combat. One can only speculate as to the effectiveness of Galen's concoction of the 'rear hooves of an Abyssinian ass, ground up, boiled in oil and flavoured with rose hips and rose petals'. However, the gladiators were not alone in using pharmacological enhancement. Ancient Olympic athletes are reported to have dined on sheep testicles (a source of testosterone) and to have liberally consumed a variety of plants (e.g. cola, cacti, hashish, fungi) and plant seeds in order to gain a competitive advantage. Clearly, the medication-fuelled ancient athletes exhibited both desirable and undesirable behaviours. Thus, it is not surprising that the ancient era of pharmacological enhancement ended with the banning of competitive 'pagan' sports including the Olympic Games in 393 AD.

What have we learned from the past? For sports physicians and athletes in ancient times, polypharmacy (the concurrent use of multiple medications) was the norm and any interactions between the 'medicines' and plant products they consumed were irrelevant as victory was paramount and lives were expendable. The probability is that some gladiators and athletes failed in the pursuit of glory simply because they may have been suffering from adverse reactions to ancient drug-plant concoctions. Times have changed and masters athletes and older exercisers are now lauded as examples of the benefits of healthy living and successful ageing. However, unlike athletes in the time of Herodicus, in the twenty-first century diet and regular exercise is complemented by the use of drugs and supplements for the treatment of acute and chronic diseases that are prevalent in the ageing population.

In the present chapter, the term 'drug' will be used to refer to prescribed, over-the counter (OTC) drugs and where applicable, illicit drugs and drugs of abuse. The term 'supplement' will, in general, refer to herbal medicines (e.g. St John's wort) and nutritional supplements (e.g. minerals and vitamins).

Globally, the majority of drugs which are prescribed are mainstream therapy used principally for the treatment of

- Infectious (microbial and parasitic) and neoplastic diseases (e.g. tumours)
- Chronic diseases (e.g. osteoporosis, rheumatoid arthritis, asthma, diabetes)
- Acute illnesses (e.g. poisoning)

Effective use of drugs has contributed to the control of both infectious diseases and acute illnesses. This has translated through to decreased mortality, increased life expectancy and better quality of life, principally in developed countries. The latter is evident from the projected increase of the world population of people aged >65 years to ~973 million by the year 2030 [3]. With this increased life expectancy, more and more of the older members of society are increasingly able to pursue physically active life styles often aided by drugs that control diseases such as ischaemic heart disease, diabetes, asthma and musculoskeletal disorders. Similarly, there has been an increase in the use of supplements. It is estimated that ~50% of the American population use prescription drugs and 54% use supplements [4]. Within the Australian population, use of supplements is comparable to the United States with an estimated use by ~50% of the Australian population [5].

With the use of both drugs and supplements, the ideal situation is one in which there is a demonstrated benefit to the individual with minimal adverse drug/supplement effects. Can we account for the physiological changes associated with ageing, increasing acute and chronic disease burden, drug/supplement use and the effect of exercise/physical exertion on the pharmacokinetics of drugs and have a 'healthy' competitive masters athlete or older exerciser? The reality is that ageing and the use of drugs and supplements is a recipe for drug-drug, drug-supplement (e.g. drug-herb, drug-nutrient, drug-vitamin interactions), drug-food, and supplement-food interactions. The incidence and clinical significance of these interactions is likely to increase with age, disease burden, drug dosage, duration of drug regimen, the number of drugs/supplements taken and the presence of malnutrition/gastrointestinal tract dysfunction. These interactions may occur through either lack of knowledge of the drugs and/or the supplements, poor labelling of medicinal products and/or accidental misuse of either the drug and/or the supplement. Importantly, several drug and drug classes are prescribed off-label (outside the licensed indication) in the older population. Therefore, the knowledge on specific adverse drug reactions and other toxic effects in this group is often limited in the pre-marketing phase.

Use of multiple drugs is common among the older population and considerable emphasis is placed on the acquisition of knowledge, currently limited as discussed above, and that identifies potential drug-drug interactions along with the subsequent clinical decisions that guide appropriate management. Unfortunately, unlike drug-drug interactions, the clinical relevance of drug-nutrient, drug-herb and drug-food interactions are less well characterised. However, with increasing awareness of the importance of drug-supplement and drug-food interactions, evidence-based reports are appearing more frequently in the literature that either document drug-nutrient and drug-supplement interactions [6–16] or report the absence of such an interaction [17,18].

In general, drug-nutrient interactions are defined as 'alterations of pharmacokinetics or pharmacodynamics of a drug or nutritional element or a compromise in nutritional status as a result of the addition of a drug' [5]. Pharmacokinetics is defined simplistically as 'what the body does to the drug' [19] and pharmacodynamics as 'what the drug does to the body' [20]. An interaction is considered clinically relevant if it significantly alters either the therapeutic response to or toxicity of the drug or compromises the nutritional status of the person. In considering drug-nutrient interactions in masters athletes and older exercisers it is essential to first consider age-related changes *per se* that can alter drug disposition; that is, the absorption, distribution, metabolism and excretion of drugs.

13.2 CHANGES IN PHARMACOKINETICS WITH AGEING

13.2.1 Drug Absorption

The majority of drug absorption occurs in the small intestine. Whether there are or are not significant changes in drug absorption with ageing is unclear due to the paucity of studies. No age-related changes in the absorption of a variety of drugs were reported by Gainsborough and others [21] but it is generally accepted that absorption of nutrients including calcium, iron, vitamin B_{12}, thiamine and folic acid may decrease with advancing age [22,23]. Relevant to drug/nutrient absorption are age-related decreases in gastric acid production, rate of gastric emptying, changes in splanchnic blood flow and intestinal motility [24]. Each of these factors may impact on drug and nutrient absorption but this may be offset by the large absorptive area available for passive diffusion of small molecular weight molecules. In the absence of overt gastrointestinal disease, the capacity for nutrient, and by inference, drug absorption in the older adult is probably sufficient [25].

13.2.2 Drug Distribution

Changes in body composition are significant with advancing age. These include

- Progressive reduction in lean body mass
- Progressive reduction in total body water (~4 L for men and 6 L for women from age 20–80 years [26])
- Relative increase in body fat

In pharmacokinetic terms, these changes lead to a change in the volume of distribution of a drug which relates the extent to which a drug is distributed to extravascular tissues throughout the body to the concentration of the drug that remains in the blood. Water-soluble drugs tend to have smaller volumes of distribution in older adults, which results in higher plasma concentrations as observed for the antidysrhythmic drug digoxin and the bronchodilator drug theophylline [23]. In contrast, if a drug is lipophilic (lipid-soluble), the volume of distribution increases because of the increase in body fat with ageing. This is important for the cardiovascular drug amiodarone which is commonly used for the treatment of dysrhythmias in the older population (e.g. atrial flutter and atrial fibrillation).

Chemically, drugs are generally considered to be either acidic (e.g. salicylic acid, warfarin) or basic (e.g. propanolol). When in blood, acidic drugs bind to albumin while basic drugs bind to alpha-1 acid glycoprotein. Age-related effects on either of these proteins are negligible but in the older adult the concentration of albumin may be reduced due to malnutrition or acute illness while the concentration of alpha-1 acid glycoprotein increases during acute illness [23]. As the effect of a drug is determined by the free (unbound) concentration of the drug, changes in the binding of drugs to albumin and alpha-1 acid glycoprotein can theoretically contribute to drug interactions or alter the physiological effect of a highly protein-bound drug. In reality clinical relevance of changes in the binding of drugs to plasma proteins is limited [27].

13.2.3 Drug Metabolism

Metabolism of orally administered drugs can occur in the small intestine and, following absorption, in the liver. This pre-systemic metabolism is often referred to as first-pass metabolism. An oral drug absorbed from the small intestine flows in the portal circulation to the liver which is the principal organ in humans that clears or extracts a drug from the blood. An active drug that escapes clearance by the liver enters into the systemic circulation, distributes to the site of action and then exerts its pharmacological effect. Subsequent passes through the liver of systemic blood containing the drug result in further metabolism until the parent drug is eliminated from the circulation.

Drug clearance by the liver depends on two factors: firstly, the capacity of the liver to extract the drug from blood (hepatic extraction ratio), and secondly, hepatic blood flow which is ~90 L/hour in a healthy 70-kg person. In general, drugs are defined by their hepatic extraction ratio into three classes: those with a high extraction (E) ratio $E > 0.7$ (e.g. glyceryl trinitrate, propanolol), intermediate extraction E 0.3–0.7 (e.g. aspirin, codeine) and low extraction ratio $E < 0.3$ (e.g. diazepam, theophylline, warfarin). When extraction is high, the clearance of the drug by the liver is dependent on liver blood flow. In contrast, for drugs with a low extraction ratio changes in blood flow have minimal impact on clearance of the drug by the liver. With ageing, reductions in liver blood flow principally affect drugs that have a high hepatic extraction ratio. More importantly, age-related reduction in liver volume may also reduce drug clearance [28].

Clearance of a drug by the liver occurs as a result of the action of hepatic enzymes that metabolise lipophilic chemicals into hydrophilic (water-soluble) metabolites that are readily eliminated in bile or urine. In the absence of metabolism, many drugs and supplements would accumulate in the body potentially causing toxicity. For the majority of drugs, the process of metabolism results in a diminution of biological activity. There are multiple enzyme families that metabolise drugs but of major importance in humans are the cytochromes P450 (CYP) and uridine 5′-diphosphoglucuronosyltransferase (UGT) enzyme families located in the endoplasmic reticulum of principally hepatocytes (liver) and enterocytes (gut). CYP catalyse functionalisation reactions (e.g. oxidation, reduction, hydrolysis reactions) that may either activate the drug in the case of inactive drugs (prodrugs) or reduce biological activity by modifying the chemical structure of the parent drug by forming a metabolite through the introduction or exposing of a functional group (e.g. $-COOH$, $-OH$, $-NH_2$ or $-SH$). Presence of specific functional groups in either the parent drug or the metabolite facilitates further metabolism by UGT enzymes that conjugate the parent drug or metabolite with glucuronic acid forming a glucuronide that is readily excreted in urine or bile. It is important to note that these enzymes, in addition to drugs, also metabolise environmental pollutants, agricultural and cosmetic products and processed food and food additives.

CYP exists as a large enzyme family that is grouped in subfamilies. There are 12 CYPs in families 1–3 (CYP1A1, 1A2, 1B1, 2A6, 2B6, 2C8, 2C9, 2C19, 2D6, 2E1, 3A4 and 3A5) that are important for drug metabolism in humans. Of these, CYP3A4 is responsible for the metabolism of ~50% of all clinically used drugs including those used to treat cardiovascular and gastrointestinal diseases commonly found in older populations. The activities of CYP enzymes are markedly altered by severe malnutrition [29]. Pharmacokinetic studies have also demonstrated age-related reduction in the clearance of many drugs metabolised by oxidation (phase I) reactions [23,30,31].

Similar to the CYP enzymes, UGTs exist as a large gene family with enzymes of the UGT1 and UGT2 families involved in the metabolism of numerous drugs and other chemicals including fatty acids and steroid hormones. In humans, the principal UGTs involved in drug metabolism are UGT1A1, 1A3, 1A4, 1A6, 1A9, 2B7 and 2B15 [32]. Similar to CYP, the activities of UGT enzymes are influenced by hormonal factors, diet, disease states, ethnicity and genetic polymorphisms in the genes encoding UGT proteins [32–34]. In contrast to the effect of advancing age on CYP activity, the situation is less clear with the activity of UGT enzymes but in general glucuronidation pathways appears to be less significantly altered [28].

13.2.4 Drug Excretion

All aspects of renal function decline with increasing age, independent of the presence or absence of co-existing disease states. These include decreases in renal blood flow, glomerular filtration, active tubular secretion and passive tubular reabsorption. On average, glomerular filtration rate (GFR) declines ~1 mL/minute each year from age 40 years onward. In healthy young adults GFR is ~120 mL/minute so by age 80 years a substantial degree of renal impairment may be present. This reduction in GFR affects the renal excretion of multiple drugs and drug metabolites including digoxin, diuretics, lithium, non-steroidal anti-inflammatory drugs and several antibiotics. For this reason, dosage adjustment is recommended for drugs with a narrow therapeutic index such as aminoglycoside antibiotics, digoxin and lithium. Reduced excretion of these drugs results in drug accumulation and the resultant higher plasma concentrations may cause serious adverse effects. There is also increasing evidence that chronic kidney disease impairs the non-renal disposition of drugs primarily metabolised by the liver [35].

Estimates of renal function are problematic with ageing as serum creatinine concentrations may be within the normal range even though renal function and lean body mass may have declined. Both the Cockcroft-Gault and Modification of Diet in Renal Disease [36] equations use serum creatinine concentrations, age, body weight and gender and could be potentially useful to calculate adjustments in drug dosage in situations of mild–moderate renal impairment. However, large-scale studies are required to test the applicability of these equations in the clinical setting and specifically in masters athletes and older exercisers.

13.3 CHANGES IN PHARMACODYNAMICS WITH AGEING

As would be expected when taking drugs or supplements, the intention is to achieve a desirable therapeutic effect while at the same time avoiding toxicity. The effect of most chemical entities occurs as a result of an interaction with a molecular target, for example a receptor (e.g. β–adrenoceptor), an enzyme (e.g. 3-hydroxy-3-methylglutaryl-coenzyme A reductase), an ion channel (e.g. calcium channels) or a transporter (e.g. the efflux transporter P-glycoprotein). When taking drugs or supplements, there is an assumed relationship between the dose taken, the concentration of the drug/supplement in blood and the effect produced. With ageing the concentration of drug in blood may be altered by changes in pharmacokinetics which in turn will alter the pharmacodynamic response to the drug/supplement [37]. In addition, age-related changes occur in molecular targets with a reduction in receptor number, the binding affinity of the drug or alterations in receptor-transduction mechanisms [38].

TABLE 13.1
Changes That Occur with Ageing in Response to Selected Drugs

Drug	Drug Class	Examples of Clinical Indications	Pharmacodynamic Effect	Age-Related Change
		Drugs Used to Treat Cardiovascular Disorders		
Adenosine	Antidysrhythmic	Acute supraventricular tachycardia	Decreased heart rate	No change [22]
Diltiazem	Calcium channel blocker	Angina, hypertension, supraventricular dysrhythmias	Vasodilation, decreased heart rate	Increased response [34]
Frusemide	Diuretic	Heart failure, renal impairment	Diuresis	Decreased response [22]
Isoprenaline	β receptor agonist	Heart block/bradycardia	Increased heart rate and increased cardiac output	Decreased response [22]
Propanolol	β receptor antagonist (β blocker)	Angina, hypertension, tachydysrhythmias	Decreased heart rate and contractility	Decreased response [35]
Verapamil	Calcium channel blocker	Angina, hypertension, supraventricular dysrhythmias	Prolongation of PR interval, decreased heart rate	Decreased response [34]
		Drugs Used to Treat or Prevent Thromboembolism		
Heparin	Anticoagulant	Treatment or prevention of venous thromboembolism	Anticoagulation	No change [22]
Warfarin	Anticoagulant	Treatment or prevention of venous thromboembolism (e.g. prevention in persons with prosthetic heart valves)	Anticoagulation	Increased response [36]

Overlaying these molecular changes are age-related alterations in homeostatic mechanisms including dysregulation of blood pressure, heart rate, blood glucose concentration, oxygen consumption and changes in haemostasis. These homeostatic changes may manifest in several ways in older exercisers including decreased response of the heart to stress and released catecholamines, decreased glycaemic control and hence an increased susceptibility to drug-induced hypoglycaemia, and decreased pulmonary function and response to hypoxia. In addition, it is well recognised that older patients are more sensitive to the anticoagulant effects of warfarin (increased risk of bleeding) but the exact mechanism is unknown [39]. Table 13.1 provides examples of changes that occur with ageing in the response to selected drugs.

13.4 EFFECT OF EXERCISE (ENDURANCE) TRAINING ON PHARMACOKINETICS

Exercise training or endurance exercise, defined as exercise repeated >3 times/week [40], has the potential to alter the pharmacokinetics of drugs. Exercise is known to decrease splanchnic blood flow thus potentially decreasing drug absorption of orally administered drugs while decrease in liver and renal blood flow may impair drug elimination. In addition, during exercise changes occur in respiratory function, gastric emptying rate and metabolic enzyme activity [41]. The interplay of various physiological systems during exercise is complex and to date there are a limited number of studies published which are not comparable because of different experimental methods including the age distribution, gender, degree of physical activity and route of administration and the type of drug studied. For further information on the impact of exercise on drug pharmacokinetics see [42–44]. The following list summarises the effect of exercise training on pharmacokinetics from a number of studies.

- Minimal change in absorption of orally administered drugs and a potential increase in absorption of drugs administered via the intramuscular or subcutaneous routes or from transdermal patches. When exercising with a glyceryl trinitrate (GTN) transdermal patch (common use) in place, increased plasma concentration of GTN has been reported both during and after exercise [45]. This may be explained by increased skin temperature, hydration and blood flow. Theoretically, the increased absorption of GTN during exercise might provide positive health benefits in patients with ischaemic heart disease because of increased coronary vasodilatation. However, this benefit might be offset by an excessive GTN-induced reduction in diastolic blood pressure and reduced coronary perfusion. Increased absorption during leg exercise (50% more than at rest) has also been reported with subcutaneous insulin. The increase in insulin absorption was observed when insulin was injected in the leg, but not when it was injected in the arm or into the abdomen [46]. When using nicotine patches, a similar increase in the plasma concentration of nicotine was reported [47].
- Plasma volume commonly decreases ~10%–15% during exercise and as a result the volume of distribution of some drugs has also been reported to vary during exercise. These changes include a decrease in the volume of distribution of the β-blocker propranolol and the calcium channel blocker verapamil, but no change with the β-blocker atenolol [48]. However, the clinical significance of these changes is unknown.
- Exercise of moderate- to high-intensity also reduces hepatic blood flow by ~60% [49] and thus it would be anticipated the extraction of high clearance drugs (E > 0.7) may be affected. The results are contradictory with some studies reporting decreases in the extraction of high-clearance drugs such as propranolol and verapamil while others failed to show a difference [44]. In terms of drug/supplement metabolism, the impact of exercise on the activity of hepatic CYP and UGT enzymes in humans is unknown [50].
- As discussed earlier in this chapter, the main route of excretion of drugs, supplements and their metabolites is principally via urine. Exercise decreases renal blood flow (~53%) and hence glomerular filtration rate. The decrement in renal function (both renal blood flow and glomerular filtration rate) is greater with intense exercise [51]. Similarly, reductions in creatinine clearance and urine volume follow the changes in renal blood flow [52]. Drugs that are excreted as parent drug with little or no hepatic metabolism are the most likely to be affected by exercise-induced changes in renal function. Limited evidence suggests physical exercise impairs the excretion of atenolol (excreted >90% as unchanged drug in urine), which causes an increase in the plasma concentration of *S*-atenolol, the clinical significance of which is unclear [43].
- Studies in young adults reported significant changes in the pharmacokinetics of theophylline, digoxin, and warfarin with increasing levels of physical exercise. A significant prolongation in the half-life of the bronchodilator theophylline and a reduced clearance were observed during and 4 hours post-exercise in six healthy volunteers [53]. This phenomenon is unlikely to be secondary to changes in liver blood flow, as theophylline has a low hepatic extraction ratio. More research is warranted to confirm these findings in view of the narrow therapeutic index of theophylline. Other studies have shown a significant reduction in serum digoxin concentrations during exercise. This phenomenon seems to be due to an increasing binding to actively working muscles as there was a concomitant increase in the skeletal muscle concentration of digoxin [54]. Finally, a significant decrease in the international normalized ratio (INR) was reported in three subjects following an increase in their physical activity levels. However, no pharmacokinetic data were collected and the mechanisms involved could not be identified [55].

It should be emphasised that many studies investigating the impact of exercise on the pharmacokinetics of drugs have used fit healthy young adults undertaking single bouts of physical exercise.

With masters athletes and older exercisers there are many unanswered questions regarding both the impact of ageing and physical exercise on the pharmacokinetics of drugs.

13.5 DRUG-NUTRIENT INTERACTIONS

Drug-nutrient interactions is a vast field especially considering the number of drugs and supplements available worldwide. In consideration of the focus of this book, only drug-nutrient interactions most likely to occur in masters athletes and older exercisers will be considered. This narrows the field principally to drug-nutrient interactions involving drugs used to treat diseases of the cardiovascular, respiratory and musculoskeletal systems. Where relevant, other drugs or supplements that may be used for acute conditions will be discussed. As previously documented, ~34% of masters athletes predominately aged >55 years take drugs for the management of cardiovascular and respiratory diseases [56]. Comparable with the general population, supplement use is higher with 60.5% of participants at the 2004 World Masters Indoor Athletic Championships indicating they took vitamins (35.4%) and minerals (29.9%) [57].

Similar to classifications schemes for adverse drug reactions, numerous schemes have been developed to aid classification of drug-nutrient interactions. No one scheme covers all drug-nutrient interactions which may have different frequencies of occurrence, different mechanisms of interaction and different clinical manifestations. In general, four types of drug-nutrient interactions (Type I–Type IV) have been described in the literature. However, they are not ideal because the types of interactions described have overlapping similarities [6,8]. In view of the complexity of ageing, disease burden and drug and supplement use interactions will be discussed in relation to effects on two of the four pharmacokinetic parameters: absorption and metabolism. The impact of either food or nutrients on either the distribution or renal excretion of drug or supplements in masters athletes or indeed the older adult remains to be documented.

It should be recognised that the evidence for many drug-food, drug-nutrient, drug-herb interactions occurring *in vivo* is very limited. Many potential interactions are based on *in vitro* data often from animal studies or are theoretical, based on the known pharmacology of the drug/supplement.

13.5.1 Absorption

13.5.1.1 Effect of Food on Drug Absorption

Food may affect both the extent and rate of absorption of a drug or supplement although the interaction may or may not be clinically important. These changes can either increase or decrease drug/supplement absorption. Both the type of food consumed and the formulation of the drug/supplement may also have an effect on absorption. At the simplest level, a direct physical interaction may occur between food and the drug/supplement. This includes food acting as a physical barrier reducing dissolution of the drug and preventing access to the mucosa of the small intestine, hence decreasing absorption, and food-induced changes in gastrointestinal motility and/or gastrointestinal secretions. The latter may be augmented by age-related changes in gastric emptying which, is ~50 minutes in young, healthy adults increasing to as much as 120 minutes in persons aged over 77 years [58]. Food-induced delays in gastric emptying rate are clinically relevant for drugs that are acid-labile (susceptible to degradation by gastric acid). These include the antibiotics erythromycin and the penicillins and the proton pump inhibitor omeprazole used in the treatment of peptic ulcer disease and gastrointestinal reflux.

Food components can infrequently bind or chelate drugs. The best example of this is the reduced absorption of the tetracycline antibiotics through chelation with calcium found in dairy products. In general, food-drug interactions are less frequent with drugs administered in solution than those administered as tablets or capsules. In addition to food-induced alteration in the extent of absorption, food can decrease the rate of absorption of a drug/supplement without having an overall effect on the total amount of drug/supplement absorbed. For these reasons it is important to remain consistent and in line with the product information as to whether the drug/supplement should be taken with food or separated from food intake by several hours.

13.5.1.1.1 Reduced Drug Absorption

A key example of a drug class where absorption is reduced by food is the bisphosphonates (e.g. alendronate) used in the treatment of osteoporosis. In general, the bioavailability of alendronate is low (<1%) but it is further reduced by food by ~40% if taken 1–2 h before food ingestion and by as much as 90% if taken up to 2 h after ingestion of food [59]. Further observation that alendronate forms insoluble complexes with calcium and magnesium led to the recommendation that alendronate should be taken after an overnight fast on an empty stomach with a full glass of water 30 minutes prior to food. The absorption of many drugs has been reported to be reduced by food but many of the studies have been conducted in healthy volunteers using a single dose of drug and the composition of the food ingested varied enormously [60].

13.5.1.1.2 Increased Drug Absorption

Often certain types of food (e.g. a high-fat meal) have been used intentionally to increase absorption of a particular drug by enhancing solubility. This is the case with the antifungal drug griseofulvin and the antiprotozoal drug atovaquone [61]. For other drugs, studies have demonstrated increased drug absorption with high-carbohydrate diets and intermediate effects on absorption with high-protein meals. For example, metoprolol and propanolol (both β-blockers) are better absorbed after meals not because food enhances absorption *per se* but rather because food increases splanchnic blood flow and reduces presystemic metabolism [62]. In masters athletes and older exercisers there are no data that specifically indicate whether food alters absorption of the commonly used drug groups.

13.5.1.2 Effect of Drugs on Nutrient Absorption

Similar to the effects of food on drug absorption, drugs can alter absorption of nutrients and these are the most commonly reported interactions. Drug-induced malabsorption can be specific for one particular nutrient or it may occur with a class of nutrients such as fat-soluble vitamins. Mechanisms underlying malabsorption include adsorption of the nutrient or of bile acids essential for nutrient solubilisation, decrease in intestinal mucosal integrity, changes in gastrointestinal motility and intraluminal pH and composition of intestinal flora. The following section details examples of drug-induced changes in nutrient absorption that may be relevant to masters athletes and older exercisers.

Non-steroidal anti-inflammatory drugs (NSAIDs) such as aspirin, diclofenac, indomethacin, ibuprofen and naproxen can all cause gastrointestinal ulceration principally as a result of inhibition of synthesis of mucosal protective prostaglandins. This adverse effect is directly related to the mechanism of action of these drugs, which is inhibition of the cyclooxygenase (COX) enzymes that are responsible for the synthesis of eicosanoids (local signalling molecules that act like local hormones). NSAID-induced perturbation of mucosal integrity, which also includes small haemorrhages, may result in iron deficiency anaemia and decreased absorption of vitamin C, glucose, xylose and amino acids [22,63]. Drugs that alter gastric acid secretion like the proton pump inhibitors (e.g. omeprazole, pantoprazole) and H_2 receptor antagonists (e.g. cimetidine, ranitidine) may alter vitamin B_{12} status [64] while chronic alcohol use is well known to alter nutrient status [65].

The bile acid binding resins (e.g. cholestyramine and colestipol) used to treat hyperlipidaemia act as their name implies by binding bile acids. These anionic-exchange resins not only bind bile salts but also bind calcium, iron, zinc, folic acid, β-carotene and vitamins A, B_{12}, D and K [66]. Thus, use of these drugs in older athletes may contribute to deficiencies of essential minerals and vitamins.

Changes in nutrient absorption also occur with many common OTC drugs including antacids and laxatives. Antacids either through a change in the pH of the stomach and/or small intestine or through the formation of non-absorbable salts can impact negatively on an individual's magnesium, phosphate, iron, copper, folic acid and riboflavin status [67,68]. Several different types of laxatives (e.g. stimulant, osmotic, bulking agents, stool softeners) are commonly used in older patients. Clinically diagnosed laxative abuse has been extensively documented from case reports to cause adverse health outcomes including deficiencies of vitamin D, vitamin B_{12}, calcium, potassium and glucose. In terms of vitamin B_{12}, oat bran as an alternative to a laxative improves vitamin B_{12} bioavailability [69].

13.5.2 Metabolism

13.5.2.1 Effect of Food on Drug Metabolism

This section will consider the interaction between dietary constituents and specific drug metabolising enzymes that are of clinical relevance. As discussed previously, the CYP enzyme of greatest importance in drug metabolism is CYP3A4. It is expressed in both the gut wall and the liver and plays an important role in both presystemic and systemic metabolism. Numerous drug-drug interactions have been reported with CYP3A4 which has a wide drug substrate and inhibitor profile. The ability of CYP3A4 to metabolise many drug substrates results from multiple substrate-binding sites within the enzyme. The differential effect of various drug inhibitors suggests that the effect of food constituents on CYP3A4 activity may not be universally predictable.

13.5.2.1.1 Grapefruit Juice

The interaction with grapefruit juice (GFJ) was first discovered when it was used to mask the taste of ethanol (used as the drug vehicle) in a study involving administration of the calcium antagonist felodipine. The investigators noted that the presystemic clearance of felodipine was reduced increasing systemic exposure and amplifying the pharmacodynamic effects of the drug [70]. Extensive investigation has determined that GFJ reduces the activity of CYP3A4 by both competitive and non-competitive interactions as well as through a true loss in activity [71]. Following ingestion of GFJ, intestinal CYP3A4 activity declines by 47% within 4 hours but the enhancing effect on the bioavailability of a drug persists for at least 24 hours [72]. Complete recovery from the effect of GFJ takes up to 72 hours after the last ingestion of the juice [73]. The active constituents in GFJ include the flavonoids naringin, narigenin, quercetin and kaempferol and the furanocoumarins bergamottin and dihydroxybergamottin. The absolute causative substance in GFJ has not been identified and it may well be a synergist effect of the flavonoids, furanocoumarins and other substances found in GFJ.

A number of the calcium channel blockers interact with GFJ and the most prominent is felodipine. Other drugs reported to show an increased plasma concentration with GFJ include cyclosporin, terfenadine, saquinavir, sirolimus, tacrolimus, simvastatin and midazolam [15,74]. In addition to the effect of CYP3A4, GFJ is also reported to be an inhibitor of the efflux transporter P-glycoprotein found in the small bowel which would increase absorption into the portal circulation [74]. Similar to GFJ, an interaction has been reported with orange juice from Seville oranges which contain similar quantities of dihydroxybergamottin as GFJ [74]. Consumption of other types of fruit juice (e.g. tangerine juice) does not appear to alter CYP3A4 activity.

13.5.2.1.2 Cranberry Juice

Anecdotal case reports led to the issue of warnings regarding a suspected interaction between cranberry juice and the anticoagulant warfarin. To date a number of randomised clinical trials have investigated whether cranberry juice affects the metabolism of warfarin. Warfarin is a racemate (an equal mixture of right- and left-handed molecules) and *S*-warfarin is more biologically active than *R*-warfarin. *S*-warfarin is metabolised by CYP2C9 while *R*-warfarin is metabolised by CYP3A4 and CYP1A2. Of seven studies conducted to date, in only one study in which 12 healthy males received concentrated cranberry extract tablets was an interaction with warfarin demonstrated. Despite the enhanced pharmacodynamics response to warfarin, the concentrated cranberry extract did not alter the metabolism of either *R*- or *S*-warfarin [75]. Of the remaining studies in which an interaction was not demonstrated, all used commercially available cranberry juice [76]. The differences in the study results may be explained by the use of a concentrated extract which does not mimic the usual practice of the consumption of cranberry juice. In addition, it is well recognised that different brands of cranberry juice vary in their composition of flavonoids and in the percentage of cranberry juice present [77]. The bulk of evidence suggest no clinically relevant interaction between warfarin and cranberry juice when consumed in limited quantities of <600 mL daily [76].

13.5.2.1.3 Cruciferous and Other Vegetables

Studies initially conducted in animals demonstrated that cruciferous vegetables (e.g. cabbage, cauliflower, broccoli, brussels sprouts) increased hepatic and intestinal CYP1A activity [74]. CYP1A2 is important in the metabolism of the bronchodilator theophylline, the analgesic phenacetin and caffeine. Results of human studies in which participants were fed the same diet for six successive days are variable with increased CYP1A2 activity demonstrated with a diet rich in cruciferous vegetables (radish sprouts, broccoli, cabbage and cauliflower), no change with allium vegetables (chives, garlic, leeks, onions) and a decrease in CYP1A2 activity with a diet supplemented with apiaceous vegetables (carrot, celery, dill weed, parsley and parsnip) [78]. The latter may be explained by the presence of furanocoumarins in apiaceous vegetables a situation analogous to the inhibitory effect on CYP3A4 by furanocoumarins found in GFJ.

13.6 EFFECTS OF NUTRIENTS/HERBAL SUPPLEMENTS ON DRUG THERAPY

13.6.1 Vitamins

It is variously reported that a single dose of vitamin C (2 g daily) decreases the bioavailability of the β-blocker propanolol [79] while supraphysiologic doses of vitamin E reduce platelet aggregation that may be additive to the antiplatelet effect of aspirin and the anticoagulant effect of warfarin [12]. Of greater importance is the diminution in the therapeutic effect of warfarin by supplements containing high quantities of vitamin K. Warfarin exerts it anticoagulant effect by inhibiting the conversion of oxidised vitamin K epoxide by the enzyme vitamin K reductase to its active reduced form, vitamin K hydroquinone. This results in the decreased synthesis of the vitamin-K-dependent coagulation factors. Increased intake of vitamin K via dietary means or by taking an additional compounded supplement may diminish the therapeutic effect of warfarin, increasing the likelihood of thromboembolic events [80]. Vitamin K is required to prevent possible reduction in bone mineral density in individuals taking warfarin chronically and it is essential to maintain a consistent intake of vitamin K that maintains a stable INR [12]. Avoiding drastic changes in vitamin K intake will assist in limiting the probability of bleeding and hence monitoring of INR is imperative.

13.6.2 Minerals

Large doses of mineral supplements (e.g. calcium, iron, magnesium, zinc) commonly used by athletes of all ages may interfere with the absorption of several antibiotics including the tetracyclines (e.g. doxycycline) and the quinolones (e.g. ciprofloxacin, norfloxacin) by forming insoluble complexes. Potassium supplements should be avoided in individuals taking angiotensin-converting enzyme inhibitors (e.g. captopril, enalapril), angiotensin receptor blockers (e.g. losartan) and

TABLE 13.2
Drug Interactions with St John's Wort

Drug	Effect of St John's Wort	Clinical Outcome
Amitriptyline (antidepressant)	Increased metabolism	Decreased antidepressant effect
Alprazolam (anxiolytic)	Increased metabolism	Increased anxiety
Cyclosporin (immunosuppressant)	Increased metabolism, increased efflux	Transplant rejection
Digoxin (cardiac glycoside)	Increased efflux	Sub-therapeutic plasma concentration
Methadone (used in opioid dependence)	Increased metabolism	Withdrawal symptoms
Oral contraceptives	Increased metabolism	Breakthrough bleeding, pregnancy
Selective serotonin uptake inhibitors (SSRIs) (antidepressants)	Increased concentration of serotonin	Serotonin syndrome (e.g. confusion, agitation)
Simvastatin (lipid lowering drug)	Increased metabolism	Decreased cholesterol lowering effect
Theophylline (bronchodilator)	Increased metabolism	Decreased bronchodilation
Warfarin (anticoagulant)	Increased metabolism	Decreased anticoagulant effect

potassium-sparing diuretics (e.g. amiloride, spironolactone) because of the risk of life-threatening hyperkalaemia.

13.6.3 St John's Wort

St John's wort (*Hypericum perforatum*) is a herbal product commonly used in the treatment of depression. Similar to all plant-derived products it is a complex mixture of dozens of constituents. The major constituent that exerts an antidepressant effect is hyperforin which inhibits neuronal reuptake of the transmitters, serotonin, noradrenaline and dopamine [81]. In addition to its effect on neurotransmitters, St John's wort (SJW) is also an inducer of CYP3A4 activity. This might reduce the bioavailability of a large number of drugs, potentially leading to reduced therapeutic efficacy (see Table 13.2) [82]. The enhanced activity of CYP3A4 persists for weeks after stopping SJW [15].

In addition to the effects on CYP3A4, SJW is also an inducer of the intestinal transporter P-glycoprotein, thus increasing efflux of drugs back into the intestine thereby decreasing bioavailability [83]. As CYP3A4 and P-glycoprotein are important regulators of the oral bioavailability of drugs, the negative impact of SJW on the intended therapeutic response can be profound. Many more herb-drug interactions have been reported from *in vitro* studies and the clinical implications of many remain to be established in humans [82].

13.7 DRUG-INDUCED CHANGES IN ELECTROLYTE STATUS

Many drugs, by virtue of either their mechanism of action or by changes in homeostasis, can alter fluid and electrolyte balance and thus the thermoregulation system in masters athletes. These changes may be clinically insignificant and no action is required in terms of either dose adjustment or ceasing drug administration. However, in some circumstances changes in electrolytes may be significant and impact negatively on the health status of the individual. Changes in electrolytes and fluid balance may be further compromised under circumstances of dehydration and sustained physical exercise especially at higher ambient temperatures. Table 13.3 provides examples of drug-induced changes in electrolytes that may occur with common drug classes used in the treatment of cardiovascular and musculoskeletal conditions.

TABLE 13.3
Examples of Drug-Induced Changes in Electrolyte Status

Drug Class	Action	Adverse Effects
	Cardiovascular Drugs	
Aldosterone antagonists Epleronone, spironolactone	Inhibition of the action of aldosterone in the kidney leads to reduced sodium reabsorption and reduced potassium excretion.	Hyperkalaemia, hyponatraemia, hypochloraemia.
Diuretics		
Loop (e.g. frusemide)	Inhibit reabsorption of sodium and chloride in ascending limb of Loop of Henle in the kidney.	Hypokalaemia, hyponatraemia, hypomagnesaemia, hyperuricaemia, hypocalcaemia.
Thiazide (e.g. hydrochlorothiazide)	Inhibit reabsorption of sodium and chloride in distal convoluted tubule of the kidney, corresponding increase in potassium excretion.	Hypokalaemia, hyponatraemia, hyperuricaemia, hypochloraemic alkalosis, hypomagnesaemia.
Potassium sparing (e.g. amiloride)	Inhibit sodium reabsorption in distal tubule of kidney, reduce potassium excretion.	Hyperkalaemia, hyponatraemia, hypochloraemia.
Angiotensin converting enzyme (ACE) inhibitors (e.g captopril, enalapril, perindopril)	Inhibit the conversion of angiotensin I to angiotensin II thereby reducing the effects of angiotensin-II-induced vasoconstriction, aldosterone release and sodium retention.	Hyperkalaemia
Sartans (e.g. candesartan, losartan, telmisartan)	Block the action of angiotensin II producing the same effects as ACE inhibitors.	Hyperkalaemia
	Musculoskeletal Drugs	
NSAIDs (e.g. celecoxib, diclofenac, ibuprofen, meloxicam, naproxen)	Inhibition of COX-1 and COX-2 thereby inhibiting synthesis of prostaglandins.	Sodium and water retention, hyperkalaemia.
Corticosteroids (e.g. betamethasone, dexamethasone, hydrocortisone, prednisolone)	Regulate expression of genes involved in inflammation and immune responses, electrolyte balance, endocrine function etc.	Sodium and water retention, hypokalaemia, hypokalaemic alkalosis, hypocalcaemia.

13.8 RULES GOVERNING MEDICATION/SUPPLEMENT USE

Use of drugs or supplements in sports at both the masters level and the internationally competitive arena is governed by the World Anti-Doping Agency (WADA) (http://www.wada-ama.org). Each year the WADA publishes a list of substances that are prohibited at all times both in and out of competition and substances that are prohibited in competition.

> A substance or method shall be considered for inclusion on the Prohibited List if WADA determines that the substance or method meets any two of the following three criteria:
> 4.3.1.1 Medical or other scientific evidence, pharmacological effect or experience that the substance or method, alone or in combination with other substances or methods, has the potential to enhance or enhances sport performance;
> 4.3.1.2 Medical or other scientific evidence, pharmacological effect or experience that the use of the substance or method represents an actual or potential health risk to the athlete;
> 4.3.1.3 WADA's determination that the use of the substance or method violates the spirit of sport described in the Introduction to the Code.
>
> **World Anti-Doping Code 2009, http://www.wada-ama.org**

The International Masters Games Association (IMGA) is a signatory to the WADA code and the IMGA Anti-Doping Rules incorporate the WADA Prohibited List. The drugs prohibited at all times includes the broad categories of

- S0: non-approved substances (e.g. drugs in development, discontinued drugs, veterinary medicines)
- S1: anabolic agents, which includes anabolic androgenic steroids and other anabolic agents including selective androgen receptor modulators (SARMs)
- S2: hormones, growth factors and related substances
- S3: beta-2 agonists
- S4: hormone and metabolic modulators
- S5: diuretics and other masking agents peptide

As well as substances prohibited in competition, including

- S6: stimulants
- S7: narcotics
- S8: cannabinoids
- S9: glucocorticoids

As well as substances prohibited in particular sports, including

- P1: alcohol
- P2: beta-blockers

In terms of the WADA prohibited list, there are many drugs that may be used chronically in the older population. These include tibolone (S1) used for the short-term treatment of menopausal symptoms and for osteoporosis; insulins (S2) for diabetes; raloxifene (S4) for post-menopausal osteoporosis and for breast cancer risk reduction; tamoxifen and toremifene (S4) for hormone receptor positive breast cancer; diuretics (S5) used in the treatment of heart failure and hypertension; glucocorticoids (S9) commonly used for acute severe asthma and autoimmune and inflammatory diseases and beta-blockers (P2) also used in the treatment of hypertension.

It is apparent that many masters athletes may be prescribed a banned substance for a chronic medical condition. Hence, the need to seek a Therapeutic Use Exemption (TUE) prior to competing in masters events. The current list does not include nutraceuticals, complementary alternative medicines, or other botanical-derived products that may contain traces of banned substances. In addition, the list does not alert masters athletes to the issues of contamination of supplements with banned substances, for example methylhexaneamine (S6). As with the ancient athletes, masters athletes should be alert to the fact that many 'natural products' contain powerful pharmacological agents that just might be on the WADA banned list. They are strongly advised to speak to their family doctor about any of the medications they use and their use in competitive sport. For a detailed discussion of the role of supplements in masters athletes, see Chapter 10.

13.9 CONCLUSION

It is widely accepted that older adults are the largest consumers of prescription drugs. A recent study conducted in the Unites States in community-dwelling residents aged 57–85 years found that 81% used at least one prescription drug, 42% used at least one OTC medication, 49% used a dietary supplement and 29% used at least five drugs concurrently [84]. Not surprisingly, the study found that overall 4% of the individuals were at risk of a major drug-drug interaction, half of which involved the use of non-prescription medications [84].

Use of supplements in masters athletes appears higher (~60%) in comparison to the older population [57] and as with drug-drug interactions, dietary supplements have the potential to interact with prescribed drugs. Thus masters athletes and older exercisers are likely to be at risk of both drug-nutrient and drug-supplement interactions that impact negatively on health outcomes. It is likely that many interactions remain unreported and are simply mistaken as either an indication of inadequate drug dosing or as an adverse drug reaction.

In the absence of a universal approach to the management of drug-nutrient and drug-supplement interactions, considerations should be given to firstly identifying the short- and long-term clinical consequences of the interaction as determined by the presence of clinical symptoms and changes in clinical chemistry/haematology laboratory parameters. Secondly, ascertain by discussion with the family doctor if dosage adjustment is required for either the drug or supplement, or whether alternative treatment options should be considered. The latter would be considerably easier if full knowledge of the mechanism of the interaction was available. However, in many instances our knowledge of drug-supplement interactions is incomplete. In the simplest situation, an interaction may occur as a result of taking both the drug and supplement at the same time and the remedy would be to separate the time of administration. In contrast, pharmacokinetic interactions may be more problematic, not easily deconstructed and a practical approach to the management of the interaction may be difficult to achieve.

Food-drug, nutrient-drug, herb-drug, dietary supplement-drug interactions are not going to cease to exist. The challenge is to increase our knowledge of how dietary factors and supplement use improve or decrease drug efficacy in the ageing adult. For sports medicine professionals, clinicians and individuals this would provide the opportunity to design programs that facilitate the use of drugs (for chronic conditions associated with ageing), dietary interventions and supplements that limit/avoid adverse interactions and promote the health and well-being of the ageing athlete.

13.10 IMPLICATIONS FOR SPORTS MEDICINE PROFESSIONALS AND CLINICIANS

- The burden of disease in the older population commonly relates to the cardiovascular, respiratory and musculoskeletal systems. These conditions generally require acute and/or long-term pharmacological management with a combination of drugs. The older population represents the main consumer of drugs in the developed world.
- There is a lack of evidence of drug-nutrient, drug-supplement interactions, and their clinical relevance, in masters athletes and older exercisers.
- For masters athletes and older exercisers with ischaemic heart disease, increased transdermal absorption of glyceryl trinitrate during exercise may be beneficial to maintain coronary perfusion during physical stress. However, this may be offset by an excessive reduction in diastolic pressure, with consequent reduction in coronary blood flow, that occurs at high ambient temperatures [85].
- Masters athletes and older exercisers may be at a higher risk of other exercise-induced changes in the pharmacokinetics of commonly prescribed drugs in this age group such as insulin, digoxin and theophylline. However, the clinical significance of the reported exercise-induced changes in pharmacokinetics remains to be established, particularly in older subjects. Health care professionals should be alert to changes in the clinical condition that may suggest insulin-related hypoglycaemia, reduced efficacy of digoxin or theophylline toxicity. A close clinical monitoring of these patients is advisable, particularly when these drugs are commenced, or their dose is changed.

13.11 IMPLICATIONS FOR MASTERS ATHLETES AND COACHES

- Masters athletes, older exercisers and coaches should be educated in recognising early symptoms related to exercise-induced changes in pharmacokinetics. For example, increased absorption of GTN and insulin with onset of dizziness, light-headedness, and paradoxical angina (GTN) or fatigue, excessive sweating, dizziness, or pre-syncope (insulin).
- It is particularly important that these symptoms are fully recognised when (a) the type or intensity of exercise is changed; (b) a specific drug is started or its dose changed, or (c) a master athlete or older exerciser is training alone.
- Information on specific drug-related symptoms during exercise should be communicated to health care professionals not aware of the patient's previous medical history (e.g. admitting doctors in case of hospital admission or new medical practitioners).

13.12 FUTURE RESEARCH DIRECTIONS

- Systematic investigation of the magnitude and clinical significance of drug-supplement interactions in different age bands of masters athletes and older exercisers with different disease burden. Ideally, such studies should investigate the effects of both acute and chronic drug therapy.
- The development of a systematic approach to elucidate the mechanisms of specific drug-supplement interactions in ageing athletes.
- The development of strategies to assist in the practical management of drug-supplement interactions that allow the treatment of disease states in the ageing athlete and avoid adverse health outcomes.

REFERENCES

1. Georgoulis, A.D., Kiapidou, I.D., Velogianni, L., Stergiou, N. and Boland, A., Herodicus, the father of sports medicine, *Knee Surg. Sports Traumatol. Arthrosc.* 15, 315–8, 2007.
2. Snook, G.A., The father of sports medicine (Galen), *Am. J. Sports Med.* 6, 128–31, 1978.
3. Centers for Disease Control and Prevention, Public health and aging: Trends in aging—United States and worldwide, *JAMA* 289(11), 1371–3, 2003.
4. Kaufman, D.W., Kelly, J.P., Rosenberg, L., Anderson, T.E. and Mitchell, A.A., Recent patterns of medication use in the ambulatory adult population of the United States; the Slone survey, *JAMA* 287, 337–44, 2002.
5. MacLennen, A.W.D. and Taylor, A., The escalating cost and prevalence of alternative medicine, *Prev. Med.* 35, 166–73, 2002.
6. Genser, D., Food and drug interaction: Consequences for the nutrition/health status, *Ann. Nutr. Metab.* 52(Suppl 1), 29–32, 2008.
7. Maka, D. and Murphy, L., Drug-nutrient interactions: A review, *AACN Clin. Issues* 11, 580–89, 2000.
8. Chan, L.-N., Drug-nutrient interaction in clinical nutrition, *Curr. Opin. Clin. Nutr. Metab. Care* 5, 327–32, 2002.
9. Sorensen, J.M., Herb-drug, food-drug, nutrient-drug, and drug-drug interactions: Mechanisms involved and their medical implications, *J. Altern. Complement. Med.* 8, 293–08, 2002.
10. Deamer, R.L., Leibovitch, E.R. and Sanderson, L.A., Careful drug selection and patient counselling can reduce the risk in older patients, *Geriatrics* 59, 19–22, 2004.
11. McCabe, B.J., Prevention of food-drug interactions with special emphasis on older adults, *Curr. Opin. Clin. Nutr. Metab. Care* 7, 21–26, 2004.
12. Boullata, J., Natural health product interactions with medication, *Nutr. Clin. Pract.* 20, 33–51, 2005.
13. Santos, C.A. and Boullata, J.L., An approach to evaluating drug-nutrient interactions, *Pharmacotherapy* 25, 1789–1800, 2005.
14. San Miguel, M.T., Martinez, J.A. and Vargas, E., Food-drug interactions in the summary of product characteristics of proprietary medicinal products, *Eur. J. Clin. Pharmacol.* 61, 77–83, 2005.
15. Mason, P., Symposium 8: Drugs and nutrition: Important drug-nutrient interactions, *Proc. Nutr. Soc.* 69, 551–57, 2010.

16. Bushra, R., Aslam, N. and Yar Khan, A., Food-drug interactions, *Oman Med. J.* 26, 77–83, 2011.
17. Mudge, D.W., Atcheson, B., Taylor, P.J. et al., The effect of oral iron administration on mycophenolatemofetil absorption in renal transplant recipients: A randomized, controlled trial, *Transplantation* 77, 206–09, 2004.
18. Gordi, T., Tan, L.H., Hong, C. et al., The pharmacokinetics of linezolid are not affected by concomitant intake of the antioxidant vitamin C and E, *J. Clin. Pharmacol.* 43, 1161–67, 2003.
19. Bryant, B. and Knights, K., Molecular aspects of drug action and pharmacodynamics, in *Pharmacology for Health Professionals*, 3rd Ed., Mosby, Sydney, Australia, 2011, p. 123.
20. Bryant, B. and Knights, K., Drug absorption, distribution, metabolism and excretions, in *Pharmacology for Health Professionals*, 3rd Ed., Mosby, Sydney, Australia, 2011, p. 129.
21. Gainsborough, N., Maskrey, V.L., Nelson, M.L. et al., The association of age with gastric emptying, *Age Ageing* 22, 37–40, 1993.
22. Couris, R.R., Gura, K.M. and Blumberg, J., Pharmacology, nutrition, and the elderly: Interactions and implications, in *Geriatric Nutrition*, R. Chernoff, ed., Jones and Bartlett, Sudbury, MA, 2006, pp. 365–405.
23. Mangoni, A., Jansen, P. and Jackson, S., Clinical pharmacology of ageing, in *Prescribing for Elderly Patients*, S. Jackson, P. Jansen, and A. Mangoni, eds., John Wiley and Sons, Ltd, Chichester, United Kingdom, 2009, pp. 1–10.
24. Bhutto, A. and Morley, J.E., The clinical significance of gastrointestinal changes with aging, *Curr. Opin. Clin. Nutr.* 11, 651–660, 2008.
25. Russell, R.M., Factors in aging that effect the bioavailability of nutrients, *J. Nutr.* 131, 1359S–61S, 2001.
26. Gille, D., Overview of the physiological changes and optimal diet in the golden age generation over 50, *Eur. Rev. Aging Phys. Act.* 7, 27–36, 2010.
27. Benet, L.Z. and Hoener, B.A., Changes in plasma protein binding have little clinical relevance, *Clin. Pharmacol. Ther.* 71, 115–21, 2002.
28. Zeeh, J. and Platt, D., The ageing liver: Structural and functional changes and their consequences for drug treatment in old age, *Gerontology* 48, 121–7, 2002.
29. Krisharwamy, K., Effects of malnutrition on drug metabolism and toxicity in humans, in *Nutritional Toxicology*, Volume II, J.N. Hathcock, ed., Academic Press Inc., New York, 1987, pp. 105–23.
30. Klotz, U., Avant, G.R., Hoyumpa, A., Schenker, S. and Wilkinson, G.R., The effects of age and liver disease on the disposition and elimination of diazepam in adult man, *J. Clin. Invest.* 55, 347–59, 1975.
31. Crooks, J., O'Malley, K. and Stevenson, I.H., Pharmacokinetics in the elderly, *Clin. Pharmacokinet.* 1, 280–85, 1976.
32. Miners, J.O., Mackenzie, P.I. and Knights, K.M., The prediction of drug-glucuronidation parameters in humans: UDP-glucuronosyltransferase enzyme-selective substrate and inhibitor probes for reaction phenotyping and *in vitro-in vivo* extrapolation of drug clearance and drug-drug interaction potential, *Drug Metab. Rev.* 42, 196–208, 2010.
33. Miners, J.O., McKinnon, R.A. and Mackenzie, P.I., Genetic polymorphisms of UDP-glucuronosyltransferases and their functional significance, *Toxicology* 181, 453–56, 2002.
34. Kiang, T.K.L., Ensom, M.H.H. and Chang, T.K.H., UDP-glucuronosyltransferases and clinical drug-drug interactions, *Pharmacol. Ther.* 106, 97–132, 2005.
35. Sun, H., Frassetto, L. and Benet, L.Z., Effects of renal failure on drug transport and metabolism, *Pharmacol. Ther.* 109, 1–11, 2006.
36. Levey, A.S., Bosch, J.P., Lewis, J.P., Graeme, T., Rogers, N. and Roth, D., A more accurate method to estimate glomerular filtration rate from serum creatinine: A new prediction equation. Modification of Diet in Renal Disease Study Group, *Arch. Intern. Med.* 130, 461–70, 1999.
37. Swift, C.G., Pharmacodynamics: Changes in homeostatic mechanisms, receptor and target organ sensitivity in the elderly, *Br. Med. Bull.* 46, 36–52, 1990.
38. Vestal, R.E., Wood, A.J.J. and Shand, D.G., Reduced beta-adrenoceptor sensitivity in the elderly, *Clin. Pharmacol. Ther.* 26, 181–6, 1979.
39. Shepherd, A.M.M., Hewick, D.S., Moreland, T.A. and Stevenson, I.H., Age as a determinant of sensitivity to warfarin, *Br. J. Clin. Pharmacol.* 4, 315–320, 1977.
40. Persky, A.M., Eddington, N.D. and Derendorf, H., A review of the effects of chronic exercise and physical fitness level on resting pharmacokinetics, *Int. J. Clin. Pharmacol. Ther.* 41, 504–16, 2003.
41. Yitalo, P., Effect of exercise on pharmacokinetics, *Ann. Med.* 23, 289–294, 1991.
42. Peng, H.T. and Cheung, B., A review of psychophysiological stressors on pharmacokinetics, *J. Clin. Pharmacol.* 51, 1499–1518, 2011.
43. Lenz, T.L., Lenz, N.J. and Faulkner, M.A., Potential interactions between exercise and drug therapy, *Sports Med.* 34, 293–306, 2004.

44. Khazaeinia, T., Ramsey, A.A. and Tam, Y.K., The effects of exercise on the pharmacokinetics of drugs, *J. Pharm. Pharmaceutical Sci.* 3, 292–302, 2000.
45. Klemsdal, T.O., Gjesdal, K. and Bredesen, J.E., Heating and cooling of nitroglycerin patch application area modify the plasma level of nitroglycerin, *Eur. J. Clin. Pharmacol.* 43, 625–8, 1992.
46. Korvisto, V.A. and Felig, P. Effects of leg exercise on insulin absorption in diabetic patients, *N. Engl. J. Med.* 298, 79–83, 1978.
47. Klemsdal, T.O., Gjesdal, K. and Zahlsen, K., Physical exercise increases plasma concentrations of nicotine during treatment with a nicotine patch, *Br. J. Clin. Pharmacol.* 39, 677–79, 1995.
48. vanBaak, M.A., Mooij, J.M.V. and Schiffers, P.M.H., Exercise and the pharmacokinetics of propranolol, verapamil, and atenolol, *Eur. J. Clin. Pharmacol.* 43, 547–50, 1992.
49. Rowell, L.B., Human cardiovascular adjustments to exercise and thermal stress, *Physiol. Rev.* 54, 75–159, 1974.
50. Dossing, M., Effect of acute and chronic exercise on hepatic drug metabolism, *Clin. Pharmacokinet.* 10, 426–31, 1985.
51. vanBaak, M.A., Influence of exercise on the pharmacokinetics of drugs, *Clin. Pharmacokinet.* 19, 32–43, 1990.
52. Suzuki, M., Sudah, M. Matsubaru, S., Kawakami, K., Shiota, M. and Ikawa, S., Changes in renal blood flow measured by radionuclide angiography following exhausting exercise in humans, *Eur. J. Appl. Physiol.* 74, 1–7, 1996.
53. Schlaeffer, F., Engelberg, I., Kaplanski, J. and Danon, A., Effect of exercise and environmental heat on theophylline kinetics, *Respiration* 45, 438–442, 1984.
54. Joreteg, T. and Jogestrand, T., Physical exercise and binding of digoxin to skeletal muscle—Effect of muscle activation frequency, *Eur. J. Clin. Pharmacol.* 27, 567–570, 1984.
55. Shibata, Y., Hashimoto, H., Kurata, C., Ohno, R., Kazui, T. and Takinami, M., Influence of physical activity on warfarin therapy, *Thromb. Haemost.* 80, 203–204, 1998.
56. Reaburn, P.R.J., Gillespie, A., Lowe, J. and Balanda, K., The World Masters Games (1994) injury study, Report to Australian Sports Commission, 1995.
57. Striegel, H., Simon, P., Wurster, C., Niess, A.M. and Ulrich, R., The use of nutritional supplements among masters athletes, *Int. J. Sports Med.* 27, 236–41, 2006.
58. Evans, M.A., Trigs, E.J. and Cheung, M., Gastric emptying in the elderly; implications for drug therapy, *J. Am. Geriatr. Soc.* 29, 201–07, 1981.
59. Gertz, B.J., Holland, S.D., Kline, W.F., Matuszewski, B.K. and Porras, A.G., Clinical pharmacology of alendronate sodium, *Osteoporosis Int.* 3(Suppl 3), S13–16, 1993.
60. Welling, P.G., Effects of food on drug absorption, *Ann. Rev. Nutr.* 16, 383–415, 1996.
61. Rolan, P.E., Mercer, A.J., Weatherley, B.C. et al., Examination of some factors responsible for food-induced increase in absorption of atovaquone, *Br. J. Clin. Pharmacol.* 37, 13–20, 1994.
62. McLean, A.J., Isbister, C., Bobik, A. and Dudley, F.J., Reduction of first-pass hepatic clearance of propanolol by food, *Clin. Pharmacol. Ther.* 30, 31–4, 1981.
63. Leonards, J.H. and Levy, G., Gastrointestinal blood loss during prolonged aspirin administration, *N. Engl. J. Med.* 289, 1020, 1973.
64. Streeter, A.M., Goulston, K.J., Bathur, F.A., Hilmer, R.S., Crane, G.G. and Pheils, M.T., Cimetidine and malabsorption of cobalamine, *Dig. Dis. Sci.* 27, 13–16, 1982.
65. Lieber, C.S., Alcohol: Its metabolism and interaction with nutrients, *Ann. Rev. Nutr.* 20, 395–430, 2000.
66. West, R.J. and Lloyd, J.K., The effect of cholestyramine on intestinal absorption, *Gut* 16, 93–8, 1975.
67. Bryant, B. and Knights, K., Drugs affecting the lower gastrointestinal tract, in *Pharmacology for Health Professionals*, 3rd Ed., Mosby, Sydney, Australia, 2011, pp. 603–8.
68. Walan, A. and Strom, M., Metabolic consequences of reduced gastric acidity, *Scand. J. Gastroenterol.* 111(Suppl), 24–30, 1985.
69. Sturtzel, B., Dietrich, A. and Wagner, K.H., The status of vitamins B6, B12, folate and homocysteine in geriatric home residents receiving laxatives or dietary fiber, *J. Nutr. Health Aging* 14, 219–23, 2010.
70. Bailey, D.G., Spence, J.D., Munoz, C. and Arnold, J.M., Interaction of citrus juices with felodipine and nifedipine, *Lancet* 337, 268–69, 1991.
71. Sica, D.A., Interaction of grapefruit juice and calcium channel blockers, *Am. J. Hypertens.* 19, 768–73, 2006.
72. Lundahl, J., Regarth, C.G., Edgar, B. and Johnsson, G., Relationship between time of intake of grapefruit juice and its effects on pharmacokinetics and pharmcodynamics of felodipine in healthy subjects, *Eur. J. Clin. Pharmacol.* 49, 61–7, 1995.

73. Lija, J.J., Kivisto, K.T. and Neuvonen, P.J., Duration of effect of grapefruit juice on the pharmacokinetics of CYP3A4 substrate simvastatin, *Clin. Pharmacol. Ther.* 68, 384–90, 2000.
74. Harris, R.Z., Jang, G.R. and Tsunoda, S., Dietary effects on drug metabolism and transport, *Clin. Pharmacokinet.* 42, 1071–88, 2003.
75. Abdul, M.I.M., Jiang, X., Williams, K.M. et al., Pharmacodynamic interaction of warfarin with cranberry but not with garlic in healthy subjects, *Br. J. Pharmacol.* 154, 1691–1700, 2008.
76. Zikria, J., Goldman, R. and Ansell, J., Cranberry juice and warfarin: When bad publicity trumps science, *Am. J. Med.* 123, 384–92, 2010.
77. Ngo, N., Zan, Z., Graf, T.N. et al., Identification of cranberry juice product that inhibits enteric CYP3A-mediated first-pass metabolism in humans, *Drug Metab. Dispos.* 37, 514–22, 2009.
78. Lampe, J.W., King, I.B., Li, S. et al., Brassica vegetables increase and apiaceous vegetables decrease cytochrome P450 1A2 activity in humans: Changes in caffeine metabolite ratios in response to controlled vegetable diets, *Carcinogenesis* 21, 1157–62, 2000.
79. Gonzalez, J.P., Valdivieso, A., Calvo, R. et al., Influence of vitamin C on the absorption and first pass metabolism of propranolol, *Eur. J. Clin. Pharmacol.* 48, 295–97, 1995.
80. Kurnik, D., Lubetsky, A., Loebstein, R., Almog, S. and Halkin, H., Multivitamin supplements may affect warfarin anticoagulation in susceptible patients, *Ann. Pharmacother.* 37, 1603–6, 2003.
81. Bilia, A.R., Gallori, S. and Vincieri, F.F., St John's wort and depression: Efficacy, safety and tolerability, an update, *Life Sci.* 70, 3077–96, 2002.
82. Hu, Z., Yang, X., Ho, P.C.L. et al., Herb-drug interactions, *Drugs* 65, 1239–82, 2005.
83. Hennessy, M., Kelleher, D., Spiers, J.P. et al., St Johns wort increases expression of P-glycoprotein: Implications for drug interactions, *Br. J. Clin. Pharmacol.* 53, 75–82, 2002.
84. Qato, D.M., Alexander, G.C., Conti, R.M., Johnson, M., Schumm, P. and Lindau, S.T.L., Use of prescription and over-the-counter medications and dietary supplements among older adults in the United States, *JAMA* 300, 2867–78, 2008.
85. Barkve, T.F., Langseth-Manrique, K., Bredesen, J.H. and Gjesdal, K., Increased uptake of transdermal glyceryl trinitrate during physical exercise and during high ambient temperature, *Am. Heart J.* 112, 537–41, 1986.

14 Training and Nutrition Needs of the Masters Endurance Athlete

Michael Leveritt and Juliet Wiseman

CONTENTS

14.1 INTRODUCTION

The number of older people involved in competitive endurance sports and activities has increased significantly in the last 20–30 years. This trend is likely to increase with a recent report on future trends in Australian sport suggesting that the number of older people involved in sports will increase and sport participation will focus on more individual and lifestyle pursuits rather than traditional team sports [1].

There are many reasons for becoming involved in sports. For many older adults, health and avoidance of disease are motivating factors, as well as success in competition with similar-aged athletes and personal improvement in performance. Sports with competitive age-group categories include triathlon, multisport, running, cycling, walking and kayaking. These sports offer opportunities for competing, training, social interaction with like-minded individuals and an identity with a sporting community.

The focus of this chapter will be the training and nutrition needs of older endurance athletes. Given that there are many different reasons for participating in endurance sports, the chapter will give consideration to training and nutrition strategies which not only maximise endurance performance but also enhance general physiological function, ensure adequate recovery from training and competition, minimise risk of injury and optimise the health benefits of active participation in endurance exercise training and competition.

Endurance sport is a generic term encompassing many different durations and intensities of exercise. For the purpose of this chapter, endurance sport will be defined as sports or events that last between approximately 30 minutes and 3 hours. This might include running events from 5 km up to the half marathon, Olympic distance or shorter triathlons, and cycling events such as criterium races. Chapter 15 provides excellent and unique insights into the training and nutrition needs of the older ultra-endurance athlete.

14.2 TRAINING NEEDS

Success in endurance sports is related to a number of physiological, biomechanical, psychological and environmental factors. The eminent US physiologist Edward Coyle developed a model in the 1990s that described how different physiological factors contributed to endurance exercise performance [2]. The model suggests that morphological characteristics such as muscle fibre type, capillary density, enzyme activity and heart function influence functional abilities including maximal oxygen consumption (VO_{2max}), rate of work at lactate threshold and the economy and efficiency of movement. These functional abilities ultimately influence performance by determining the power output or velocity of movement during an endurance event. Sports physiologists have used this model extensively to identify the training strategies that improve physiological parameters that are most closely related to endurance performance. The model is also useful for older endurance athletes to identify which physiological factors are most at risk of decline with ageing and which factors can be improved through training and nutrition.

Declining physiological function has long been considered to be an inevitable consequence of ageing. The deterioration in endurance sport performance with age tends to occur after the age of 35 years. Modest decrements in performance are seen until age 50 years followed by a more rapid decline at older ages [3]. It should not automatically be assumed that decrements in performance are a result of declining physiological function with ageing. It is possible that the time devoted to training activities declines as people age due to other lifestyle-related factors such as occupational and/or family commitments. For example, a longitudinal study of individuals undertaking run training for up to 33 years after the age of 45 years suggested that some age-related cardiovascular changes can be reduced by high-intensity endurance training [4]. However, the impact of training in offsetting the usual age-related reduction in VO_{2max} is highly dependent on the continued magnitude of the training stimulus [5]. In fact, older athletes that stop training have a very rapid decline in VO_{2max} as they age and quickly return to levels that match their sedentary counterparts [5]. Therefore, maintaining training intensity and duration appears crucial in order to reduce the age-related declines in physiological function commonly observed in older endurance athletes.

Although training can offset some of the commonly observed age-related decline in physiological function, endurance performance does clearly decrease with age. The decrease in performance is most likely to be associated with a decline in VO_{2max}, maximal heart rate, active muscle mass, fast-twitch muscle fibre size and blood volume [3,6]. Therefore, it is important to identify training strategies that facilitate adaptation in these physiological parameters.

Endurance training philosophies and approaches are many and varied. Training intensity, volume and frequency can all be manipulated to modify the adaptive response. The impact of different combinations of intensity, volume and frequency of training on physiological adaptation and subsequent changes in performance has been studied and debated for decades among scientists, athletes and coaches. Perhaps surprisingly there is rarely universal agreement on the 'best' approach to endurance training. This is because people use a mix of information from scientific studies, anecdotal reports and personal experience when deciding on the most ideal training prescription.

Each source of information has strengths and limitations. For example, scientific studies are excellent for answering specific questions in well-controlled environments. However, the findings don't always apply to individual situations and athletes. Anecdotal reports can often capture information missed by science because studies in that area may not have been conducted to date. However, these reports may not be reliable without objective evaluation. Personal experience should always be used when adjusting training modifications because there is significant individual variability in training responses. However, training prescription solely by trial and error may take considerable time to identify the most effective approach. The following paragraphs will provide a brief review of scientific studies into how manipulating training intensity, volume and frequency can impact on endurance performance. Recommendations below will discuss how to use this information to adapt training programs for the individual requirements of older endurance athletes.

Although many exercise training studies have been conducted in older adults, most focus on the use of exercise to promote health and/or manage disease conditions. Few studies actually compare the effect of manipulating intensity, volume and frequency of training on changes in endurance performance in masters endurance athletes. Nevertheless, it has been shown that physiological adaptation to training in older adults is similar to changes observed in younger adults [7]. Therefore, many of the findings from studies of younger adults are likely to be applicable to older athletes.

Endurance athletes tend to self-select training volumes and intensity that include mostly long-duration continuous training at low intensity [8]. This type of training is often called long slow distance (LSD) training. More recently, attention has been given to the value of high-intensity interval training (HIT) for endurance athletes [9,10]. HIT involves intermittent bouts of exercise at intensities above lactate threshold separated by periods of rest. HIT has become popular because it has been shown to result in greater improvement in VO_{2max} than LSD training or training at an intensity close to the lactate threshold [9]. HIT has also been shown to improve cycling time trial performance in highly trained endurance athletes [10]. Therefore, it is recommended to include HIT training in the training programs of older endurance athletes who have been pre-screened by medical practitioners and who have progressively improved their endurance fitness over time. HIT training is also important because it is likely to stimulate and develop fast-twitch muscle fibres which appear to be most at risk of deterioration during the ageing process. However, including HIT needs to be done carefully because this type of training is likely to induce higher training stress than LSD or threshold training.

Stephen Seiler has suggested that several training intensity zones be used in the prescription of training for endurance athletes [11]. Both a three-zone and a five-zone model were proposed with both models having common anchor points around the lactate threshold. For simplicity, the three-zone model will be discussed here. Seiler describes the three training intensity zones with reference to blood lactate concentrations of below 2 $mmol{\cdot}L^{-1}$, between 2 and 4 $mmol{\cdot}L^{-1}$ and above 4 $mmol{\cdot}L^{-1}$ [11]. The first zone includes traditional LSD training; the second zone is described as threshold training; and HIT training is performed in the third and highest intensity zone.

Interestingly, when training loads are monitored across a variety of sports, training intensity appears to be distributed in a manner that 80% of training is performed in the LSD zone and the remaining 20% as either threshold or HIT training [11]. Training in lower-intensity zones is typically thought to facilitate metabolic and morphological adaptations in the muscle and cardiovascular system, while HIT training develops the ability to tolerate the accumulation of metabolic by-products associated with high-intensity exercise. Therefore, it is clear that endurance athletes require training in each intensity zone. The split of 80% LSD and 20% threshold/HIT appears to be appropriate given that manipulating this ratio seems to have equivocal effect on exercise performance [12]. Therefore, it is recommended that older endurance athletes include some training in each of the three training zones and a balance of 80% LSD and 20% threshold/HIT is suggested.

Endurance athletes often overlook resistance training as part of their overall training load. However, there may be benefits associated with increasing muscular strength for endurance athletes [13]. Resistance training has been shown to increase both running and cycling economy in younger athletes [14,15]. These studies have shown that adding resistance training to the normal endurance training program of both runners and cyclists can improve muscle strength and reduce the oxygen cost at a given exercise intensity. The enhanced economy associated with increased muscular strength is likely to result in improved performance, particularly in longer duration events. In addition, in older individuals, resistance training is effective at off-setting the usual age-related decline in skeletal muscle mass [16]. Consequently, resistance training is likely to have both performance and overall health benefits for older endurance athletes and should be included in an overall training regime.

14.3 NUTRITION

Nutrition plays an important role in enhancing endurance performance. Good nutrition has the potential to provide energy during exercise, offset fatigue, enhance recovery and improve adaptation to training. The purpose of the next section is to select key aspects of nutrition that relate specifically to endurance events that last between approximately 30 minutes and 3 hours. These include carbohydrate, protein, fluid and ergogenic aids.

14.3.1 Carbohydrate

Carbohydrate is an important nutrient for older endurance athletes. High muscle glycogen levels have been shown to enhance performance in events lasting longer than 90 minutes [17]. Muscle glycogen stores of older healthy adults are lower than younger individuals [18]. While this might initially seem concerning for older endurance athletes, endurance training can increase muscle glycogen stores in older adults [19] and this response is similar to that seen in younger athletes [20]. In addition, exercise can ameliorate the usual impaired glucose tolerance that is commonly observed with age [21]. Therefore, although changes in carbohydrate metabolism are evident with increasing age, the influence of regular training offsets this and carbohydrate recommendations are likely to be similar for older endurance athletes as those for younger athletes.

Recent carbohydrate recommendations (see Table 14.1) suggest endurance athletes training 1–3 hours each day should consume 6–10 g/kg/day of carbohydrate to ensure sufficient fuel for training and adequate restoration of muscle and liver glycogen between training sessions [22]. The wide range in recommended intake is provided in Table 14.1 because carbohydrate requirements vary considerably among individuals depending on both training intensity and volume [23]. Increasing carbohydrate intake from ~10 to ~13 g/kg/d has been shown to further enhance muscle glycogen storage, but not result in any increase in performance [24].

Extreme and excessive intake of carbohydrate may not be desirable because the extra glycogen is also stored with additional water, which may contribute to additional body weight carried during exercise. Unfortunately, generic one size fits all guidelines for daily carbohydrate may be too simplistic to account for marked variations in daily training load and body composition of individual athletes. Therefore, more contemporary recommendations for carbohydrate intake are moving away from daily ranges in favour of a more individualised approach that may vary on a daily basis to accommodate variations in training intensity and volume.

The provision of carbohydrate immediately before and during exercise has been demonstrated to elicit an ergogenic effect due to a number of mechanisms, which may be different depending on the duration of the exercise task. These include the provision of an exogenous muscle fuel source, muscle glycogen sparing, prevention of low blood glucose concentrations and possible effects on the central

TABLE 14.1
Summary of Guidelines for Daily Carbohydrate Intake

	Situation	Carbohydrate Target
Light	Low-intensity or skill-based activities	3–5 g/kg/day
Moderate	Moderate exercise program (~1 h per day)	5–7 g/kg/day
High	Endurance training program including moderate- to high-intensity exercise for 1–3 hours per day	6–10 g/kg/day
Very high	Endurance training program including moderate- to high-intensity exercise for >4–5 hours per day	8–12 g/kg/day

Source: Modified from Burke, L. M. et al., *J. Sports Sci.*, 29, S17–27, 2011.

nervous system [22]. During exercise, the maximal rate of exogenous carbohydrate oxidation appears to be ~1.0 g/minute when glucose is ingested [25]. However, this rate can be increased by up to 65% when additional sugars such as fructose are added to glucose. This increase is due to other sugars using different intestinal transport pathways [26]. Consuming carbohydrate during exercise in amounts greater than maximal rates of exogenous oxidation can result in the accumulation of unabsorbed carbohydrate and potential gastrointestinal discomfort [27]. Therefore, current recommendations for carbohydrate intake during endurance exercise are often conservative to ensure a fine balance between optimal fuel provision and gastrointestinal comfort. However, it is likely that 80–90 g/h of carbohydrate with a glucose:fructose ratio of 2:1 will provide the best opportunity for maximal exogenous carbohydrate oxidation during events lasting longer than 1 hour [25]. Given that there is little evidence of significant changes in intestinal carbohydrate transport mechanisms with age [28], these guidelines should be applicable to older endurance athletes. Older endurance athletes should experiment during training with these high intakes as they may not always be well tolerated by all individuals, particularly during running events. See Chapter 4 for a detailed discussion of the carbohydrate needs of masters athletes.

The availability and use of different macronutrients such as fat and carbohydrate during exercise has the potential to influence biochemical signalling pathways in the muscle that regulate adaptations to training [29]. For example, metabolic adaptation to training has the potential to be enhanced when muscle glycogen availability is low [30]. This creates somewhat of a dilemma when formulating carbohydrate recommendations for training. On one hand, endurance training quality is enhanced when carbohydrate is readily available. On the other hand, training adaptation may be better if carbohydrate availability is restricted. This has led to the suggestion that carbohydrate intake could be cycled and periods of 'training low' in which training is undertaken with reduced carbohydrate availability might be included in a periodised training plan to provide stimulus for enhanced adaptation [31]. However, periods of 'training high' in which training is undertaken with high carbohydrate availability are also undertaken to maximise the quality of training and prepare athletes for immediate competition [31].

This concept of carbohydrate periodisation is relatively new and, as with most aspects of sports nutrition, individual responses are likely to be quite variable. In addition, training with low carbohydrate availability for extended periods of time is potentially both physically and mentally challenging for many athletes. Therefore, embarking on a program of carbohydrate periodisation should be done with caution and careful monitoring of individual responses should be conducted. Nevertheless, in well-trained older endurance athletes, cycling periods of high- and low-carbohydrate intake may well provide the stimulus necessary to enhance adaptation and ultimately provide small, but significant, improvements in performance.

14.3.2 Protein

Protein is often not considered to be a particularly important macronutrient for endurance athletes [32]. However, it may be more significant for older endurance athletes for a number of reasons. Firstly, older individuals experience a progressive loss of muscle mass which can have significant negative impacts on neuromuscular function [33]. Secondly, although protein contributes a relatively small proportion of energy use during exercise, this may be significant if long periods of exercise training are undertaken. Finally, the oxidation of leucine is elevated during endurance exercise [34]. Leucine is an important amino acid trigger for protein synthesis [35] and increased oxidation of this amino acid by older endurance athletes has the potential to cause interference with muscle recovery and regeneration during periods of heavy training.

Protein requirements for young endurance athletes have been suggested to be around 1.6 g/kg/d largely due to increased oxidation during exercise [36]. Given that very little empirical data exist to allow estimates of protein requirements of older endurance athletes, recommendations are usually based on an extrapolation from the requirements of younger endurance athletes. Surprisingly, it has been recommended that older endurance athletes may require slightly less protein than younger athletes [20]. This recommendation is largely based on the assumption that training load in older athletes is unlikely to be as high as younger athletes and therefore less protein may be oxidised during exercise. However, given that higher protein intakes may be protective against the age-related loss of muscle mass, it might be more prudent to recommend a similar protein intake for older endurance athletes as their younger counterparts even if training load is slightly lower. A protein intake of 1.6 g/kg/d is almost twice that recommended for non-athletes, although intake at this level is still relatively easy to achieve if following a typical Western diet.

Current protein guidelines have been criticised because achieving recommended intakes each day may not provide optimal intake to maintain body composition and support bone health if protein intake is not evenly distributed across each meal of the day [37]. Muscle protein synthesis is greatest after consumption of meals containing protein. However, the rate of muscle protein synthesis reaches a maximum after consumption of approximately 30 g of protein and intakes greater than 30 g do not appear to cause further increases in protein synthesis, at least in younger individuals [37]. If protein intake is distributed in a manner that sees small amounts consumed in the early meals of the day and larger amounts consumed in the evening, muscle protein synthesis for the whole day is likely to be less than if protein was distributed evenly across the meals of the day. This is even more important for older individuals because they may have some resistance to the effects of some anabolic hormones that stimulate protein synthesis [38]. Therefore, in addition to increased total intake of protein, it is also recommended that the protein intake of older endurance athletes be evenly distributed throughout the day. For a more detailed discussion on the protein needs of masters athletes from various sport disciplines, see Chapter 6.

14.3.3 Fluid

Older individuals undertaking endurance exercise are potentially at greater risk of dehydration during exercise because of a reduced thirst response, lower total body water and declining kidney function [39]. Moreover, endurance exercise performance begins to decline when fluid losses of approximately 2% of body weight occur during exercise [40]. Therefore, it is recommended that athletes of all ages consume fluids during exercise in sufficient amounts to prevent fluid losses of greater than 2% of body weight [40].

These guidelines have recently been challenged by studies suggesting that endurance performance is only be impaired by dehydration when time to fatigue rather than time trial tests are evaluated [41] and when exercise is conducted in windless laboratory conditions which do not replicate outdoor environments [42]. Timothy Noakes argues that encouraging athletes to only drink when thirsty during exercise is sufficient to maintain optimal performance and is likely to better prevent the adverse effects associated with fluid overload [43]. However, it is not clear if this is appropriate for older individuals with impairments in the thirst response. Excessive fluid ingestion during exercise also has the potential to cause gastrointestinal distress and/or hypernatremia (see Chapter 9) in masters endurance athletes; however, these symptoms can vary widely between individuals.

Given that fluid ingestion during exercise is currently a relatively controversial area of sport science, it is prudent to be conservative with recommendations in this area. Older endurance athletes should be encouraged to drink according to their thirst during exercise. However, monitoring fluid losses by measuring body weight changes in training may be necessary for individuals to determine if different rates of fluid intake are likely to result in benefits or decrements in endurance performance. It is likely that optimal fluid intake during exercise will vary significantly between individual athletes. For more detailed discussion on the fluid needs of masters athletes, see Chapter 9.

14.3.4 Supplements and Ergogenic Aids

Dietary supplements and purported ergogenic aids are widely available in for endurance athletes. Unfortunately, very few of these supplements have been investigated thoroughly to determine their effectiveness at improving performance. There are even fewer studies investigating the effects of dietary supplements and ergogenic aids on endurance performance in older athletes. In light of this relative lack of research, this section will focus on only two ergogenic aids that have the potential to benefit endurance performance in older endurance athletes. These two supplements are caffeine and nitrates.

Caffeine is one of the most widely used pharmacologically active substances in the world and has been shown to improve endurance performance by approximately 3% when consumed before and/or during exercise [44]. The dose required to achieve optimal performance gains appears to be 3 mg per kg body mass [45]. This dose is equivalent to approximately 600 ml of energy drink or two cups of coffee. Caffeine can improve performance when consumed in tablet form or in coffee [46]. However, it is recommended to consume it in tablet form because the amount of caffeine in coffee can vary significantly [47]. Caffeine is most effective when consumed 1 hour prior to exercise [48], although studies have shown that small amounts of caffeine consumed in cola beverages can enhance performance when consumed in the concluding stages of an endurance performance task [49].

Contrary to popular belief, caffeine consumption during exercise does not cause dehydration and it has even been shown to enhance performance when consumed before exercise performed in hot conditions [50]. The effectiveness of caffeine is most likely related to its effects on the central nervous system which increase arousal and reduce the perception of effort during exercise [51].

The effects of caffeine on performance are less impressive in studies on older healthy individuals [52]. However, very few studies have been conducted to specifically evaluate the effects of caffeine on performance in well-trained older endurance athletes. Nevertheless, the age range of participants in many caffeine studies is quiet broad and studies showing performance benefits often include participants over 30 years of age. Therefore, it is reasonable to assume that caffeine, in relatively low doses, is likely to be ergogenic in older endurance athletes when consumed approximately 1 hour before exercise.

Dietary nitrate has received recent attention from researchers due to its potential to reduce the oxygen cost of exercise [53], which in turn, improves exercise economy and ultimately endurance performance. Nitrate supplementation, usually in the form of nitrate-rich beetroot juice, has the potential to improve the function of many physiological systems in the body by increasing nitric oxide content after nitrate is converted to nitrite and subsequently nitric oxide by bacteria in the mouth. Nitric oxide is a potent chemical able to influence many physiological processes, but it is best known for its ability to dilate blood vessels, which has the potential to reduce blood pressure and possibly enhance oxygen supply to tissues. Indeed, short periods (up to 2 weeks) of dietary nitrate supplementation has recently been shown to produce significant reductions in systolic blood pressure [54]. Given that vascular function is often less than optimal in older adults, dietary nitrate supplementation may have the potential to be beneficial for overall cardiovascular function in addition to any improvements in exercise performance.

Results of studies investigating nitrate supplementation on endurance performance have been mixed with many studies showing improvement, but some also showing no significant effect. A recent systematic review and meta-analysis collated the results of 17 studies involving 184 participants that all investigated the effect of dietary nitrate supplementation on endurance exercise performance in younger individuals [55]. The authors concluded that nitrate supplementation provided only a small benefit to exercise performance; however, this small benefit was considered meaningful in many sporting situations. Unfortunately, no studies were conducted on older endurance athletes which makes it difficult to determine if nitrate supplementation is also effective for older athletes. However, given that nitrate supplementation can improve vascular function and reduce blood pressure in older individuals [54], it is reasonable to assume that nitrate supplementation is also likely to benefit performance in older endurance athletes.

Nitrate supplementation used in many research studies involves the consumption of around 500 ml of beetroot juice (equivalent to approximately 350 mg of nitrate) daily for a week before an endurance performance test or event. Unfortunately, the nitrate content of beetroot can vary due to growing conditions and consumption of nitrate via beetroot juice cannot guarantee optimal intake of nitrate. Fortunately there are now concentrated shots of beetroot juice with known nitrate concentration commercially available and these are recommended rather than juicing fresh beetroot. Athletes supplementing with dietary nitrate are also advised to cease the use of any oral antibacterial mouthwash products as these may limit the conversion of nitrates to nitrites and ultimately nitric oxide in the mouth. Consumption of concentrated beetroot juice also has the potential to cause discolouration of urine and faeces and athletes should be aware of this before undertaking a period of supplementation. For more detailed discussion on supplement use and ergogenic aids for masters athletes, see Chapters 10 and 11, respectively.

14.4 CONCLUSION

In conclusion, older endurance athletes should include high-intensity interval and threshold training in addition to base training involving LSD exercise. Resistance training also has the potential to improve running economy and reduce the commonly observed age-related loss of muscle mass and should be considered an important component of training for an older endurance athlete.

Carbohydrate and protein are the most important macronutrients for older endurance athletes. Carbohydrate intake should be individually manipulated on a daily basis to accommodate variations in training intensity and duration and periods of training with low carbohydrate availability should be considered to enhance metabolic adaptations to training. Protein needs of older endurance athletes are likely to be double those of their age-matched sedentary counterparts and should be evenly distributed throughout the day to ensure as much as possible dietary protein is utilised for tissue repair and resynthesis.

Fluid needs of older endurance athletes during exercise should be dictated initially by thirst, but careful monitoring of body mass losses in both training and performance should be undertaken to determine ideal requirements for individuals. Caffeine and nitrate supplements are two ergogenic aids likely to benefit older endurance athletes.

Readers interested in increasing their knowledge in this area are encouraged to look at a number of published reviews [56–63].

14.5 IMPLICATIONS FOR SPORTS MEDICINE PROFESSIONALS AND CLINICIANS

- The evidence base for recommendations on training and nutrition for older endurance athletes is relatively scant with many recommendations based on extrapolations from studies conducted on younger individuals.
- Given the scant evidence base, careful monitoring of individual response to training and nutrition is recommended to ensure advice and guidance provided to older endurance athletes is optimal.

14.6 IMPLICATIONS FOR MASTERS ATHLETES AND COACHES

- Optimal training strategies for older endurance athletes should include high-intensity interval training mixed with LSD training. Resistance training should also be considered in order to maintain lean body mass, which is likely to benefit both health and performance.
- Carbohydrate intake should be individually manipulated to accommodate variations in training intensity and duration.
- Protein requirements are likely to be significantly higher for older endurance athletes compared with non-exercising individuals of similar age.
- Caffeine and nitrate supplements are two ergogenic aids likely to benefit older endurance athletes.

14.7 FUTURE RESEARCH DIRECTIONS

- Identification of the optimal mix of high-intensity interval training and LSD training to maximise performance while minimising risk of injury and illness in older endurance athletes.
- Exploring the effect of periodising carbohydrate intake where some training sessions are conducting with low carbohydrate availability on both physiological adaptation to training and changes in endurance performance.
- Examining the influence of ergogenic aids such as caffeine and nitrates on endurance performance in older endurance athletes to see if the benefits observed in younger athletes are also applicable to masters athletes.

REFERENCES

1. Hajkowicz, S.A., Cook, H., Wilhelmseder, L. and Boughen, N., *The Future of Australian Sport: Megatrends Shaping the Sport Sector Over the Coming Decades*, CSIRO Publishing, Melbourne, Australia, 2013, http://www.csiro.au/Portals/Partner/Futures/Future-of-Australian-Sport.aspx, accessed 24 January 2014.
2. Coyle, E.F., Integration of the physiological factors determining endurance performance ability, *Exerc. Sport. Sci. Rev.* 23, 25–64, 1995.
3. Reaburn, P. and Dascombe, B., Endurance performance in masters athletes, *Eur. Rev. Aging Phys. Act.* 5, 31–42, 2008.
4. Kasch, F.W., Boyer, J.L., Schmidt, P.K. et al., Ageing of the cardiovascular system during 33 years of aerobic exercise, *Age Ageing* 28, 531–6, 1999.
5. Katzel, L.I., Sorkin, J.D. and Fleg, J.L., A comparison of longitudinal changes in aerobic fitness in older endurance athletes and sedentary men, *J. Am. Geriatr. Soc.* 49, 1657–64, 2001.
6. Faulkner, J.A., Davis, C.S., Mendias, C.L. and Brooks, S.V., The aging of elite male athletes: Age-related changes in performance and skeletal muscle structure and function, *Clin. J. Sport Med.* 18, 501–7, 2008.
7. Harber, M.P., Konopka, A.R., Undem, M.K. et al., Aerobic exercise training induces skeletal muscle hypertrophy and age-dependent adaptations in myofiber function in young and older men, *J. Appl. Physiol.* 113, 1495–1504, 2012.
8. Billat, V., Lepretre, P.-M., Heugas, A.-M., Laurence, M.-H., Salim, D. and Koralsztein, J.P., Training and bioenergetic characteristics in elite male and female Kenyan runners, *Med. Sci. Sports Exerc.* 35, 297–304, 2003.
9. Helgerud, J., Bach, R., Hoff, J. et al., Aerobic high-intensity intervals improve VO_{2max} more than moderate training, *Med. Sci. Sports Exerc.* 39, 665–71, 2007.
10. Laursen, P.B., Shing, C.M., Peake, J.M., Coombes, J.S. and Jenkins, D.G., Interval training program optimization in highly trained endurance cyclists, *Med. Sci. Sports Exerc.* 34, 1801–7, 2002.
11. Seiler, S., What is best practice for training intensity and duration distribution in endurance athletes? *Int. J. Sports Physiol. Perf.* 5, 276–91, 2010.
12. Ingham, S.A., Carter, H., Whyte, G.P. and Doust, J.H., Physiological and performance effects of low-versus mixed-intensity rowing training, *Med. Sci. Sports Exerc.* 40, 579–84, 2008.
13. Jung, A.P., The impact of resistance training on distance running performance, *Sports Med.* 33, 539–52, 2003.
14. Storen, O., Helgerud, J., Stoa, E.M. and Hoff, J., Maximal strength training improves running economy in distance runners, *Med. Sci. Sports Exerc.* 40, 1087–92, 2008.
15. Sunde, A., Støren, Ø., Bjerkaas, M., Larsen, M.H., Hoff, J. and Helgerud, J., Maximal strength training improves cycling economy in competitive cyclists, *J. Strength Cond. Res.* 24, 2157–65, 2010.
16. Campbell, W.W. and Leidy, H.J., Dietary protein and resistance training effects on muscle and body composition in older persons, *J. Am Coll. Nutr.* 26, 696S–703S, 2007.
17. Hawley, J.A., Schabort, E.J., Noakes, T.D. and Dennis, S.C., Carbohydrate-loading and exercise performance. An update, *Sports Med.* 24, 73–81, 1997.
18. Cartee, G.D., Influence of age on skeletal muscle glucose transport and glycogen metabolism, *Med. Sci. Sports Exerc.* 26, 577–85, 1994.
19. Cox, J.H., Cortright, R.N., Dohm, G.L. and Houmard, J.A., Effect of aging on response to exercise training in humans: Skeletal muscle glut-4 and insulin sensitivity, *J. Appl. Physiol.* 86, 2019–25, 1999.

20. Tarnopolsky, M.A., Nutritional consideration in the aging athlete, *Clin. J. Sport Med.* 18, 531–8, 2008.
21. Elahi, D. and Muller, D.C., Carbohydrate metabolism in the elderly, *Eur. J. Clin. Nutr.* 54, S112–20, 2000.
22. Burke, L.M., Hawley, J.A., Wong, S.H. and Jeukendrup, A.E., Carbohydrates for training and competition, *J. Sports Sci.* 29, S17–27, 2011.
23. Jeukendrup, A.E., Nutrition for endurance sports: Marathon, triathlon, and road cycling, *J. Sports Sci.* 29, S91–9, 2011.
24. Coyle, E.F., Jeukendrup, A.E., Oseto, M.C., Hodgkinson, B.J. and Zderic, T.W., Low-fat diet alters intramuscular substrates and reduces lipolysis and fat oxidation during exercise, *Am. J. Physiol. Endocrinol. Metab.* 280, E391–8, 2001.
25. Jeukendrup, A.E., Carbohydrate and exercise performance: The role of multiple transportable carbohydrates, *Curr. Opin. Clin. Nutr. Metab. Care* 13, 452–7, 2010.
26. Jentjens, R.L., Moseley, L., Waring, R.H., Harding, L.K. and Jeukendrup, A.E., Oxidation of combined ingestion of glucose and fructose during exercise, *J. Appl. Physiol.* 96, 1277–84, 2004.
27. de Oliveira, E.P. and Burini, R.C., Food-dependent, exercise-induced gastrointestinal distress, *J. Int. Soc. Sports Nutr.* 8, 12, 2011.
28. Saltzman, J.R. and Russell, R.M., The aging gut. Nutritional issues, *Gastroenterol. Clin. North Am.* 27, 309–24, 1998.
29. Coffey, V.G. and Hawley, J.A., The molecular bases of training adaptation, *Sports Med.* 37, 737–63, 2007.
30. Hansen, A.K., Fischer, C.P., Plomgaard, P., Andersen, J.L., Saltin, B. and Pedersen, B.K., Skeletal muscle adaptation: Training twice every second day vs. training once daily, *J. Appl. Physiol.* 98, 93–9, 2005.
31. Burke, L.M., Fueling strategies to optimize performance: Training high or training low? *Scand. J. Med. Sci. Sports* 20(Suppl 2), 48, 2010.
32. Burke, L.M., Millet, G. and Tarnopolsky, M.A., Nutrition for distance events, *J. Sports Sci.* 25, S29–38, 2007.
33. Doherty, T.J., Invited review: Aging and sarcopenia, *J. Appl. Physiol.* 95, 1717–27, 2003.
34. Phillips, S.M., Dietary protein for athletes: From requirements to metabolic advantage, *Appl. Physiol. Nutr. Metab.* 31, 647–54, 2006.
35. Crozier, S.J., Kimball, S.R., Emmert, S.W., Anthony, J.C. and Jefferson, L.S., Oral leucine administration stimulates protein synthesis in rat skeletal muscle, *J. Nutr.* 135, 376, 2005.
36. Tarnopolsky, M., Protein requirements for endurance athletes, *Eur. J. Sports Sci.* 4, 1–15, 2004.
37. Layman, D.K., Dietary guidelines should reflect new understandings about adult protein needs, *Nutr. Metab.* 6, 12, 2009.
38. Fry, C.S. and Rasmussen, B.B., Skeletal muscle protein balance and metabolism in the elderly, *Curr. Aging Sci.* 4, 260–8, 2011.
39. Kenney, W.L., Thermoregulation at rest and during exercise in healthy older adults, *Exerc. Sport Sci. Rev.* 25, 41–76, 1997.
40. Sawka, M.N., Burke, L.M., Eichner, E.R. et al., American College of Sports Medicine position stand. Exercise and fluid replacement, *Med. Sci. Sports Exerc.* 39, 377, 2007.
41. Goulet, E.D., Effect of exercise-induced dehydration on endurance performance: Evaluating the impact of exercise protocols on outcomes using a meta-analytic procedure, *Br. J. Sports Med.* 47, 679–86, 2013.
42. Wall, B., Watson, G., Peiffer, J., Abbiss, C.R., Siegel, R. and Laursen, P.B., Current hydration guidelines are erroneous: Dehydration does not impair exercise performance in the heat, *Br. J. Sports Med.* 2013, doi:10.1136/bjsports-2013-092417.
43. Noakes, T.D., Is drinking to thirst optimum? *Ann. Nutr. Metab.* 57(Suppl 2), 9–17, 2010.
44. Ganio, M.S., Klau, J.F., Casa, D.J., Armstrong, L.E. and Maresh, C.M., Effect of caffeine on sport-specific endurance performance: A systematic review, *J. Strength Cond. Res.* 23, 315–24, 2009.
45. Desbrow, B., Biddulph, C., Devlin, B., Grant, G.D., Anoopkumar-Dukie, S. and Leveritt, M.D., The effects of different doses of caffeine on endurance cycling time trial performance, *J. Sports Sci.* 30, 115–20, 2012.
46. Hodgson, A.B., Randell, R.K. and Jeukendrup, A.E., The metabolic and performance effects of caffeine compared to coffee during endurance exercise, *PLoS One* 8, e59561, 2013.
47. Desbrow, B., Hughes, R., Leveritt, M. and Scheelings, P., An examination of consumer exposure to caffeine from retail coffee outlets, *Food Chem. Toxicol.* 45, 1588–92, 2007.
48. Skinner, T.L., Jenkins, D.G., Taaffe, D.R., Leveritt, M.D. and Coombes, J.S., Coinciding exercise with peak serum caffeine does not improve cycling performance, *J. Sci. Med. Sport* 16, 54–9, 2013.

49. Cox, G.R., Desbrow, B., Montgomery, P.G. et al., Effect of different protocols of caffeine intake on metabolism and endurance performance, *J. Appl. Physiol.* 93, 990–9, 2002.
50. Pitchford, N.W., Fell, J.W., Leveritt, M.D., Desbrow, B. and Shing, C.M., Effect of caffeine on cycling time-trial performance in the heat, *J. Sci. Med. Sport* 17(4), 445–9, 2014.
51. Doherty, M. and Smith, P.M., Effects of caffeine ingestion on rating of perceived exertion during and after exercise: A meta-analysis, *Scand. J. Med. Sci. Sports* 15, 69–78, 2005.
52. Jensen, M., Norager, C., Fenger-Gron, M. et al., Caffeine supplementation had no effect on endurance capacity in elderly subjects who had abstained from caffeine-containing nutrition for 8 hours, *J. Caff. Res.* 1, 109–16, 2011.
53. Bailey, S.J., Fulford, J., Vanhatalo, A. et al., Dietary nitrate supplementation enhances muscle contractile efficiency during knee-extensor exercise in humans, *J. Appl. Physiol.* 109, 135–48, 2010.
54. Siervo, M., Lara, J., Ogbonmwan, I. and Mathers, J.C., Inorganic nitrate and beetroot juice supplementation reduces blood pressure in adults: A systematic review and meta-analysis, *J. Nutr.* 143, 818, 2013.
55. Hoon, M.W., Johnson, N.A., Chapman, P.G. and Burke, L.M., The effect of nitrate supplementation on exercise performance in healthy individuals: A systematic review and meta-analysis, *Int. J. Sport Nutr. Exerc. Metab.* 23, 522–32, 2013.
56. Buchheit, M. and Laursen, P., High-intensity interval training, solutions to the programming puzzle: Part I: Cardiopulmonary emphasis, *Sports Med.* 43(5), 313–38, 2013.
57. Buchheit, M. and Laursen, P., High-intensity interval training, solutions to the programming puzzle: Part II: Anaerobic energy, neuromuscular load and practical applications, *Sports Med.* 43(10), 927–54, 2013.
58. Beattie, K., Kenny, I.C., Lyons, M. and Carson, B.P., The effect of strength training on performance in endurance athletes, *Sports Med.* Feb. 15 (Epub ahead of print), 2014.
59. Gist, N.H., Fedewa, M.V., Dishman, R.K. and Cureton, K.J., Sprint interval training effects on aerobic capacity: A systematic review and meta-analysis, *Sports Med.* 44(2), 269–79, 2014.
60. Ronnesetad, B.R. and Mujika, I., Optimizing strength training for running and cycling endurance performance: A review, *Scand. J. Med. Sci. Sports* Aug. 5 (Epub ahead of print), 2013.
61. Stellingwerff, T., Conteporary nutrition approaches to optimize elite marathon performance, *Int. J. Sports Physiol. Perform.* 8(5), 573–8, 2013.
62. Garth, A.K. and Burke, L.M., What do athletes drink during competitive sporting activities?, *Sports Med.* 43(7), 539–64, 2013.
63. Brisswalter, J. and Nosaka, K., Neuromuscular factors associated with decline in long-distance running performance in masters athletes, *Sports Med.* 43(1), 51–63, 2013.

15 Training and Nutritional Needs of the Masters Ultra-Endurance Athlete

Paul B. Laursen

CONTENTS

15.1 INTRODUCTION

Our innate desire to explore the boundaries of our own individual physical abilities, along with increased opportunities in Western-world societies, has lead to increased participation levels in endurance events that extend over very long distances and durations. When the exercise duration in these long-distance events lengthen beyond 4 hours, exercise physiologists no longer term these as endurance events; instead they are put into a category of their own, known as 'ultra-endurance' events. This is because the energy demands of such events are so significant that they create their own unique nutritional and training requirements which will be explored throughout this chapter.

There are now many popular modern-day ultra-endurance challenges. These include ultra-marathon running events, long-distance triathlons like the Ironman, ultra-distance cycling or randonneur events, marathon swims and other multi-sport adventure races. It may take a number of years to develop the endurance capacity, mental stamina, and fatigue defence systems necessary to complete or compete in these events safely. Thus, it is not surprising that the majority of participants, and often sometimes the overall winners of such events, are masters athletes [1].

As with shorter-duration events, age has an influence on ultra-endurance performance. Figure 15.1 shows the mean finish times of the top 10 competitors in different age groups of both genders from the 2006 to 2008 Hawaiian Ironman World Championships [2]. This reveals that ultra-endurance performance begins to slow after age 35, with more marked reductions occurring after age 55 [2]. In alignment with other definitions presented throughout this book, a masters ultra-endurance athlete will be subsequently defined as an athlete that is older than 35 years of age, and who systematically trains for, and competes in, ultra-endurance events [2,3].

The purpose of this chapter is to explore the specific challenges inherent in ultra-endurance events, and make recommendations to masters athletes for how they might train, fuel and perform in an ultra-endurance event. Subsequently, the chapter is divided into three parts. The first part takes a practitioner's approach, performing a needs-analysis, and highlights the physiological requirements of an ultra-endurance event for masters athletes by assessing energy and water requirements, thermoregulatory demands, muscle damage levels and cramping that often occur in such events. Second, the chapter describes the preparation and accompanying nutritional practices required to create the physiological defense systems to limit each fatigue-causing factor outlined. Finally, the chapter offers strategies for maximising race day ultra-endurance performance for the masters ultra-endurance athlete; approaches that include heat acclimation, tapering, pacing, carbohydrate ingestion, caffeine supplementation and using thirst to optimise hydration during the event. Throughout the chapter, consideration for the specific requirements of masters athletes are addressed.

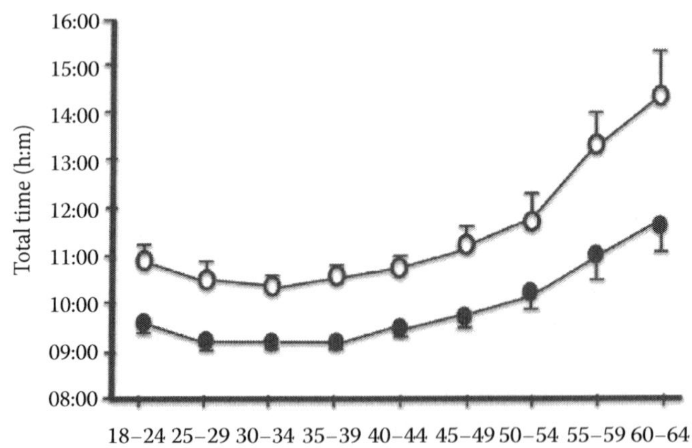

FIGURE 15.1 Mean (±SD) age group performance times for male (solid circles) and female (open circles) at the Hawaii Ironman Triathlon World Championships (2006–2008). (Modified from Lepers, R. and Maffiuletti, N.A., *Med. Sci. Sports Exerc.* 43(1), 134–9, 2011.)

15.2 DEMANDS OF AN ULTRA-ENDURANCE EVENT

In the context of this chapter, and to reiterate the point, an ultra-endurance event is one defined as moderate to high-intensity (below anaerobic threshold intensity) exercise performed for durations longer than 4 hours. Such events include the half- (1.9-km swim, 90-km bike, 21.1-km run) and full-distance Ironman (3.8-km swim, 180 km-bike, 42.2 km-run) triathlons, ultra-marathon running events, ultra-cycling events and multi-sport adventure races. Importantly however, it is not the distance *per se* that defines an event as being ultra-endurance vs. endurance, but more the duration that it takes an individual to complete the required distance. This duration will be dictated by both the imposed demands of the course (hills, ambient temperature, wind) coupled with an individual's performance ability. To illustrate, a marathon run would typically not be considered an ultra-endurance event for top finishers able to complete the event in under 2 hours 20 minutes, but most certainly becomes an ultra-endurance event for individuals that take over 4 hours to finish.

Performing such work for long durations at relatively high intensities (~80% maximum heart rate) [4] requires high energy expenditures, elicits a rise in core temperature and causes generally large water turnover rates, muscle damage and a high incidence of muscle cramping.

15.2.1 Bioenergetics

Estimates of energy expenditure in ultra-endurance events are considerable. A half-Ironman triathlon may require 4500 kcal (1076 kJ) [5], a full Ironman triathlon may require 8500 to 11,500 kcal (2032 to 2075 kJ) [6,7], and very prolonged extreme feats such as the Race Across America cycle race have been estimated at 179,650 kcal (42,937 kJ) ~17,965 kcal (4294 kJ) per day [8]. Quite simply, the longer you are out there working, the more energy it requires.

With energy contribution from the immediate adenosine triphosphate–creatine phosphate (ATP-CP) and short-term (anaerobic glycolytic) energy systems considered relatively insignificant, performance in ultra-endurance events will be dependent on both the rate and efficiency of oxygen-derived ATP) repletion. As protein oxidation is relatively small during exercise (see Chapter 6), carbohydrate and lipid oxidation rates become a main determinant of race success in ultra-endurance events. As outlined by Hawley and Hopkins [9], the pathways for carbohydrate and lipid oxidation in muscle mitochondria include the aerobic glycolytic and lipolytic systems, respectively. The aerobic glycolytic system refers to one's capacity to use carbohydrate (breakdown of glucose to pyruvate, to acetyl CoA, through the Krebs cycle and electron transport chain) to derive ATP aerobically, while the aerobic lipolytic system describes one's capacity to break down triglycerides to fatty acids (lipolysis), to acetyl CoA (β-oxidation), to be also run through the Krebs cycle and electron transport chain to derive ATP aerobically.

With ultra-endurance exercise, there is a progressively greater use of fat as a fuel over the duration of the event, until it can contribute up to 80% of the total energy expenditure [10]. Cross-sectional studies on trained versus untrained athletes show that endurance training increases the ability to use fat stores from both intramuscular triglycerides and adipocytes [11]. While muscle mitochondrial respiratory capacity may diminish slightly with age, even in subjects matched for VO_{2max}, [12], the principles surrounding effective training for ultra-endurance exercise remain the same for masters athletes as they do for their younger counterparts. That is, endurance training loads should be progressively juggled so that the training-induced protein signaling is maximised around recovery that facilitates autonomic balance [6]. These issues are expanded on in Section 15.3.

15.2.2 Core Temperature

The chemical energy conversion of macronutrients to the mechanical energy that powers an ultra-endurance masters athlete elicits an accompanying release of energy in the form of heat (~75%).

While this energy gives us our warm-blooded temperatures required for life, it can also lead to problems when our heat-producing metabolic rate becomes greater than our ability to remove it from our body. This imbalance is usually seen as a rise in core temperature.

Core temperature measured in ultra-endurance events has been shown to vary. In an ultra-endurance multi-sport adventure race (Southern Traverse), core temperature was reported to range from 36.0° to 39.2°C [13]. In various Ironman triathlons, core temperature was reported to range from between 34.2° and 40.5°C [14–17]. Thus, both hypothermia [14,15] and hyperthermia can be experienced; the latter occurrence particularly in hot races and/or with higher work rates [17]. Such high body temperatures may also induce fatigue-related reductions in speed [17]. For example, Laursen et al. presented a case study of a masters Ironman triathlete performing in a hot (35°C) Ironman Western Australia race, where the triathlete's pace slowed markedly after reaching a core temperature of 39.4°C [17].

Heat transfer in the body occurs through the processes of radiation, conduction, convection and evaporation. The most powerful of these heat removal processes (~75%) for the exercising human is the evaporation of sweat, which releases 580 kcal (139 kJ) per litre of sweat evaporated from the skin. While there is some evidence to suggest that the skin vasodilation response to heat may be partially diminished in older adults [18], the high heat removal aspects of sweat evaporation should be adequate to facilitate a thermal balance in ultra-endurance masters athletes. Nevertheless, while we humans are well-evolved to perform ultra-endurance exercise, our high sweat rate capacity means that water can be removed from our body at high rates, and must therefore be replaced at appropriate rates. What exactly is an appropriate fluid replacement rate will be the topic of the next section.

15.2.3 Body Weight Changes, Water Balance and Hyponatremia in Ultra-Endurance Events

Body mass change following different ultra-endurance events has been shown to vary quite substantially. For example, ultra-endurance cyclists competing in the 720-km Swiss Cycling Marathon lost 1.5% of their body mass [19], ultra-endurance swimmers competing over 12 hours showed no change in body mass [20], while ultra-marathon runners competing in a 100-km footrace lost 3% of body mass [21]. In the Ironman triathlon, body mass change has been reported to have a vast range from between −10.7% and +3.7% [14,16,22,23]. While it is often thought that the main contributor to body mass loss during an ultra-endurance event will be the aforementioned sweat rate, another significant source of body mass loss, not always appreciated, will be the mass lost in the form of oxidised substrate (stored carbohydrate, lipid and protein), generally thought to be in the range of 1–2 kg [24]. Another potential source of body mass loss is the water that is lost when glycogen is oxidised because 1 g of glycogen is stored in skeletal muscle with approximately 3 g of water [25]. Once muscle glycogen stores (~450 g) are oxidised during an ultra-endurance event, the water that was stored with it (~1 L) must be released and returned to the circulation. While it might be argued that an age-related lower level of lean body mass (sarcopenia) could reduce the degree to which water-bound glycogen is lowered during such an event, in general, ultra-endurance masters athletes have likely maintained muscle mass [26], and should still expect to lose between 2–3 kg of mass in the form of stored substrate and water over the course of ultra-endurance event [24,27,28]. For example, Laursen et al. showed that well-trained Ironman triathletes (age 34.7 ± 4.8 years), performing a ~10-hour Ironman Western Australia lost 2.3 ± 1.2 kg (~3%). Moreover, none of these athletes required medical attention [16]. Thus, masters ultra-endurance athletes should expect to lose about 3% of their body mass (~2–3 kg) over the course of their event, without any adverse health or performance consequences.

In fact, masters athletes that either do not lose much body mass, or gain mass during the course of an ultra-endurance event from drinking, are more likely to develop a dilutional hyponatremia [22,28,29], defined as a serum sodium concentration less than 135 mEq L^{-1}. For example, Speedy et al. showed an inverse relationship between post-race sodium concentrations and percentage change in body weight ($r = -0.63$) in the New Zealand Ironman [22].

Hyponatremia has been reported as a common medical occurrence in ultra-endurance events since the early 1980s. For example, Hiller et al. showed that 27% (17/64) of studied athletes requiring medical care in the 1982–1985 Hawaii Ironman triathlons were hyponatremic following the race [30]. Initial attempts to lower the occurrence of hyponatremia were to supplement with sodium tablets during the race, but these studies showed no effect of salt supplementation [31,32]. While fluid overload appears to be the main cause of hyponatremia [22,29], it can still occur when athletes lose body mass. For example, in the aforementioned case study [17], the masters athlete (age 35 years) lost 2% of his body mass during a hot (33.1°C) Ironman, but still became hyponatremic at the halfway point of the marathon run (131 $mEq \cdot L^{-1}$). While a high fluid consumption during the cycle phase (1.71 $L \cdot h^{-1}$), which exceeded this athletes' sweat rate (1.42 $L \cdot h^{-1}$), was a potential cause of the hyponatremia, another could have been a heat- and/or exercise-induced over-secretion of arginine vasopressin (AVP) [33]. Thus, the peak high core temperature (39.4°C) mentioned previously that likely caused the ultra-endurance masters athlete to slow in pace may also have stimulated a nonosmotic AVP secretion, leading to fluid retention and a dilutional hyponatremia [17]. Indeed, Speedy et al. have also shown that hyponatremia can develop with modest levels of fluid intakes [28]. Recently however, Hew-Butler et al. showed that plasma volume and serum sodium concentrations were maintained in Ironman triathletes, despite significant (3.8%) body weight loss during the course of the event [34].

Thus, it is important to appreciate that body weight is not an accurate predictor of fluid balance and should be viewed with caution when being used as a regulatory tool for monitoring water and sodium balance during ultra-endurance events.

15.2.4 Muscle Cramps

Exercise-associated muscle cramping is defined as involuntary painful skeletal muscle spasms that occur during or immediately after physical exercise [35]. In land-based ultra-endurance athletes, while it depends on the specific form of locomotion, these tend to be localised in the calf, hamstring or quadriceps muscles. While this is a common occurrence found during or after an ultra-endurance race, the cause(s) and risk factors for cramping remain somewhat unclear and controversial. Traditional hypotheses state that heat [36], along with dehydration and electrolyte imbalances [37], are the cause of such cramping. However, a number of studies have now convincingly shown no relationship between the occurrence of such cramping and either dehydration or electrolyte changes in marathon runners or Ironman triathletes [38–40].

More recently, a study by Schwellnus et al. showed that a history of muscle cramping and an overall faster race time were the main predictors of exercise-associated muscle cramping in 210 triathletes competing in the South African Ironman [40]. In this study, athletes who cramped also tended to predict faster overall cycle and run times before the race, and attempted to cycle and run faster during the race compared with non-cramping athletes who reported similar past performances [40]. These findings support the case study by Laursen et al. that showed a masters triathlete performing the first 60 minutes of the marathon run phase at a high intensity (14 $km \cdot h^{-1}$) that caused his core temperature to reach critical levels (39.4°C), before he slowed, cramped severely at the halfway point of the marathon run and walked the remaining 21 km [17]. This athlete had a history of faster races and a desire to finish much faster than he did [17]. In ultra-marathon runners competing in a 56-km footrace, athletes that tended to experience cramping had a past history of cramping (i.e. it was a common occurrence), paced inappropriately with a faster running pace at the early stage of the race and tended to begin with pre-race muscle damage (see next section) likely due to training sessions completed too close to competition without adequate recovery. Interestingly, age is not necessarily associated with muscle cramping [40,41], so special considerations are not needed for masters athletes *per se* with respect to cramping. However, masters athletes that have gone faster at ultra-endurance events in earlier years need to appreciate their present physical ability and pace according to speeds practiced in training.

All of these above-mentioned findings support Schwellnus et al.'s muscle fatigue cramping model, suggesting that various neuromuscular fatigue elements leads to abnormal neuromuscular control, namely an increase in muscle spindle afferent activity, a reduction in Golgi tendon organ afferent activity and a resulting increase in alpha motor neuron activity leading to the muscle spasm [42]. The practical application is that ultra-endurance athletes need to pace themselves at speeds closer to, or slightly below, those that are practiced, so as to avoid excessive fatigue and resulting muscle cramps. This suggestion will be expanded on in both the subsequent training and pacing sections of the current chapter.

15.2.5 Muscle Damage

One of the revealing signs of the physical toll placed on the run-based ultra-endurance athlete (runners and triathletes) is the degree of muscle damage the activity inflicts [43]. This has been characterised by muscle soreness, loss of muscle function, and reductions in performance [44]. For example, Suzuki et al. showed reductions in muscle strength and jump height, with accompanying increases in muscle soreness, blood markers of muscle damage, and inflammation in the 24-hour period following an Ironman triathlon [44].

Thus, for run-based ultra-endurance athletes, training appropriately to run long-distances is important. Specific run training results in adaptations that reduce muscle damage following subsequent bouts of exercise. In time, fibres are regenerated, and adaptations in the connective tissue provide greater resilience to insult during the critical long-distance event [45]. Such adaptations create more resilient muscle fibres and tendons, lessen muscle damage and pain and improve run performance ability. Of course, significant muscle damage may occur irrespective of training level, and may actually be higher in well-trained athletes due to the higher run speeds, greater muscle mass engaged and reduced amount of walking relative to less-trained athletes. Regardless, a well-trained ultra-endurance athlete of any age can recover from this muscle damage within approximately one week [46]. For example, Nosaka et al. showed in a well-trained 35-year-old triathlete that physiological and psychological markers of recovery and muscle damage returned to baseline measures after 8 days following completion of an Ironman triathlon [46].

15.3 PREPARATION FOR ULTRA-ENDURANCE RACING

The earlier-outlined demands of ultra-endurance competition form the basis for the preparation goals that should occur beforehand to combat the various fatigue-inducing stressors. The high energy requirements, along with high incidence of cramping and significant muscle damage levels known to occur, highlight that training and nutritional aspects will have the greatest impact on reducing these stressors and improving performance in the masters ultra-endurance athlete during competition.

15.3.1 Bioenergetic Goals

The large energy requirements of ultra-endurance competition identify that success in such events will stem from the ability of the athlete to oxidise macronutrients at high rates and to transfer this energy to the mechanical energy needed to power the athlete over the ultra-distance. The energy required will be mainly provided through oxidative phosphorylation in the mitochondria of the active muscles, and the three inputs include oxygen, free adenosine diphosphate and inorganic phosphate and reducing equivalents. The reducing equivalents are derived from the metabolism of fat and carbohydrate, which are mobilised from intramuscular stores, adipose tissue, liver and exogenously ingested carbohydrate [47]. The efficiency at which the human body can transfer chemical to mechanical energy is influenced highly by the exercise training program, which creates a cascade of signals [48] that put into motion an up-regulation of defence systems that permit (1) an increase in the rate of energy production from both aerobic pathways, (2) a tighter metabolic control (i.e. matching ATP production with ATP hydrolysis), (3) an increased economy of motion and therefore (4) less fatigue in working muscles during exercise [49].

While physical training makes the largest contribution towards impacting these endogenous bioenergetic efficiencies, nutritional aspects applied during an ultra-endurance event are also important. To illustrate, Kimber et al. showed in recreational triathletes (age 35 ± 8 years) competing in an Ironman triathlon that total energy expenditure approximated 10,000 kcal (2390 kJ) and that energy intake during the event was around 4000 kcal (956 kJ) (94% carbohydrate) [7]. Thus, in the case of this event, about 6000 kcal (1434 kJ) of energy would have been oxidised from endogenous (stored) macronutrient sources [7]. This example highlights the obvious need for high rates of fat and carbohydrate oxidation during ultra-distance events and training.

Carbohydrate stores in the body are limited with a typical well-trained male athlete storing around 450 g of carbohydrate (~350 g as muscle glycogen, ~95 g as liver glycogen and ~5 g as circulating blood glucose). This approximates 1800 kcal (430 kJ) of energy. Thus, to determine fat and protein oxidation needs when considering any ultra-endurance event, ~1800 kcal (430 kJ) can be subtracted from the estimated energy requirement. Using the prior example, ~1800 kcal (430 kJ) of endogenous carbohydrate subtracted from the pre-calculated 6000 kcal (1434 kJ) energy deficit leaves ~4200 kcal (1004 kJ) that must be oxidised from endogenous protein and lipid sources and exogenously consumed carbohydrate. While oxidation of amino acids from endogenous protein stores is thought to be minimal, the ability to oxidise endogenous fat and both endogenous and exogenous carbohydrate sources at high rates will contribute highly to ultra-endurance event success. Thus, the key to performance success for the ultra-endurance masters athlete lies in an intelligent and demanding training program, coupled with the ability to consume and then maximise carbohydrate absorption and oxidation.

15.3.2 Training Principles for Ultra-Endurance Events

With respect to training for an ultra-endurance event, there are probably a number of different ways one could go about it [50]. Regardless, the basic principles of training include progressive overload, specificity, frequency, duration, intensity and recovery [51]. The foundation of any exercise training program is the principle of progressive overload. This could be achieved by progressively increasing how long you train for in a session (duration), how hard you perform that session (intensity), how often you perform your training (frequency) and how much (or little) recovery or rest is inserted between your sessions. The principle of specificity states simply that you get what you train for. For the masters ultra-endurance athlete, time spent performing the specific exercise mode being prepared for needs to be relatively high despite possible family and work demands. With respect to training frequency, this will depend on the level of the masters athlete and the stage of the training program, but it is not unusual for high-level ultra-endurance athletes to perform two or more training sessions on a given day, on multiple days, so long as adequate recovery is also programmed [52].

Training for long durations is a critical component of the training program for any ultra-endurance athlete, regardless of age. When exercise is prolonged, this depletes carbohydrate reserves, and the continuation of exercise relies more on fat as a fuel source. Such training elicits important adaptations during the recovery phase that will permit more fat to be used earlier on in a subsequent training session, thereby reducing the formation of lactic acid, slowing the rate of glycogen breakdown and reducing phosphocreatine use [53]. This adaptation plays a major role in the increased endurance ability shown following endurance training. Training intensity also has a profound effect on acute changes in fitness levels [54]. While the acute benefits of high-intensity training are impressive, the ability to perform such training is limited, and too much high-intensity training can lead to overtraining [55].

15.3.3 Practical Training Recommendations

The above principles of any exercise training program are important to appreciate for the high-performing ultra-endurance masters athlete. The systematic way upon which these principles are organised and put into practice fall under the concept of periodisation which is the art of varying the training session—its intensity, its duration, how often it is performed and how much rest and recovery is performed in between sessions [51]. In terms of the distribution of intensity and volume in the program of any endurance athlete's training program, it is becoming increasingly clear that an 80:20 distribution of training, in terms of the percentage of training completed below and above the first ventilatory (aerobic; ~70% of maximal heart rate) threshold, may be optimal [50,56]. While it is unclear why this distribution may be optimal, it may be that such a training intensity distribution elicits an appropriate degree of molecular signalling to the genes that transcribe the proteins responsible for mitochondrial biogenesis, substrate handling and anatomical structuring, while at the same time preserving autonomic balance of the organism [50,56].

Interestingly, the training practices of ultra-endurance athletes and their beliefs regarding the program that best achieves success tend to vary [52,57]. Nevertheless, if we assume that a polarised distribution of intensity could be optimal for the masters ultra-endurance athlete, this can be achieved by determining the event-specific heart rate, speed or power output associated with the first ventilatory (aerobic) threshold [58], and monitoring the quantity of training performed above and below this threshold. Practically speaking, this intensity usually sits around 70% of maximal heart rate (±5%). Thus, daily/weekly training should be manipulated so that training loads progressively build and also fluctuate with recovery weeks to achieve the desired adaptation, always keeping in mind the demands of the ultra-endurance event outlined in Section 15.2.

15.4 ULTRA-ENDURANCE EVENT PREPARATION AND PERFORMANCE

The final section of this chapter deals with the activities that can be performed in the final few weeks leading into an ultra-endurance event, as well as those actions that can assist with performance during the event itself.

15.4.1 Pre-Event Preparation

While the previous section was centred on long-term preparation for an ultra-endurance event, the following section will focus on the final 2 weeks leading into an ultra-endurance event. Short-term pre-race strategies that have shown success at improving performance include tapering, heat acclimation and ensuring adequate carbohydrate, fluid and caffeine ingestion.

15.4.1.1 Tapering

The taper is the phase of the training program characterised by reduced training load in the final days leading up to major competition [59]. The aim of this phase is to lower accumulated fatigue of the prior intensive training block, maximise physiological adaptations, and consequently improve ultra-endurance performance. This is generally achieved by reducing the number of training sessions or shortening the duration of the training session. While studies specifically investigating the influence of a taper on ultra-endurance performance for masters athletes are lacking, it is logical to reduce training load in the week preceding a major event to allow for the best performance possible. In ultra-marathon runners competing in a 56-km footrace, athletes that developed muscle cramp tended to begin their race with higher levels of muscle damage, most likely due to training sessions completed too close to competition without adequate recovery [41]. The challenge for the older ultra-endurance athlete and coach is to design a taper that avoids detraining, retains or improves adaptations and subsequent performance, but without causing excessive muscle damage leading into the event. An 8-day to 3-week taper, characterised by a reduction in training volume and a maintenance of training intensity, is generally considered best practice leading into most endurance events [59]; a practice that should also serve well for the ultra-endurance masters athlete.

15.4.1.2 Heat Acclimation

Ultra-endurance events often take place in summer months and as a result tend to be performed in conditions of high ambient temperatures and/or humidity. These warm environments create a unique physiological challenge. Not only must blood be distributed to working muscles to power the athlete over the ultra-distance course, but substantial blood must also be diverted to the skin to dissipate excess heat. One strategy that has been found to successfully improve performance is the act of heat acclimation [60].

Heat acclimation has been shown to induce a number of positive physiological adaptations, including reduced oxygen uptake at a given power output, muscle glycogen sparing, reduced blood lactate at a given power output, plasma volume expansion, improved myocardial efficiency and increased ventricular compliance. Using a 10-day heat acclimation program (90-minute cycling at 50% VO_{2max} in 40°C, 30% relative humidity [RH]), Lorenzo et al. showed 8% improvements in 1-hour time trial performance in hot (38°C, 30% RH) and 5% in cool conditions (13°C, 30% RH) in well-trained young cyclists [60]. Heat acclimation also increased plasma volume, power output at lactate threshold, maximal cardiac output and VO_{2max} relative to the control group that performed the same 10-d exercise protocol under cool conditions [60]. These findings suggest that heat acclimation could be of benefit for the ultra-endurance masters athlete irrespective of whether or not it happens to be hot on race day.

Although it may be difficult to find the facilities needed to create the warm environment required for heat acclimation, the ultra-endurance athlete may be able to perform a modified version of the protocol used by Lorenzo et al. by completing light exercise in the heat over the final days leading up to their event [60]. Other practical and less-expensive methods of increasing the body's heat load during exercise could include wearing heavy clothing, wearing non-breathable clothing or exercising in poorly ventilated rooms or heated indoor swimming pools.

15.4.1.3 Carbohydrate Loading

The availability of carbohydrate as a substrate for muscle metabolism and central nervous system support is a critical contributor to ultra-endurance performance [61]. As mentioned earlier in this chapter, total body carbohydrate stores are limited and are substantially less than the fuel requirements of the ultra-endurance athlete. Therefore, in an effort to boost these limited stores, carbohydrate loading by consuming carbohydrate intakes of 10–12 g kg^{-1} d^{-1} over the 36–48 hours leading up to competition are often promoted to improve performance [61]. For example, Rauch et al. showed that 3 days of carbohydrate loading improved power output during a 3-hour high-intensity cycling trial in eight young endurance-trained cyclists [62]. In line with this study, it seems prudent to endorse similar recommendations and for masters athletes to consume 10–12 g kg^{-1} d^{-1} over the 36–48 hours leading up to an ultra-endurance event. For a detailed discussion on the carbohydrate needs of masters athletes before, during and after training, see Chapter 4.

15.4.1.4 Hydration and Drinking Guidelines for Ultra-Endurance Events

Guidelines for drinking have been heavily debated in recent years. Earlier recommendations based on laboratory studies recommended that athletes should drink early in training or competition, and as much fluid as tolerable [63], or at levels that match sweat rate during the event [64]. This message, promoted heavily in the media and through commercial interests, created a fear of dehydration for athletes and practitioners that continues to resonate throughout the media to this day [65].

Over recent years, well-respected sport scientist Tim Noakes argues that athletes can safely gauge fluid replacement using their innate serum osmolality-based thirst mechanism [66]. This means that athletes will drink to a level of thirst which is governed by hypothalamic osmoreceptors that relay information pertaining to the level of blood osmolality. What may happen in some athletes performing ultra-endurance events, especially during the latter stages of an event, is that the pain, fatigue and slowing of pace that generally occurs [67] may be interpreted incorrectly as a sign of dehydration by some athletes fearful of this condition, which could prompt an athlete to drink beyond their needs and confound the problem. One initiative put in place by both New Zealand and South African Ironman triathlon race organisers has been to reduce the number of drink stations available on the course and thus lower the opportunity to drink. This action successfully lessened the occurrence of hyponatremia in ultra-endurance triathlon racing, and is an action that should be followed by ultra-endurance event race organisers throughout the world [14,15,68].

As mentioned earlier in this chapter, the importance of hydration status on exercise performance may have been previously overstated [65]. Nevertheless, it seems prudent to ensure adequate hydration to the level of one's thirst [66]. Adequate water levels are also required to store the glycogen goals of carbohydrate loading. This was shown indirectly in the study by Laursen et al. where ultra-endurance triathletes began their event 1 kg heavier 30 minutes prior to starting their Ironman event than when weighed just 2 days prior, likely due to the added water that gets stored with glycogen [16].

In summary, there is no reason why athletes need specific recommendations for fluid volumes, as these will depend largely on sweat rates that will be influenced by environmental temperatures, metabolic rates and resulting core temperatures. Thus, the best advice for masters athletes competing in ultra-endurance events is to ensure there is availability of fluids, but to drink according to thirst. For more detailed discussion on the fluid, electrolyte and hydration needs of masters athletes, see Chapter 9.

15.4.1.5 Caffeine

In 2004, caffeine was removed from the list of prohibited substances of the World Anti-Doping Agency, meaning that athletes can consume caffeine either in their background diets or for the specific purposes of performance enhancement without fear of sanctions. Not surprisingly, caffeine was reported to have been used by 89% of athletes competing in the 2005 Hawaii Ironman triathlon, and at levels that would be considered to be performance-enhancing [69]. While the mechanisms of how caffeine enhances prolonged performance are not entirely clear, the potentially beneficial effects include the mobilisation of fat from adipose tissue and the muscle cell, stimulation of epinephrine release, direct effects on cardiac muscle, direct changes to muscle contractility, and alterations to the central nervous system to change perceptions of effort or fatigue [70].

With performance-enhancing levels shown to be around the 3 mg kg^{-1} dose level, this seems an appropriate dose to recommend for masters ultra-endurance athletes. Pill or tablet form tends to be the best way to ensure that the appropriate dosage is taken, as certain products that claim to have caffeine in them also contain other substances that could compete with caffeine's effect. As levels tend to peak about an hour after consumption, this seems an appropriate period to ingest caffeine prior to race start. Furthermore, re-ingestion of this dose every 3–4 hours during the event seems logical to balance the body's caffeine removal rates. Of course, there are a number of side effects [70], and masters athletes need to experiment with their chosen dosage in training before using caffeine in an important ultra-endurance event.

15.4.2 Considerations during the Ultra-Endurance Event

The training is completed, the pre-race preparation is in place and the race has begun. What practices now might assist to give the masters ultra-endurance athlete the best performance they can achieve on the day of the event? The final ingredients towards optimising ultra-endurance performance may now come down to appropriate nutrition in the form of carbohydrate and fluid consumption, along with an appropriate pacing strategy.

15.4.2.1 Carbohydrate Assimilation

As established throughout this chapter, the energy demands of an ultra-endurance event are high. Once the race has begun, it is important to supplement the muscle cells with a source of exogenous carbohydrate to provide the reducing equivalents required for the high aerobic metabolic rates needed. High carbohydrate ingestion rates have been shown to be related to ultra-endurance performance. For example, in male Ironman triathletes, Kimber et al. showed that Ironman finishing time was inversely related to carbohydrate intake ($g{\cdot}kg^{-1}{\cdot}h^{-1}$) during the marathon run ($r = -0.75$, $p < 0.05$) [7]. As such, increasing carbohydrate intake during an ultra-endurance event may be a useful strategy for improving performance, likely by providing the much-needed energy during the later stages of the event.

Just how much carbohydrate an ultra-endurance athlete should ingest during an event has received an increase in research interest of late. Previously, it was found that carbohydrate (glucose) oxidation was limited to 1 g min^{-1} due to a saturation of SGLT1 glucose transporters in the small intestine [71]. However, through the use of a mixed carbohydrate solution of glucose and fructose, it was subsequently shown that carbohydrate delivery and oxidation could be increased by as high as 1.75 g min^{-1} [72]. This increased carbohydrate absorption occurs via fructose absorption through the GLUT5 transporter, with the ingested fructose subsequently converted to glucose in the liver. The increased carbohydrate oxidation with multiple transportable carbohydrates is also accompanied by increased fluid delivery and improved oxidation efficiency, and with this, a reduced likelihood of gastrointestinal distress [73].

Recent studies have also shown reduced fatigue and improved exercise performance with multiple transportable carbohydrates compared with single carbohydrate sources. For an extensive review of this area, the reader is referred to the recent work of Jeukendrup [73]. Based on this research, it seems prudent for ultra-endurance masters athletes to attempt to consume carbohydrate during ultra-endurance exercise at a rate of at least 1.5 g min^{-1}, in a 2:1 ratio of glucose to fructose in order to maintain higher exercise intensities throughout their ultra-endurance event and improve subsequent ultra-endurance event performance.

15.4.2.2 Hydration Guidelines

Guidelines for drinking have been discussed earlier in this chapter and will not be extended further. Hydration requirements will fluctuate with variations in both environmental conditions and metabolic rate. It appears that the most prudent advice is to drink throughout an ultra-endurance event in accordance with one's thirst [66]. Because environmental conditions are sometimes not known until after the race begins, a potential strategy may be to have a variety of more (gels, cola) and less (weak carbohydrate-electrolyte, water) concentrated drinks available for use during the event (if possible), and to self-administer carbohydrate and fluid levels according to requirements. It is more than likely that most athletes, especially masters athletes with years of experience, do this intuitively during long-distance racing.

15.4.2.3 Pacing

The pacing strategy, or how fast or slow one chooses to perform an event, is known to have an influence on performance outcome in endurance events [67]. For example, O'Toole showed that faster finishers in the Hawaii Ironman Triathlon were able to maintain their training paces throughout all three activities of the triathlon [52]. Typically, ultra-endurance athletes perform a positive pacing strategy, characterised by a fast initial pace, and then a reduction in pace throughout the remainder of event [4,74]. This has been shown as a decline in heart rate at an average rate of 1%–2% per hour during an ultra-endurance event [4]. It is believed that this progressive reduction in exercise intensity may be the result of glycogen depletion, neuromuscular fatigue, and/or psychological factors associated with the perception of fatigue [67]. While it is difficult to do so, ultra-endurance masters athletes are advised to attempt to perform an even pacing strategy, and to perform their event at a pace that is similar to that which is performed in training [52].

15.5 SUMMARY

In summary, ultra-endurance events require prolonged (>4-hour) durations of moderate- to high-intensity exercise which mostly use energy from the oxidation of fat and carbohydrate. Ultra-endurance training programs for masters athletes generally consist of long-duration training, but optimally this should be completed with progressive overload using an 80:20 polarised blend of training with intensities below (80%) and above (20%) the first ventilatory (aerobic) threshold (~70% of maximum heart rate). Research suggests that such training improves fat oxidation rates, lowers lactate production, spares glycogen and increases fatigue resistance. Pre-event preparation strategies include the taper, ensuring adequate hydration, carbohydrate loading, acclimating to the heat and consuming 3 mg kg^{-1} of caffeine 1 hour prior to race start. During ultra-endurance racing, masters athletes should pace themselves by performing at speeds that resemble those practiced in training, consuming up to 1.75 g min^{-1} of carbohydrate using a mix of fructose and glucose in a 1:2 ratio, and drink according to thirst.

Little research has examined the physical and nutritional preparation of athletes for ultra-endurance events. Readers interested in these areas may wish to read some peer-reviewed studies and literature reviews [75–81].

15.6 IMPLICATIONS FOR SPORTS MEDICINE PROFESSIONALS AND CLINICIANS

- Appreciate that the energy demands of ultra-endurance events are significant.
- The large energy demands require highly efficient energy production, mostly from fat and carbohydrate sources.
- An individual's endogenous fat and carbohydrate oxidation rates will result from their applied endurance training program.
- Monitoring body weight is not an accurate predictor of fluid balance and should be viewed with caution when being used as a regulator tool for monitoring water and sodium balance in ultra-endurance events.

15.7 IMPLICATIONS FOR MASTERS ATHLETES AND COACHES

- Training for ultra-endurance events should generally consist of prolonged training, but the classic principles of exercise training including aspects of progressive overload and recovery should be adhered to.
- An 80:20 polarised balance of training performed below and above the first ventilatory (aerobic) threshold (~70% of maximum heart rate) may be a good training strategy in masters athletes who have the luxury of time given family and work commitments.
- A 3-mg kg^{-1} dose of caffeine ingested 1 hour prior to an ultra-endurance event is likely to enhance performance.
- Carbohydrate in the forms of drinks, gels and so forth should be consumed during ultra-endurance exercise at a rate of 1.5 $g.min^{-1}$ in a 2:1 ratio of glucose to fructose.
- As hyponatremia due to over-drinking can occur in some individuals during ultra-endurance events, the masters athlete should be encouraged to drink to thirst requirements throughout their event.

15.8 FUTURE RESEARCH DIRECTIONS

- Is a polarised model of training optimal for masters ultra-endurance athletes?
- As ultra-endurance events are long, what length of training session should be progressed to in the weeks prior to a major ultra-endurance event for a masters athlete?
- Are the current carbohydrate intake guidelines for younger athletes, before, during and after exercise the same for older athletes?
- Are the current fluid intake guidelines for younger athletes, before, during and after exercise the same for older athletes?

REFERENCES

1. Knechtle, B., Rust, C.A., Rosemann, T. and Lepers, R., Age-related changes in 100-km ultra-marathon running performance, *Age* 34(4), 1033–45, 2011.
2. Lepers, R. and Maffiuletti, N.A., Age and gender interactions in ultraendurance performance: Insight from the triathlon, *Med. Sci. Sports Exerc.* 43(1), 134–9, 2011.
3. Reaburn, P. and Dascombe, B., Endurance performance in masters athletes, *Eur. Rev. Aging Phys. Act.* 5(1), 31–42, 2008.
4. Laursen, P.B., Knez, W.L., Shing, C.M., Langill, R.H., Rhodes, E.C. and Jenkins, D.G., Relationship between laboratory-measured variables and heart rate during an ultra-endurance triathlon, *J. Sports Sci.* 23(10), 1111–20, 2005.
5. Gillum, T.L., Dumke, C.L. and Ruby, B.C., Muscle glycogenolysis and resynthesis in response to a half Ironman triathlon: A case study, *Int. J. Sports Physiol. Perf.* 1(4), 408–13, 2006.
6. Laursen, P.B. and Rhodes, E.C., Factors affecting performance in an ultraendurance triathlon, *Sports Med.* 31(3), 195–209, 2001.
7. Kimber, N.E., Ross, J.J., Mason, S.L. and Speedy, D.B., Energy balance during an ironman triathlon in male and female triathletes, *Int. J. Sport Nutr. Exerc. Metab.* 12(1), 47–62, 2002.
8. Knechtle, B., Enggist, A. and Jehle, T., Energy turnover at the Race Across America (RAAM)—A case report, *Int. J. Sports Med.* 26(6), 499–503, 2005.
9. Hawley, J.A. and Hopkins, W.G., Aerobic glycolytic and aerobic lipolytic power systems. A new paradigm with implications for endurance and ultraendurance events, *Sports Med.* 19(4), 240–50, 1995.
10. Gollnick, P.D., Metabolism of substrates: Energy substrate metabolism during exercise and as modified by training, *Fed. Proc.* 44(2), 353–7, 1985.
11. Coggan, A.R., Raguso, C.A., Gastaldelli, A., Sidossis, L.S. and Yeckel, C.W., Fat metabolism during high-intensity exercise in endurance-trained and untrained men, *Metabolism* 49(1), 122–8, 2000.
12. Larsen, S., Hey-Mogensen, M., Rabol, R., Stride, N., Helge, J.W. and Dela, F., The influence of age and aerobic fitness: Effects on mitochondrial respiration in skeletal muscle, *Acta Physiol.* 205(3), 423–32, 2012.
13. Lucas, S.J., Anglem, N., Roberts, W.S. et al., Intensity and physiological strain of competitive ultra-endurance exercise in humans, *J. Sports Sci.* 26(5), 477–89, 2008.
14. Sharwood, K.A., Collins, M., Goedecke, J.H., Wilson, G. and Noakes, T.D., Weight changes, medical complications, and performance during an Ironman triathlon, *Br. J. Sports Med.* 38(6), 718–24, 2004.
15. Sharwood, K., Collins, M., Goedecke, J., Wilson, G. and Noakes, T., Weight changes, sodium levels, and performance in the South African Ironman Triathlon, *Clin. J. Sports Med.* 12(6), 391–9, 2002.
16. Laursen, P.B., Suriano, R., Quod, M.J. et al., Core temperature and hydration status during an Ironman triathlon, *Br. J. Sports Med.* 40(4), 320–5, 2006.
17. Laursen, P.B., Watson, G., Abbiss, C.R., Wall, B.A. and Nosaka, K., Hyperthermic fatigue precedes a rapid reduction in serum sodium in an ironman triathlete: A case report, *Int. J. Sports Physiol. Perf.* 4(4), 533–7, 2009.
18. Sagawa, S., Shiraki, K., Yousef, M.K. and Miki, K., Sweating and cardiovascular responses of aged men to heat exposure, *J. Gerontol.* 43(1), M1–8, 1988.
19. Rust, C.A., Knechtle, B., Knechtle, P. and Rosemann, T., No case of exercise-associated hyponatraemia in top male ultra-endurance cyclists: The 'Swiss Cycling Marathon', *Eur. J. Appl. Physiol.* 112(2), 689–97, 2011.
20. Knechtle, B., Knechtle, P., Kaul, R. and Kohler, G., No change of body mass, fat mass, and skeletal muscle mass in ultraendurance swimmers after 12 hours of swimming, *Res. Q. Exerc. Sport* 80(1), 62–70, 2009.
21. Knechtle, B., Wirth, A., Knechtle, P. and Rosemann, T., Increase of total body water with decrease of body mass while running 100 km nonstop—Formation of edema? *Res. Q. Exerc. Sport* 80(3), 593–603, 2009.
22. Speedy, D.B., Faris, J.G., Hamlin, M., Gallagher, P.G. and Campbell, R.G., Hyponatremia and weight changes in an ultradistance triathlon, *Clin. J. Sport Med.* 7(3), 180–4, 1997.
23. Hew-Butler, T., Collins, M., Bosch, A. et al., Maintenance of plasma volume and serum sodium concentration despite body weight loss in ironman triathletes, *Clin. J. Sports Med.* 17(2), 116–22, 2007.
24. Pastene, J., Germain, M., Allevard, A.M., Gharib, C. and Lacour, J.R., Water balance during and after marathon running, *Eur. J. Appl. Physiol.* 73(1–2), 49–55, 1996.
25. Jeukendrup, A.E. and Gleeson, M., *Sport Nutrition: An Introduction to Energy Production and Performance*, 2nd Ed., Human Kinetics, Champaign, IL, 2010.

26. Wroblewski, A.P., Amati, F., Smiley, M.A., Goodpaster, B. and Wright, V., Chronic exercise preserves lean muscle mass in masters athletes, *Phys. Sportsmed.* 39(3), 172–8, 2011.
27. Brouns, F., Heat-sweat-dehydration-rehydration: A praxis oriented approach, *J. Sports Sci.* 9(S1), 143–52, 1991.
28. Speedy, D.B., Noakes, T.D., Kimber, N.E. et al., Fluid balance during and after an ironman triathlon, *Clin. J. Sport Med.* 11(1), 44–50, 2001.
29. Noakes, T.D., Changes in body mass alone explain almost all of the variance in the serum sodium concentrations during prolonged exercise. Has commercial influence impeded scientific endeavour? *Br. J. Sports Med.* 45(6), 475–7, 2011.
30. Hiller, W.D., O'Toole, M.L., Fortess, E.E., Laird, R.H., Imbert, P.C. and Sisk, T.D., Medical and physiological considerations in triathlons, *Am. J. Sports Med.* 15(2), 164–7, 1987.
31. Speedy, D.B., Thompson, J.M., Rodgers, I., Collins, M., Sharwood, K. and Noakes, T.D., Oral salt supplementation during ultradistance exercise, *Clin. J. Sports Med.* 12(5), 279–84, 2002.
32. Hew-Butler, T.D., Sharwood, K., Collins, M., Speedy, D. and Noakes, T., Sodium supplementation is not required to maintain serum sodium concentrations during an Ironman triathlon, *Br. J. Sports Med.* 40(3), 255–9, 2006.
33. Hew-Butler, T., Arginine vasopressin, fluid balance and exercise: Is exercise-associated hyponatraemia a disorder of arginine vasopressin secretion? *Sports Med.* 40(6), 459–79, 2010.
34. Hew-Butler, T., Jordaan, E., Stuempfle, K.J. et al., Osmotic and nonosmotic regulation of arginine vasopressin during prolonged endurance exercise, *J. Clin. Endocrinol. Metab.* 93(6), 2072–8, 2008.
35. Schwellnus, M.P., Derman, E.W. and Noakes, T.D., Aetiology of skeletal muscle 'cramps' during exercise: A novel hypothesis, *J. Sports Sci.* 15(3), 277–85, 1997.
36. Armstrong, L.E., Casa, D.J., Millard-Stafford, M., Moran, D.S., Pyne, S.W. and Roberts, W.O., American College of Sports Medicine position stand. Exertional heat illness during training and competition, *Med. Sci. Sports Exerc.* 39(3), 556–72, 2007.
37. Eichner, E.R., The role of sodium in 'heat cramping', *Sports Med.* 37(4–5), 368–70, 2007.
38. Schwellnus, M.P., Nicol, J., Laubscher, R. and Noakes, T.D., Serum electrolyte concentrations and hydration status are not associated with exercise associated muscle cramping (EAMC) in distance runners, *Br. J. Sports Med.* 38(4), 488–92, 2004.
39. Sulzer, N.U., Schwellnus, M.P. and Noakes, T.D., Serum electrolytes in Ironman triathletes with exercise-associated muscle cramping, *Med. Sci. Sports Exerc.* 37(7), 1081–5, 2005.
40. Schwellnus, M.P., Drew, N. and Collins, M., Increased running speed and previous cramps rather than dehydration or serum sodium changes predict exercise-associated muscle cramping: A prospective cohort study in 210 Ironman triathletes, *Br. J. Sports Med.* 45(8), 650–6, 2011.
41. Schwellnus, M.P., Allie, S., Derman, W. and Collins, M., Increased running speed and pre-race muscle damage as risk factors for exercise-associated muscle cramps in a 56 km ultra-marathon: A prospective cohort study, *Br. J. Sports Med.* 45(14), 1132–6, 2011.
42. Schwellnus, M.P., Cause of exercise associated muscle cramps (EAMC)—Altered neuromuscular control, dehydration or electrolyte depletion? *Br. J. Sports Med.* 43(6), 401–8, 2009.
43. Farber, H.W., Schaefer, E.J., Franey, R., Grimaldi, R. and Hill, N.S., The endurance triathlon: Metabolic changes after each event and during recovery, *Med. Sci. Sports Exerc.* 23(8), 959–65, 1991.
44. Suzuki, K., Peake, J., Nosaka, K. et al., Changes in markers of muscle damage, inflammation and HSP70 after an Ironman Triathlon race, *Eur. J. Appl. Physiol.* 98(6), 525–34, 2006.
45. Ebbeling, C.B. and Clarkson, P.M., Exercise-induced muscle damage and adaptation, *Sports Med.* 7(4), 207–34, 1989.
46. Nosaka, K., Abbiss, C.R., Watson, G., Wall, B., Suzuki, K. and Laursen, P., Recovery following an Ironman triathlon: A case study, *Eur. J. Sports Sci.* 10(3), 159–65, 2010.
47. Spriet, L.L., Regulation of substrate use during the marathon, *Sports Med.* 37(4–5), 332–6, 2007.
48. Coffey, V.G. and Hawley, J.A., The molecular bases of training adaptation, *Sports Med.* 37(9), 737–63, 2007.
49. Hawley, J.A. and Spargo, F.J., Metabolic adaptations to marathon training and racing, *Sports Med.* 37(4–5), 328–31, 2007.
50. Laursen, P.B., Training for intense exercise performance: High-intensity or high-volume training? *Scand. J. Med. Sci. Sports* 20(Suppl 2), 1–10, 2010.
51. Lambert, M.I., Viljoen, W., Bosch, A., Pearce, A.J. and Sayers, M., General principles of training, in *The Olympic Textbook of Medicine in Sport. Volume of the Encyclopaedia of Sports Medicine*, M.P. Schwellnus, ed., Blackwell Publishing Ltd., West Sussex, United Kingdom, 2008.
52. O'Toole, M.L., Training for ultraendurance triathlons, *Med. Sci. Sports Exerc.* 21(5 Suppl), S209–13, 1989.

53. Hawley, J.A., Adaptations of skeletal muscle to prolonged, intense endurance training, *Clin. Exp. Pharmacol. Physiol.* 29(3), 218–22, 2002.
54. Laursen, P.B. and Jenkins, D.G., The scientific basis for high-intensity interval training: Optimising training programmes and maximising performance in highly trained endurance athletes, *Sports Med.* 32(1), 53–73, 2002.
55. Billat, V.L., Flechet, B., Petit, B., Muriaux, G. and Koralsztein, J.P., Interval training at VO_{2max}: Effects on aerobic performance and overtraining markers, *Med. Sci. Sports Exerc.* 31(1), 156–63, 1999.
56. Seiler, S., What is best practice for training intensity and duration distribution in endurance athletes? *Int. J. Sports Physiol. Perf.* 5(3), 276–91, 2010.
57. Gulbin, J.P. and Gaffney, P.T., Ultraendurance triathlon participation: Typical race preparation of lower level triathletes, *J. Sports Med. Phys. Fit.* 39(1), 12–5, 1999.
58. Lucia, A., Hoyos, J., Perez, M. and Chicharro, J.L., Heart rate and performance parameters in elite cyclists: A longitudinal study, *Med. Sci. Sports Exerc.* 32(10), 1777–82, 2000.
59. Mujika, I., Intense training: The key to optimal performance before and during the taper, *Scand. J. Med. Sci. Sports* 20(Suppl 2), 24–31, 2010.
60. Lorenzo, S., Halliwill, J.R., Sawka, M.N. and Minson, C.T., Heat acclimation improves exercise performance, *J. Appl. Physiol.* 109(4), 1140–7, 2010.
61. Burke, L.M., Hawley, J.A., Wong, S.H. and Jeukendrup, A.E., Carbohydrates for training and competition, *J. Sports Sci.* 29(Suppl 1), S17–27, 2011.
62. Rauch, L.H., Rodger, I., Wilson, G.R. et al., The effects of carbohydrate loading on muscle glycogen content and cycling performance, *Int. J. Sport Nutr.* 5(1), 25–36, 1995.
63. Sawka, M.N. and Coyle, E.F., Influence of body water and blood volume on thermoregulation and exercise performance in the heat, *Exerc. Sport Sci. Rev.* 27, 167–218, 1999.
64. Convertino, V.A., Armstrong, L.E., Coyle, E.F. et al., American College of Sports Medicine position stand. Exercise and fluid replacement, *Med. Sci. Sports Exerc.* 28(1), i–vii, 1996.
65. Noakes, T.D., Oral fluids: How pseudoscience gulls the gullible, *Sth. Afr. Med. J.* 98(6), 410, 2, 2008.
66. Noakes, T.D., Is drinking to thirst optimum? *Ann. Nutr. Metab.* 57(Suppl 2), 9–17, 2010.
67. Abbiss, C.R. and Laursen, P.B., Describing and understanding pacing strategies during athletic competition, *Sports Med.* 38(3), 239–52, 2008.
68. Wharam, P.C., Speedy, D.B., Noakes, T.D., Thompson, J.M., Reid, S.A. and Holtzhausen, L.M., NSAID use increases the risk of developing hyponatremia during an Ironman triathlon, *Med. Sci. Sports Exerc.* 38(4), 618–22, 2006.
69. Desbrow, B. and Leveritt, M., Awareness and use of caffeine by athletes competing at the 2005 Ironman Triathlon World Championships, *Int. J. Sport Nutr. Exerc. Metab.* 16(5), 545–58, 2006.
70. Burke, L.M., Caffeine and sports performance, *Appl. Physiol. Nutr. Metab.* 33(6), 1319–34, 2008.
71. Jeukendrup, A.E. and Jentjens, R., Oxidation of carbohydrate feedings during prolonged exercise: Current thoughts, guidelines and directions for future research, *Sports Med.* 29(6), 407–24, 2000.
72. Jentjens, R.L. and Jeukendrup, A.E., High rates of exogenous carbohydrate oxidation from a mixture of glucose and fructose ingested during prolonged cycling exercise, *Br. J. Nutr.* 93(4), 485–92, 2005.
73. Jeukendrup, A.E., Carbohydrate and exercise performance: The role of multiple transportable carbohydrates, *Curr. Opin. Clin. Nutr. Metab. Care* 13(4), 452–7, 2010.
74. Laursen, P.B., Rhodes, E.C., Langill, R.H., McKenzie, D.C. and Taunton, J.E., Relationship of exercise test variables to cycling performance in an Ironman triathlon, *Eur. J. Appl. Physiol.* 87(4–5), 433–40, 2002.
75. Costa, R.J., Crockford, M.J., Moore, J.P. and Walsh, N.P., Heat acclimation responses of an ultra-endurance running group preparing for hot desert-based competition, *Eur. J. Sport Sci.* 14(Suppl. 1), S131–41, 2014.
76. Costa, R.J., Teixeira, A., Rama, L. et al., Water and sodium intake habits and status of ultra-endurance runners during a multi-stage ultra-marathon conducted in a hot ambient environment: An observational field based study, *Nutr. J.* 12, 13, 2013.
77. Whyte, G., Age, sex and (the) race: Gender and geriatrics in the ultra-endurance age, *Extrem. Physiol. Med.* 3(1), 1–3, 2014.
78. Lazzer, S., Salvadego, D., Rejc, E., Buglione, A., Antonutto, G. and di Prampero, P.E., The energetics of ultra-endurance running, *Eur. J. Appl. Physiol.* 112(5), 1709–15, 2012.
79. Klapcinsak, B., Waskiewicz, Z., Chrapusta, S.J., Sadowska-Krepa, E., Czuba, M. and Langfort, J., Metabolic responses to a 48-h ultra-marathon in middle-aged male amateur runners, *Eur. J. Appl. Physiol.* 113(11), 2781–93, 2013.
80. Ranchordas, M.K., Nutrition for adventure racing, *Sports Med.* 42(11), 915–27, 2012.
81. Knechtle, B., Nutrition in ultra-endurance racing—Aspects of energy balance, fluid balance and exercise-associated hyponatremia, *Med. Sportiva*, 17(4), 200–10, 2013.

16 Training and Nutritional Needs of the Masters Sprint Athlete

Marko T. Korhonen, Marko Haverinen and Hans Degens

CONTENTS

16.1 INTRODUCTION

Over the past decades, there have been increasing numbers of middle-aged and older people taking part in masters (>35 years) track and field competitions. Sprint running, especially the 100-m, has been a very popular competitive event from the beginning of the first international master athletics championships in the 1970s. With large numbers of serious competitive masters athletes, the current standard of sprint running is extremely high in many countries. Although the achievement of success at the highest level is largely dependent on superior genetic endowment, training-related adaptations in various attributes of sprinting ability are of considerable importance [1]. In order to reach their full potential, the training of ageing athletes must be regarded as a long-term systematic process where biomechanical, physiological and nutritional characteristics are developed together.

This chapter will review the research examining the effects of ageing on short sprint running performance (60 and 100 m) and its determinants in highly competitive male runners with special emphasis on practical aspects of training and nutrition. Because data in many areas are very limited, the literature is supplemented with information found in young sprinters and older non-athletes.

16.2 CHANGES IN SPRINT PERFORMANCE WITH AGEING

16.2.1 Competition Performance Times

Athletic records provide the basis for understanding the effect of ageing on the ability to run fast. The current world records for the men's 100-m sprint suggest that the peak performance occurs between the ages of 20 to 30 years (see Figure 16.1 [2,3]). Thereafter, the age-based record performances (in m/s) decrease almost linearly at a rate about 0.6% per year until approximately 80 years of age. However, the determination of the effects of ageing on record performances in sprinting is complicated by cohort differences and may produce a different pattern of change than longitudinal trends. In a retrospective study, Conzelmann [4] examined the best German male runners with repeated participation in sprinting competition over many years. The average rate of longitudinal decline in 100-m performance from age 20–25 to ages 70–75 years was approximately 0.3%–0.4%/year and smaller than the cross-sectional decline (~0.6%/year) of the 10 highest-ranked all time

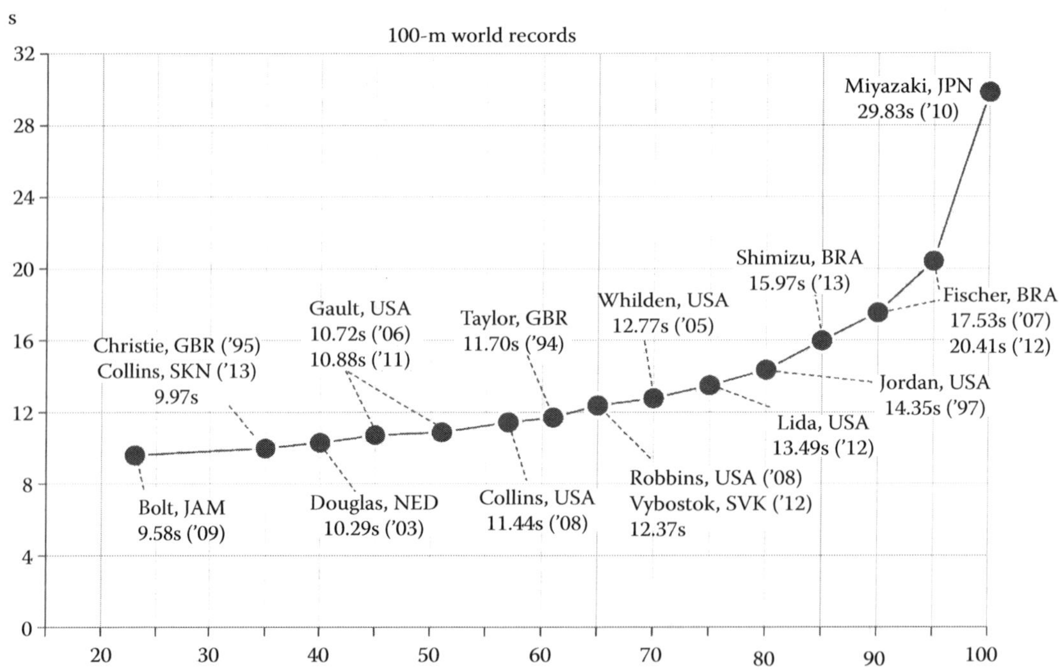

FIGURE 16.1 The official 100-m world records (year 2013) in open and each 5-year (>35 years) classes in men. The year when the record was made is in brackets. (From World Masters Athletics, Records. Available at http://www.world-masters-athletics.org/records, accessed 30 January 2014; IAAF Athletics, Senior Indoor Records. Available at http://www.iaaf.org/statistics/records, accessed 30 January 2014.)

national performances [4]. However, it is probable that longitudinal change in sprinting ability may be influenced by changes in training practices and competitive status.

In systematically trained runners who have reached their full athletic potential during adulthood, the rate and magnitude of sprint performance decline could be greater than in those with a lower-level training and performance at young adult age. Merlene Ottey presents a unique example of an athlete who has been able to continue her career as an elite-level international sprinter until her early 50s. Her personal best 100-m times have over 16 years declined from 10.74 seconds (36 years) to 11.82 seconds (52 years) corresponding to a decline in running velocity of about 0.57%/year. Given that she is at a stable, optimal level of training (still trying to qualify for major championships), the decrement in sprint running performance may reflect the smallest possible rate of change in sprint performance due to biological ageing *per se*.

16.2.2 Velocity Curve

Success in sprint running events requires not only high maximum velocity but also an efficient starting action, running acceleration and speed endurance. The 100-m competitive sprint running performance of young elite athletes has frequently been evaluated by a velocity curve [5–8] which describes acceleration from a resting position to maximum velocity and deceleration at the end of the run. During the European Veterans Athletics Championships in 2000, we investigated for the first time the velocity curve characteristics of the 100-m races in master sprinters using video analysis. In male finalists (40–89 years, $n = 37$) the age-associated differences in velocity were similar—approximately 5%–6% per decade in early acceleration (0–10 m), maximum velocity and deceleration (90–100 m) phases. One apparent difference between runners of different ages was the length of the acceleration phase. In the oldest runners (80–89 years) it took only about 25 m to reach the maximum velocity of 6.7 m/s whereas the athletes in the youngest age group (40–49 years) attained their maximum velocity of 10.2 m/s at around 45 m. Reports from major championships have shown that young elite athletes achieve very steep initial acceleration and could continue to accelerate up to about 60–70 m to increase speed to a maximum of ~11.8–12.0 m/s during a competitive sprint run performance [5–8]. Another major finding in our competition analysis was that the relative loss in velocity from the peak velocity sequence to the end of the race became greater with age (from 5.4% at age 40–49 years to 10.6% at age 80–89 years). These values were somewhat greater when compared to the decreases of about 2%–7% in velocity in young elite sprint runners [5–8]. On the other hand, in older sprint runners, maximum speed is achieved earlier so there is greater potential to decelerate towards end of the race.

16.2.3 Stride Parameters

At the first level of mechanical analysis, running velocity is determined by a product of stride rate and stride length. In the competition analyses above, the effect of age on the stride variables was examined during different phases of the 100-m race [9]. The results showed age-related declines in both acceleration and maximum velocity were primarily related to a reduction in stride length. In maximum velocity phase, stride length declined from about 2.19 m in the 40–49-year-old runners to 1.60 m in runners over 80 years (Table 16.1). Stride rate showed a small age-related decline from 4.66 to 4.23 steps per second and was explained by a progressive increase in contact time while flight time did not show any significant decrease until the oldest age group.

The same trends for stride characteristics during maximum speed phase were observed earlier by Hamilton et al. [10] who studied 83 elite-level male sprinters aged 30–94 years in competition conditions. They also found age-related decreases in range of motion in both the hip and knee joints, while leg swing time remained virtually unchanged with age. Similarly, Roberts and co-workers [11] reported that 60–65-year-old male runners had decreased range of motion and angular velocities at lower limb joints but comparable swing duration to that observed in 20–22-year-old runners.

TABLE 16.1
Step Parameters during Maximum Velocity Phase of the 100-m Race Measured on World-Class Young Adult and Master Male Sprinters

	Velocity (m/s)	Step Length (m)	Step Rate (Hz)	Flight Time (s)	Contact Time (s)
Young	12.55	2.70	4.63	0.128	0.087
40–49 years	10.20	2.19	4.66	0.121	0.098
50–59 years	9.32	2.02	4.64	0.121	0.102
60–69 years	8.90	1.96	4.54	0.116	0.109
70–79 years	7.89	1.79	4.42	0.111	0.118
80–89 years	6.74	1.60	4.23	0.097	0.141

Sources: Based on data from Mann, R., *The Mechanics of Sprinting and Hurdling*, Create Space, Lexington, KY, 2011 (young athletes); Korhonen, M.T. et al., *Med. Sci. Sports Exerc.* 41(4), 844–856, 2009 (masters athletes).

However, the authors suggested that the age-related decline in swing limb kinetics is not necessarily due to reduction in force generating potential, but rather reflect a strategy to match the swing limb timing to the reduced stride length and increased contact time.

16.2.4 Ground Reaction Forces

Ground-leg interaction is the major factor in sprint running because it is during the contact phase of the step cycle that segmental forces can act on and thus influence horizontal speed. Therefore, the measurement of ground reaction forces (GRF) can provide valuable information about the effect of age on performance. However, to our knowledge, the effects of age on GRF have only been examined once. In a laboratory-based study on Finnish sprint runners ranging in age from 17 to 82 years, force production during maximum velocity sprinting was described using average net resultant GRF (i.e. combination of horizontal and vertical force) as a specific force indicator [12]. The magnitude of both the braking and push-off forces declined progressively with age and was reflected in changes in step length, contact time and consequently in maximum velocity. Along with the 27% age-related decline in sprint running velocity (from 9.7 to 7.1 m/s), braking force and push-off forces decreased by 20% and 32%, respectively. In addition to decreased force production, the mean angle of push-off resultant force became more vertically oriented that may impair the acceleration of the body in the optimal horizontal direction and thus affecting stride length. A notable finding was also greater age-related increase in contact time in braking than push-off phase (Figure 16.2). It could be hypothesized that high eccentric impact loads are less well tolerated in older ages resulting in a longer braking phase and this could impair elastic energy/force potentiation during concentric phase of the contact [13].

Mechanical stiffness during contact (eccentric phase) is thought to be an important determinant of optimal reactive force production in sprint running. In the study on ageing Finnish sprint runners, stiffness regulation of whole body and contact leg was predicted by spring-mass models (ratio of peak GRF to vertical length change of the centre of mass or to leg length) [12]. It was found that vertical stiffness and leg stiffness decreased by 41% and 21%, respectively, from the 17–33-year-old runners to runners over 70 years. In addition, stiffness values were strongly related to braking phase contact time, suggesting that high stiffness is a prerequisite for tolerating higher impact loads and can lead to faster transition from the braking to the push-off phase.

The exact process by which stiffness during running is regulated is not fully understood, but may reflect a complex interaction of centrally programmed prelanding activation and reflex potentiation after the impact phase [14], stiffness of tendons and other connective tissues [15], and muscle force-generating capacity. A 20-week training program emphasising maximum strength and explosive strength training exercises increased sprint running leg stiffness by 14% in a group of elite masters

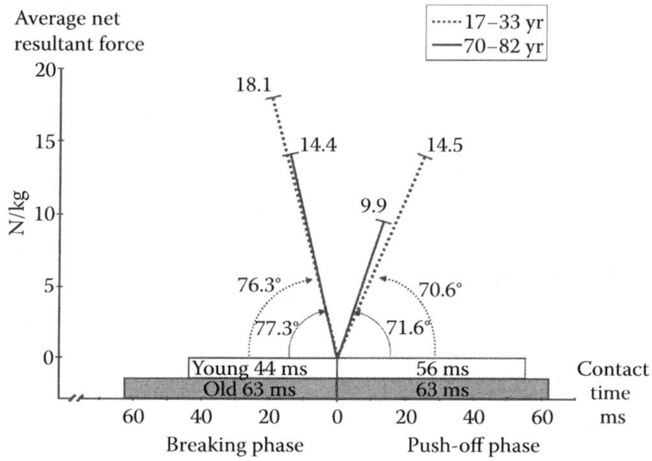

FIGURE 16.2 Resultant force production characteristics of maximum speed running in the youngest and oldest athlete groups. There was a greater relative age-group difference in push-off than braking forces as well as greater age-related increase in braking than push-off ground contact time. Further, the mean angle of push-off force increased with age. (From Korhonen, M.T., *Effects of Aging and Training on Sprint Performance, Muscle Structure and Contractile Function in Athletes*, Ph.D. thesis, Studies in Sport, Physical Education and Health, No. 137, University of Jyväskylä, Finland, 2009.)

male sprint runners (52–78 years) with limited or no prior strength training experience [16]. Thus, it might be hypothesised that muscle force-generating capacity is an important factor determining age-related declines in stiffness and reactive force production during sprint running. However, a limitation of the vertical and leg stiffness calculations are that they do not provide information about joint-specificity and the interaction of muscle and tendon function. Studies in young athletes have suggested that stiffness in the ankle joint rather than knee joint determines ground contact time in sprinting [17].

16.3 LIMITING FACTORS IN SPRINT PERFORMANCE WITH AGEING

16.3.1 Maximal and Explosive Muscle Strength

Several studies in young adult athletes have reported significant correlations between sprint running ability and explosive muscle strength/power defined by various jumping tests and isometric rate of force development [18–20]. In addition, many investigations have shown positive relationships between measures of sprint running performance and maximum strength [18,19,21]. The advantage of higher maximum strength is likely to be connected to its influence on power production (power = force × velocity). For stronger runners, the inertia of body weight represents a smaller percentage of maximum strength and it is thus easier to accelerate. Masters sprint and strength/power athletes have been found to experience progressive age-related reductions in both maximal and explosive strength characteristics, the decrease being somewhat larger for rapid force production capacity [22–24]. We have previously observed that in sprinters between 17 and 82 years of age the maximum load that can be lifted one time (1-RM) using concentric half squat exercise reduced from approximately 2.5 to 1.6 times body weight (BW) (–36%) while counter-movement jump height declined from 52 to 23 cm (–56%) [12]. With regard to sprint performance, the squat 1-RM and vertical jump heights measured in our study correlated positively with both sprinting speed and stride frequency, and negatively with contact time of maximum velocity phase. The squat 1-RM was positively associated with vertical and leg stiffness [12].

In an ongoing study we have tried to identify the importance of different lower extremity muscles in the age-related decline in maximum sprinting speed. Muscle moments and powers at the ankle, knee and hip joints were evaluated during maximum-speed phase at 30–40 m in young (26 ± 6 years), upper middle-aged (61 ± 5 years) and old (78 ± 4 years) male sprinters (n = 13 in each group). The preliminary data indicate that a significant age-related decline in muscular output occurred at the level of hip and ankle joints, but surprisingly, not at knee joint level. In regression analysis, power generation of the ankle plantarflexors explained 80% of the total variance, with knee power absorption being other factor (5%) to appear in the model. Although the decline in overall sprinting performance (start, acceleration, maximum-speed phase) with age is probably linked to the function of multiple muscle groups, the ankle plantarflexors may become the important weak link in the force production chain during the maximum-speed phase. This should be taken into consideration for the design of sprint training programs for masters sprinters.

16.3.2 Muscle Mass and Contractility

A major factor affecting rapid-force production capacity is the inherited muscle fibre composition. Analyses of muscle fibre contractile properties have shown that shortening velocity and power of fast type IIA and IIB muscle fibres is ~4- and ~10-fold higher, respectively, than that of slow type I fibres [25,26] in young and middle-aged untrained men. In successful young sprint runners, fast fibres (IIA+B) have been found to account for about 60% (range 50%–75%) of the fibres in the vastus lateralis thigh muscle [27]. However, in young sprinters the proportion of the total muscle cross-sectional area occupied by fast fibres is likely to be greater because the training-induced muscle fibre enlargement (hypertrophy) is typically much more pronounced in the fast compared to slow fibres [28,29]. Another factor that could influence contractile velocity is muscle fibre length and pennation angle (the angle at which fibres insert into the aponeurosis) [30]. A greater fibre length (more sarcomeres in series) enhances to contraction velocity, whereas increased pennation angle and muscle thickness (more sarcomeres in parallel) enhances the contractile force potential.

In our study, various muscle characteristics were examined in 18- to 84-year-old sprint runners [28]. The results implied that the decline in contractile force and velocity potential of quadriceps muscle with age were mainly attributable to reductions in muscle thickness (mass) and size of fast-contracting type II fibres, because the muscle fibre distribution, fascicle length as well as single-fibre contractile force and velocity remained largely unchanged with ageing. The percentage decline in cross-sectional area of fast type II fibres was 6.9% per decade, while type I fibre area remained unaltered (Figure 16.3). Our findings of selective atrophy of fast fibres agree with the results of master sprint runners and jumpers [31,32] and ageing endurance-trained athletes [33–35]. However, the size of fast fibres appears to be far above the age norms in masters athletes exposed to long-term strength training [32–34], suggesting that resistance training in masters sprinters be encouraged.

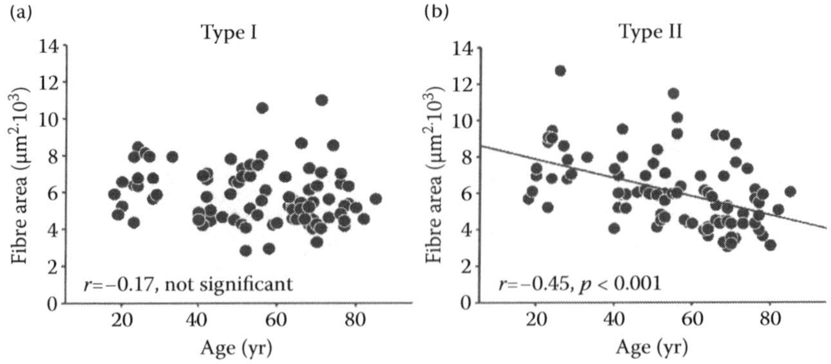

FIGURE 16.3 Association between age and mean fibre cross-sectional area of type I (a) and type II muscle fibres (b) of the vastus lateralis muscle. (Adapted from Korhonen, M.T. et al., *J. Appl. Physiol.* 101[3], 906–917, 2006.)

In addition to muscle fibre atrophy, the major factor underlying the ageing-related decrease in muscle mass is a loss of muscle fibre number due to the age-related reduction in number of functioning motor units. In human vastus lateralis muscle, the decrease in fibre number has been reported to be about 50%, from 650,000 to 325,000 fibres between age 20 and 80 years [37]. Whether the loss of motor units and fibres can be slowed or prevented by systematic exercise is one of the most important unanswered questions relating to deterioration in muscle function in older ages.

There is preliminary evidence from masters endurance runners that exercise may counteract muscle from motor unit loss. Power and co-workers [38] measured the number of functioning motor units (MUs) in lower leg tibialis anterior muscle and found that MU number was higher in habitually trained 65-year-old male runners (140 ± 53 MU) than age-matched controls (91 ± 22 MU) but similar to those of 25-year-old recreationally active controls (150 ± 43 MU). Their recent subsequent study [39] showed that the number of functioning MU was lower in the upper limb biceps muscles in both endurance-trained (185 ± 69 MU) and untrained (133 ± 69 MU) older men compared with the young men (354 ± 113 MU) suggesting that the life-long exercise might provide neuroprotective effects only in muscle groups that are directly over-loaded by exercise.

As regards to relationships between muscle structural properties and sprint running performance, we found that combined knee extensor and plantar flexor muscle thickness was significantly associated with maximum running speed and 60-m running times in runners aged between 17 and 82 years [12]. Moreover, the muscle thickness correlated with both leg and vertical stiffness and, in a regression analysis, muscle thickness was the strongest predictor of GRF during the braking phase. In other words, it seems that the larger the leg muscles, the higher the stiffness and ability to produce/tolerate high eccentric forces. These findings appear to be in line with Weyand et al. [40] who estimated the vertical force requirement for different velocities in young runners and concluded that the greater body masses of faster sprint runners are directly associated with the greater ground support forces required to reach faster running speeds. Figure 16.4 presents a simplified model of

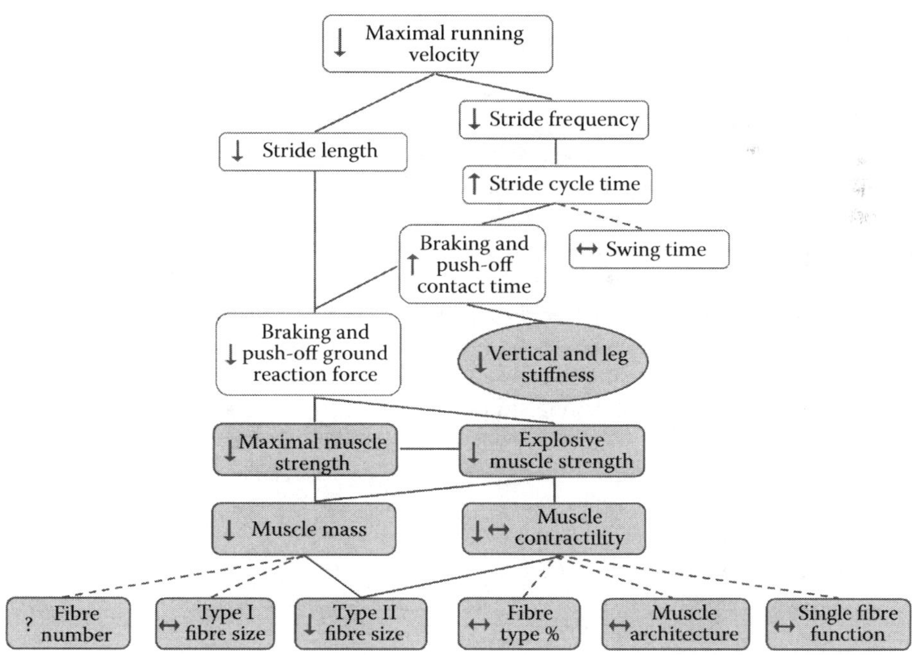

FIGURE 16.4 Schematic diagram of the skeletal muscle and biomechanical factors that may determine age-related decline in sprint running performance. Arrows denote significant decrease (↓), increase (↑) and no alteration (↔). (Adapted from Korhonen, M.T. et al., *Med. Sci. Sports Exerc.* 41[4], 844–856, 2009.)

some of the structural and functional changes in skeletal muscle with age that may be connected to decline in sprinting performance.

16.3.3 Tendon Properties

Tendons can play an important role as power amplifiers during sprint running. Some recent studies have examined the association of tendon compliance (elongation of tendon and aponeurosis at given tendon force in isometric contractions) on sprint performance in young runners [41,42]. These studies suggest that the stiffness of the tendon that is optimal for performance is dependent on the specific joint/muscle group. For example, Stafilidis and Arampatzis [41] and Kubo et al. [42] have found more compliant tendon structures at the knee extensors were related to better 100-m sprint times. A major suggested advantage of increased tendon compliance at the knee extensor muscles for sprinters is that it allows muscle fibres to generate force at lower shortening velocities that augment the muscle force potential as a result of the force-velocity relation (the faster a muscle shortens the less force it can produce). However, the compliance of tendon structures at the calf muscle was not associated with sprint run performance [42] and sprinters showed considerably higher stiffness compared to endurance-trained and untrained subjects [43].

Earlier studies have shown that in sprint running, minimum contact time is determined, at least in young runners, by stiffness of the ankle joint [17]. Therefore, one could assume that stiffer tendon structures at plantar flexors are best suited for the fast contact pattern. It has been suggested that age-related changes in tendon properties (e.g. loss of Achilles tendon stiffness) play a role in the age-related decline in sprint running performance by compromising the rate of force development and elastic storage capacity [44]. However, the currently available scientific data on muscle-tendon behaviour is from untrained people using isometric contractions. Therefore, to verify the assumptions above, studies in physically highly active masters sprinters during actual sprint running conditions are warranted.

16.3.4 Flexibility

Training of flexibility is commonly recommended for sprint athletes for reducing the risk of injury [45]. In addition, good flexibility is thought to be an important prerequisite to perform technically correct sprint running stride and is an especially important issue in sprint hurdling [45,46]. Ageing is associated with a degeneration and hardening of soft tissue leading to functional loss of joint flexibility [47]. The age-related changes in flexibility are evident for both untrained and athletic people and can start in the 20s. In a study on amateur soccer players of three different age levels of competition (19–44 years, $n = 24$), McHugh et al. [48] found that players over 30 years of age had less lumbar flexion and hip rotation static flexibility than players in their thirties (19–29 years). In our studies, we have measured static range of motion (ROM) in the hip, knee and ankle goniometrically (with modified Thomas test [49,50]) to estimate the flexibility of quadriceps and iliopsoas hamstrings (straight leg raise) and calf muscles in 68 male sprinters ranging in age from 17 to 82 years (unpublished data). There was a progressive age-related decline in flexibility values for hamstrings (r with age = -0.33, $p < 0.01$) and quadriceps ($r = -0.40$, $p < 0.001$), but no significant age effect was found in iliopsoas and calf muscle flexibility. The difference in average range of motion between the youngest (17–29 years) and oldest group (70–82 years) was 11.6° (95.4° vs. 83.8°) for hamstring flexibility and 16.0° (66.9° vs. 50.9°) for quadriceps flexibility.

The association between flexibility and sprint performance measures was analysed in a pooled sample using partial correlation analysis, controlling for age ($n = 52$). Interestingly, the flexibility of the hamstring muscles was inversely related to running speed ($r = -0.36$, $p < 0.05$) and stride frequency ($r = -0.50$, $p < 0.001$) of maximum speed phase (30–40 m) and showed a strong trend for direct association with 60-m sprint running times ($r = 0.26$, $p = 0.059$). These findings suggest possible performance benefits in runners with lower compliance of the hamstring muscle group.

Although the above data should be interpreted cautiously due to non-sport-specific static flexibility measurements, they raise questions as to what is an optimal flexibility from a sprint running performance standpoint. There are some theories that if muscles and tendons become easily lengthened and stretched this could lead to suboptimal stiffness and decreased rate of force development that is a critical factor for sprint run performance [51]. Therefore, some researchers have suggested that the focus on the development of flexibility in athletes might not be to exceed but rather to maintain normal physiological range of motion that allow good body positions to perform an effective movement pattern [52]. In addition, it is recommended that because acute stretching can decrease force output, pre-event stretching should be limited to stretching within available ROM and performed at least 45–60 minutes before an event [52]. Nevertheless, it is plausible that soft tissue may become more injury-prone with ageing [53] and thus the importance of flexibility and stretching from an injury prevention point of view may increase in masters athletes. Clearly, more scientific evidence is needed about the effects of flexibility and stretching on injury rates and sprint performance in ageing athletes.

16.3.5 Energy Metabolism

In sprint running, the ability to produce force over a long period of time is affected by adenosine triphosphate (ATP) supply to the muscles. Due to the requirement for rapid production of energy, the major ATP contribution to sprinting comes from anaerobic processes of phosphocreatine (PCr) breakdown and degradation of glycogen to lactate (anaerobic glycolysis). Intramuscular PCr is a very rapid energy source but is limited in quantity and reduced considerably during the first 5 seconds of maximal sprinting [54]. Anaerobic glycolysis, which is also activated at the beginning of exercise, reaches a maximal rate by about 5 seconds of maximal sprinting but can be maintained for a longer time [54]. It has been estimated that in world-class 100-m performance (10 s) the energy production is 50% from both PCr and anaerobic glycolysis, whereas in the 400 m, the relative energy contribution is about 62.5% from anaerobic glycolysis, 12.5% from PCr and 25% from aerobic processes [55]. Increased anaerobic glycolytic stress with increasing sprint distance is reflected in peak post-exercise blood lactate concentrations, $[La]_{b\ peak}$. In young high-performance male sprinters $[La]_{b\ peak}$ following 100-, 200- and 400-m sprint races have been found to be about 12–14 mmol/l, 17–20 mmol/l and 20–25 mmol/l, respectively [56–59].

Muscle fatigue is a complex performance-limiting phenomenon in sprinting. A muscle biopsy study in seven young male sprint runners (100-m records: 10.60–10.99 s) has suggested that PCr depletion is the main factor for the loss of speed towards the end of the 100 m sprint, because the energy transfer from glycogen may not be fast enough to maintain the high rates of ATP utilisation needed for sprinting [54]. Fatigue in sprinting may also be related to the lactic acid-induced accumulation of H^+ ions (fall in pH) that may impair contractile function either directly (inhibition of cross-bridge kinetics) or indirectly (via glycolytic inhibition) [60]. Some investigations have connected fatigue to other components of the metabolism, such as increased inorganic phosphate from PCr breakdown and potassium ion concentrations [61]. Nevertheless, the exact mechanism of fatigue during sprint running remains unclear.

Our current understanding of the effects of age on energy production during sprinting is restricted to $[La]_{b\ peak}$ measurements that provide a rough indirect measure about anaerobic glycolytic energy production. We studied $[La]_{b\ peak}$ in competition conditions in 81 male sprint runners aged 40 to 88 years [62]. The results showed an age-associated decline in $[La]_{b\ peak}$ following 100-m (from 14.6 to 10.9 mmol/l), 200-m (17.4 to 15.4 mmol/l) and 400-m (17.0 to 14.1 mmol/l) events, the age-group differences becoming significant after 70 years of age. Moreover, the decline in $[La]_{b\ peak}$ with age was related to increases in running times and thus slowing of sprint run performance. These data support the view that reduced energy production via anaerobic glycolysis in older ages may be a factor in the curvilinear deterioration in overall sprint run performance [63]. Our results also agree with the recent study by Benelli et al. [64] who studied blood lactate response to competitive swimming in 52 male swimmers (40–79 years) using the same analytical method. They found an age-related decline in $[La]_{b\ peak}$ following competitive 50–400-m events (from 14.2 to 8.2 mmol/l) with the age-related difference becoming most salient after 70 years of age. However, Reaburn and Mackinnon [65] reported no significant age differences in the capillary $[La]_{b\ peak}$ following a 100-m freestyle swimming test when comparing groups of male swimmers aged 25–35, 36–45, 46–55, and 56+ years ($n = 4$ in each group), but their differing findings may relate to the small number of elderly athletes.

The exact causative factors explaining age-related decline in $[La]_{b\ peak}$ have not been distinguished, but some hypotheses could be suggested. Total lactic acid production is highly correlated with both the contractile muscle mass [66,67] and the size and number of fast fibres [68,69]. Therefore the age-related reduction in muscle mass via preferential atrophy and loss of fast fibres could play a major role in the observed age-related decreases in $[La]_{b\ peak}$. It is also known that high-intensity sprint training increases both muscle [70,71] and blood lactate accumulation [72] together with increases in glycolytic enzyme activities [70,71]. Because older sprinters in general exhibit an age-related reduction in the volume of high-intensity exercise they undertake [62], this could in part contribute to an age-related decline in anaerobic metabolic capacity. In addition, on the basis of studies on untrained people, other factors such as preferential reliance on oxidative metabolism during exercise [73] could potentially play a role in reduced lactate production. However, a problem when interpreting the findings of general ageing population is that the physiological changes may reflect sedentary lifestyle and decreased physical activity rather than ageing process *per se*.

16.4 TRAINING METHODS TO IMPROVE SPRINT PERFORMANCE

To improve sprint performance both hard and persistent physical training over a long period is required. Optimisation of training is therefore highly desirable, but little is known about how to best train older sprint athletes. Many masters sprint runners have adopted their training methods through personal experience rather than application of research-based practices. The purpose of this section is to provide scientific and practical knowledge of sprint running that will help the design of effective training programs. Examples of training practices employed by successful master sprinter will be given.

16.4.1 Basic Training Principles

The basic principles of training include progressive overload, training specificity, accommodation and individuality [74]. Progressive overload suggests that in order to allow physiological systems to systematically adapt to physical training, the intensity and duration of that training should increase progressively over time. Compared to younger exercisers, the older athletes may need more time to recover after hard training sessions [75]. Therefore, the frequency of high-intensity or high-volume training bouts may need to be reduced to avoid overtraining and/or injury. Training specificity refers to the concept that adaptation to exercise is specific to the type of loading. In the case of enhancing sprint performance, the training practices should reflect the physiological and biomechanical demands (e.g. energy systems, muscle groups, force production characteristics) of the competitive event. In practical terms, this means that a mixture of sprint, strength and plyometric exercises should be employed when training for sprint running. If the same exercise with the same training load is used over an extended period of time, the adaptation occurs only during the early part of training. In other words the response to a constant stimulus decreases over time, which is referred to as accommodation. Therefore, the intensity and volume of the training sessions should be progressively increased and the types of exercises varied to maximise adaptation. Periodisation of training into different training cycles (weekly, monthly and yearly cycles) ensures variation in overall training load and optimises adaptation before major competitions. According to the principle of individuality, athletes may respond differently to training stimuli, partly due to the genetic differences [76]. For example, the volume of training that is optimal for one athlete can lead to overtraining in others. Coaches should be aware of the individual differences and plan training considering characteristics, such as the age, training years, strengths and weaknesses, health status and recovery rate of the individual athlete.

16.4.2 Speed Training

Many successful master sprinters apply only speed exercises during training. Their success is proof of the effectiveness of the event-specific training in maintenance of sprinting ability with ageing. Sprint exercises form the basis for developing explosive power and anaerobic energy production. In addition, fast cyclical sprint movements require a high level of neuromuscular coordination/skill, which can be achieved only by regular sprinting. For speed development, the training sessions with short sprints should be done in a fully recovered state. In maximal speed efforts, psychological factors such as willpower and concentration are thought to be essential to achieve an optimal training response especially in terms of recruiting maximum number of fast motor units [77].

The intensity of the sprint training remains high throughout the training year while the distances in running drills increase as the competition season approximates (Figure 16.5). This principle is referred to as the short to long approach and it is widely used in speed training for short sprint events (100–200 m, short sprint hurdles). When it comes to long sprints (400-m flat and hurdles) typically a long to short approach is utilised simultaneously. In this approach the speed of the training sessions is increased and the length of running distances decreased gradually as the training year progresses towards the competition season.

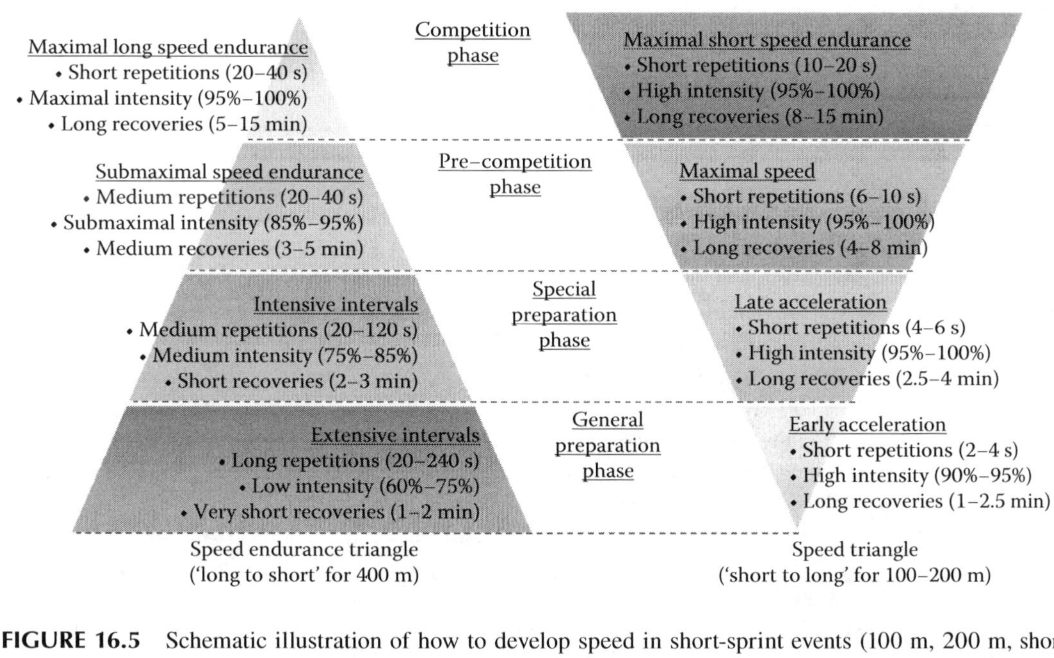

FIGURE 16.5 Schematic illustration of how to develop speed in short-sprint events (100 m, 200 m, short sprint hurdles) in different parts of the training year according to the 'short to long' approach, accompanied by the principles of simultaneous speed endurance development in long sprints (400-m flat and hurdles) according to the 'long to short' approach.

16.4.3 Strength Training

Both running and plyometric (jumping) exercises are essential to develop anaerobic metabolic properties of skeletal muscles, sprint-specific neuromuscular coordination, and both tendon strength and elastic properties. However, training regimens consisting solely of running and plyometric exercise are ineffective to increase muscle mass and strength that are essential attributes for a good sprinting ability. Therefore, optimal training regimens to enhance sprint performance in master sprinters also require high-intensity weight training. One of the most significant impacts of strength training in master sprint athletes could be an effective overload of the fast-contracting type II fibres that are known to be particularly at risk of age-related atrophy [28,78].

The success of strength training to optimise sprint performance in masters sprinters is indicated by a number of studies. For example, Cristea et al. [16] examined the effects of combined strength and speed training (4×/week) in world-class male sprinters (52–78 years, n = 7 and 4 controls) who had limited or no previous experience in weight training. The 20-week periodised training program increased type II fibre size by 17%–20%. This was accompanied by significant improvements in maximal (21%–40%) and explosive (4%–29%) strength, maximum speed (4%) and 60-m sprint times (2%). Running mechanics were also altered with significant increases in propulsive ground reaction forces (8%), rate of force development (12%–14%), stride length (3%) and a decrease in ground contact time (5%–9%). Reaburn and co-workers [79,80] found that an 8-week combined sprint (2×/week) and hypertrophic strength (3×/week) training program in male sprinters (55 ± 6 years, n = 6 and 4 controls) resulted not only in an increased maximal leg strength (10%–25%) but also improvements in 100-m (4%) and 300-m (2%) sprint performances. Taken together, these studies strongly suggest that combined resistance and sprint training is clearly more effective than sprint training alone.

In sprint events one can distinguish a start, acceleration, maximum speed and speed maintenance phase. Each of these phases places different demands on strength and power-generating capacities of the various muscle groups. The acceleration phase requires particularly a high maximum and explosive force production in the hip extensor muscles, while the maximum speed phase depends especially on the ability to produce high reactive power by the plantar and knee flexors and hip extensors. Figure 16.6 shows an example of sprint and strength exercises that are planned using the information on force production and technique requirements of a 100-m sprint run event.

16.4.4 Structure of the Training Programs

To avoid overtraining and to reach maximum performance during important competitions, the annual planning based on short- and long-term objectives is an important aspect of training for the athlete [81]. Most young and masters sprinters concentrate on both indoor and outdoor competitions and thus an annual training program with double-peak periodisation models could be optimal. Tables 16.2 through 16.4 show this approach developed and employed by a successful male masters sprinter (100–200 m) with a long-term personal experience in coaching of young elite athletes. The indoor season represents the phase I and the outdoor season phase II with general and pre-competition phases in both. The type of exercises and rhythm (hard/easy) are fundamentally similar in both indoor and outdoor seasons, with deviations in the length of the training phases. The training program contains a mixture of aerobic, speed endurance, acceleration and maximum speed and strength exercises. The aim is to preserve sprint performance at a relatively high level throughout the year. Within weeks, there are two–three developing heavy training sessions and two–three maintenance or recovery sessions. The muscle conditioning, daily flexibility practices and injury prevention strategies are also central elements in training of this successful sprinter.

The annual training hours of 438 (8.4 hours/week) and training sessions of 222 (4.3 sessions/week) is lower than that normally observed in young sprint athletes. This may be attributable to

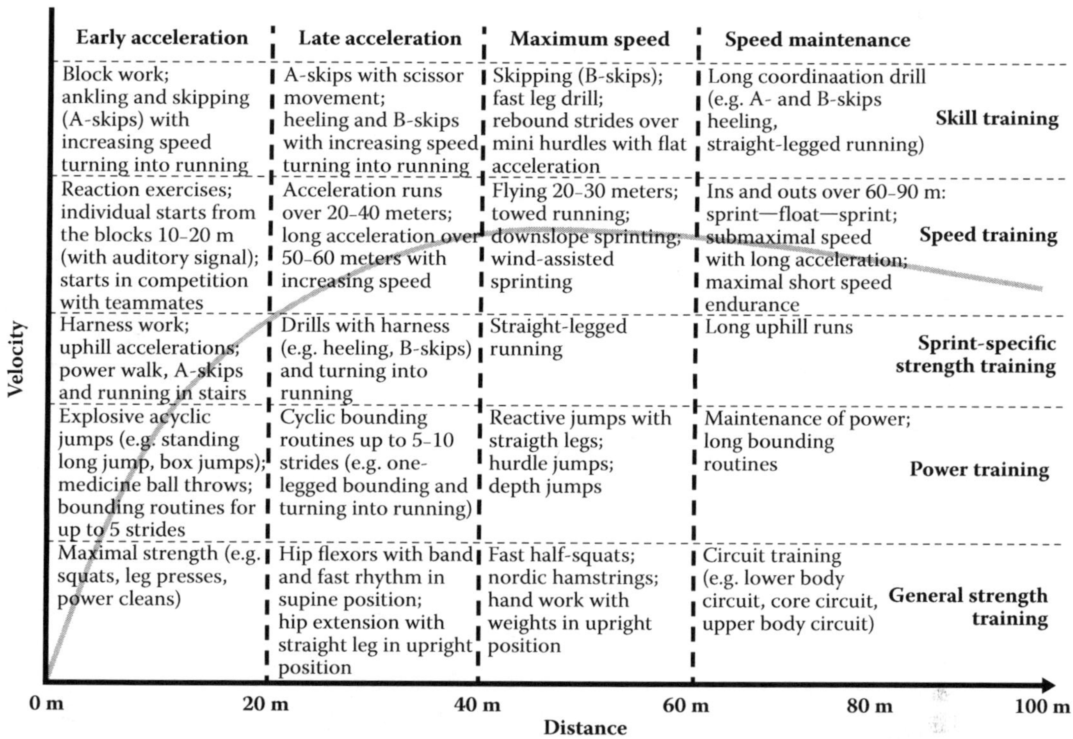

FIGURE 16.6 The different sections of a sprint running event (100 m in this example) and how these sections are emphasised in selection of skill, speed, sprint-specific strength, power and general strength-training exercises. The grey line represents a typical velocity curve of an elite master sprinter.

differences in recovery potential, which reduces the optimal training frequency and consequently the training volume in masters versus younger sprinters. There is some evidence that highly trained masters sprinters are susceptible to fatigue and/or overtraining. For example, Heazlewood [82] studied training and performance characteristics of 40–60-year-old elite Australian masters male sprinters who used a traditional single-peak periodisation model. Many of the sprinters reported chronic fatigue after the competition phase and hence needed a rest period before resumption of training. The generalised fatigue and overtraining in masters sprinters could partially be related to age-related changes in circulating hormones, which could affect also the rapidity and magnitude of the training response [75].

16.5 NUTRITION FOR THE MASTERS SPRINT RUNNER

16.5.1 Energy Needs

Dietary energy and the intakes of macro- and micronutrients and fluids can have an important influence on both health and performance characteristics. The first important consideration is an energy balance that depends on energy intake and expenditure. In all athletes, total energy intake should be raised to meet the increased energy expended during training and to maintain body weight. Insufficient amount of energy intake can result in illness and/or the onset of physical and psychological symptoms of overtraining. However, the energy expenditure can vary considerably in different sports as discussed at length in Chapter 3.

As a general rule it can be said that energy expenditure is higher in submaximal endurance training than in strength, speed or skill-based athletic training and this is reflected in nutritional intake

TABLE 16.2
Structure of Training Program of World-Champion Male Sprinter Aged 65 years[a]

Type of Training	General Preparation I 15.10–31.12 11 Weeks	Competition Preparation I 1.1–31.1 4 Weeks	Indoor Competitions 1.2–28.2 4 Weeks	General Preparation II 1.3–30.4 8 Weeks	Competition Preparation II 1.5–30.6 8 Weeks	Outdoor Competitions 1.7–31.8 8 Weeks
Aerobic work (50%–70% of maximum heart rate)	Steady state jogging and light interval runs, and cross-country skiing can be an alternative form at wintertime. Aerobic work is also incorporated into warming-up and cooling-down exercises and coordination drills.					
Speed endurance						
• Sprint drills (length of runs)	100–300 m	60–200 m	60–150 m	200–400 m	60–300 m	60–150 m
• Range of speeds (% max)	70%–75%	80%–85%	85%–90%	65%–70%	75%–80%	85%–95%
• Weekly volume	800 m	1000 m	800 m	1000 m	800 m	600 m
Speed						
• Start/acceleration/max speed	30–60 m	30–80 m	30–60 m	30–60 m	30–150 m	30–150 m
• Range of speeds (% max)	90%–95%	90%–98%	90%–100%	90%–95%	95%–103%	90%–100%
• Weekly volume	200–300 m	400–500 m	300–400 m	200–300m	400–500 m	200–300 m
Technique	Starting practice and general technique drills as a part of speed exercise.					
Maximum, explosive and hypertrophy weight training	5–10 exercises, 4–6 sets of 1–10 reps at 60–100% maximum load (often with pyramid method)					
Sprint-specific explosive strength	Hill sprints, vertical and horizontal forward jumps and hops, sled pulls, weight throws					
% of total amount of strength training	50%	70%	90%	50%	70%	90%
Muscle conditioning and flexibility	Aerobic circuit, stretching	Aerobic circuit, stretching	Aerobic circuit, stretching	Aerobic circuit, stretching	Aerobic circuit, stretching	Aerobic circuit, stretching

Notes: Weight training exercises

1. One- and two-leg squats (with barbell and Smith machine)
2. One- and two-leg lying leg (knee) curls
3. One- and two-leg (knee) extensions
4. Gluteus exercise
5. Pull-up (without and with extra weights up to 30 kg)
6. Standing and seated calf raise (varied foot positions/angles)
7. Bent-knee sit-ups
8. Back extensions

[a] 100-m record 12.50 seconds at age 65 years.

TABLE 16.3
Structure of Training Program of World-Champion Male Sprinter Aged 65 Years

	General Preparation I 15.10–31.12 11 Weeks	Competition Preparation I 1.1–31.1 4 Weeks	Indoor Competitions 1.2–28.2 4 Weeks	General Preparation II 1.3–30.4 8 Weeks	Competition Preparation II 1.5–30.6 8 Weeks	Outdoor Competitions 1.7–31.8 8 Weeks
Number of competitions	0	1–2	1–2	0	5–6	5–6
Times of exercise	55	20	18	40	36	28
Type of training						
• Aerobic work	11	2	2	10	4	4
• Speed endurance	11	4	4	6	8	8
• Speed/technique	11	6	6	6	12	10
• Weight training	11	2	2	10	4	2
• Sport-specific explosive strength	11	6	4	8	8	4
• Muscle conditioning and flexibility	Daily	Daily	Daily	Daily	Daily	Daily
Rhythm (hard/easy)	2:1	Based on training (recovery)	Based on competition schedule	2:1	Based on training (recovery)	Based on competition schedule
Performance tests	Sprint 20, 30, 60 m (flying starts). Stride length and frequency. Standing long and triple jumps	Sprint 20, 30, 60 m (flying starts). Stride length and frequency. Standing long and triple jumps	Sprint 20, 30, 60 m (flying starts). Stride length and frequency. Standing long jump	Sprint 20, 30, 60 m (flying starts). Stride length and frequency. Standing long jump	Sprint 20, 30, 60 m (flying starts). Stride length and frequency. Standing long jump	Sprint 20, 30, 60 m (flying starts). Stride length and frequency. Standing long jump
Injury prevention strategies	Sports massage and physiotherapy (1 time/3 weeks)	Sports massage and physiotherapy (1 time/2 weeks)	Sports massage and physiotherapy (if needed)	Sports massage and physiotherapy (1 time/3 weeks)	Sports massage and physiotherapy (1 time/10 days)	Sports massage and physiotherapy (if needed)

TABLE 16.4
Summary of Yearly Training Volume of World-Champion Male Sprinter Aged 65 Years

Type of Training	Training Sessions	Training Hours	Percentage of Total
Aerobic work	33	41	9
Speed endurance	41	62	14
Speed/technique+	51	114	26
Competitions/starts	25		
Maximum, explosive and hypertrophy weight training	31	47	11
Sport-specific explosive strength	41	62	14
Muscle conditioning and flexibility	(225)	112	26
Total	222	438	100

of athletes [83,84]. One study assessed the dietary intake by 3-d food records of 62 elite young adult Japanese track and field athletes [83]. It was found that the mean daily energy intake was 2653 kcal (40.0 kcal/kg) for male sprinters and 3628 kcal (59.9 kcal/kg) for male long-distance runners. These findings are in line with those obtained in young adult Finnish track and field athletes [85]. After examining 5-d food records in this study, Mero and co-workers found that male sprinters and hurdlers (n = 15) consumed an average 2848 kcal/day (38.4 kcal/kg) while male endurance runners (n = 5) averaged 3578 kcal (53.6 kcal/kg). Mero has recommended a daily energy intake of about 2000–3000 kcal (25–45 kcal/kg) for young adult sprint and power athletes, 2500–4000 kcal (35–55 kcal/kg) for ball sports athletes and 3000–6000 kcal (45–70 kcal/kg) for endurance athletes during training season depending on the energy expenditure of an individual [86].

The research of dietary patterns of ageing athletes has focused on endurance-trained athletes [87–89] while the information for masters sprint runners or strength athletes [90] is very limited. As a part of our larger veteran athlete project, Malmberg [91] evaluated dietary intake of 54 male sprinters, 40–85 years of age, during their winter training season (Table 16.5 [92]). The absolute daily energy intake declined ~15% ($p < 0.05$) from 2430 kcal/day in the youngest to 2070 kcal/day in the oldest athlete group. However, when energy intake was expressed as kcal/kg/day, the groups were similar. Although the values for masters sprint runners were about 10% higher than in age-matched general population [93], they were well below those reported for masters endurance runners [87–89] and young adult sprinters [83,84]. Compared to young sprint athletes, the masters sprinters may need lower absolute amount of energy for body weight maintenance due to decreasing lean body mass which is the main determinant of energy expenditure [94]. Moreover, the lower training volumes observed in older athletes in general is likely to decrease the need for energy in masters athletes. However, it should be emphasised that food diaries are characterised by underreporting [95] and that the true energy requirements of masters sprinters may perhaps be somewhat higher than our results indicate. However, this should be verified with more accurate assessments of energy intake and expenditure in future studies.

16.5.2 Macronutrients

Carbohydrates are the major energy source of muscle during physical activity and are critical for proper function of the brain and nervous system. In typical sprint training, the reliance on carbohydrate utilisation (blood glucose, muscle and liver glycogen) is high. However, since the overall effective training volume is relatively low, the availability of carbohydrates is not as critical as that in longer-duration aerobic exercise as discussed in Chapter 14. The guidelines for young athletes suggest that in sprint runners, carbohydrates should provide approximately 50%–60% of the daily energy intake to meet the needs of activity and recovery from training. When adjusted to body mass the carbohydrate intake of 3–7 g/kg/day is suggested to be sufficient when training 1–2 hours daily

TABLE 16.5
Anthropometric Characteristics and Average Daily Dietary Intake of Male Masters Sprinters and Basic Recommendations for Male Sprint and Strength Athletes

		Age				
		40–49 (n = 10)	50–59 (n = 13)	60–69 (n = 19)	70–84 (n = 12)	Recommendations
Height	cm	183 ± 8	174 ± 4	172 ± 4	171 ± 5	
Body mass	kg	84 ± 8	74 ± 6	72 ± 6	70 ± 10	
Body fat	%	21 ± 3	20 ± 3	21 ± 4	23 ± 5	
LBM	kg	67 ± 6	58 ± 4	57 ± 4	54 ± 5	
Energy	kcal	2430 ± 390	2230 ± 410	2370 ± 290	2070 ± 210	2000–3000
	Kcal/kg	29.8 ± 4.2	31.2 ± 6.0	32.6 ± 5.2	29.6 ± 4.1	25–45
Protein	E%	15.9 ± 2.9	17.6 ± 1.6	17.1 ± 2.5	16.1 ± 2.0	15–20
	g/kg	1.14 ± 0.18	1.34 ± 0.29	1.43 ± 0.30	1.20 ± 0.22	1.2–1.8
Carbohydrates	E%	50.0 ± 3.2	50.4 ± 6.2	51.7 ± 8.4	51.0 ± 5.4	40–60
	g/kg	3.61 ± 0.65	3.88 ± 1.09	4.31 ± 0.93	3.83 ± 0.72	5–6
Total fat	E%	30.9 ± 4.7	29.3 ± 4.8	28.6 ± 5.3	31.6 ± 5.8	25–35
	g/kg	0.99 ± 0.20	0.99 ± 0.25	1.06 ± 0.27	1.04 ± 0.18	
Saturated fat	E%	12.0 ± 2.9	11.2 ± 2.7	11.0 ± 2.9	12.2 ± 3.0	<10
Monounsaturated fat	E%	10.5 ± 1.6	10.1 ± 2.3	9.4 ± 2.2	10.6 ± 2.2	10–15
Polyunsaturated fat	E%	4.7 ± 0.6	4.6 ± 1.1	4.9 ± 1.6	4.9 ± 1.2	5–10
Alcohol	E%	1.8 ± 1.2	2.3 ± 2.1	2.9 ± 4.0	1.0 ± 0.7	
	g	10.8 ± 7.0	13.0 ± 14.0	18.4 ± 25.0	5.1 ± 3.7	
Cholesterol	mg	304 ± 106	284 ± 111	318 ± 118	252 ± 76	<300
Dietary fibre	g	29 ± 11	32 ± 10	34 ± 10	25 ± 7	25–35
Water	L	2.5 ± 0.7	2.4 ± 0.6	2.2 ± 0.4	2.2 ± 0.6	>2

Sources: Modified from Malmberg, K., *Dietary Patterns of Masters Sprinters Aged 40 to 85 Years*, unpublished thesis (in Finnish), University of Jyväskylä, Finland, 2003; Mero, A., Nutrition coaching, in *Sport Coaching* (in Finnish), A. Mero, A. Nummela, K. Keskinen and K. Häkkinen, eds., VK Kustannus Oy, Lahti, Finland, 2004, pp. 179–209; Borg, P., Fogelholm, M. and Hiilloskorpi, H., *Nutrition for Exerciser* (in Finnish), Edita Publishing, Helsinki, Finland, 2004.

Notes: Values are means ± SD. Statistical significance of the trend in the data was examined using analysis of variance. Group effect was significant for body height, body mass, and LBM (all $p < 0.001$) and absolute energy intake ($p < 0.05$). LBM, lean body mass; n, number of subjects.

[96]. In our research [91], masters sprinters consumed an average 4.0 ± 0.9 g/kg/day (51% ± 6%) carbohydrate that could adequately meet the need given that they were undertaking run-based training of about 1 hour per day (Table 16.5) [12].

The timing of carbohydrate intakes is important to consider since the glycogen-depleted state might have negative effects on both muscle strength and short-term high-intensity exercise [97]. A carbohydrate-containing meal approximately 3–4 hours before exercise should elevate muscle and liver glycogen levels to enable maximum intensity training. Consuming small amounts of carbohydrate (sports drinks) during exercise could help to maintain blood glucose concentration but may be needed only in the intensive training sessions lasting more than 1 hour. If rapid recovery is needed from training or events during a competition, carbohydrate feeding should start immediately after exercise since the speed of muscle glycogen synthesis is maximal during the first 2 hours of recovery [98]. Carbohydrates with moderate to high glycaemic index (i.e. sports drinks, white bread, potatoes) induce fast muscle glycogen synthesis and could hasten carbohydrate replenishment and thus recovery for the next event or training bout [99]. However, in masters sprinters there is typically one training session per day and immediate recovery is not critical. Therefore, for these athletes, post-exercise and other dietary carbohydrate should come primarily from healthy low-glycaemic carbohydrate foods (i.e. fruits, vegetables, whole grain bread, brown rice) that provide also important micronutrients and dietary fibre for health. The carbohydrate needs of masters athletes are discussed in detail in Chapter 4.

The recommended dietary allowance for protein intake is 0.8 g/kg/day. However, based on the findings of maintenance of muscle mass (instead of nitrogen balance), a higher protein intake of about 1.1 g/kg/day may be needed to prevent sarcopenia [100]. Protein recommendations for masters athletes are higher than for non-athletes but could vary somewhat depending on the nature of the sport. Older endurance athletes are advised to consume 1.2–1.4 g/kg/day while in strength-trained athletes the need for protein intake may be as high as 1.5–1.7 g/kg/day [101]. In strength-trained athletes the increased protein (amino acid) intake can be a prerequisite for tissue repair and hypertrophy whereas in endurance athletes long duration of exercise may also increase the use of amino acids for energy production. The development of muscle mass is also a significant training focus in older sprint athletes and during periods of hard training it may be important to increase and target protein intake at 1.5–1.7 g/kg/day for maximum benefit (Table 16.5). Consuming protein at these levels may not increase the risk for metabolic, cardiac, renal, bone or liver diseases in healthy individuals [102].

The quality of protein in food, as determined by its essential amino acid content, is thought to be an important factor for training-induced anabolic response of muscle [103,104]. Consuming protein from animal sources may optimise the growth or maintenance of muscle mass, a view also supported by a large prospective cohort study in older community-dwelling adults [100]. Lean pork and beef, poultry, fish, eggs and dairy products are good examples of high-quality protein sources containing all essential amino acids and in amounts adequate to sustain protein synthesis. Of the different amino acids, the branched-chain amino acid leucine is thought to be particularly important for muscle protein synthesis [103,104]. Recent studies suggest that whey protein (component of milk) that has a high rate of absorption and is rich in branched-chain amino acids (including leucine) may provide a good protective effect against age-related muscle atrophy [105–107]. Therefore, it has been suggested that older athletes could benefit from consuming dietary supplements with whey protein. Casein (major component of milk) has also been widely promoted to strength trainers especially due to its slow absorption qualities being optimal between meals or before bed [103].

The influence of timing of protein intake to stimulate resistance exercise-induced muscle anabolism has been studied extensively in recent years. Although not all studies agree [108,109], a number of investigations suggest that the anabolic effect of protein intake (with or without carbohydrate stimulates) is increased when taken before or immediately after exercise than at other times of the day [103,110,111]. During and within the first 2 hours following exercise, the physiological state of the body appears to be more suitable for rapid protein resynthesis than in a delayed condition (3 hours), possibly because of increases in muscle blood flow, insulin sensitivity and delivery of amino acids to muscle [112].

Of potential importance for older athletes are studies demonstrating that with ageing muscle may become less sensitive to lower doses of amino acids and thus may require a higher quantity of protein to obtain a similar anabolic response to that of young muscle. It has been found that, while in the young, exercise-induced rate of muscle protein synthesis plateaus with ingestion of 20 g of high-quality protein, elderly may require 40 g of protein to achieve maximal stimulation of protein synthesis after exercise [113]. Thus it has been suggested that to optimise muscle anabolism, older exercisers should eat a sufficient amount of high-quality, leucine-rich protein preferably with three or more daily meals [114]. The protein needs of masters athletes are discussed in detail in Chapter 6.

A commonly overlooked issue is that the recovery and trainability of athletes may be influenced by fatty acids. A low-fat diet has found to be associated with reduced testosterone in men [115,116] and a reduction in oestrogen levels in women [117]. Testosterone is known to be a strong mediator of acute and long-term responses and adaptations to physical training and it is possible that too little fat intake may have indirect negative influence on trainability. Evidence from our masters sprinters study [118] and research on untrained elderly individuals [119,120] suggests that of the different fat subtypes, it is saturated fat that may increase biologically active testosterone concentrations, probably by affecting serum sex hormone-binding globulin (SHBG) concentrations. In the masters sprint runners in our study, the relative fat intake was an average 30% with saturated fat contributing 11.5% (Table 16.5). Based on a national survey [121], the diet of the general population (35–74 years) in Finland is quite similar in the total fat intake (32.4%) and saturated fat intake (12.5%) to that of the masters sprinters in our study.

According to some dietary guidelines, this level of fat intake could be of nutritional concern. However, a number of large research studies have failed to substantiate the view that consuming fat at this level is detrimental to health. For example, a recent population-based, prospective cohort study showed that receiving more than 30% of daily energy from fat and more than 10% from saturated fat did not increase all-cause mortality [122]. Indeed, men in the highest quartile of total fat intake, receiving 48% of their total energy intake from fat, had the lowest cardiovascular mortality. Nevertheless, the use of mono- and polyunsaturated fats should be recommended due to their numerous beneficial health effects such as lowered cholesterol and triglyceride levels in blood. For a more detailed discussion on the fat needs of masters athletes and the importance of nutrients for health and chronic disease prevention, see Chapters 5 and 12, respectively.

Interestingly, recent research [123] suggests omega-3 polyunsaturated fats (found in fish oil and some plants such as flaxseed) can increase the rate of muscle protein synthesis in older men and might therefore promote muscle adaptations. Hence, to ensure an optimal anabolic environment, a moderate-fat diet with sufficient protein and energy is advisable for older sprint athletes. Overall, it appears that in most master sprinters we studied, normal dietary habits provided an adequate intake of proteins, fats and carbohydrates as also reflected by normal glucose and lipid profiles, except for relatively high cholesterol levels (Table 16.6 [124]). Moreover, in the masters athletes, total testosterone concentrations were within normal physiological range (ref.values for 51–70 years: 8–29

TABLE 16.6
Blood Biochemical Values of Male Masters Sprinters and Recommended Levels for Men

		Age				
		40–49 (n = 10)	**50–59 (n = 13)**	**60–69 (n = 19)**	**70–84 (n = 10)**	**Recommendations**
Serum total cholesterol	(mmol/L)	5.5 ± 0.8	5.6 ± 1.1	5.5 ± 1.2	5.6 ± 0.9	<5.0[a]
Serum HDL cholesterol	(mmol/L)	1.1 ± 0.3	1.3 ± 0.3	1.3 ± 0.3	1.1 ± 0.3	>1.1[a]
Fasting blood glucose	(mmol/L)	4.8 ± 0.7	4.6 ± 0.5	4.7 ± 0.4	4.7 ± 0.5	<5.5[b]
Hemoglobin	(g/L)	148 ± 5	146 ± 4	144 ± 5	148 ± 5	132–164[a]
Hematocrit	(%)	46 ± 2	45 ± 1	45 ± 1	46 ± 2	0.38–0.49[a]
Total testosterone	nmol/L	16.2 ± 7.3	14.2 ± 1.9	16.4 ± 4.3	17.1 ± 7.3	
SHBG	nmol/L	37.5 ± 12.5	35.3 ± 10.7	41.7 ± 12.3	64.4 ± 18.5	
FAI	nmol/nmol	0.43 ± 0.12	0.42 ± 0.10	0.42 ± 0.16	0.28 ± 0.12	

Sources: Modified from Malmberg, K., *Dietary Patterns of Masters Sprinters Aged 40 to 85 Years*, Unpublished thesis (in Finnish), University of Jyväskylä, Finland, 2003; Korhonen, M.T., *Effects of Aging and Training on Sprint Performance, Muscle Structure and Contractile Function in Athletes*, Ph.D. thesis, Studies in Sport, Physical Education and Health, No. 137, University of Jyväskylä, Finland, 2009.

Notes: Values are means ± SD; group effect was significant for SHBG ($p < 0.001$) and FAI ($p < 0.05$). FAI, free androgen index (total testosterone/SHBG); n, Number of subjects; SHBG, sex hormone-binding globulin.

[a] Borg, P., Fogelholm, M. and Hiilloskorpi, H., *Nutrition for Exerciser*, (in Finnish), Edita publishing, Helsinki, Finland, 2004.

[b] Ceriello, A. and Colagiuri, S., International Diabetes Federation guideline for management of postmeal glucose: A review of recommendations, *Diabet. Med.* 25(10), 1151–6, 2008.

nmol/L; for 70+ years: 6–25 nmol/L) and the estimated prevalence of hypogonadism was only 2%, defined as having a free androgen index (total testosterone/SHBG) below 0.153 [125].

16.5.3 Micronutrients

In the above section we concluded that an adequate fat intake is important to realise an optimal anabolic environment. In addition to this, fats are crucial for the uptake of the fat soluble vitamins A, D, E and K. Even though the intake of macronutrients and the caloric intake appear adequate in masters athletes, a large proportion, including sprint runners, has a lower than the daily recommended intake of one or more micronutrients, among them some of the fat-soluble vitamins [83,126]. One of the most commonly observed nutritional deficiencies in older people is a vitamin D deficiency [126]. Only 20%–50% of masters sprinters exceeded 100% of the RDI of D vitamin, and 15%–50% had less than two-thirds of RDI (Table 16.7 [127]), a level associated with likelihood of inadequate intake of micronutrients [128]. Studies have suggested that inadequate vitamin D intake with age may not only increase the risk of various diseases and bone loss but could also contribute to the deterioration of muscle characteristics including loss and atrophy of fast type II fibres [129,130].

TABLE 16.7
Percent of Male Masters Sprinters Meeting ≥100% and (≥67%) of the RDAs for Vitamins and Minerals for Healthy Male Population

	Age			
	40–49 (*n* = 10)	**50–59 (*n* = 13)**	**60–69 (*n* = 19)**	**70–84 (*n* = 12)**
Vitamin A	50 (90)	54 (92)	53 (79)	75 (92)
Vitamin D	20 (50)	31 (85)	32 (63)	50 (67)
Vitamin E	30 (90)	46 (100)	58 (95)	58 (75)
Thiamin (B_1)	70 (90)	69 (100)	95 (100)	58 (100)
Riboflavin (B_2)	80 (90)	85 (100)	100	100
Niacin	100	100	100	100
Folate	70 (90)	77 (100)	68 (95)	50 (100)
Cobalamin (B_{12})	100	100	100	100
Vitamin C	60 (90)	92 (100)	68 (84)	92 (100)
Calcium	90 (100)	92 (92)	89 (95)	92 (100)
Potassium	80 (90)	100	89 (95)	75 (100)
Magnesium	80 (90)	85 (100)	89 (95)	92 (100)
Iron	90 (100)	100	100	83 (100)
Zinc	90 (100)	100	100	100
Selenium	100	100	100	100

Sources: Modified from Malmberg, K., *Dietary Patterns of Masters Sprinters Aged 40 to 85 Years*, Unpublished thesis (in Finnish), University of Jyväskylä, Finland, 2003; RDAs from Hasunen, K., Heiskanen, S., Packalén, L. et al., *Finnish Nutrition Recommendations* (in Finnish), National Nutrition Council, Ministry of Agriculture and Forestry, Edita, Helsinki, Finland, 2005.

Notes: Recommended Dietary Allowances (RDAs): Vitamin A = 900 RE; vitamin D = 7.5 μg for ages 31–60 years, 10.0 μg for ages ≥61 years; vitamin E = 10 mg α-toko; thiamin =1.4 mg for ages 31–60 years, 1.3 mg for ages 61–74 years, 1.2 mg for ages ≥75 years; riboflavin = 1.7 mg for ages 31–60 years, 1.5 mg for ages 61–74 years, 1.3 mg for ages ≥75 years; niacin = 19 mg for ages 31–60 years, 17 mg for ages 61–74 years, 15 mg for ages ≥75 years; folate = 300 μg; vitamin B12 = 2 μg; vitamin C = 75 mg; calcium = 800 mg; potassium = 3500 mg; magnesium = 350 mg; iron = 9 mg; zinc = 9 mg.

The use of vitamin and mineral supplements is common among masters athletes [131]. In a recent review, Brisswalter and Louis [132] addressed the role of vitamin supplementation on recovery, inflammation and muscle performance in athletes. There remains a lot of uncertainty regarding potential benefits of these supplements. One concern is that high-dose vitamin supplementation may prevent training-induced adaptations, perhaps by interfering reactive oxygen species (ROS)-mediated physiological processes, such as insulin signalling. Therefore, the authors argue that use of supplementations is questionable and the antioxidant micronutrients intake should follow the daily recommendations. While Chapters 7 and 8 examine the vitamin and mineral needs respectively of masters athletes, clearly further research of specific needs of highly trained masters athletes is needed.

Although not a micronutrient, maintaining an adequate hydration status is important for optimal performance during both training and competition. On the basis of studies in young adult athletes, there is greater negative effect of body water deficit (dehydration) for aerobic exercise performance than muscular strength and anaerobic (sprint) performance [133]. It has been reported that while dehydration of as little as 2% body mass due to sweat loss may be enough to cause a measurable reduction in aerobic performance, dehydration of up to 3%–5% may not impair anaerobic or strength performance [133]. To our knowledge, no investigators have documented the effect of dehydration on performance in older athletes. However, maintenance of optimal hydration status may become challenging in older athletes (see Chapter 9) since ageing could bring physiological changes such as reduced thirst sensation, less ability to concentrate urine (increase urine formation) and reduced potential to dissipate heat [134].

In addition, due to the well-observed age-related loss of muscle mass, decreases in total body water increase the susceptibility to exercise-induced dehydration and subsequent harmful influences on thermoregulation and performance [135]. Apart from acute effects on performance, long-term dehydration can cause several symptoms and health problems such as increased blood pressure, tiredness and diarrhoea. Because of these risks, older athletes should be careful to obtain enough water during the day. Fluid intake of athletes is dependent on various individual, training and environmental factors and no firm recommendation can be provided. It has been estimated that one should consume over 1–1.5 L of water a day (in addition to other fluids) and 0.4–0.8 L/hour during exercise, but thermally stressful environments and exercise intensity can increase this need. The fluid, electrolytes and hydration needs of masters athletes are discussed in detail in Chapter 9.

16.5.4 Nutrition for Sprint Racing

Unlike long-distance running, sprint running performance from 60–400 m is not limited by muscle glycogen stores [60] so there is no need for carbohydrate loading before competition. In addition, pre-race intakes of proteins or fats are unlikely to result in an acute improvement in performance. Therefore, sprinter's performance is more related to long-term dietary practices than the acute influence of nutritional intake. The major goal of the precompetition food consumption of all athletes is to stay hydrated (but avoid overdrinking), maintain adequate blood glucose levels and prevent gastrointestinal distress [136].

Caffeine could have some beneficial effect on sprint performance [136,137]. However, capsules or tablets are considered a better form of taking caffeine than strong coffee since the latter is more likely to cause gastrointestinal distress [136]. In order to avoid abdominal discomfort during the stress of competition, a common strategy is to eat 3–4 hours before events and ingest a small amount of sport drink and/or water 1–2 hours before event. Clearly, the optimal timing as well as amount and types of food and fluids for race day nutrition can vary greatly from athletes to athletes and no detailed recommendations can be provided. Fine-tuning of precompetition nutrition should be based on personal preference and food tolerance.

As discussed in Section 16.3.5, a significant proportion of the ATP supply during a sprint is derived from immediate PCr breakdown. We might therefore expect that oral creatine supplementation may enhance anaerobic performance by increasing intracellular creatine and PCr in muscle. The results of studies in young sprinters appear conflicting with some studies showing significant positive effect [138,139] and others no effect [140–142] on sprint performance following creatine supplementation. The potential benefit of creatine supplementation could be the most evident in repetitive sprint performance with not enough time for full recovery of phosphagen pool between sprints [143–145].

The use of creatine supplements is also widespread among masters athletes [131]. However, there appears to be only one study that has examined the effect of creatine loading on sprint performance in masters athletes. Wiroth et al. [146] supplemented elderly male masters cyclists (66 years, $n = 14$) with creatine for five days (3×5 g/day) which resulted in no improvements in anaerobic cycling test (five all-out 10-s sprints separated by 60-s passive recovery). However, improvements in performance were observed in young (26 years, $n = 14$) and elderly (70 years, $n = 14$) sedentary controls suggesting that habitual physical activity level may influence the response to creatine supplementation.

Several, but not all, studies indicate muscular benefit from creatine supplementation during strength training in young athletes [147,148] and this could have an indirect influence on sprint performance. The creatine supplementation has found to increase total training load and amplify training-induced muscle fibre growth possibly by increasing myofibrillar protein synthesis [149] and the number of satellite cells and myonuclei [150]. However, again, data on masters athletes are not available and the evidence from well-controlled studies on untrained older people is inconclusive to support the beneficial effects of creatine supplementation during strength training on muscle characteristics [151–155].

Some data suggest that the response to creatine supplementation is high in individuals with faster fibre type profile and greater muscle mass [156] and thus ageing-related decreases in type II muscle fibre number and size could reduce the effectiveness of creatine supplementation. On the other hand, older masters sprinters have demonstrated considerably larger size of fast fibres than untrained people [28] and may theoretically possess favourable physiological profile to respond the supplementation. To clarify this issue, new research with assessment of intramuscular creatine stores among masters sprinters is warranted. Finally, it is noteworthy that in some persons creatine supplementation may lead to weight gain (~1%–3%) due to water retention [144,157] that may have small negative effect on mass-dependent sprint running performance. Another important consideration is that although there typically are no adverse effects on health, a number of studies have linked creatine supplementation to muscle cramping, dehydration, diarrhoea and dizziness [158].

During sprint running, acidification of both the blood and muscles (decrease in pH) take place that can compromise contractile function leading to muscular fatigue. Extra- and intracellular buffering agents such as sodium bicarbonate and carnosine may enhance sprint performance by attenuating this acidification [136,159]. The consumption of sodium bicarbonate is known to increase pH and bicarbonate concentrations in the blood that increases the rate of H+ and lactate ions efflux from active muscles [159]. Theoretically this would keep the muscle pH within normal levels to maintain contractile capacity and delay the onset of fatigue during long-term anaerobic performance such as 400-m sprint runs. In support of this assumption, several, but not all, studies have found positive effect of bicarbonate loading (200–300 mg/kg, 1–2 hours before exercise) on longer sprint and middle-distance performances lasting 1–7 minutes (i.e. 400 m–3 km) [159]. However, the predominance of research indicates that bicarbonate loading has no beneficial effects for shorter efforts (30–40 seconds or less) [159].

While sodium bicarbonate helps maintain pH outside the cell, carnosine can act as an intracellular buffer slowing the drop in pH. Inside the muscle cells, carnosine is synthesised from beta-alanine and histidine with the help of enzyme carnosine synthethase. However, of these two amino acids it is beta-alanine that drives carnosine synthesis. Supplementation with beta-alanine for 4 and 10 weeks has been shown to elevate carnosine levels by about 60% and 80%, respectively, in physically active young men [160]. As to performance benefits, a recent meta-analysis of studies showed that beta-alanine supplementation (mean daily dose 5.12 g/day) may produce improvement in maximal performance lasting 60–240 seconds and over 240 seconds [161]. However, no significant benefit of beta-alanine was found for exercise lasting less than 60 seconds. There could be some mild acute side effects with both sodium bicarbonate (gastrointestinal discomfort) and beta-alanine (skin irritation and prickly sensation) ingestion and no information exists about the effects of long-term use of beta-alanine on health. We are not aware of any studies examining the influence of sodium bicarbonate or beta-alanine/carnosine in masters athletes and it is questionable whether the same effects exist in this cohort. The use and efficacy of both supplements and ergogenic aids in masters athletes are discussed in detail in Chapters 10 and 11.

16.6 CONCLUSIONS

Sprint running ability is determined by multiple biomechanical and neuromuscular factors. In this chapter we have presented some of the major biomechanical and physiological changes that may be associated with decline in sprint performance with age in male runners. In addition, we have provided information about fundamental principles of training applied to ageing sprinters. In order to maximise sprinting potential, athletes of all ages should adhere to training practices in which demands of the sport and athlete's individual strength and weaknesses are carefully considered.

Because age-related loss of muscle mass seems to be primarily responsible for the changes in sprint running ability, care must be taken to design exercises which promote muscle growth with special emphasis to increase the size of fast-contracting type II fibres. Therefore, heterogeneous training program containing components of high-intensity strength training together with run-based training is essential for optimal maintenance of sprinting ability in masters athletes. Furthermore, older age can lead to impaired recovery and may require modifications in short- and long-term periodisation of training (variation of volume, intensity and exercise selection) to optimise adaptation and peak performance before important competitions.

Nutritional factors are also important for effective training. Masters sprinters may not be concerned about adequate energy intake from carbohydrates due to relatively low energy requirements of sprint training. However, combined sprint and strength training may increase protein needs and older sprinters should pay attention to quality protein consumption to aid in muscle recovery.

16.7 IMPLICATIONS FOR MASTERS ATHLETES AND COACHES

- Although success in sprinting is largely affected by inherited physiological characteristics such as muscle fibre type composition, the determinants of sprint performance can be improved significantly by proper training in athletes of all ages.
- Age-related slowing of maximum running speed is associated with reduction in stride length and an increase in contact time, while stride frequency shows a minor decline and swing time remains unaffected. The changes in stride length and contact times are directly related to decreased ability to produce high-magnitude ground reaction forces.
- Sprint running is a complex neuromuscular skill that must be constantly rehearsed. Only with frequent practices and many repetitions can correct movement pattern remain effective and stable. Accordingly, the best way to maintain sprinting ability is to sprint. In short-sprint events (60–100 m) all speed phases are critical for overall performance and need to be focused on in training. Optimal sprint technique can be impaired by insufficient flexibility. Inclusion of flexibility exercises in the training schedule is necessary.
- Strength is a critical element of sprint running and the importance of weight training for masters runners cannot be overstated. Improved strength levels will enable the ability to generate a higher magnitude of ground reaction force more quickly, resulting in increased stride length and frequency. Weight training is the only exercise mode for effective maintenance of muscle mass and fast fibre size that plays a critical role in sprint running performance with age. Consider doing strength training at least two times per week throughout the year including both maximal and explosive strength and plyometric (jump) exercises.

- Advancing age is known to be associated with a slower rate of recovery from exercise. To optimise recovery-adaptation there is need for modifications in intensity and volume of training within weeks and months.
- All athletes must consume an adequate amount of calories to meet the increased energy demands of exercise. Insufficient energy intake reduces the benefits of training and can lead to weight loss and a higher risk of illness and overtraining. The diet for sprint athletes should provide approximately 10%–20% (1.2–1.7 g/kg) of daily energy intake from protein, about 50%–60% from carbohydrates (3–7 g/kg) and the remaining 30% should be provided by fat.
- Protein is essential for repair and building of new muscle tissue in response to training and during periods of hard training it may be important to target protein intake at 1.5–1.7 g/kg/day for maximum benefit. Consuming high-protein before, during and immediately after training rather than other times of day may enhance protein metabolism and muscle growth.
- There is published and anecdotal evidence that some masters sprinters use sports supplements such as creatine, beta-alanine and sodium bicarbonate to enhance sprinting performance. However, based on the few available studies in older and younger athletes, the ergogenic effect of sports supplements for older sprint runners can be questioned. In addition, since the supplementation may induce some adverse health effects, the use any nutritional aids should be done under the guidance of a qualified nutrition or health professional. Verify that any types of supplements or pharmaceuticals you are planning to take are not on a banned list.

16.8 IMPLICATIONS FOR SPORTS MEDICINE PROFESSIONALS AND CLINICIANS

- Whereas athletes and coaches are largely interested in improving the performance, sports medicine professionals and clinicians are primarily concerned about the health and secondarily in maintaining the performance of the masters athlete. In many cases the recommendations that improve performance are equally beneficial for the health of the athlete and the advice above for athletes and coaches thus also applies to the sports medicine practitioner.
- Masters athletes are more prone to various types of injuries than young athletes. It is therefore particularly important to monitor any impact of demanding resistance and run/jump training on the integrity of the trained muscles, tendons, cartilage and bones and impact on blood pressure that rises considerably during particular weight lifting exercises. For masters athletes having structural problems (e.g. knee and lower back), certain typical sprint-training exercises such as intensive jumping, bounding and deep squat exercises should be avoided.
- Consider that recovery from training bouts is slower and longer in the older athlete and pay special attention to recovery from injuries or tissue damage incurred during training; if no special heed is given to this advice the older athlete may suffer from lasting fatigue and overtraining consequences.
- Although many masters sprint athletes appear to have quite healthy food behaviours, they need more information about the most appropriate energy and nutrient intake to sustain the specific demands of training. Annual monitoring of dietary intake is useful to ensure that diet contains an adequate amount of energy and nutrients. In addition, regular assessment of blood profiles may be advisable to detect as early as possible any mineral and vitamin deficiencies.
- The use of legal nutritional supplements should be closely supervised with a particular emphasis on the specific complications that may arise from the use of particular nutritional aids. It must be recognised that some medications and even pharmaceuticals sold without

prescription (e.g. prohormones) are classified as performance-enhancing drugs and their use is banned by anti-doping committees around the world. See Chapters 10 and 13 for a more detailed discussion these areas.

16.9 FUTURE RESEARCH DIRECTIONS

- Most previous studies on the effect of age on sprint performance are based on cross-sectional design that is limited in its ability in determining causality between performance/physiological changes and ageing. To define the true effect of ageing on sprint performance and its determinants, there is need for more longitudinal studies where athletes are followed for several years.
- Perhaps the most fundamental impact of ageing on physical performance is the progressive loss of muscle fibres, especially fast type II fibres. Although this change is commonly thought to be inevitable, recent studies have suggested that the muscle fibre loss can be prevented or slowed by regular endurance exercise. This issue clearly warrants further exploration in masters athletes from various sports.
- Studies should be conducted to evaluate muscle-tendon behaviour and elastic energy utilisation in ageing athletes. Due to exercise-type and intensity specificity, the muscle-tendon interaction should be measured *in vivo* during the contact phase of fast running. In addition, because older sprinters show variability in foot strike pattern (forefoot, midfoot, rearfoot), we need also to know how the landing strategy affect the spring-like bouncing mechanism.
- To date, the studies on the effect of ageing on anaerobic metabolic characteristics such as muscle enzyme activities and ATP, PCr and lactate concentrations have focused on non-athletes. However, well-trained masters sprinters may have very different metabolic capabilities than normal age-matched individuals. More research on muscle metabolism and its role in age-related differences in sprint performance in masters sprint athletes is needed.
- Decreased ability to tolerate heavy training may be a key factor for age-related performance losses. However, the physiological bases of diminishing trainability with age is still unclear. More studies on the possible effects of anabolic hormonal and nutrition factors on trainability in masters athletes should be undertaken.
- Although the values for various performance and musculoskeletal properties in masters sprint athletes are maintained far above the age norms, the available evidence for potential training-related risks are still very limited. New information about the benefits and risks of demanding strength-, run- and jump-based exercises is needed not only to counsel the masters athletes themselves but also to develop modified training programs for non-athletes in whom the improvement of rapid force and musculoskeletal characteristics with age has good potential to enhance functional well-being.
- With very few exceptions, most of the studies on the effects of ageing on sprint performance have used male participants. More research is needed to learn how the physiological factors related to sprint performance are affected by gender.

REFERENCES

1. Ross, A. and Leveritt, M., Long-term metabolic and skeletal muscle adaptations to short-sprint training: Implications for sprint training and tapering, *Sports Med.* 31(15), 1063–82, 2001.
2. World Masters Athletics, Records, http://www.world-masters-athletics.org/records, accessed 30 January 2014.
3. IAAF Athletics, Senior Indoor Records, http://www.iaaf.org/statistics/records, accessed 30 January 2014.
4. Conzelmann, A., The plasticity of courses of physical performance in the second part of life, in *Healthy Aging, Activity, and Sports (Proceedings, PAAS IV)*, G. Huber, ed., Health Promotion Publications, Gamburg, Germany, 1997, pp. 435–45.
5. Ae, M., Ito, A. and Suzuki, M., The men's 100 meters, *New Stud. Athlet.* 7(1), 47–52, 1992.

6. Ritzdorf, W., 100 meters—Biomechanical Research Project at the VIth World Championships in Athletics, Athens 1997: Preliminary report, *New Stud. Athlet.* 12(1), 43–73, 1997.
7. Bruggemann, G.-P. and Glad, B., Time analysis of the sprint events, in *Scientific Research Project at the Games of the XXIVth Olympiad-Seoul 1988, Final Report*, G.-P. Bruggemann and B. Glad, eds., International Athletic Foundation/International Amateur Athletic Federation, London, 1990, pp. 11–89.
8. Kersting, U.G., Biomechanical analysis of the sprinting events, in *Biomechanical Research Project Athens 1997, Final Report*, G.P. Bruggemann, D. Koszewski, and H. Muller, eds., Meyer & Meyer, Oxford, United Kingdom, 1999, pp. 12–72.
9. Korhonen, M.T., Mero, A. and Suominen, H., Age-related differences in 100-m sprint performance in male and female master runners, *Med. Sci. Sports Exerc.* 35(8), 1419–28, 2003.
10. Hamilton, N., Changes in sprint stride kinematics with age in master's athletes, *J. Appl. Biomech.* 9(1), 15–26, 1993.
11. Roberts, E.M., Cheung, T.K., Abdel Hafez, A.M. and Hong, D., Swing limb biomechanics of 60- to 65-year-old male runners, *Gait Posture* 5(1), 42–53, 1997.
12. Korhonen, M.T., Mero, A.A., Alen, M. et al., Biomechanical and skeletal muscle determinants of maximum running speed with aging, *Med. Sci. Sports Exerc.* 41(4), 844–56, 2009.
13. Mero, A., Komi, P.V. and Gregor, R.J., Biomechanics of sprint running. A review, *Sports Med.* 13(6), 376–92, 1992.
14. Dietz, V., Schmidtbleicher, D. and Noth, J., Neuronal mechanisms of human locomotion, *J. Neurophysiol.* 42(5), 1212–22, 1979.
15. Butler, R.J., Crowell, H.P. and Davis, I.M., Lower extremity stiffness: Implications for performance and injury, *Clin. Biomech.* 18(6), 511–7, 2003.
16. Cristea, A., Korhonen, M.T., Hakkinen, K. et al., Effects of combined strength and sprint training on regulation of muscle contraction at the whole-muscle and single-fibre levels in elite master sprinters, *Acta Physiol.* 193(3), 275–89, 2008.
17. Kuitunen, S., Komi, P.V. and Kyrolainen, H., Knee and ankle joint stiffness in sprint running, *Med. Sci. Sports Exerc.* 34(1), 166–73, 2002.
18. Young, W., McLean, B. and Ardagna, J., Relationship between strength qualities and sprinting performance, *J. Sports Med. Phys. Fitness* 35(1), 13–9, 1995.
19. Mero, A., Luhtanen, P., Viitasalo, J.T. and Komi, P.V., Relationships between the maximal running velocity, muscle fiber characteristics, force production and force relaxation in sprinters, *Scand. J. Sports Sci.* 3(1), 16–22, 1981.
20. Cronin, J.B. and Hansen, K.T., Strength and power predictors of sports speed, *J. Strength Cond. Res.* 19(2), 349–57, 2005.
21. Wisloff, U., Castagna, C., Helgerud, J., Jones, R. and Hoff, J., Strong correlation of maximal squat strength with sprint performance and vertical jump height in elite soccer players, *Br. J. Sports Med.* 38(3), 285–8, 2004.
22. Pearson, S.J., Young, A., Macaluso, A. et al., Muscle function in elite master weightlifters, *Med. Sci. Sports Exerc.* 34(7), 1199–206, 2002.
23. Ojanen, T., Rauhala, T. and Häkkinen, K., Strength and power profiles of the lower and upper extremities in master throwers at different ages, *J. Strength Cond. Res.* 21(1), 216–22, 2007.
24. Anton, M.M., Spirduso, W.W. and Tanaka, H., Age-related declines in anaerobic muscular performance: Weightlifting and powerlifting, *Med. Sci. Sports Exerc.* 36(1), 143–7, 2004.
25. Larsson, L. and Moss, R.L., Maximum velocity of shortening in relation to myosin isoform composition in single fibres from human skeletal muscles, *J. Physiol.* 472(1), 595–614, 1993.
26. Bottinelli, R., Canepari, M., Pellegrino, M.A. and Reggiani, C., Force-velocity properties of human skeletal muscle fibres: Myosin heavy chain isoform and temperature dependence, *J. Physiol.* 495(2), 573–86, 1996.
27. Andersen, J.L., Muscle fiber type characteristics of the runner, in *Running & Science*, J. Bangsbo and H.B. Larsen, eds., Munksgaard, Copenhagen, Denmark, 2001, pp. 49–65.
28. Korhonen, M.T., Cristea, A., Alen, M. et al., Aging, muscle fiber type, and contractile function in sprint-trained athletes, *J. Appl. Physiol.* 101(3), 906–17, 2006.
29. Sjöström, M., Johansson, C. and Lorentzon, R., Muscle pathomorphology in m. quadriceps of marathon runners. Early signs of strain disease or functional adaptation? *Acta Physiol. Scand.* 132(4), 537–41, 1988.
30. Blazevich, A.J., Effects of physical training and detraining, immobilisation, growth and aging on human fascicle geometry, *Sports Med.* 36(12), 1003–17, 2006.

31. Reaburn, P.R.J., The lifetime athlete—Physical work capacities and skeletal muscle characteristics, unpublished Ph.D. thesis, The University of Queensland, Australia, 1993.
32. Iwaoka, K., Funato, K., Takatoh, S., Mutoh, Y. and Miyashita, M., Characteristics of leg extensor muscle in a world champion masters jumper. A case study, *J. Sports Med. Phys. Fitness* 29(4), 394–7, 1989.
33. Proctor, D.N., Sinning, W.E., Walro, J.M., Sieck, G.C. and Lemon, P.W., Oxidative capacity of human muscle fiber types: effects of age and training status, *J. Appl. Physiol.* 78(6), 2033–8, 1995.
34. Klitgaard, H., Mantoni, M., Schiaffino, S. et al., Function, morphology and protein expression of ageing skeletal muscle: A cross-sectional study of elderly men with different training backgrounds, *Acta Physiol. Scand.* 140(1), 41–54, 1990.
35. Aagaard, P., Magnusson, P.S., Larsson, B., Kjaer, M. and Krustrup, P., Mechanical muscle function, morphology, and fiber type in lifelong trained elderly, *Med. Sci. Sports Exerc.* 39(11), 1989–96, 2007.
36. Brown, M.B. and Coggan, A., Is muscle wasting inevitable with aging? *Med. Sci. Sports Exerc.* 22(2), S73, 1990.
37. Lexell, J., Taylor, C.C. and Sjostrom, M., What is the cause of the ageing atrophy? Total number, size and proportion of different fiber types studied in whole vastus lateralis muscle from 15- to 83-year-old men, *J. Neurol. Sci.* 84(2–3), 275–94, 1988.
38. Power, G.A., Dalton, B.H., Behm, D.G., Vandervoort, A.A., Doherty, T.J. and Rice, C.L., Motor unit number estimates in masters runners: Use it or lose it?, *Med. Sci. Sports Exerc.* 42(9), 1644–50, 2010.
39. Power, G.A., Dalton, B.H., Behm, D.G., Doherty, T.J., Vandervoort, A.A. and Rice, C.L., Motor unit survival in lifelong runners is muscle dependent, *Med. Sci. Sports Exerc.* 44(7), 1235–42, 2012.
40. Weyand, P.G. and Davis, J.A., Running performance has a structural basis, *J. Exp. Biol.* 208(14), 2625–31, 2005.
41. Stafilidis, S. and Arampatzis, A., Muscle-tendon unit mechanical and morphological properties and sprint performance, *J. Sports Sci.* 25(9), 1035–46, 2007.
42. Kubo, K., Kanehisa, H., Kawakami, Y. and Fukunaga, T., Elasticity of tendon structures of the lower limbs in sprinters, *Acta Physiol. Scand.* 168(2), 327–35, 2000.
43. Arampatzis, A., Karamanidis, K., Morey-Klapsing, G., De Monte, G. and Stafilidis, S., Mechanical properties of the triceps surae tendon and aponeurosis in relation to intensity of sport activity, *J. Biomech.* 40(9), 1946–52, 2007.
44. Arampatzis, A., Degens, H., Baltzopoulos, V. and Rittweger, J., Why do older sprinters reach the finish line later?, *Exerc. Sport Sci. Rev.* 39(1), 18–22, 2011.
45. Blazevich, A.J., Flexibility training for sprint runners, *Natl. Strength Cond. J.* 23(4), 42–49, 2001.
46. Mann, R., *The Mechanics of Sprinting and Hurdling*, Create Space, Lexington, KY, 2011.
47. Holland, G.J., Tanaka, K., Shigematsu, R. and Nakagaichi, M., Flexibility and physical functions of older adults: A review, *J. Aging Phys. Act.* 10(1), 169–206, 2002.
48. McHugh, M.P., Gleim, G.W., Magnusson, S.P. and Nicholas, J.A., A cross-sectional study of age-related musculoskeletal and physiological changes in soccer players, *Med. Exerc. Nutr. Health* 2(1), 261–68, 1993.
49. Witvrouw, E., Danneels, L., Asselman, P., D'Have, T. and Cambier, D., Muscle flexibility as a risk factor for developing muscle injuries in male professional soccer players. A prospective study, *Am. J. Sports Med.* 31(1), 41–6, 2003.
50. Harvey, D., Assessment of the flexibility of elite athletes using the modified Thomas test, *Br. J. Sports Med.* 32(1), 68–70, 1998.
51. Wilson, G.J., Murphy, A.J. and Pryor, J.F., Musculotendinous stiffness: Its relationship to eccentric, isometric, and concentric performance, *J. Appl. Physiol.* 76(6), 2714–9, 1994.
52. Haff, G.G., Roundtable discussion: Flexibility training, *Strength Cond. J.* 28(2), 64–85, 2006.
53. Galloway, M.T. and Jokl, P., Age and sports participation: the effect of aging on muscle function and athletic performance, *Sports Med. Arthrosc. Rev.* 4(3), 221–34, 1996.
54. Hirvonen, J., Rehunen, S., Rusko, H. and Harkonen, M., Breakdown of high-energy phosphate compounds and lactate accumulation during short supramaximal exercise, *Eur. J. Appl. Physiol.* 56(3), 253–9, 1987.
55. Newsholme, E.A., Blomstrand, E., MacAndrew, E. and Parry-Billings, M., Biochemical causes of fatigue and overtraining, in *Endurance in Sport*, R.J. Shephard and P.-O. Åstrand, eds., Blackwell Scientific, Oxford, United Kingdom, 1992, pp. 351–64.
56. Hirvonen, J., Physiology of anaerobic performance, unpublished report (in Finnish), University of Jyväskylä, Finland, 1984.
57. Kindermann, W. and Keul, J., *Anaerobe Energiebereitstellung im Hochleistungssport [Anaerobic capacity in elite sports]*, Verlag Karl Hofmann, Schondorf, Germany, 1977.

58. Locatelli, E., The importance of anaerobic glycolysis and stiffness in the sprints (60, 100 and 200 metres), *New Stud. Athlet.* 11(3), 121–5, 1996.
59. Lacour, J.R., Bouvat, E. and Barthelemy, J.C., Post-competition blood lactate concentrations as indicators of anaerobic energy expenditure during 400-m and 800-m races, *Eur. J. Appl. Physiol.* 61(3–4), 172–6, 1990.
60. Hirvonen, J., Nummela, A., Rusko, H., Rehunen, S. and Harkonen, M., Fatigue and changes of ATP, creatine phosphate, and lactate during the 400-m sprint, *Can. J. Sport Sci.* 17(2), 141–4, 1992.
61. Westerblad, H., Allen, D.G. and Lannergren, J., Muscle fatigue: Lactic acid or inorganic phosphate the major cause?, *News Physiol. Sci.* 17(1), 17–21, 2002.
62. Korhonen, M.T., Suominen, H. and Mero, A., Age and sex differences in blood lactate response to sprint running in elite master athletes, *Can. J. Appl. Physiol.* 30(6), 647–65, 2005.
63. Reaburn, P. and Dascombe, B., Anaerobic performance in master athletes, *Eur. Rev. Aging. Phys. Act.* 6(1), 39–53, 2009.
64. Benelli, P., Ditroilo, M., Forte, R., De Vito, G. and Stocchi, V., Assessment of post-competition peak blood lactate in male and female master swimmers aged 40–79 years and its relationship with swimming performance, *Eur. J. Appl. Physiol.* 99(6), 685–93, 2007.
65. Reaburn, P.R. and Mackinnon, L.T., Blood lactate responses in older swimmers during active and passive recovery following maximal sprint swimming, *Eur. J. Appl. Physiol.* 61(3–4), 246–50, 1990.
66. Jensen-Urstad, M., Svedenhag, J. and Sahlin, K., Effect of muscle mass on lactate formation during exercise in humans, *Eur. J. Appl. Physiol.* 69(3), 189–95, 1994.
67. Stainsby, W.N. and Brooks, G.A., Control of lactic acid metabolism in contracting muscles and during exercise, *Exerc. Sport Sci. Rev.* 18(1), 29–63, 1990.
68. Essen, B. and Haggmark, T., Lactate concentration in type I and II muscle fibres during muscular contraction in man, *Acta Physiol. Scand.* 95(3), 344–6, 1975.
69. Tesch, P., Sjodin, B. and Karlsson, J., Relationship between lactate accumulation, LDH activity, LDH isozyme and fibre type distribution in human skeletal muscle, *Acta Physiol. Scand.* 103(1), 40–6, 1978.
70. Linossier, M.T., Denis, C., Dormois, D., Geyssant, A. and Lacour, J.R., Ergometric and metabolic adaptation to a 5-s sprint training programme, *Eur. J Appl. Physiol.* 67(5), 408–14, 1993.
71. MacDougall, J.D., Hicks, A.L., MacDonald, J.R., McKelvie, R.S., Green, H.J. and Smith, K.M., Muscle performance and enzymatic adaptations to sprint interval training, *J. Appl. Physiol.* 84(6), 2138–42, 1998.
72. Mero, A., Rusko, H., Peltola, E., Pullinen, T., Nummela, A. and Hirvonen, J., Aerobic characteristics, oxygen debt and blood lactate in speed endurance athletes during training, *J. Sports Med. Phys. Fitness* 33(2), 130–6, 1993.
73. Lanza, I.R., Larsen, R.G. and Kent-Braun, J.A., Effects of old age on human skeletal muscle energetics during fatiguing contractions with and without blood flow, *J. Physiol.* 583(3), 1093–105, 2007.
74. Bompa, T.O. and Haff, E., *Periodization: Theory and Methodology of Training*, Human Kinetics, Champaign, IL, 2009.
75. Foster, C., Wright, G., Battista, R.A. and Porcari, J.P., Training in the aging athlete, *Curr. Sports Med. Rep.* 6(3), 200–6, 2007.
76. Bouchard, C., Malina, R. and Perusse, L., *Genetics of fitness and Physical Performance*, Human Kinetics, Champaign, IL, 1997.
77. Mero, A., Training principles for mature athlete, in *Different Way to Age* (in Finnish), K. Viiru, J. Manninen, M. Nieminen, H. Suominen, C. Sundqvist, A. Tiihonen, and R. Taponen, eds., KS Paino, Kajaani, Finland, 2011, pp. 67–90.
78. Aagaard, P., Suetta, C., Caserotti, P., Magnusson, S.P. and Kjaer, M., Role of the nervous system in sarcopenia and muscle atrophy with aging: Strength training as a countermeasure, *Scand. J. Med. Sci. Sports* 20(1), 49–64, 2010.
79. Reaburn, P., Logan, P. and Mackinnon, L., Serum testosterone response to high-intensity resistance training in male veteran sprint runners, *J. Strength Cond. Res.* 11(4), 256–60, 1997.
80. Reaburn, P. and Mackinnon, L., The effect of high-intensity isotonic training on anaerobic work capacity in veteran sprint runners, Report for Coaches—Australian Sports Commission Applied Sports Research Program, unpublished, 1995.
81. Williams, C. and Gandy, G., Physiology and nutrition for sprinting, in *Perspectives in Exercise Science and Sports Medicine Volume 7: Physiology and Nutrition for Competitive Sport*, D.R. Lamb, H.G. Knuttgen, and R. Murray, eds., Cooper, Travers City, MI, 2001, pp. 55–98.
82. Heazlewood, I., Training programs of elite veteran track and field athletes, in *Healthy Aging, Activity, and Sports (Proceedings, PAAS IV)*, G. Huber, ed., Health Promotion Publications, Gamburg, Germany, 1997, pp. 446–9.

83. Sugiura, K., Suzuki, I. and Kobayashi, K., Nutritional intake of elite Japanese track-and-field athletes, *Int. J. Sport Nutr.* 9(2), 202–12, 1999.
84. Fogelholm, G.M., Himberg, J.J., Alopaeus, K. et al., Dietary and biochemical indices of nutritional status in male athletes and controls, *J. Am. Coll. Nutr.* 11(2), 181–91, 1992.
85. Mero, A., Tuomala, I. and Rantala, T., Nutrition for track and field athletes, unpublished (in Finnish), University of Jyväskylä, Finland, 1994.
86. Mero, A., Nutrition coaching (in Finnish), in *Sport Coaching,* A. Mero, A. Nummela, K. Keskinen, and K. Häkkinen, eds., VK Kustannus Oy, Lahti, Finland, 2004, pp. 179–209.
87. Chatard, J.C., Boutet, C., Tourny, C., Garcia, S., Berthouze, S. and Guezennec, C.Y., Nutritional status and physical fitness of elderly sportsmen, *Eur. J. Appl. Physiol.* 77(1–2), 157–63, 1998.
88. Blair, S.N., Ellsworth, N.M., Haskell, W.L., Stern, M.P., Farquhar, J.W. and Wood, P.D., Comparison of nutrient intake in middle-aged men and women runners and controls, *Med. Sci. Sports Exerc.* 13(5), 310–5, 1981.
89. van Pelt, R.E., Dinneno, F.A., Seals, D.R. and Jones, P.P., Age-related decline in RMR in physically active men: Relation to exercise volume and energy intake, *Am. J. Physiol. Endocrinol. Metab.* 281(3), E633–9, 2001.
90. Sallinen, J., Ojanen, T., Karavirta, L., Ahtiainen, J.P. and Hakkinen, K., Muscle mass and strength, body composition and dietary intake in master strength athletes vs untrained men of different ages, *J. Sports Med. Phys. Fitness* 48(2), 190–6, 2008.
91. Malmberg, K., *Dietary Patterns of Masters Sprinters Aged 40 to 85 Years*, unpublished thesis (in Finnish), University of Jyväskylä, Finland, 2003.
92. Borg, P., Fogelholm, M. and Hiilloskorpi, H., *Nutrition for Exerciser*, (in Finnish), Edita Publishing, Helsinki, Finland, 2004.
93. Männistö, S., Ovaskainen, M-L. and Valsta, L., The National Findiet 2002 Study, Publications of the National Public Health Institute Report No B3/2003 (in Finnish), National Public Health Institute, Helsinki, Finland, 2003.
94. Wilson, M.M. and Morley, J.E., Invited review: Aging and energy balance, *J. Appl. Physiol.* 95(4), 1728–36, 2003.
95. Buzzard, M., 24-hour dietary recall and food record methods, in *Nutritional Epidemiology*, W. Willett, ed., Oxford University Press, New York, 1998, pp. 51–73.
96. Rodriguez, N.R., Di Marco, N.M. and Langley, S., American College of Sports Medicine position stand. Nutrition and athletic performance, *Med. Sci. Sports Exerc.* 41(3), 709–31, 2009.
97. Conley, M.S. and Stone, M.H., Carbohydrate ingestion/supplementation or resistance exercise and training, *Sports Med.* 21(1), 7–17, 1996.
98. Ivy, J.L., Katz, A.L., Cutler, C.L., Sherman, W.M. and Coyle, E.F., Muscle glycogen synthesis after exercise: Effect of time of carbohydrate ingestion, *J. Appl. Physiol.* 64(4), 1480–5, 1988.
99. Walton, P. and Rhodes, E.C., Glycaemic index and optimal performance, *Sports Med.* 23(3), 164–72, 1997.
100. Houston, D.K., Nicklas, B.J., Ding, J. et al., Dietary protein intake is associated with lean mass change in older, community-dwelling adults: The Health, Aging, and Body Composition (Health ABC) Study, *Am. J. Clin. Nutr.* 87(1), 150–5, 2008.
101. Campbell, W.W. and Geik, R.A., Nutritional considerations for the older athlete, *Nutrition* 20(7–8), 603–8, 2004.
102. Hoffman, J.R. and Falvo, M.J., Protein—which is the best?, *J. Sports Sci. Med.* 3(1), 118–130, 2004.
103. Hulmi, J.J., Lockwood, C.M. and Stout, J.R., Effect of protein/essential amino acids and resistance training on skeletal muscle hypertrophy: A case for whey protein, *Nutr. Metab.* 7(Jun), 51, 2010.
104. Phillips, S.M., Tang, J.E. and Moore, D.R., The role of milk- and soy-based protein in support of muscle protein synthesis and muscle protein accretion in young and elderly persons, *J. Am. Coll. Nutr.* 28(4), 343–54, 2009.
105. Dangin, M., Guillet, C., Garcia-Rodenas, C. et al., The rate of protein digestion affects protein gain differently during aging in humans, *J. Physiol.* 549(2), 635–44, 2003.
106. Katsanos, C.S., Chinkes, D.L., Paddon-Jones, D., Zhang, X.J., Aarsland, A. and Wolfe, R.R., Whey protein ingestion in elderly persons results in greater muscle protein accrual than ingestion of its constituent essential amino acid content, *Nutr. Res.* 28(10), 651–8, 2008.
107. Burd, N.A., Yang, Y., Moore, D.R., Tang, J.E., Tarnopolsky, M.A. and Phillips, S.M., Greater stimulation of myofibrillar protein synthesis with ingestion of whey protein isolate v. micellar casein at rest and after resistance exercise in elderly men, *Br. J. Nutr.* 108(6), 958–62, 2012.
108. Verdijk, L.B., Jonkers, R.A., Gleeson, B.G. et al., Protein supplementation before and after exercise does not further augment skeletal muscle hypertrophy after resistance training in elderly men, *Am. J. Clin. Nutr.* 89(2), 608–16, 2009.

109. Hoffman, J.R., Ratamess, N.A., Tranchina, C.P., Rashti, S.L., Kang, J. and Faigenbaum, A.D., Effect of protein-supplement timing on strength, power, and body-composition changes in resistance-trained men, *Int. J. Sport Nutr. Exerc. Metab.* 19(2), 172–85, 2009.
110. Kerksick, C., Harvey, T., Stout, J. et al., International Society of Sports Nutrition position stand: Nutrient timing, *J. Int. Soc. Sports Nutr.* 5(8), 17–18, 2008.
111. Candow, D.G. and Chilibeck, P.D., Timing of creatine or protein supplementation and resistance training in the elderly, *Appl. Physiol. Nutr. Metab.* 33(1), 184–90, 2008.
112. Biolo, G., Tipton, K.D., Klein, S. and Wolfe, R.R., An abundant supply of amino acids enhances the metabolic effect of exercise on muscle protein, *Am. J. Physiol.* 273(1), E122–9, 1997.
113. Yang, Y., Breen, L., Burd, N.A. et al., Resistance exercise enhances myofibrillar protein synthesis with graded intakes of whey protein in older men, *Br. J. Nutr.* 108(10), 1780–8, 2011.
114. Breen, L. and Phillips, S.M., Skeletal muscle protein metabolism in the elderly: Interventions to counteract the 'anabolic resistance' of ageing, *Nutr. Metab.* 8(Oct), 68, 2011.
115. Hamalainen, E.K., Adlercreutz, H., Puska, P. and Pietinen, P., Decrease of serum total and free testosterone during a low-fat high-fibre diet, *J. Steroid Biochem.* 18(3), 369–70, 1983.
116. Volek, J.S., Kraemer, W.J., Bush, J.A., Incledon, T. and Boetes, M., Testosterone and cortisol in relationship to dietary nutrients and resistance exercise, *J. Appl. Physiol.* 82(1), 49–54, 1997.
117. Holmes, M.D., Spiegelman, D., Willett, W.C. et al., Dietary fat intake and endogenous sex steroid hormone levels in postmenopausal women, *J. Clin. Oncol.* 18(21), 3668–76, 2000.
118. Korhonen, M.T., *Effects of Aging and Training on Sprint Performance, Muscle Structure and Contractile Function in Athletes*, Ph.D. thesis, Studies in Sport, Physical Education and Health, No.137, University of Jyväskylä, Finland, 2009.
119. Key, T.J., Roe, L., Thorogood, M., Moore, J.W., Clark, G.M. and Wang, D.Y., Testosterone, sex hormone-binding globulin, calculated free testosterone, and oestradiol in male vegans and omnivores, *Br. J. Nutr.* 64(1), 111–9, 1990.
120. Allen, N.E., Appleby, P.N., Davey, G.K. and Key, T.J., Lifestyle and nutritional determinants of bioavailable androgens and related hormones in British men, *Cancer Causes Control* 13(4), 353–63, 2002.
121. Paturi, M., Tapanainen, H., Reinivuo, H. and Pietinen, P., *The National Findiet 2007 Survey. Publications of the National Public Health Institute Report No B23/2008* (in Finnish), National Public Health Institute, Helsinki, Finland, 2008.
122. Leosdottir, M., Nilsson, P.M., Nilsson, J.A., Mansson, H. and Berglund, G., Dietary fat intake and early mortality patterns—Data from The Malmo Diet and Cancer Study, *J. Intern. Med.* 258(2), 153–65, 2005.
123. Smith, G.I., Atherton, P., Reeds, D.N. et al., Dietary omega-3 fatty acid supplementation increases the rate of muscle protein synthesis in older adults: A randomized controlled trial, *Am. J. Clin. Nutr.* 93(2), 402–12, 2011.
124. Ceriello, A. and Colagiuri, S., International Diabetes Federation guideline for management of postmeal glucose: A review of recommendations, *Diabet. Med.* 25(10), 1151–6, 2008.
125. Harman, S.M., Metter, E.J., Tobin, J.D., Pearson, J. and Blackman, M.R., Longitudinal effects of aging on serum total and free testosterone levels in healthy men. Baltimore Longitudinal Study of Aging, *J. Clin. Endocrinol. Metab.* 86(2), 724–31, 2001.
126. Rosenbloom, C.A. and Dunaway, A., Nutrition recommendations for masters athletes, *Clin. Sports Med.* 26(1), 91–100, 2007.
127. Hasunen, K., Heiskanen, S., Packalén, L. et al., *Finnish Nutrition Recommendations* (in Finnish), National Nutrition Council, Ministry of Agriculture and Forestry, Edita, Helsinki, Finland, 2005.
128. Mullins, V.A., Houtkooper, L.B., Howell, W.H., Going, S.B. and Brown, C.H., Nutritional status of U.S. elite female heptathletes during training, *Int. J. Sport Nutr. Exerc. Metab.* 11(3), 299–314, 2001.
129. Hamilton, B., Vitamin D and human skeletal muscle, *Scand. J. Med. Sci. Sports* 20(2), 182–90, 2009.
130. Verhaar, H.J., Samson, M.M., Jansen, P.A., de Vreede, P.L., Manten, J.W. and Duursma, S.A., Muscle strength, functional mobility and vitamin D in older women, *Aging (Milano)* 12(6), 455–60, 2000.
131. Striegel, H., Simon, P., Wurster, C., Niess, A.M. and Ulrich, R., The use of nutritional supplements among master athletes, *Int. J. Sports Med.* 27(3), 236–41, 2006.
132. Brisswalter, J. and Louis, J., Vitamin supplementation benefits in master athletes, *Sports Med.* 44(3), 311–8, 2014.
133. Sawka, M.N., Burke, L.M., Eichner, E.R., Maughan, R.J., Montain, S.J. and Stachenfeld, N.S., American College of Sports Medicine position stand. Exercise and fluid replacement, *Med. Sci. Sports Exerc.* 39(2), 377–90, 2007.
134. Sawka, M.N. and Montain, S.J., Fluid and electrolyte supplementation for exercise heat stress, *Am. J. Clin. Nutr.* 72(2 Suppl), 564S–72S, 2000.
135. Schoeller, D.A., Changes in total body water with age, *Am. J. Clin. Nutr.* 50(5 Suppl), 1176–81, 1989.

136. Tipton, K.D., Jeukendrup, A.E. and Hespel, P., Nutrition for the sprinter, *J. Sports Sci.* 25(1 Suppl), S5–15, 2007.
137. Glaister, M., Howatson, G., Abraham, C.S. et al., Caffeine supplementation and multiple sprint running performance, *Med. Sci. Sports Exerc.* 40(10), 1835–40, 2008.
138. Bosco, C., Tihanyi, J., Pucspk, J. et al., Effect of oral creatine supplementation on jumping and running performance, *Int. J. Sports Med.* 18(5), 369–72, 1997.
139. Skare, O.C., Skadberg, and Wisnes, A.R., Creatine supplementation improves sprint performance in male sprinters, *Scand. J. Med. Sci. Sports* 11(2), 96–102, 2001.
140. Delecluse, C., Diels, R. and Goris, M., Effect of creatine supplementation on intermittent sprint running performance in highly trained athletes, *J. Strength Cond. Res.* 17(3), 446–54, 2003.
141. Javierre, C., Barbany, J.R., Bonjorn, V.M., Lizarraga, M.A., Ventura, J.L. and Segura, R., Creatine supplementation and performance in 6 consecutive 60 meter sprints, *J. Physiol. Biochem.* 60(4), 265–71, 2004.
142. Javierre, C., Lizarraga, M.A., Ventura, J.L., Garrido, E. and Segura, R., Creatine supplementation does not improve physical performance in a 150 m race, *Rev. Esp. Fisiol.* 53(4), 343–8, 1997.
143. Branch, J.D., Effect of creatine supplementation on body composition and performance: A meta-analysis, *Int. J. Sport. Nutr. Exerc. Metab.* 13(2), 198–226, 2003.
144. Schedel, J.M., Terrier, P. and Schutz, Y., The biomechanic origin of sprint performance enhancement after one-week creatine supplementation, *Jpn. J. Physiol.* 50(2), 273–6, 2000.
145. Bishop, D., Edge, J., Davis, C. and Goodman, C., Induced metabolic alkalosis affects muscle metabolism and repeated-sprint ability, *Med. Sci. Sports Exerc.* 36(5), 807–13, 2004.
146. Wiroth, J.B., Bermon, S., Andrei, S., Dalloz, E., Hebuterne, X. and Dolisi, C., Effects of oral creatine supplementation on maximal pedalling performance in older adults, *Eur. J. Appl. Physiol.* 84(6), 533–9, 2001.
147. Volek, J.S. and Rawson, E.S., Scientific basis and practical aspects of creatine supplementation for athletes, *Nutrition* 20(7–8), 609–14, 2004.
148. Nissen, S.L. and Sharp, R.L., Effect of dietary supplements on lean mass and strength gains with resistance exercise: A meta-analysis, *J. Appl. Physiol.* 94(2), 651–9, 2003.
149. Willoughby, D.S. and Rosene, J., Effects of oral creatine and resistance training on myosin heavy chain expression, *Med. Sci. Sports Exerc.* 33(10), 1674–81, 2001.
150. Olsen, S., Aagaard, P., Kadi, F. et al., Creatine supplementation augments the increase in satellite cell and myonuclei number in human skeletal muscle induced by strength training, *J. Physiol.* 573(2), 525–34, 2006.
151. Gotshalk, L.A., Volek, J.S., Staron, R.S., Denegar, C.R., Hagerman, F.C. and Kraemer, W.J., Creatine supplementation improves muscular performance in older men, *Med. Sci. Sports Exerc.* 34(3), 537–43, 2002.
152. Chrusch, M.J., Chilibeck, P.D., Chad, K.E., Davison, K.S. and Burke, D.G., Creatine supplementation combined with resistance training in older men, *Med. Sci. Sports Exerc.* 33(12), 2111–7, 2001.
153. Bermon, S., Venembre, P., Sachet, C., Valour, S. and Dolisi, C., Effects of creatine monohydrate ingestion in sedentary and weight-trained older adults, *Acta Physiol. Scand.* 164(2), 147–55, 1998.
154. Eijnde, B.O., Van Leemputte, M., Goris, M. et al., Effects of creatine supplementation and exercise training on fitness in men 55–75 yr old, *J. Appl. Physiol.* 95(2), 818–28, 2003.
155. Bemben, M.G., Witten, M.S., Carter, J.M., Eliot, K.A., Knehans, A.W. and Bemben, D.A., The effects of supplementation with creatine and protein on muscle strength following a traditional resistance training program in middle-aged and older men, *J. Nutr. Health Aging* 14(2), 155–9, 2010.
156. Syrotuik, D.G. and Bell, G.J., Acute creatine monohydrate supplementation: A descriptive physiological profile of responders vs. nonresponders, *J. Strength Cond. Res.* 18(3), 610–7, 2004.
157. Hultman, E., Soderlund, K., Timmons, J.A., Cederblad, G. and Greenhaff, P.L., Muscle creatine loading in men, *J. Appl. Physiol.* 81(1), 232–7, 1996.
158. Graham, A.S. and Hatton, R.C., Creatine: a review of efficacy and safety, *J. Am. Pharm. Assoc.* 39(6), 803–10, 1999.
159. Requena, B., Zabala, M., Padial, P. and Feriche, B., Sodium bicarbonate and sodium citrate: Ergogenic aids?, *J. Strength Cond. Res.* 19(1), 213–24, 2005.
160. Hill, C.A., Harris, R.C., Kim, H.J. et al., Influence of beta-alanine supplementation on skeletal muscle carnosine concentrations and high intensity cycling capacity, *Amino Acids* 32(2), 225–33, 2007.
161. Hobson, R.M., Saunders, B., Ball, G., Harris, R.C. and Sale, C., Effects of beta-alanine supplementation on exercise performance: A meta-analysis, *Amino Acids* 43(1), 25–37, 2012.

17 Training and Nutrition Needs of the Masters Strength/Power Athlete

Michael D. Roberts, Vincent J. Dalbo and Thomas W. Buford

CONTENTS

17.1 INTRODUCTION

Sports nutrition practices have existed for numerous centuries. For instance, Pythagoras of Samos (580–500 B.C.) recognised the need for nutritional adequacy to support the demands of rigorous training and implemented diets with a high-meat content for his athletes [1]. In the modern era, the field of sports nutrition blossomed in the early twentieth century largely due to the joint efforts of scientists and practitioners in elucidating the importance of various nutrients on adaptations to physical training. The advent of modern sports nutrition was marked by studies of carbohydrate and fat metabolism conducted by Swedish scientists in the 1930s. The field of evolved in the 1960s when the emphasis of athletic performance became centred on skeletal muscle glycogen utilisation. In the 1970s the sports nutrition field continued to grow when numerous university laboratories across the world began studying trained endurance athletes, and further expanded in the 1980s when exercise physiologists and nutritionists began collaborating on research projects [2].

Sports nutrition research in the resistance training area gained widespread notoriety in the 1990s. Since then, scientists have utilised numerous molecular techniques to examine the effects of nutritional supplements on skeletal muscle adaptations to physical training [3–5]. Despite the overwhelming amount of sports nutrition research that has been or is currently being performed with athletes in general, a paucity of research still exists regarding how various macronutrients, supplements and/or exercise affect older resistance-trained strength/power athletes.

Compared to younger peers, older adults have a reduced ability to physically recover following a resistance training workout [6]. This finding strongly suggests the need for optimal sports nutrition in this cohort.

It should be noted, however, that there is no one optimal dietary prescription for the masses to ascribe to. Instead, new evidence suggests that individuals respond differently to both diet and exercise. For example, researchers from Stanford University recently discovered that females possessing a particular genotype, or genetic make-up, responded differently to low-fat versus a low-carbohydrate diet [7]. According to this study, a given genotype may predispose an individual to lose anywhere from 4 lb (if she was a non-responder based upon her genetic profile) to 13 lb (if her genes enabled her to respond favourably to either a low-fat or low-carbohydrate diet). Thus, one can imagine the challenges in recommending an 'optimal' diet given that nutritional needs of master athletes likely vary on a person to person basis.

While numerous studies on dietary contributions to aerobic adaptations of older adults exist, research examining the relationship between diet and training adaptations with older strength/power athletes is sparse. For example, a search query in *SciVerse Scopus* (a bibliographic database of research journals) yields four peer-reviewed research journal articles published on this topic. Nonetheless, researchers and practitioners alike have made great advances in determining optimal nutritional regimens for athletes in different disciplines. Thus, the bases for the recommendations discussed throughout this chapter are adopted from several scientific viewpoints ranging from online articles written by renowned nutritionists to scientific journal position statements from organisations such as the International Society of Sports Nutrition, the American Dietetic Association and the American College of Sports Medicine. Our aim for this chapter is that readers can apply some of the knowledge presented in this chapter in order to optimise their own diets or the diets of the older athletes under their care with an end-goal of complementing their athletic performance.

17.2 PHYSIOLOGICAL DIFFERENCES IN TRAINING ADAPTATIONS TO STRENGTH TRAINING BETWEEN YOUNGER AND OLDER ATHLETES

Prior to making dietary recommendations for masters strength/power athletes, it is necessary to discuss what is currently known with regard to ageing, muscle physiology and resistance training adaptations. In general, it is well known that both muscle mass and strength decrease with ageing. For example, Jan Lexell performed classic work whereby he used autopsy analyses to demonstrate that aged men (70–73 years old) possessed approximately 110,000 less muscle fibres in the vastus lateralis leg muscle compared to 19–37-year-old men; representing a 23% decline in muscle fibre content with ageing [8]. Furthermore, older men possessed 30% less type II (force- and power-producing) muscle fibres compared to their younger cohort [8]. More recent data revealed that approximately 20%–30% of whole-body lean body mass (most of which is muscle mass) is lost between the third and eighth decade of life [9]. Thus, the scientific literature has demonstrated a clear association between ageing and decrements in muscle mass and strength [10,11]. Figure 17.1 highlights the rate of age-related loss in both muscle mass and strength.

In general, the acute and chronic responses to resistance training are composed of multiple phases which can be fit to a paradigm coined by scientist Hans Selye as the general adaptation syndrome [12]. In this paradigm (see Figure 17.2), the initial alarm phase can be thought of as the physiological response to the first few resistance training bouts whereby muscle damage and inflammation are subsequently followed by muscle repair mechanisms resulting in an increase in protein synthesis and the stimulation of muscle stem cell activity to enhance muscle growth. Of note, muscle strength is typically lost during the alarm phase due to extensive muscle damage that is incurred from the first few workouts. However, weight-trained muscle subsequently undergoes the resistance phase whereby strength and muscle size increase during subsequent weeks and months of consistent training. Finally, the exhaustion phase may occur when athletes reach stagnation and either plateau in their training adaptations or begin experiencing strength decrements. While this latter phase is difficult to discern in strength/power athletes of any age, there is a large body of evidence suggesting that incremental variations in training load and volume can prevent stagnation, increase performance variables and/or increase muscle mass gains [13,14]. Likewise, research studies presented throughout this chapter suggests that optimising one's diet can play a major role in preventing stagnation and optimising training adaptations.

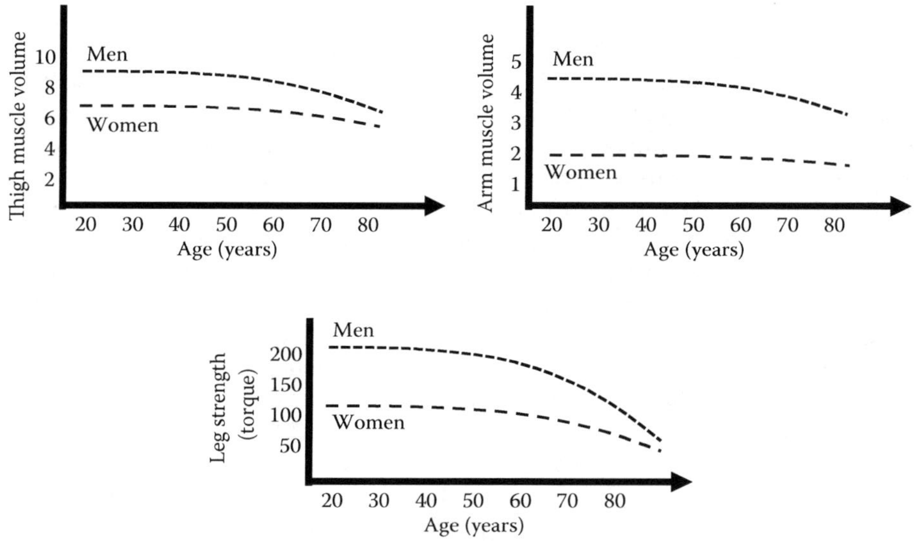

FIGURE 17.1 Trends demonstrating losses in thigh muscle volume, arm muscle volume and leg strength with aging.

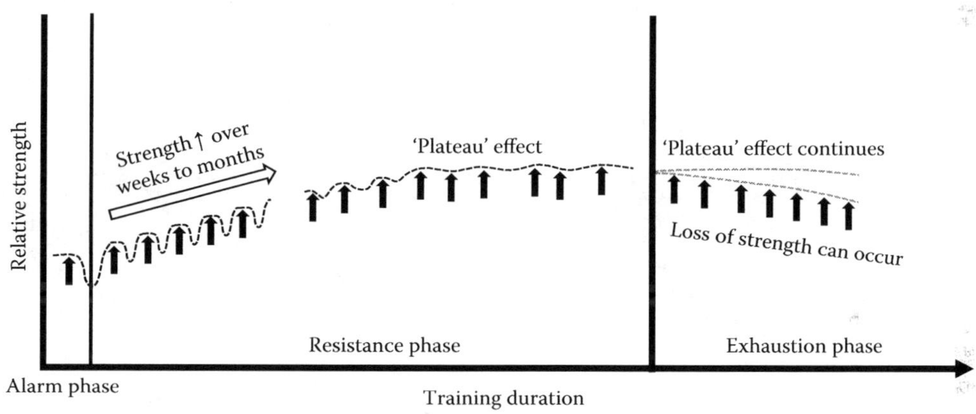

FIGURE 17.2 Demonstration outlining the general adaptation syndrome.

Currently, the existing body of literature suggests that older individuals can gain strength and muscle mass through resistance training [16,17]. However, in general it appears that older individuals generally respond less favourably to training sessions when compared to younger individuals. For example, Kumar et al. reported that intramuscular anabolic signalling mechanisms and myofibrillar protein synthesis (which is indicative of muscle rebuilding) were dampened among healthy but non-athletic men in their 70s compared to those in their 20s [18]. Older individuals also present an impaired inflammatory response within skeletal muscle tissue following a resistance training bout [19,20].

The activation of inflammatory immune cells after a muscle-damaging resistance training bout is integral to muscle repair and growth because immune cells have been shown to stimulate muscle stem cell replication [21,22] and possibly muscle protein synthesis [23] since muscle stem cells are important in the recovery process following resistance training. Therefore, the diminished ability of older individuals to elicit an intramuscular immune cell response following resistance exercise is likely unfavourable with regard to muscle fibre repair and subsequent muscle rebuilding mechanisms.

When examining training adaptations following 16 weeks of resistance training, Petrella et al. determined that muscle fibre growth was significantly greater in 20–35-year-old males and females versus their 60–75-year-old counterparts [24]. In explaining these findings, the investigators suggested that the diminished ability of older individuals to recruit muscle stem cells to donate more muscle nuclei with chronic training likely dampened their ability to experience muscle growth. For a schematic representation of these phenomena, refer to Figure 17.3.

Skeletal muscle samples analysed from older and younger individuals also suggest that tissue from older individuals possess genes that are turned on which are indicative of cellular ageing [25]. However, in this same study, 6 months of resistance training in the older cohort turned off these ageing genes making the older muscle genetically similar to the younger cohort. The 6-month program consisted of two workouts per week with three sets of 10 repetitions for each of the following exercises: leg press, chest press, leg extension, leg flexion, shoulder press, lat pull-down seated row, calf raise, abdominal crunch and back extension and 10 repetitions for arm flexion and arm extension. Training progressed from one set of each exercise at 50% of the initial 1 repetition maximum (1RM) to three sets at 80% of 1RM over the training period.

Finally, it is noteworthy that recovery periods between resistance training sessions likely differ between younger and older individuals. In support of this hypothesis, Roth et al. determined that a 3-day per week training regimen for 9 weeks produced significantly more muscle damage in 65–75-year-old women versus 20–30-year-old women [6]. Specifically, microscopic data revealed that 2%–4% of muscle cells were damaged in the young group whereas 5%–17% of muscle fibres were damaged in the older group [6]. Taking all of this data into consideration along with the aforementioned evidence suggesting that older individuals possess impairments in post-exercise

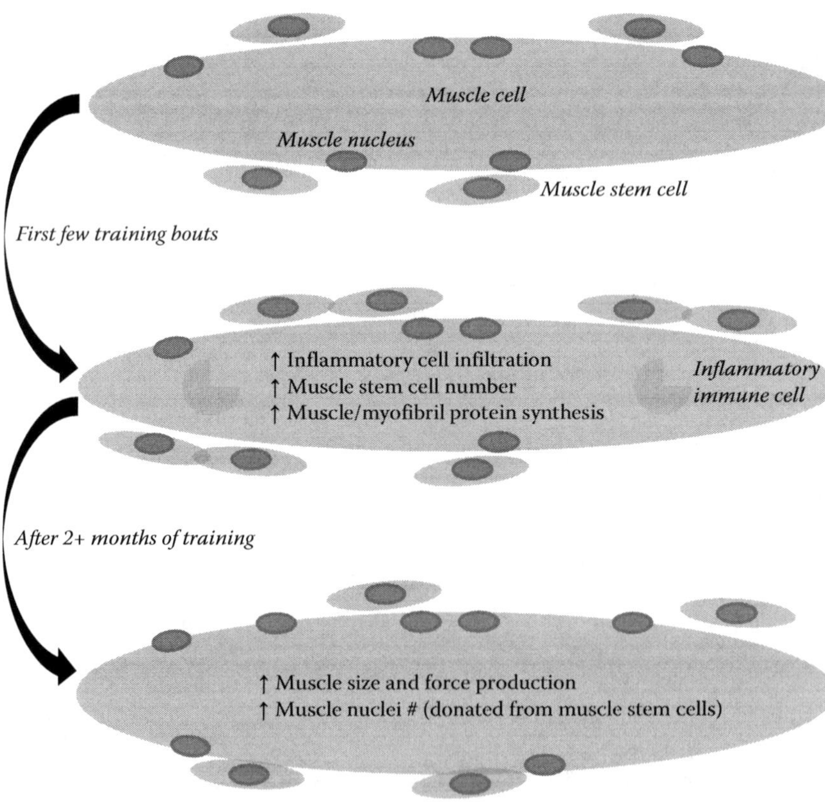

FIGURE 17.3 Depiction of acute post-exercise and chronic post-exercise adaptations at the cellular level.

muscle inflammation/repair implies that training volume should be relatively lower in older individuals over chronic training periods in order to ensure that adequate neuromuscular recovery occurs between exercise bouts.

In summary, the combination of an impaired muscle rebuilding response to resistance exercise, a diminished capacity of muscle stem cells to become activated after exercise, and the different genetic environment of skeletal muscle in older individuals are likely to reduce an older person's capabilities to gain muscle mass with resistance training [26].

While the above studies have provided strong evidence to suggest that hypertrophic potential of older muscle is impaired, studies do exist to suggest that lifelong resistance training maintains skeletal muscle in a youth-like state at both the molecular and functional levels. As mentioned above, there is evidence suggesting that 6 months of resistance training makes older muscle more similar to younger muscle at the messenger RNA (mRNA) level. Furthermore, data published by Verdijk et al. suggests that older muscle possesses less type II fibre-specific muscle stem cells [27]. However, 12 weeks of resistance training significantly increased type II muscle fibre size by 28% and remarkably increased type II fibre stem cells to a level similar to younger individuals [28].

In earlier research undertaken on masters weightlifters, Pearson et al. compared 54 elite-level masters weightlifters (40–87 years old) with a similar number of aged-matched, healthy untrained individuals [29]. Masters weightlifters were able to generate 32% more lower-body peak power and 32% more knee extensor force than the untrained individuals, and 85-year-old weightlifters were as powerful as 65-year-old control subjects. Therefore, it appears that long-term weight-training is able to maximise muscle strength while preventing or even reversing age-related muscle loss. In summary, the above section of the chapter highlights the following:

- Both the number of motor units (nerve fibres and the muscle fibres that they innervate) and muscle strength is lower in older versus younger individuals.
- Older individuals present a dampened acute anabolic response to resistance exercise as evidenced by decreased muscle protein synthesis and anabolic signalling.
- Relative to younger individuals, older individuals exhibit a lessened acute immune response to resistance training which likely contributes to the impaired recovery observed between resistance training bouts.
- Older individuals are able to increase muscle fibre size and strength in response to chronic resistance training, although their ability to do so is impaired relative to younger counterparts.
- Decades of resistance training by masters athletes may keep skeletal muscle in a youth-like physiological state and thus make the ageing muscle more resilient to injury as well as stronger.

17.3 GENERAL DIETARY RECOMMENDATIONS FOR MASTERS STRENGTH/POWER ATHLETES

Skeletal muscle is a dynamic tissue as muscle proteins are constantly broken down prior to being re-synthesised [4]. In general, resistance exercise accelerates intramuscular protein turnover (muscle/myofibrillar protein synthesis and muscle protein breakdown). Hence, when athletes of any age consume extra supplemental protein in conjunction with resistance training, muscle protein synthesis rates exceed muscle protein breakdown rates. Chronically, this results in an increase in both muscle mass and strength [4]. Evidence presented later in this chapter also suggests that higher volume resistance training depletes up to 30% of intramuscular glycogen stores for energy production which also demonstrates the need for glycogen replenishment through dietary carbohydrate intake. Finally, more recent research is beginning to elucidate how skeletal muscle uses dietary fatty acids to promote skeletal muscle growth and recovery in response to resistance training. The remainder of this section will discuss what the current evidence suggests regarding the intake recommendations of these macronutrients.

17.3.1 Protein Intake Recommendations

According to renowned muscle physiologist and sports nutrition researcher Stuart Phillips, 'there is likely no other dietary component that inspires as much debate, insofar as athletes are concerned, as protein' [30]. However, most experts in the field agree that strength/power athletes need to consume more protein than a non-athlete given that (a) beyond intramuscular fluid content, skeletal muscle is mostly comprised of protein, (b) intramuscular protein synthesis is bolstered and muscle protein breakdown is decreased following protein ingestion, and (c) bodybuilders and strength athletes typically consume disproportionately more protein in their diets.

The International Society of Sports Nutrition recommends that athletes should obtain 1.4–2.0 g of protein per kg of bodyweight (0.63–0.91 g per lb) per day [31]. The American College of Sports Medicine, American Dietetic Association and the Dieticians of Canada recently published a joint statement claiming that athletes should obtain 1.2–1.7 g of protein per kg of bodyweight (0.54–0.77 g per lb) per day [32].

It has been suggested that athletes who do not eat foods rich in essential amino acids such as vegans and/or athletes who want to gain muscle mass should consume more protein on a day-to-day basis (2.0+ g of protein per kg of bodyweight or 0.91 g/lb) in order to ensure that enough essential amino acids are ingested [33,34]. However, Phillips et al. argue that athletes and populations such as Canadian and Alaskan Inuit routinely consume up to 3.0 g/kg of protein per day and that these intakes have not led to maladies such as decrements in kidney function and/or decrements in bone mass as some would suggest occur [30]. Therefore, in spite of the current recommendations for protein adequacy, more research is needed to examine the quantities of protein intake that are optimal for strength/power athletes, particularly in masters athletes.

Leucine has been suggested to be an integral amino acid for the stimulation of muscle protein synthesis [35]. Thus, protein sources with more leucine content are widely suggested to be more beneficial for muscle growth. In this regard, milk-based foods contain 10% (milk isolate, casein) to 12% (whey) leucine content, meat and egg-based products contain approximately 8%–9% leucine and plant-based products such as wheat protein contain less than 8% leucine which makes the latter protein sources less suitable for optimal stimulation of muscle growth [36].

Given that whey and/or casein protein is a rich source of leucine, supplementation of these protein forms has become a common practice amongst strength/power athletes. Kerksick et al. demonstrated that young resistance-trained males ingesting a supplemental protein beverage containing 40 g of whey protein and 8 g of casein protein exhibited a 4.2-lb (1.9-kg) increase in muscle mass following 12 weeks of resistance training [37]. Findings from our own laboratory also demonstrated that resistance-trained males between the ages of 18 and 30 years exhibited a 2.4-lb (1.1-kg) increase in muscle mass, an 18–25-lb (8–11-kg) increase in bench press strength, and a 50–55-lb (23–25-kg) increase in leg press strength after a 50-day intervention whereby they supplemented with an 580 extra calories per day (90 g protein, 48 g carbohydrate, 2 g fat) with two meal replacement supplements containing whey protein [38]. Similarly, Phillips and colleagues reviewed numerous research studies and determined that individuals that resistance-trained for 8–16 weeks while consuming milk or a whey protein supplement exhibited the greatest gains in muscle mass (~3.0 kg or 6.5 lb) [39]. Conversely, those that consumed a soy protein supplement while training gained less muscle mass (~1.5 kg or 3.3 lb) and those that consumed a carbohydrate/placebo drink gained the least amount of muscle mass (~1.0 kg or 2.2 lb).

Thus, it is evident that bolstering whey/casein protein intake, whether through diet or supplementation, yields beneficial training effects in resistance-trained athletes. Although quantity recommendations for protein supplementation in resistance-trained athletes have not been established, particularly in masters athletes, researchers have demonstrated that consuming roughly 20 g of milk/whey/casein-based protein sources within 1 hour of working out increases anabolic muscle rebuilding mechanisms following exercise [40].

It is widely acknowledged that both muscle mass and strength loss accompany ageing. However, conflicting evidence exists suggesting that older adults may or may not possess impairments in being able to utilise amino acids from protein-rich foods for muscle-building mechanisms. For example, Katsanos et al. determined that 68-year-old healthy but non-athletic subjects were less able to transport amino acids into skeletal muscle after ingesting 7 g of essential amino acids compared to 31-year-old subjects [41].

Previous literature also established that older individuals present impairments in muscle-building mechanisms in response to the infusion of insulin and amino acids (which mimics conditions after a meal) [42]. However, in an research paper titled 'Aging does not impair the anabolic response to a protein-rich meal', Symons et al. demonstrated that muscle protein synthesis increased similarly in 70-year-old and 41-year-old subjects up to 5 hours following the ingestion of 4 oz of lean beef which contained 10.1 g of essential amino acids [43]. A subsequent study by the same research group replicated their previous finding and discovered that 8 oz of lean beef did not further stimulate muscle protein synthesis within or between age groups [44]. Therefore, it seems that, independent of exercise, older individuals are able to disseminate and utilise amino acids from dietary protein sources similarly to younger individuals so long as the protein sources are rich in essential amino acids.

With regard to protein requirements for older individuals that undertake resistance training, few studies have adequately supported the suggestion that consuming more dietary protein is advantageous for optimising training adaptations. For instance, Campbell et al. determined that older adults who resistance-trained while consuming a meat-containing mixed diet presented larger increases in muscle mass and type II muscle fibre size relative to those who trained and consumed a lacto-ovo-vegetarian diet over a 12-week period [45]. A more recent study also determined that supplementing with a protein-containing drink (10 g protein + 7 g carbohydrate + 3 g fat) immediately after resistance exercise resulted in greater muscle mass and strength gains following 12 weeks of resistance exercise training in older adults [46]. Importantly, those that supplemented with the protein-containing drink 2 hours following exercise did not experience increases in leg-kicking strength and/or muscle mass which emphasises the importance of consuming a protein source within 30 minutes of the cessation of each training bout.

In this regard, Singh and colleagues demonstrated that supplementing older men and women who resistance trained over a 10-week period with a 360-calorie beverage (15 g soy protein, 54 g carbohydrates, 9 g fat) doubled their muscle strength compared to those who trained without the supplemental beverage (250% increase versus a 100% increase, respectively) [47]. However, statistical analysis from the Singh et al. study revealed that changes in both muscular strength and muscle cell size were prominently due to the increase in caloric intake and not necessarily due to increased protein consumption.

Supplementing older men with 20 g of protein prior to and following every resistance training bout for 12 weeks has also been shown to have no additive effects on muscle mass and/or strength gains when compared to older men that consumed a placebo drink [48]. However, the older individuals consuming the protein supplement still only consumed 1.1 g/kg/day of protein. Some argue that adequate protein intakes for older, non-exercising individuals should be at least 1.0 g/kg/day (versus the current recommendation of 0.8 g/kg/day) since older individuals are more metabolically stressed than younger individuals as a result of more wound-healing, pressure ulcers, and the gradual losses in muscle mass [49].

In summary, the above evidence supports the suggestion that older strength/power athletes may benefit from increased protein and energy consumption, especially if protein and/or calorie intakes are suboptimal during training. The following points summarise the current body of literature regarding protein intakes suggestions for older strength/power athletes:

- Scientific position stands recommend that protein intakes for strength/power should be 1.2–2.0 g per kg of bodyweight (0.54–0.91 g per lb) per day (refer to Table 17.1 for protein sources). For a 200-lb (90.6-kg) athlete, this recommendation equals 100–180+ g protein per day.

TABLE 17.1
Sources of Macronutrients

Food (Serving Size)	Protein (g)	CHO (g)	Fat (g)	Calories
Dietary Protein Sources				
Lean ground beef, 4%–7% fat (3 oz)	18	0	~3	~120
Ground beef, 20% fat (3 oz)	15	0	18	210
Sirloin steak, fat trimmed (3 oz)	26	0	5	156
Chicken: white meat, no skin (3 oz)	18	0	0	93
Chicken: dark meat, no skin (3 oz)	24	0	9	174
Turkey: white meat (3 oz)	24	0	0	114
Salmon (3 oz)	18	0	12	174
Halibut, tilapia, cod (3 oz)	18	0	2	93
Tuna, canned in water (3 oz)	21	0	0	96
Eggs: whole (1 medium)	6	0	5	71
Eggs: whites only (1 large)	4	0	0	16
Skim milk (1 cup or 8 fl oz)	8	12	0	83
Tofu (3 oz)	6	3	3	51
Cheese: made from whole milk (1 oz)	6	0	9	105
Yogurt: low fat (1 cup, 8 oz)	13	17	4	154
Cottage cheese: low fat (1 cup, 8 oz)	28	2	6	163
Ham: sliced, lean (3 oz)	15	0	3	90
Pork loin: lean meat only (3 oz)	15	0	6	132
Dietary Carbohydrate Sources				
Pasta: spaghetti, macaroni, etc. (1 cup, cooked)	8	43	1	220
White/wheat bread or rolls (1 roll, 1 oz)	2	13	2	76
Baked potato: plain (medium)	4	46	0	200
Sweet potato: plain (large)	4	37	0	162
White rice (1 cup)	4	45	0	205
Brown rice (1 cup)	5	45	2	216
Bagel: plain (regular size)	11	56	2	290
Beans: red, black, pinto (1 cup)	16	40	0	220
Oatmeal (1 cup, cooked)	6	29	3	160
Low-fat granola: bar or cereal (1 oz)	2	23	2	109
Corn (1 cup)	4	46	1	184
Apple, medium size	0	25	0	95
Orange, medium size	1	17	0	69
Banana, medium size	1	27	0	105
Grapes (1 cup, 30 grapes)	1	27	0	104
Berries: blueberries, cranberries, blackberries, strawberries, etc. (1 cup)	1	13–21	0	53–84
Tomatoes (1 cup, chopped)	2	5	0	25
Carrots, beets, turnips (1 cup)	1	12	0	52
Cruciferous vegetables: greens, broccoli, cauliflower, cabbage, etc. (1 cup cooked)	2–3	6–7	0	30–40
Dietary Fat Sources				
Butter (1 oz)	1	0	15	140
Whole milk (1 cup or 8 fl oz)	8	13	8	146
2% milk (1 cup or 8 fl oz)	8	12	5	120
Peanuts (1 oz)	5	7	14	166
Almonds (1 oz)	4	6	17	177

(continued)

TABLE 17.1 (Continued)
Sources of Macronutrients

Food (Serving Size)	Protein (g)	CHO (g)	Fat (g)	Calories
Peanut butter: commercial, sweetened (1 oz)	7	6	14	165
Cream cheese (1 oz)	2	1	10	96
Salad dressing: ranch, bleu cheese, Italian (1 oz)	0	2	14	136
Avocado (1/2)	1.5	6	10.5	114

Note: Caloric and macronutrient data was obtained from http://www.nutritiondata.com.
Measurements:
3 oz = size of a deck of playing cards or a Dixie cup.
1 oz = 2 tablespoons, except for rolls or bread which is porous.
8 oz or 8 fl oz = approximately 3 small Dixie cups.

- Masters athletes striving to build muscle should consume roughly 2+ g/kg/day of protein [30,33]. Hence, a 200-lb (90.6-kg) masters athlete should consume upwards of 180–200 g protein per day.
- It is important to obtain protein frequently throughout the day in order to keep muscle in an anabolic state. Thus, ensure each meal (breakfast, lunch, dinner and snacks) contain roughly 20–30 g of protein.
- While supplementation with protein shakes (whey/casein-based) are not necessary for athletes (i.e. muscle gains have been shown to occur independently of protein supplementation), protein supplements offer a rich source of amino acids and have been shown to offer the greatest benefit to resistance-trained athletes when compared to other protein or energy sources according to a recent review of literature [39].
- A protein supplement containing 20 g of whey protein has been shown to positively affect muscle-building mechanisms when taken within 1 hour following a resistance training bout.

For a detailed discussion on the protein needs of masters athletes from a range of sport disciplines, see Chapter 6.

17.3.2 Carbohydrate Intake Recommendations

Carbohydrates are integral to endurance athletes such as long-distance swimmers, runners, cyclists, triathletes and soccer players given that they are the preferred fuel source for energy production during exercise. In fact, endurance athletes that are carbohydrate-deprived begin breaking down muscle protein for fuel almost immediately during prolonged exercise. For example, Lemon and Mullin demonstrated that serum urea (a surrogate marker of intramuscular muscle protein breakdown) increases within 15 minutes of moderate cycling during a 60-minute cycling bout [50]. However, in the same study, endurance athletes in a well-fed state (not carbohydrate or glycogen-depleted) did not exhibit signs of protein catabolism during exercise.

Much less is known regarding carbohydrate requirements for strength/power athletes. However, it is well established that weight training decreases intramuscular carbohydrate stores (muscle glycogen). In this regard, it largely depends upon the amount of weight training performed per training session. For example, muscle biopsy analyses revealed that 20 sets of lower body exercises (averaging nine reps per set) performed within a 30-minute period decreased intramuscular glycogen stores by 27% in young healthy individuals [51]. A similar study conducted by Haff et al. examined young men that resistance-trained in the morning while ingesting a 250-g carbohydrate supplement versus a non-caloric placebo [52]. The men were instructed to perform light-intensity squats to exhaustion 4 hours following either supplement or placebo consumption. Those that ingested the carbohydrate supplement performed more repetitions and exercised 30 minutes longer than those who did not consume carbohydrate.

Current research suggests it is likely that consuming substantially less carbohydrate following a resistance training workout is equally as effective in replenishing lost glycogen stores. For example, Roy and Tarnopolsky demonstrated that consuming either 1 g/kg of carbohydrate (which is 91 g for a 200-lb athlete) or isocaloric amounts of a carbohydrate-protein-fat (66%–23%–11%, or 66 g of carbohydrate for a 200-lb athlete) shake similarly increased skeletal muscle glycogen stores following a 27-set workout [53]. These findings suggest that consuming anywhere from 66–250 g of carbohydrate upon the completion of a high-volume resistance training workout (i.e. 9+ sets at 6–12 reps per set) appears sufficient to replenish lost glycogen stores after a resistance training bout.

In spite of the above literature, it is unlikely that Olympic lifters and power-lifters performing substantially less volume during workouts experience decrements in intramuscular glycogen stores. Furthermore, if too much carbohydrate is consumed by a strength/power athlete then the chances for unwanted weight gain (fat) may result. In this regard, exercise physiologist Tim Noakes recently wrote a commentary suggesting that the overconsumption of carbohydrates can be 'toxic' for the body [54]. In this commentary, Noakes makes the following points:

- The most recent US Dietary Guidelines (2010) promotes that individuals consume 6–11 daily servings of breads, cereals and pasta. Americans seem to follow these recommendations in spite of the fact that obesity has become the largest medical problem in the United States.
- High-protein weight loss regimens have been researched and shown to produce results that are at least equally effective to reduced-energy diets with no harmful side effects from high-protein diets having been noted.
- Some very large industries, including the soft drink, sugar and confectionary industries, do not want people to know that lower-carbohydrate diets are healthier than people may expect.

To further explore the effects that low- vs. high-carbohydrate diets have on various health markers is beyond the realm of this chapter. However, it is an important topic to be familiar with when making carbohydrate recommendations to strength/power athletes of any age. Readers interested in more literature regarding the chronic overconsumption of high-glycaemic carbohydrates potentially leading to increases in body fat and other obesity-related diseases (insulin resistance, fatty liver disease, etc.) are encouraged to read two papers in the reference list at the end of this chapter [55,56].

It is evident that carbohydrate intake recommendations for masters strength/power athletes can substantially vary. According to a publication by the Food and Nutrition Board, a generalised recommended dietary reference intake for healthy but inactive males and females aged 19–70 years is approximately 130 g of carbohydrate per day [57]. However, some research advises that athletes should consume roughly 5–7 g/kg per day for 'general training needs' [58]. The latter recommendation would be equivalent to 455–637 g of carbohydrate per day which is roughly 90–130 g of carbohydrates per meal if spread over five meals per day. Since scientific literature is particularly lacking in this area, we would suggest for masters strength/power athletes to aim for 3–5 g/kg (1.4–2.3 g/lb) per day as a compromise between the two earlier suggestions. If these carbohydrate intakes result in lethargy and decrements in workout volume and/or intensity then intakes can be increased to 5–7 g/kg (2.3–3.2 g/lb) per day. Athletes of any age should obtain carbohydrate from relatively unprocessed foods including fruits, vegetables, steel-cut oatmeal, quinoa, beans and legumes and whole grain pasta or brown rice which are both unprocessed and contain bran. Table 17.1 lists other sources of carbohydrates that are unprocessed.

In summary, the following summarises the current body of literature regarding carbohydrate intake suggestions for older strength/power athletes:

- Carbohydrates are an essential macronutrient given their role in intramuscular energy production during exercise.
- The overconsumption of carbohydrates can potentially increase weight gain and body fat in strength/power athletes that expend minimal energy outside of the gym.
- High-volume resistance exercise can deplete glycogen stores in exercised muscle by roughly 30%, although it is likely that strength/power athletes performing low-volume/high-intensity training (Olympic and power lifters) likely experience marginal losses in muscle glycogen.
- In general, masters strength/power athletes can likely sustain muscle glycogen stores by consuming 3–5 g/kg (1.4–2.3 g/lb) per day of carbohydrate. If these intakes result in lethargy and decrements in workout volume and/or intensity then intakes should be increased to 5–7 g/kg (2.3–3.2 g/lb) per day.

For a detailed discussion of the carbohydrate needs of masters athletes from a range of sport disciplines, see Chapter 4.

17.3.3 Fat Intake Recommendations

Dietary fats are a rich source of essential fatty acids which cannot be synthesised by the body and aid in the digestion and bodily absorption of vitamins A, D, E and K. Fatty acids are also used by cells throughout the body for energy production, fuel storage and cell membrane formation. Furthermore, dietary fat and cholesterol derived from animal-based foods are used for hormone synthesis. Indeed, there is scientific evidence suggesting that low-fat diets can depress testosterone levels by as much as 15% [59] which is obviously not optimal for older weight-training athletes. More recent evidence supports the role of dietary fats in sustaining higher testosterone levels in strength athletes. For instance, Sallinen et al. reported that testosterone levels are positively correlated with fat intakes in young strength-training athletes [60].

As with the carbohydrate intake recommendations made above, literature examining dietary fat needs in strength/power athletes of any age is lacking. In a review article titled 'Nutritional practices of elite athletes. Practical recommendations', Economos et al. claim that elite athletes typically consumed between 25%–30% of their energy intake in the form of dietary fat [61]. Hence, for master strength/power athletes consuming 2000–2500 calories per day, these figures are equivalent to 55–83 g of fat per day.

According to the 2009 Joint Position Stand written by the American College of Sports Medicine, American Dietetic Association and the Dieticians of Canada, athletes should strive to take in 20%–35% of their daily energy intake from dietary fats [32] which is approximately 1.0–1.5 g per kg (0.5–0.7 g per lb) of fat per day. Hence, we currently know that (a) athletes in general should consume roughly 20%–35% of their energy intake from fat, (b) restricting fat intakes below these aforementioned recommendations can potentially impair normal bodily homeostasis including decreases in the production of anabolic hormones and (c) the effects of consuming too much fat in athletes is not known, albeit given that dietary fat is energy dense, it is likely that nonfunctional weight gain will occur.

With regard to the essential fatty acids obtained from dietary fat, there are two of major importance: alpha-linolenic acid (an omega-3 fatty acid) and linoleic acid (an omega-6 fatty acid). As mentioned earlier in this chapter, exercise induces an inflammatory response within skeletal muscle which subsequently increases protein synthesis. One interesting fact about linoleic acids is that skeletal muscle uses these fatty acids to produce inflammatory signallers (termed prostaglandins) after exercise in order to increase muscle-rebuilding mechanisms. Two studies by Trappe et al. determined that providing 1200 mg of ibuprofen to subjects after performing ~120 eccentric leg extensions blunted the intramuscular prostaglandin and muscle protein synthesis responses 24 hours following exercise [23,62]. However, Trappe et al. recently published a study examining 64–67-year-old men and demonstrated that the taking of acetaminophen or ibuprofen (both which blunt intramuscular prostaglandin production) during 12 weeks of leg extensor resistance-training, actually increased muscle growth (acetaminophen: ↑ 12.5%; ibuprofen: ↑ 10.9%; placebo: ↑ 8.6%) and muscle strength (acetaminophen: ↑ 19 kg; ibuprofen: ↑ 19 kg; placebo: ↑ 15 kg) compared to a placebo group [63].

These recent findings suggest that older strength-training athletes may potentially benefit from increasing their dietary intake of omega-3 fatty acids (alpha-linolenic acid, eicosapentaenoic acid and/or docosahexaenoic acid) which counteract omega-6 fatty acids and are putatively used by skeletal muscle and other tissues to produce metabolites that counteract inflammation. In this regard, a recent study examined the effects of supplementing the diets of 65-year-old resistance training subjects with 14 g per day of alpha-linolinic acid [64]. Interestingly, the researchers discovered that knee flexor muscle strength increased in subjects and blood interleukin-6 (a marker of low-grade inflammation during ageing) decreased after 12 weeks compared to a placebo group of the same age. Hence, it is apparent that intramuscular fatty acids obtained through the diet, especially those involved with prostaglandin synthesis, may exhibit major influences on the skeletal muscle repair to resistance training. Figure 17.4 models a theoretical role of some of the dietary fatty acids in facilitating resistance training adaptations.

Foods rich in omega-3 fatty acids include flaxseed oil and fish oil (salmon, sardine). Foods rich in omega-6 fatty acids include vegetable/sunflower/soybean oils, mayonnaise, walnuts and salad dressings. Nonetheless, more research is needed regarding which types of dietary fats are more advantageous for younger and older strength/power athletes to consume in order to optimise training adaptations and promote recovery between workouts.

The following summarises the current body of literature regarding dietary fat intake suggestions for older strength/power athletes:

- Essential fatty acids (derived from dietary fats) cannot be synthesised by the body and (a) aid in the digestion and bodily absorption of vitamins A, D, E and K, and (b) are integral for energy production, fuel storage and cell membrane formation.
- Omega-3 and omega-6 fatty acids play a role in post-exercise inflammation and recovery. In older athletes, diets lower in omega-6 fatty acids and more rich in omega-3 fatty acids may optimise training adaptations and recovery.
- In general, masters strength/power athletes should consume anywhere from 20%–35% of their energy intake from fat. This is approximately 1.0–1.5 g per kg (0.5–0.7 g per lb) of fat per day.

Chapter 5 examines in detail the fat needs of masters athletes.

Readers interested in increasing their knowledge in this area are encouraged to look at a number of published reviews [65–74].

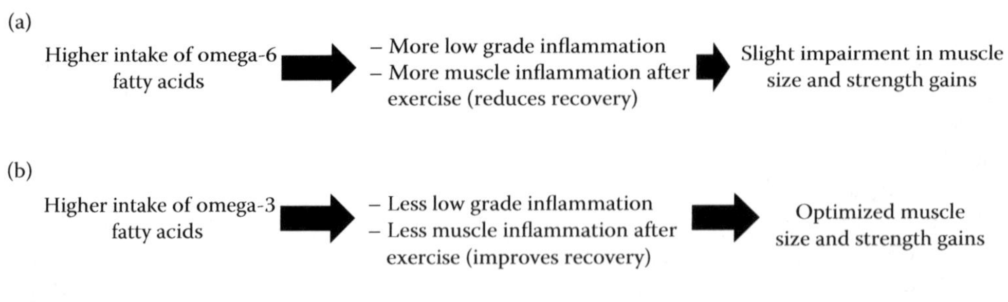

FIGURE 17.4 Depiction of how different dietary fats affect inflammation and recovery from exercise.

17.4 IMPLICATIONS FOR SPORTS MEDICINE PROFESSIONALS, CLINICIANS, MASTERS ATHLETES AND COACHES

As emphasised in the introduction of this chapter, each person responds differently to different dietary and workout regimens. Therefore, it is of the upmost importance that each masters strength/power athlete be in tune with their body when experimenting with the dietary practices presented in this chapter. In this regard, if following the intake recommendations from this chapter lead to (a) weight fluctuations which, in turn, impair performance, or (b) lethargy which, again, impairs performance, then it is imperative to make alterations. Nonetheless, the scientific literature cited in this chapter provides a template for coaches and athletes to follow when formulating diet plans. For meal-planning ideas, the reader should refer to Tables 17.1 and 17.2 as well as the following sources:

- http://www.nutritionadata.com: this website offers nutrition information on a vast variety of foods and provides tools which enable users to determine how foods affect their health.

TABLE 17.2
Sample Meal Plan for Masters Strength and Power Athletes

Meal	Protein (g)	CHO (g)	Fat (g)	Calories
Meal 1 (7:00 AM)				
• 2 large eggs, scrambled	12	0	10	142
• 1 piece whole-grain toast	2	13	2	76
• Butter (1/2 tbsp)	1	27	0	105
• 1 banana				
Subtotals	15	40	12	323
Snack (10:00 AM)				
• 1 apple	0	25	0	95
• Almonds (1 oz)	4	6	17	177
Subtotals	4	31	17	272
Meal 3 (1:00 PM)				
• Chicken breast (4 oz)	24	0	0	124
• Black beans (1/2 cup)	8	20	0	110
• Chopped strawberries (1 cup)	1	15	0	64
Subtotals	54	70	0	298
Snack (3:00 PM)				
• Low-fat granola bar (3 oz)	6	69	6	327
Subtotals	6	69	6	327
Post-exercise whey with water (after exercise) *w/optional 3–5 g creatine monohydrate*	20	0	0	80
Meal 4 (8:00 PM)				
• Sirloin steak (6 oz)	52	0	10	312
• Green beans (1 cup)	3	7	0	40
• Corn (2 cups)	8	92	2	368
Subtotals	63	99	12	720
Snack 2 (10:00 PM)				
• Cottage cheese (1/2 cup)	14	1	3	81.5
• Chopped pineapple (1 oz)	1	22	0	82
Subtotals	15	23	3	163.5
Totals	177	332	50	2185

Note: CHO = carbohydrates; tbsp = tablespoon.

- http://www.webmd.com/diet/default.htm: this WebMD-based interactive website offers a variety of food suggestions and recipes based upon fitness goals.
- http://www.gssiweb.com: sponsored by the Gatorade Sports Science Institute, this website assists athletes in optimising health and performance by providing a plethora of research-based information regarding sports nutrition.

17.5 FUTURE RESEARCH DIRECTIONS

As emphasised throughout this chapter, research is lacking which examines how various macronutrients, supplements and/or exercise stressors affect older resistance-trained strength/power athletes. In this regard, addressing the following research questions may greatly enhance our understanding:

- How much dietary protein is essential for masters strength/power athletes to sustain muscle mass?
- How much dietary protein is needed to increase muscle mass and/or improve recovery in masters strength/power athletes?
- What are the carbohydrate requirements needed to sustain strength and energy levels in masters strength/power athletes during both training and competition?
- What types of fatty acids (obtained through the diet as well as with supplementation) promote the most favourable recovery and training adaptations from resistance training in masters athletes?
- While this will be a challenging endeavour, will genomics research result in masters strength/power athletes being able to be genotyped by their physician in order to better ascertain dietary guidelines that fit their training needs?

While these questions require vast resources and will be challenging to answer, research laboratories around the world are continuing to work around the clock to further the knowledge in the sports nutrition field.

REFERENCES

1. Grivetti, L.E. and Applegate, E.A., From Olympia to Atlanta: A cultural-historical perspective on diet and athletic training, *J. Nutr.* 127(5 Suppl), 860S–868S, 1997.
2. Dunford, M., ed. *Fundamentals of Sport and Exercise Nutrition*, Human Kinetics, Champaign, IL, 2010.
3. Roberts, M.D., Dalbo, V.J., Hassell, S.E., Brown, R. and Kerksick, C.M., Effects of preexercise feeding on markers of satellite cell activation, *Med. Sci. Sports Exerc.* 42(10), 1861–9, 2010.
4. Elliot, T.A., Cree, M.G., Sanford, A.P., Wolfe, R.R. and Tipton, K.D., Milk ingestion stimulates net muscle protein synthesis following resistance exercise, *Med. Sci. Sports Exerc.* 38(4), 667–74, 2006.
5. Cribb, P.J. and Hayes, A., Effects of supplement timing and resistance exercise on skeletal muscle hypertrophy, *Med, Sci, Sports Exerc.* 38(11), 1918–25, 2006.
6. Roth, S.M., Martel, G.F., Ivey, F.M. et al., High-volume, heavy-resistance strength training and muscle damage in young and older women, *J. Appl. Physiol.* 88(3), 1112–8, 2000.
7. Nelson, M.D., Prabhakar, P., Kondragunta, V., Kornman, K.S. and Gardner, C., Genetic phenotypes predict weight loss success: The right diet does matter, in American Heart Association's Joint Conference—50th Cardiovascular Disease Epidemiology and Prevention and Nutrition, Physical Activity and Metabolism, San Francisco, 2010.
8. Lexell, J., Henriksson-Larsen, K., Winblad, B. and Sjostrom, M., Distribution of different fiber types in human skeletal muscles: Effects of aging studied in whole muscle cross sections, *Muscle Nerve* 6(8), 588–95, 1983.
9. Kyle, U.G., Genton, L., Hans, D., Karsegard, L., Slosman, D.O. and Pichard, C., Age-related differences in fat-free mass, skeletal muscle, body cell mass and fat mass between 18 and 94 years, *Eur. J.Clin. Nutr.* 55(8), 663–72, 2001.

10. Janssen, I., Heymsfield, S.B., Wang, Z.M. and Ross, R., Skeletal muscle mass and distribution in 468 men and women aged 18–88 yr., *J. Appl. Physiol.* 89(1): 81–8, 2000.
11. Lindle, R.S., Metter, E.J., Lynch, N.A. et al., Age and gender comparisons of muscle strength in 654 women and men aged 20–93 yr, *J. Appl. Physiol.* 83(5), 1581–7, 1997.
12. Perdrizet, G.A., Hans Selye and beyond: Responses to stress, *Cell Stress Chaperones* 2(4), 214–9, 1997.
13. Kraemer, W.J., Ratamess, N., Fry, A.C. et al., Influence of resistance training volume and periodization on physiological and performance adaptations in collegiate women tennis players, *Am. J. Sports Med.* 28(5), 626–33, 2000.
14. Hoffman, J.R., Ratamess, N.A., Klatt, M. et al., Comparison between different off-season resistance training programs in Division III American college football players, *J. Strength Cond. Res.* 23(1), 11–19, 2009.
15. Baechle, T.R. and Earle, R.W., eds., *Essentials of Strength and Conditioning.* 2nd Ed., Human Kinetics, Champaign, IL, 2000.
16. Evans, W.J., Exercise training guidelines for the elderly, *Med. Sci. Sports Exerc.* 31(1), 12–17, 1999.
17. Hakkinen, K., Alen, M., Kallinen, M., Newton, R.U. and Kraemer, W.J., Neuromuscular adaptation during prolonged strength training, detraining and re-strength-training in middle-aged and elderly people, *Eur. J. Appl. Physiol.* 83(1), 51–62, 2000.
18. Kumar, V., Selby, A., Rankin, D. et al., Age-related differences in the dose-response relationship of muscle protein synthesis to resistance exercise in young and old men, *J. Physiol.* 587(Pt 1), 211–7, 2009.
19. Przybyla, B., Gurley, C., Harvey, J.F. et al., Aging alters macrophage properties in human skeletal muscle both at rest and in response to acute resistance exercise, *Exp. Gerontol.* 41(3), 320–7, 2006.
20. Peake, J., Della Gatta, P. and Cameron-Smith, D., Aging and its effects on inflammation in skeletal muscle at rest and following exercise-induced muscle injury, *Am. J. Physiol. Regul. Integr. Comp. Physiol.* 298(6), R1485–95, 2010.
21. Toumi, H., F'Guyer, S. and Best, T.M., The role of neutrophils in injury and repair following muscle stretch, *J. Anat.* 208(4), 459–70, 2006.
22. Chazaud, B., Sonnet, C., Lafuste, P. et al., Satellite cells attract monocytes and use macrophages as a support to escape apoptosis and enhance muscle growth, *J. Cell. Biol.* 163(5), 1133–43, 2003.
23. Trappe, T.A., White, F., Lambert, C.P., Cesar, D., Hellerstein, M. and Evans, W.J., Effect of ibuprofen and acetaminophen on postexercise muscle protein synthesis, *Am. J. Physiol. Endocrinol. Metab.* 282(3), E551–6, 2002.
24. Petrella, J.K., Kim, J.S., Cross, J.M., Kosek, D.J. and Bamman, M.M., Efficacy of myonuclear addition may explain differential myofiber growth among resistance-trained young and older men and women, *Am. J. Physiol. Endocrinol. Metab.* 291(5), E937–46, 2006.
25. Melov, S., Tarnopolsky, M.A., Beckman, K., Felkey, K. and Hubbard, A., Resistance exercise reverses aging in human skeletal muscle, *PLoS One* 2(5), e465, 2007.
26. Petrella, J.K., Kim, J.S., Mayhew, D.L., Cross, J.M. and Bamman, M.M., Potent myofiber hypertrophy during resistance training in humans is associated with satellite cell-mediated myonuclear addition: A cluster analysis, *J Appl Physiol.* 104(6): 1736–42, 2008.
27. Verdijk, L.B., Koopman, R., Schaart, G., Meijer, K., Savelberg, H.H. and van Loon, L.J., Satellite cell content is specifically reduced in type II skeletal muscle fibers in the elderly, *Am. J. Physiol. Endocrinol. Metab.* 292(1), E151–7, 2007.
28. Verdijk, L.B., Gleeson, B.G., Jonkers, R.A. et al., Skeletal muscle hypertrophy following resistance training is accompanied by a fiber type-specific increase in satellite cell content in elderly men, *J. Gerontol. A Biol. Sci. Med. Sci.* 64(3), 332–9, 2009.
29. Pearson, S.J., Young, A., Macaluso, A. et al., Muscle function in elite master weightlifters, *Med. Sci. Sports Exerc.* 34(7), 1199–206, 2002.
30. Phillips, S.M., Moore, D.R. and Tang, J.E., A critical examination of dietary protein requirements, benefits, and excesses in athletes, *Int. J. Sport Nutr. Exerc. Metab.* 17(Suppl), S58–76, 2007.
31. Campbell, B., Kreider, R.B., Ziegenfuss, T. et al., International Society of Sports Nutrition position stand: Protein and exercise, *J. Int. Soc. Sports Nutr.* 4, 8, 2007.
32. Rodriguez, N.R., Di Marco, N.M. and Langley, S., American College of Sports Medicine position stand. Nutrition and athletic performance, *Med. Sci. Sports Exerc.* 41(3), 709–31, 2009.
33. Lambert, C.P., Frank, L.L. and Evans, W.J., Macronutrient considerations for the sport of bodybuilding, *Sports Med.* 34(5), 317–27, 2004.
34. McArdle, W.D., Katch, F.I. and Katch, V.L., *Exercise Physiology: Energy, Nutrition, and Human Performance*, 5th Ed., *Series Exercise Physiology: Energy, Nutrition, and Human Performance,* Lippincott Williams & Wilkins, Philadelphia, 2001.

35. Jefferson, L.S. and Kimball, S.R., Translational control of protein synthesis: Implications for understanding changes in skeletal muscle mass, *Int. J. Sport Nutr. Exerc. Metab.* 11(Suppl), S143–9, 2001.
36. Kim, J.S., Wilson, J.M. and Lee, S.R., Dietary implications on mechanisms of sarcopenia: Roles of protein, amino acids and antioxidants, *J. Nutr. Biochem.* 21(1), 1–13, 2010.
37. Kerksick, C.M., Rasmussen, C.J., Lancaster, S.L. et al., The effects of protein and amino acid supplementation on performance and training adaptations during ten weeks of resistance training, *J. Strength Cond. Res.* 20(3), 643–53, 2006.
38. Roberts, M.D., Iosia, M., Kerksick, C.M. et al., Effects of arachidonic acid supplementation on training adaptations in resistance-trained males, *J. Int. Soc. Sports Nutr.* 4, 21, 2007.
39. Phillips, S.M., Tang, J.E. and Moore, D.R., The role of milk- and soy-based protein in support of muscle protein synthesis and muscle protein accretion in young and elderly persons, *J. Am. Coll. Nutr.* 28(4), 343–54, 2009.
40. Tipton, K.D., Elliott, T.A., Cree, M.G., Wolf, S.E., Sanford, A.P. and Wolfe, R.R., Ingestion of casein and whey proteins result in muscle anabolism after resistance exercise, *Med. Sci. Sports Exerc.* 36(12), 2073–81, 2004.
41. Katsanos, C.S., Kobayashi, H., Sheffield-Moore, M., Aarsland, A. and Wolfe, R.R., Aging is associated with diminished accretion of muscle proteins after the ingestion of a small bolus of essential amino acids, *Am. J. Clin. Nutr.* 82(5), 1065–73, 2005.
42. Guillet, C., Prod'homme, M., Balage, M. et al., Impaired anabolic response of muscle protein synthesis is associated with S6K1 dysregulation in elderly humans, *FASEB J.* 18(13), 1586–7, 2004.
43. Symons, T.B., Schutzler, S.E., Cocke, T.L., Chinkes, D.L., Wolfe, R.R. and Paddon–Jones, D., Aging does not impair the anabolic response to a protein-rich meal, *Am. J. Clin. Nutr.* 86(2), 451–6, 2007.
44. Symons, T.B., Sheffield-Moore, M., Wolfe, R.R. and Paddon-Jones, D., A moderate serving of high-quality protein maximally stimulates skeletal muscle protein synthesis in young and elderly subjects, *J. Am. Diet. Assoc.* 109(9), 1582–6, 2009.
45. Campbell, W.W., Barton, M.L., Jr., Cyr-Campbell, D. et al., Effects of an omnivorous diet compared with a lactoovovegetarian diet on resistance-training-induced changes in body composition and skeletal muscle in older men, *Am. J. Clin. Nutr.* 70(6), 1032–9, 1999.
46. Esmarck, B., Andersen, J.L., Olsen, S., Richter, E.A., Mizuno, M. and Kjaer, M., Timing of postexercise protein intake is important for muscle hypertrophy with resistance training in elderly humans, *J. Physiol.* 535(Pt 1), 301–11, 2001.
47. Singh, M.A., Ding, W., Manfredi, T.J. et al., Insulin-like growth factor I in skeletal muscle after weight-lifting exercise in frail elders, *Am. J. Physiol.* 277(1 Pt 1), E135–43, 1999.
48. Verdijk, L.B., Jonkers, R.A., Gleeson, B.G. et al., Protein supplementation before and after exercise does not further augment skeletal muscle hypertrophy after resistance training in elderly men, *Am. J. Clin. Nutr.* 89(2), 608–16, 2009.
49. Chernoff, R., Protein and older adults, *J. Am. Coll. Nutr.* 23(6 Suppl), 627S–630S, 2004.
50. Lemon, P.W. and Mullin, J.P., Effect of initial muscle glycogen levels on protein catabolism during exercise, *J. Appl. Physiol.* 48(4), 624–9, 1980.
51. Tesch, P.A., Colliander, E.B. and Kaiser, P., Muscle metabolism during intense, heavy-resistance exercise, *Eur. J. Appl. Physiol. Occup. Physiol.* 55(4), 362–6, 1986.
52. Haft, G.G., Stone, M.H., Warren, B.J. et al., The effect of carbohydrate supplementation on multiple sessions and bouts of resistance exercise, *J. Strength Cond. Res.* 13(2), 111–117, 1999.
53. Roy, B.D. and Tarnopolsky, M.A., Influence of differing macronutrient intakes on muscle glycogen resynthesis after resistance exercise, *J. Appl. Physiol.* 84(3), 890–6, 1998.
54. Noakes, T. Against the grains, http://www.discovery.co.za/email_za/mailers/pdfs/general/noakes.pdf, accessed 28 January 2014.
55. Brand-Miller, J.C., Holt, S.H., Pawlak, D.B. and McMillan, J., Glycemic index and obesity, *Am. J. Clin. Nutr.* 76(1), 281S–5S, 2002.
56. Browning, J.D., Baker, J.A., Rogers, T., Davis, J., Satapati, S. and Burgess, S.C., Short-term weight loss and hepatic triglyceride reduction: Evidence of a metabolic advantage with dietary carbohydrate restriction, *Am. J. Clin. Nutr.* 93(5), 1048–52, 2011.
57. United States Department of Agriculture. National Agricultural Library, http://fnic.nal.usda.gov/, accessed 28 January 2014.
58. Burke, L.M., Cox, G.R., Culmmings, N.K. and Desbrow, B., Guidelines for daily carbohydrate intake: Do athletes achieve them? *Sports Med.* 31(4), 267–99, 2001.
59. Hamalainen, E.K., Adlercreutz, H., Puska, P. and Pietinen, P., Decrease of serum total and free testosterone during a low-fat high-fibre diet, *J. Steroid Biochem.* 18(3), 369–70, 1983.

60. Sallinen, J., Pakarinen, A., Ahtiainen, J., Kraemer, W.J., Volek, J.S. and Hakkinen, K., Relationship between diet and serum anabolic hormone responses to heavy-resistance exercise in men, *Int. J. Sports Med.* 25(8), 627–33, 2004.
61. Economos, C.D., Bortz, S.S. and Nelson, M.E., Nutritional practices of elite athletes. Practical recommendations, *Sports Med.* 16(6), 381–99, 1993.
62. Trappe, T.A., Fluckey, J.D., White, F., Lambert, C.P. and Evans, W.J., Skeletal muscle PGF(2)(alpha) and PGE(2) in response to eccentric resistance exercise: Influence of ibuprofen acetaminophen, *J. Clin. Endocrinol. Metab.* 86(10), 5067–70, 2001.
63. Trappe, T.A., Carroll, C.C., Dickinson, J.M. et al., Influence of acetaminophen and ibuprofen on skeletal muscle adaptations to resistance exercise in older adults, *Am. J. Physiol. Regul. Integr. Comp. Physiol.* 300(3), R655–62, 2011.
64. Cornish, S.M. and Chilibeck, P.D., Alpha-linolenic acid supplementation and resistance training in older adults, *Appl. Physiol. Nutr. Metab.* 34(1), 49–59, 2009.
65. Perez-Gomez, J. and Calbert, J.A., Training methods to improve vertical jump performance, *J. Sports Med. Phys. Fitness* 53(4), 339–57, 2013.
66. Storey, A. and Smith, H.K., Unique aspects of competitive weightlifting: Performance, training and physiology, *Sports Med.* 42(9), 769–90, 2012.
67. Isner-Horobeti, M.E., Dufour, S.P., Vautravers, P., Geny, B., Coudeyre, E. and Richard, R., Eccentric exercise training: Modalities, applications and perspectives, *Sports Med.* 43(6), 483–512, 2013.
68. McMaster, D.T., Gill, N., Cronin, J. and McGuigan, M., The development, retention and decay rates of strength and power in elite rugby union, rugby league and American football: A systematic review, *Sports Med.* 43(5), 367–84, 2013.
69. Cadore, E.L. and Izquierdo, M., How to simultaneously optimize muscle strength, power, functional capacity, and cardiovascular gains in the elderly: An update, *Age (Dordr)* 35(6), 2329–44, 2013.
70. Reid, K.F. and Fielding, R.A., Skeletal muscle power: A critical determinant of physical functioning in older adults, *Exerc. Sport Sci. Rev.* 40(1), 4–12, 2012.
71. Steib, S., Schoene, D. and Pfeifer, K., Dose-response relationship of resistance training in older adults: A meta-analysis, *Med. Sci. Sports Exerc.* 42(5), 902–14, 2010.
72. Raymond, M.J., Bramley-Tzerefos, R.E., Jeffs, K.J., Winter, A. and Holland, A.E., Systematic review of high-intensity progressive resistance strength training of the lower limb compared with other intensities of strength training in older adults, *Arch. Phys. Med. Rehab.* 94(8), 1458–72, 2013.
73. Stellingwerff, T., Maughan, R.J. and Burke, L.M., Nutrition for power sports: Middle-distance running, track cycling, rowing, canoeing/kayaking, and swimming, *J. Sports Sci.* 29(Suppl. 1), S79–89, 2011.
74. Kilduff, L.P., Finn, C.V., Baker, J.S., Cook, C.J. and West, D.J., Preconditioning strategies to enhance physical performance on the day of competition, *Int. J. Sports Physiol. Perform.* 8(6), 677–81, 2013.

18 Training and Nutritional Needs of the Masters Team Sport Athlete

Aaron J. Coutts, Amy E. Mendham and Rob Duffield

CONTENTS

18.1 INTRODUCTION

Team sports are organised activities that require well developed decision-making and sport-specific skill proficiency, whilst incorporating a wide range of physical and physiological capacities of each individual on the team. The social cohesion that comes from working in a group to achieve a common goal makes team sports popular activities for people of all ages.

Opportunities for participation in team sports for masters athletes are many, and whilst there are several national and international competitions for both men and women, the majority of team sport participants in masters sport compete at the recreational, non-elite level. Despite the popularity of team sports amongst masters athletes, there is only a relatively small body of literature that has examined issues surrounding the competition, training demands and specific nutritional concerns for the masters athlete playing team sports.

The goal of this chapter is to overview the competition and physiological demands of team sports for masters athletes, including recommendations on training and nutrition. This chapter is divided into three sections. The first will examine the generic physical and physiological demands of field-based, team sports—with particular reference to the older athlete. The second section will provide training, nutrition and recovery recommendations that will allow the masters team sport athlete to best prepare for and recover from the demands of competitions. The final section will discuss the role of team sports in maintaining health in masters athletes and provide a summary of recommendations for coaches, sports medicine professionals and clinicians working in this area.

18.2 PHYSICAL AND PHYSIOLOGICAL DEMANDS OF TEAM SPORTS

Team sports are generally described as moderate-to-long duration sports that involve many irregular bouts of brief but intense periods that are interspersed with periods of rest and lower intensity activity [1,2]. These stochastic and intermittent work demands result in a continuous change in the contribution of the body's various energy production pathways [3,4]. Whilst the general activity profile in many team sports have common threads (i.e. prolonged, high-intensity intermittent exercise) [1], there are very specific technical and tactical demands of the various sports that are essential for high-level performance. Figure 18.1 shows a theoretical model of the interrelationships between the generic qualities that underpin performance in team sports.

Figure 18.2 expands on this model to show a schematic of the proposed relationships between team sport athletes, their physical characteristics, technical/tactical abilities and performance. Whilst complex, these relationships allow us to understand the interactions between physiological capacities and team sport performance, to then appreciate the training demands relevant to the masters athlete.

Whilst a detailed discussion of the technical and tactical requirements for specific sports is beyond the scope of this chapter, recent research has shown a complicated relationship between technical abilities of teams and the physical activity of the players within that team. The link between increased technical/tactical proficiency and reduced activity profiles is supported by research that has shown increased technical proficiency reduces physical match demands in both professional soccer [5,6] and Australian Rules football players [7]. To date there has been only one study to describe the tactical aspects of soccer match play in masters athletes. This study demonstrated that these masters players tended to play in a co-operative manner [8], which may explain their relatively lower activity profile compared to younger players. For example, it was reported that 42% of the

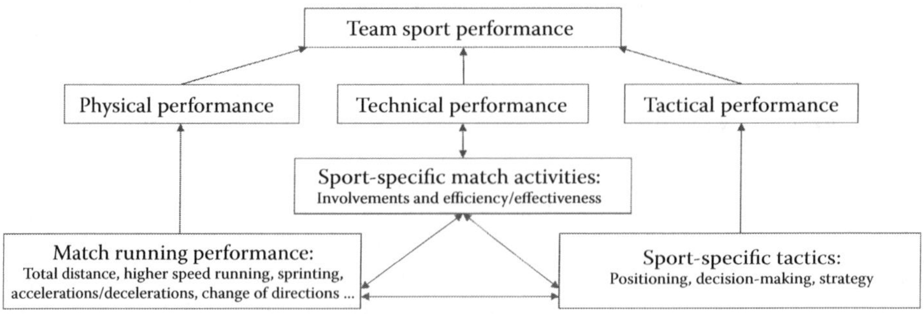

FIGURE 18.1 General factors that underpin performance in team sports.

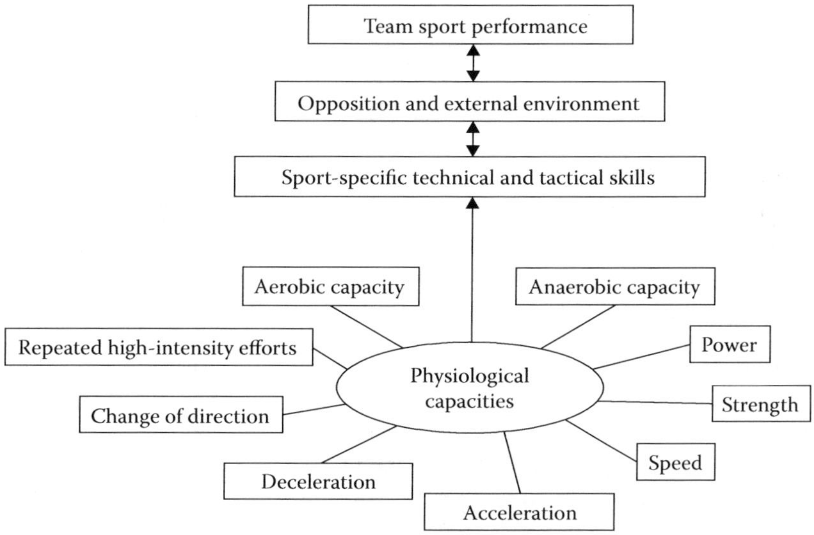

FIGURE 18.2 Theoretical model of relationships between physiological capacities and match performance demands in team sports.

passing sequences in masters-friendly games involved three or more possessions and the older players completed fewer tackles than younger players. From these observations, it was suggested that masters soccer players benefit from the increased soccer playing experience through improved tactical approaches. Their experience and ability to integrate tactically with teammates is demonstrated through longer passing sequences which reduce their need to run greater distances. It was also suggested that these players reduced their tackle rates to avoid unnecessary injuries. These findings suggest that there is a complex interrelationship between the technical, tactical and physical requirements of team sports, but these relationships may be specific to a particular sport and influenced by player experience and physical characteristics.

18.2.1 Physical Characteristics

There have only been a few studies that have described the physical characteristics in masters team sport athletes. Similar to research from other sports [9–11], these studies have shown that masters team sport athletes often gain a health protective benefit from the effects of ageing, and have increased physical capacities compared to age- and gender-matched individuals with these adaptations being specific to the training demands of each sport. For example, Tessitore et al. reported that masters soccer players but not basketball players had an improved VO_{2max} compared to age-matched sedentary individuals [12,13]. The authors suggested that the increased match demands with soccer (related to pitch size) and the larger training volumes completed by the older soccer players (i.e. soccer: trained and played a 70-min friendly match twice a week; basketball: 1.5 h training and a 60-min friendly match once a week) explained the differences between the sports. Similarly, these studies showed increased countermovement jump performance in both the older basketball [12] and soccer players [13] compared to similarly aged, physically active men [14]. Notably however, the basketball players had greater jump capacity than the soccer players but both were less than values reported for trained younger athletes.

In most team sports, the ability to sprint and rapidly accelerate are fundamental characteristics required for successful match play. There have only been a few reports of sprint characteristics in masters team sports athletes [12,13,15] with each study showing poorer sprint performance compared to younger sport-matched athletes. Notably however, the basketball athletes were slower than the soccer players over a 10-m sprint.

Unfortunately, there is little data to provide a consensus on the influence of team sport training on physical characteristics in older athletes. The limited available evidence suggests a likely beneficial health protective effect against ageing of team sport training. However, it appears that these effects are related to training dose (i.e. volume and intensity), and the specific training content for each sport. Future studies are required to examine the link between training content and the changes in health and performance characteristics in masters team sport athletes.

18.2.2 Body Composition

While the anthropometrical requirements of team sports vary, both between sports and between playing positions within the same sport, there are some fundamental characteristics that assist physical performance in team sports. Indeed, team sports that require higher energetic demands (i.e. those that cover longer distances during competition and training) and many rapid changes in activity and direction would be suited to athletes with a lighter and lean physique. Moreover, with the exceptions of team sports such as ice hockey, rugby union and rugby league that have regular heavy collisions, most team sport athletes benefit from lower levels of body fat. Whilst the body fat levels do not reach the levels of high-performance endurance athletes such as triathletes, middle- and long-distance runners and cyclists, younger team sport athletes typically have lower proportions of fat compared to the untrained population. There is little information on the body composition of older team sport athletes; however, age-related losses on lean mass appear inevitable.

It well known that as humans age, lean muscle tissue is reduced, most notably through the atrophy of type II motor units [10,16]. Unfortunately for team sport athletes, higher total lean mass and a relatively higher proportion of type II muscle fibres is considered advantageous [1]. Indeed, between 25–50 years, there is a ~5%–10% reduction in muscle size, which accelerates thereafter. This loss of muscle mass has significant impact on the team sport athlete where lean muscle mass and more specifically, recruitment of type II muscle fibres form the basis of the intense actions (i.e. sprinting, acceleration, tackling, changing direction etc.) that are important for team sport performance. Accordingly, nutritional and training strategies that assist with protecting loss of lean mass are of specific importance for this group. For more detailed discussion on the physiological changes that affect nutrition and performance in masters athletes, see Chapters 1 and 2, respectively.

Due to its relationship with muscle power production [17–19], it is generally understood that lean mass influences physical performance in team sports more directly than endurance sports [20,21]. While there are no studies that have examined the relationships between lean mass and team sport performance, there have been numerous studies showing that maximal voluntary strength [22–24], peak power output [19] and maximal running velocity [25] are well related to muscle cross-sectional area. These observations likely explain in part why athletes that participate in higher levels of team sport competition tend to have greater lean mass and lower body fat [26]. To achieve optimal body composition, masters team sport athletes should undertake regular strength training and eat a well-balanced diet that consists of high-quality foods. As will be discussed later, an optimal diet in team sport athletes should meet the energy requirements of their sport and have appropriate timing and dosing of food intake.

18.2.3 Physical Demands

The physiological characteristics of athletes are often explained by the demands of competition. The typical activity profile of team sports shows that a large period of matches is spent at low intensity interspersed by short periods of high-intensity effort, with changes in activity every 3–4 seconds. During most team sports, less than 2% of the total distance covered is performed at a high intensity, with sprints lasting on average ~2 s [27–29]. Additionally, there are many changes in accelerations from various speeds [30] that also add to the energetic demands of sports [31]. High-intensity activities are important in team sports for any age group and are defined as any activity requiring a near maximal effort such as high-speed running, accelerating tackling, jumping, kicking, passing, changing direction and sprinting [3,32,33]. Whilst these activities make up only a small percentage of workload during team sports, they are considered to be important for involvement in play and are often decisive to the match outcome [3,32].

To date, there have been few reports on the physical activity profiles during competitions in masters team sport athletes [12,13,15]. For example, Tessitore et al. demonstrated a reduction in time spent at high intensities in the second half of a friendly masters soccer game in 12 older male players (age range 53–72 years, mean 62.8 ± 5.9 years), with an increase in time spent walking and a reduction in time spent running as the game progressed [13]. These authors also showed that older soccer players have a reduced capacity to recover from periods of high-intensity activity and tend to spend more time at lower intensities compared to younger soccer players. This group also later reported that masters basketball players tend to adopt a more conservative physical activity profile compared to younger players during matches [12]. It was suggested that older players adopt this conservative behaviour through adjusting tactical approaches, by adopting a zone defensive pattern, avoiding demanding three-point shots and ending efforts quickly rather than continuing the effort. This approach might have been adopted as a pacing strategy to adjust for lower fitness levels or to avoid contact and risk of injury. The friendly nature of these games may also explain these findings. Unfortunately however, whilst physical fitness of these players were relatively low (i.e. VO_{2max} – soccer: 36.3 ± 11.3 ml/kg/min; basketball: 22.9 ± 2.2 ml/kg/min), the designs of these studies prevents us from attributing the reduction in activity profile to the decreased fitness. Regardless of the exact cause, it is logical that the physiological changes that occur with ageing (i.e. decreased VO_{2max}, reduced anaerobic capacity and decreased lean mass) would cause a reduction in match work capacity compared to younger athletes. With the recent developments in microtechnologies (i.e. Global Positioning Systems [GPSs] and accelerometers), it has become easier for scientists to assess the physical activity demands of team sports, and this may allow more research to provide a better understanding of the demands of competition in masters team sports.

18.3 PHYSIOLOGICAL REQUIREMENTS AND FATIGUE

There have only been a small number of studies that have examined the physiological requirements of match play in masters team sports [12,13,15]. Whilst not entirely clear, it seems that masters team sport athletes show increased evidence of fatigue toward the end of matches than younger, fitter counterparts, despite competing at lower intensities. Given such juxtaposition, special attention needs to be given to issues such as energy substrate depletion, neuromuscular fatigue, muscle soreness and recovery to better understand the foundations of fatigue in masters team sport athletes.

18.3.1 Energy Substrate Depletion

Team sports often result in a significant depletion of intramuscular carbohydrate stores. Muscle biopsy data collected from national soccer players during simulated matches reveals a progressive reduction (~50%) in muscle glycogen during competition [34,35]. In particular, most glycogen depletion occurs in the type I fibres (50% empty or nearly empty), with smaller reductions (20%–40% nearly empty) in type II fibres [35,36]. At present, no studies have examined changes in muscle glycogen content in masters team sport athletes during competition. However, the age-related reduction in type II fibres suggest that there will be a greater reliance on muscle glycogen content in type I muscle fibres in team sport—this will likely be at the consequence of reduced higher-speed activities. Similar to research in masters sprint running [37], it seems that these reductions may also blunt lactate and pH responses in masters athletes compared to younger team sport participants. Regardless, the intermittent nature of team sports has been shown to be taxing on both glycolytic and oxidative energy pathways, and as such substantial carbohydrate depletion is likely to exist in masters team sport matches. Accordingly, carbohydrate is an important component of the masters team sport athlete's diet both leading into team sport competition and during the recovery period.

18.3.2 Thermoregulation and Hydration

There are a number of physiological adjustments that occur with ageing that impact upon the thermoregulatory functioning in athletes. Due to reduced cardiovascular functioning, lower cardiac output, diminished skin blood flow and decreased thirst sensations, older athletes (i.e. >50 years) have an increased risk of heat stress than younger athletes [38]. Of particular concern are the altered thirst sensations which may further compromise thermoregulation during training and competition, especially in hot conditions. These physiological adjustments increase the need for careful hydration and cooling practices which reduce the risk of heat stress. At present there are no specific guidelines for fluid replacement or heat policies for ageing athletes. In absence of specific recommendations, it is proposed that general advice for the younger athletic populations be adopted [39]. A detailed discussion of the fluid, electrolyte and hydration needs of masters athletes is presented in Chapter 9.

The paucity of research describing the hydration responses or hydration status of masters team sport athletes is surprising. Nonetheless, results from studies that describe the change in mass before and after a team sport match in younger trained professional athletes [40–42] show that the normal post-game reductions in body mass is around 2–3 kg, resulting in fluid loss of 1–2 kg/hour, depending on match duration and environmental conditions [43]. How these data relate to masters athletes is unknown. However, the typical decrease in total body water with ageing and subsequent decrease in blood plasma volume and VO_{2max} would suggest that masters athletes may be at greater risk of performance reductions and heat illness sooner than younger counterparts. Importantly though, if older athletes maintain their training status and aerobic capacity they can prevent this reduction in thermoregulatory tolerance during exercise in the heat [44].

The exercise-related heat stress, demonstrated through heart rate, skin blood flow responses and evaporative heat loss, may be exacerbated in older athletes if aerobic capacity is not maintained [44]. Moreover, the decreased osmoreceptors responsible for thirst sensation [45] and reduced sweat response with ageing [46] may further compromise thermoregulation capacity in older athletes. To adjust for these losses, we recommend that masters team sport athletes ensure euhydration prior to competition and training, drink regularly during training and competition and rehydrate following competition. Indeed, there is a case that older athletes should follow the guidelines for fluid pre-hydration, hydration during exercise and recovery more aggressively than their younger counterparts to off-set the age-related physiological adjustments. However, we also recognise that the reduced demands of many team sports competitions in master athletes (i.e. lower activity profile) may not necessitate the higher fluid consumption demands of younger athletes.

In team sports, these practices are particularly important when competing in a tournament or twice-a-day training or competition scenarios (e.g. masters games or state, national or international events) where athletes are at increased risk of dehydration. Specifically, if training or matches exceed 1 hour, it is suggested that sports drinks containing 6%–8% carbohydrate (CHO) and electrolytes be consumed to defend these losses of fluid and also help maintain blood glucose levels. Additionally, given that masters athletes may have lower blood and plasma volumes relative to younger athletes, which may be then further decreased by training and competing in team sports, there is likely to be a significant reduction in the hydration status. The specific fluid needs of masters athletes are discussed in detail in Chapter 9.

18.3.3 Neuromuscular Fatigue

Studies examining the neuromuscular performance changes following match play in younger team sport athletes have shown a small but potentially important suppression of peak power [15,47,48].

Indeed, data from younger team sport athletes show reduced contractile function, peak power and force following amateur rugby league [49], tennis [50] and soccer matches [51], with a greater decrease in higher-level players. Similarly, repeated 30-m sprint times have been reported to be 2%–3% slower following match-play [48]. In contrast, recent research on masters soccer players (52.3 ± 10.2 years) demonstrated that explosive power (i.e. counter-movement jump and repeated jumps), 10-m sprint performance and various inter-limb co-ordination tests were not negatively affected following a friendly soccer match, whilst repeated jump test performance actually increased [15]. These results were surprising as older athletes are reported to have a reduced volume of type II muscle fibres and an increased perception of fatigue following intense exercise [52]. Possible reasons for these differences were that the masters football match was 70 min in duration, compared to the matches in the other studies on younger individuals that were from 90–180 min in duration. Additionally, whilst speculative, it may be that the speed of match play in the masters games were not sufficient to induce substantial neuromuscular fatigue, though more data on match demands of master athletes is still required. As such, additional studies are required to understand the extent of neuromuscular fatigue in masters team sports; particularly because it has been suggested that recovery from neuromuscular fatigue may be reduced in older athletes.

18.3.4 Muscle Soreness and Recovery

In most team sports there are many activities that involve eccentric muscle contractions and induce muscle damage, soreness, injury and reduced physical performance. Actions such as changes in direction, accelerations and decelerations are particularly damaging to muscle. Accordingly, an important part of the training week in team sports is devoted to recovering from these stressors [53]. Moreover, when there is only a relatively short period of time between matches (e.g. <5 days) or in tournament scenarios such as masters games or high-level competitions where many games are played within a relatively short period of time, players may have inadequate recovery which can impact upon performance [54–56]. Indeed, it has been shown that when recovery is compromised though increased training and muscle damage between simulated matches, sprint performance in the following match may be reduced [54].

Similarly, other studies reported reduced match running performance and vertical jump performance and increased muscle damage markers during a 4-day tournament where a match was played each day in younger well-trained soccer players [57,58]. Moreover, reduced exercise performance and increased match injury rates have been shown during periods of heavy competition of training in younger professional soccer players [59,60]. Collectively, these findings suggest that team sport athletes are at risk of incomplete recovery when there is little time between matches. Whilst similar data on masters athletes are lacking, it is suggested this may be a greater problem for masters athletes as the rate of recovery following intense exercise in this group is often delayed.

Older athletes require a longer period than younger athletes to recovery from similar fatiguing exercise stimulus [61]. The two reported explanations for the delayed recovery in masters athletes are that ageing leads to a greater amount of exercise-induce damage or fatigue, and that the state of repair following exercise is impaired [62]. Whilst there are no examples from team sport interventions *per se*, Fell, Reaburn and Harrison reported that veteran cyclists reported a greater increase in muscle soreness following 3 days of high-intensity training compared to training-matched younger [52]. In contrast however, several other studies have shown no differences in markers of muscle damage (i.e. soreness, creatine kinase, oxidative damage etc.) between older and younger groups with matched training [63,64].

Nonetheless, anecdotally, older athletes often report slower recovery following intensive training and this may be due to diminished regeneration kinetics. These reduced recovery kinetics in masters athletes may be due to reduced recovery of muscle glycogen [65,66] and the time taken to repair damaged muscle fibres via reduced myofibrillar protein synthesis and anabolic signalling [67]. However, because of these mechanisms, masters athletes should be aware that recovery from intense exercise, such as training and competitions in team sports, may be compromised. On the basis of these observations, we suggest that additional focus is given to appropriate recovery nutrition and recovery strategies (i.e. cryo- and hydrotherapies, compression) to assist recovery for masters athletes during periods of regular competition, sometimes twice a day, as in tournament scenarios.

18.4 TRAINING AND RECOVERY RECOMMENDATIONS FOR OLDER TEAM SPORT ATHLETES

Similar to other sports, team sport athletes of all ages benefit from a systematic approach to training. Appropriate periodisation of the stress applied to athletes is important to obtain optimal training results, allowing adequate recovery between each training dose [68]. At present however, there are few published examples of training periodisation in the various team sports [53,69–71] and none in masters team sport athletes. Nonetheless, the concept of periodisation is generally well accepted amongst the coaching community and is commonly recommended to be used in team sports.

18.4.1 Preseason Training

Preseason training is often designed to provide a strong aerobic base with less focus spent developing anaerobic capacity, speed and the ability to improve repeat speed. The preseason for professional team sports can range from 6–20 weeks depending on the sport and competitive level. Whilst there are no published data on the preseason training programs for masters team sport athletes, it is likely that the older athlete would complete shorter preparatory phases of training, or alternatively complete a lower volume of year-round consistent training and competition as many older competitors participate for recreation rather than competitive reasons. It likely, however, that masters team sport athletes would increase training and competition loads prior to competing in important tournaments (e.g. World Masters Games, National Championships etc.).

Aerobic conditioning, which is typically the primary goal of preseason training, can be applied through a number of ways but generic interval training, small-sided games and cross-training are most common [72,73]. Additionally, resistance training also plays an important role in the developing lean muscle mass during the preparation period. Given the well-documented age-related decrease in muscle mass that accompanies ageing, resistance training is even more important for the masters team sport athlete. Depending on the sport and goals of the athlete, it is common that younger team sport athletes would complete two–five resistance training sessions per week during the preseason. While work and family commitments may make this difficult for masters athletes, two–three resistance training sessions a week are highly recommended.

Another focus of preseason training is to refine and develop sport-specific technical skill and tactics. Whilst these sessions are typically of lower intensity than generic fitness training, they form the foundation of individual and team performance in team sports. The few studies that have reported on training undertaken by master team sport athletes suggest that these lower-intensity skills sessions or friendly games form the basis of most training regimes [12,13,15]. Regardless of the content of training, it is likely that training volume is decreased in masters team sport athletes compared to their younger counterparts. To maximise training outcomes from preseason training, we recommend a mixed-methods approach for master team sport athletes, including various periodised skill, aerobic and resistance training. However, to reduce injury risk, we also suggest that care be taken to ensure gradual load progression to prevent training overload and ensure adequate recovery between high-intensity training sessions.

In the later stages of preseason it is recommended that specific fitness qualities be developed through an increase in skill sessions that incorporate higher-intensity training that often simulates match play. The implementation of well-designed, sport-specific small-sided games and shorter repeated effort high-intensity intervals are recommended [72,73]. We also recommend that these sessions be completed in a well recovered state and after a sufficient general preparatory period of lower-intensity and lower-volume training. The focus in resistance training also shifts towards increasing strength and power to best prepare players to remain strong and powerful throughout the season. Towards the end of the specific preparatory phase, training volume decreases as practice matches are incorporated into the training schedule to further prepare the athletes for the season ahead.

18.4.2 In-Season Training

There are no scientific reports of typical in-season training programs undertaken by masters team sport athletes. However, Tessitore et al. reported in a study of the physiological and match demands of 12 masters soccer players (age: 62.8 ± 5.9 years) that this group typically maintained their fitness through playing two friendly games per week [13]. This group also reported that 10 masters basketball players (age: 55 ± 5 years) typically trained for 1.5 h/week and a friendly match during the past 10 years [12]. More recent studies have reported that older soccer players typically train twice a week (~1.5-h/session) without coach supervision [74]. These training periodisations and doses are remarkably different (i.e. lower) from those typically seen in younger or professional team sports, and suggest that different periodisation is needed for these older groups. It is possible that these differences in training intensity may partly explain the physical changes that occur with ageing in older sprint athletes [37]. Nonetheless, it has been shown that the moderate training doses of team sport training (i.e. soccer) can help preserve strength, power and interlimb coordination compared to age-matched sedentary counterparts [15,74]. Therefore, until further empirical evidence is available, it is difficult to provide precise recommendations on optimal training periodisation for the in-season period for older team sport athletes, other than to infer from practices from younger team sport groups.

Unfortunately, there is very little evidence that describes current or optimal training practices for team sport athletes of any age. However, like other sports, older team sport athletes typically complete lower training loads than younger counterparts. There are some basic rules that can be used to avoid poor periodisation during the in-season period. These include

- Ensure proper recovery from previous match.
- Avoid sudden increases in training dose, especially after poor performances.
- Avoid large training session in the 24 hours before matches.
- Main training session between match should be completed following 72 hours' recovery.
- Alternate hard and easy training days.
- Train specifically—fitness work can mostly be done with the ball in the form of small-sided games (SSGs).
- Avoid overreaching close to the commencement of the season or during the in-season.

18.4.3 Post-Match Recovery

It is established that the perceived recovery of masters athletes may be compromised compared to younger counterparts following high-intensity training sessions or competitions [52,61]. Based on these findings, it seems logical to suggest that the time course of recovery from games and intense training is delayed in older team sport athletes. During team sport matches there is substantial disruption to various physiological systems and these may take 4–5 days for homeostasis to return [55,56,75–77]. Figure 18.3 below shows the theoretical model of recovery kinetics in these physiologic systems.

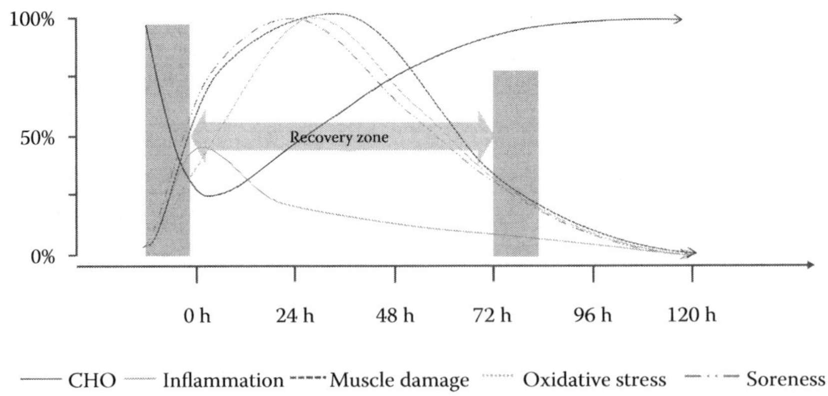

FIGURE 18.3 Modelled time course of recovery in various psycho-physiological aspects of recovery following a team sport match.

From a practical perspective, we recommend that nutritional intake, cold water immersion, sleeping, active recovery, stretching, compression garments, and massage can be used to assist in the recovery process for masters athletes [78]. Simple strategies such as appropriate hydration, diet and sleep are effective in their ability to counteract the disruption to the physiological systems and increased perceptions of fatigue, soreness and stress that often observed following competition. Practical interventions such as providing fluid and meals containing high-glycaemic carbohydrate and essential amino acids within the hour following the match are effective in counteracting the muscle damage and facilitating muscle carbohydrate restoration [79,80]. Sleep is also an essential part of recovery as disturbance after a match is common and can negatively impact on the recovery [81]. Cold water immersion is effective during acute periods of tournament play in order to regain performance levels faster and repress the acute inflammatory process [57,58] and possibly improve sleep [82]. Each of these interventions are recommended for masters athletes. However, it is advised that athletes of all ages are guided by their perceptions of soreness and fatigue before returning to high-intensity training. This is especially important when returning to sport after a lay-off or during periods of increased competition.

18.5 NUTRITION FOR MASTERS TEAM SPORT ATHLETES

18.5.1 Nutrition for Training and Competition

There are a number of nutrition-related factors that are associated with fatigue during training in team sport. The major concerns for the team sport athlete are ensuring that energy needs are being met during both training and competition and to avoid high levels of body fluid losses. Whilst the energy requirements of younger athletes is determined by a myriad of factors (e.g. body composition, mode of exercise, training intensity, duration and load), these requirements are typically lower in older athletes due to the age-related reductions in energy expenditure and training volume. The energy needs of masters athletes are met through consumption of carbohydrates, fats, proteins and alcohol. Similar to younger athletes, the recommended macronutrient intakes are 55%–58% carbohydrates, 12%–15% protein and 25%–30% fats [83].

Many studies in younger athletes have examined muscle carbohydrate changes in team sports such as soccer and shown significant depletion in muscle (in both type I and II fibres) carbohydrate content and significant relationships between carbohydrate depletion and reduced physical performances in the match [35,79,84]. It has also been reported that since masters athletes have an

TABLE 18.1
Carbohydrate Intake Goals for Team Sport Athletes

	Daily Requirements	Carbohydrate Goals
Low	Low-intensity physical or technical session	3–5 g/kg/day
Moderate	Moderate training session (~1 hour/day)	5–7 g/kg/day
High	1–3 hours/day of moderate- and/or high-intensity training	6–10 g/kg/day
Very high	>4–5 hours/day of moderate- and/or high-intensity training	10–12 g/kg/day

Source: Modified from Mujika, I. and Burke, L.M., *Ann. Nutr. Metab.* 57(Suppl 2), 26–35, 2010.

age-related loss in lean mass and lower resting metabolic rate they may have a reduced demand for energy compared to younger counterparts. Therefore, it is important that masters team sport athletes maintain sufficient energy to meet the energetic demands of training and competition and to prevent lean muscle loss resulting from insufficient energy intake. Specifically, appropriate rehydration, muscle glycogen replenishment and replacement of essential amino acids are critical to ensuring optimal protein resynthesis following exercise.

In addition to the general recommendations for carbohydrate intake during various levels of physical training, there are specific adjustments to carbohydrate intake that masters athletes should make to prevent fatigue or increase recovery (Table 18.1). For example all team sport athletes, regardless of their age, may encounter circumstances where specific adjustments to carbohydrate intake may be required, including maximal post-event refuelling (10–12 g/kg/day), fast between session (hourly repeats of 1.0–1.2 g/kg/day until normal meals are returned), pre-game fuelling (1–4 g/kg consumed in the 4 hours prior to games), and during game fuelling (small amounts, 30–60 g/hour for games <90 min, up to 90 g/hour for longer games) [80]. The carbohydrate needs of masters athletes are discussed in detail in Chapter 4.

Importantly for the masters team sport athlete, refuelling and rehydration during games are essential for delaying fatigue, particularly in hot conditions. The intermittent nature of team sports allows players with opportunities to refuel. Indeed, breaks in play (i.e. quarter/half-time, time outs and substitutions) provide excellent opportunities for both rehydration and refuelling. Therefore, older team sport athletes are encouraged to practice intermittent rehydration during training.

18.5.2 Supplements and Ergogenic Aids

Whilst a well-balanced diet of appropriate macronutrients, mineral and vitamins are essential for effective sports training, older team sport athletes may gain ergogenic benefit through nutritional supplementation. There is now evidence emerging that supports some marketing claims that dietary supplements can improve team sport performance. As a complement to a well-balance diet, several supplements have been shown to provide ergogenic benefit to team sport athletes. Table 18.2 provides a summary of the supplements reported to improve physical performance and health status in team sport athletes. Importantly however, masters athletes should be aware that supplements should not be used as a shortcut to replace a well-balanced diet, a well-structured training program, appropriate sleep and recovery and a healthy lifestyle away from training. Current evidence suggests that once athletes of any age have healthy and balanced eating habits, specific supplementation with agents such as creatine, alkalising agents and caffeine and possibly β-alanine, can help improve team sport performance. The use and efficacy of supplements and ergogenic aids in masters athletes is discussed in detail in Chapters 10 and 11, respectively.

TABLE 18.2
Supplements That May Improve Performance and Health in Masters Team Sports Athletes

	Supplements for Achieving Nutrient Goals
Sports drinks	Used to refuel after long training sessions and competition.
Gels	Electrolytes replace sweat losses.
Bars	Portable and convenient source of CHO, protein and micronutrients for pre-match, recovery or travelling.
Liquid meal replacements	Portable and convenient source of CHO, protein and micronutrients for pre-match, recovery or travelling.
	Supplements with Potential Ergogenic Benefit
Creatine	Supplementation increases the muscle content of creatine phosphate which promotes ATP resynthesis via the phosphagen system. Typical loading protocols include a 5-day loading dose of 20–30 g usually delivered in multiple smaller doses (i.e. 4 × 5 g), followed by a maintenance dose of 2–5 g/day. A notable side effect of creatine loading is an increase in body mass (~1 kg) secondary to increased water retention.
Caffeine	The ergogenic benefits of caffeine are likely due to facilitation of the nervous system, Na^+/K^+ATPase activity, increase intracellular (calcium), increased (catecholamine) and blocking of adenosine receptors. Whilst exact loading protocols for caffeine are not clear, it seems that ~2–3 mg/kg is sufficient to produce an ergogenic effect and loading can occur prior to warm-up for a match.
Bicarbonate	Alkalising agents such as $NaHCO_3$ increase the extracellular buffer capacity, assisting efflux of H^+ from the muscle to the blood and preserving muscle pH during intense exercise. Optimal ingestion protocols for team sports are 0.2–0.3 g/kg of $NaHCO_3$ taken 60–120 min before matches. Sodium citrate has also been used as an alkalising agent by some athletes. There is a risk of gastrointestinal problems if taken with large volumes of fluid.
β-Alanine	β-Alanine supplementation can increase muscle carnosine concentrations, improve muscle buffering capacity and high-intensity exercise performance. Studies have shown that 4.8–6.4 g/day delivered in six–eight smaller doses during a day increases muscle carnosine by ~40–60%.
	Supplements with Potential Health Benefit
Multi-vitamins	Source of micronutrients when food quality is low or unreliable.

Source: Modified from Mujika, I. and Burke, L.M., *Ann. Nutr. Metab.* 57(Suppl 2), 26–35, 2010.
Note: ATP = adenosine triphosphate; CHO = carbohydrate; $NaHCO_3$ = sodium bicarbonate.

18.6 ROLE OF TEAM SPORTS IN THE HEALTH OF THE MASTERS ATHLETE

Over the last century, progressive changes in behavioural and lifestyle habits have been observed which may contribute to physical inactivity, excessive nutritional intake and resultant increase in obesity [85]. Such changes coincide with an increased prevalence of chronic diseases such as type 2 diabetes, cardiovascular disease and some cancers [85–87]. Consequently, there is a need for a population-wide approach to increase physical activity levels aimed at improving quality of life; potentially, through improvements in functional ability, cognitive functioning, weight management and the overall prevention of chronic diseases [86]. Hence the current challenge is to encourage practical exercise interventions that will promote an active lifestyle within sedentary population groups [88] and provide motivation to continue with an active lifestyle.

Given the popularity of many team sports (e.g. rugby, hockey, soccer, netball, Australian Rules football, basketball etc.), these activities may be a popular and effective exercise intervention for reducing chronic disease. Indeed, since current position stands from peak industry bodies suggest that older adults should include both aerobic and muscle strengthening exercises in their regular exercise regimes [89], team sports could be an ideal activity since they are characterised by moderate-to-high-intensity aerobic training, punctuated by periods of very intense activities such as accelerations, jumps, changes of directions and sprints [12,13,15,74]. Furthermore, engagement in socially oriented team sports is reported to provide positive motivation and facilitate individual compliance and persistence, contributing to improved physically activity and lifestyle choices [90,91].

Previous research has often focused on the cardiovascular, metabolic and body composition responses in relation to strength (e.g. free weights and machine weights) and/or aerobic training such as running, cycling, jogging and walking [92]. However, in recent years SSGs applied to football- and rugby-specific activities have become a popular team sport training approach. Moreover, such exercise modes have recently been applied to older sedentary populations as a therapeutic exercise modality to assess acute inflammatory and glucose regulatory responses [93] and chronic metabolic, cardiovascular and body composition adaptations [90,91,94–96].

Sport-specific SSGs are increasingly being used as an alternative aerobic stimulus to interval training [73]. During training for team sports it is common to manipulate both the number of players and the size of the playing field to prescribe the relative exercise intensity. As such, these SSGs are a common strategy adopted by coaches as an alternative training method [73,97]. Previously, SSGs were used to develop technical and tactical abilities; however, they are now used by many amateur teams (trained/untrained) as an effective tool for aerobic training, capable of improving cardiovascular and musculoskeletal health in both trained and untrained populations [94,97]. Moreover, SSGs can elicit heart rate responses ranging up to 80%–95% of maximal heart rate when used for physical conditioning [92,98] and have been shown to meet the American College of Sports Medicine guidelines for appropriate exercise intensity for increasing cardiorespiratory fitness [99]. The chronic adaptations to such intensities are reported to result in improvements in maximum aerobic power, blood pressure, postural balance, bone mineral density, leg strength, muscle capillarisation and intermittent exercise performance within middle-aged sedentary males and females [92,96,100].

Team sports involve high- and low-intensity aerobic and anaerobic training including sprints and specific actions with high eccentric loading on the muscle and impact on bone [92,101]. Indeed, 12 weeks of football (soccer) training were shown to decrease blood pressure (6%), decrease total cholesterol (5%), decrease fat mass percentage (12%), increase lean body mass (3%), increase leg bone mass (3%) and increase oxygen consumption (13%) compared to non-training control group, in sedentary middle-aged men and were often equal to or better than conventional aerobic fitness (running) training [92,96]. These studies suggest that recreational football can improve musculoskeletal, metabolic and cardiovascular adaptations important for health and disease prevention [88,92,102].

The popularity of team sports provides a potential vehicle for physical activity to promote awareness and prevention of preventable chronic disease [88]. Previous research suggests team-sport-based activities may provide older sedentary adults with an alternative exercise mode capable of improving factors related to cardiac health, physical functioning and body composition management. However, further research is required to assess the chronic physiological adaptations of clinical markers associated with disease development alongside adaptations in fitness, strength and body composition. Additionally, such research should focus on a wider range of popular teams sports (netball, rugby, basketball, hockey etc.) as a stimulus to complement traditional exercise modes of exercise prescription (i.e. stationary cycling, machine weights) within older, sedentary and high-disease risk populations.

18.7 CONCLUSIONS

Performance in team sports is determined by a myriad of physical, technical and tactical factors. In this chapter we have examined some of the physical and physiological factors that underpin performance in team sports, and discussed the changes that may be associated with the age-related decline in these factors. In addition, we have provided new information around the training and competition demands of masters team sport athletes.

In order to maximise performance, team sport athletes should adhere to training practices in which the physical and physiological demands of the sport are met. However, more importantly training should also allow athletes to develop the technical and tactical demands of the sport. Accordingly, much of the physical training in team sports is completed through team-based match play and SSGs. We suggest that the masters athlete can gain physical advantage through developed independent aspects of their physiological profile (e.g. strength, power, speed, aerobic fitness etc.) that are determined to be under developed.

Like many athletic pursuits, the age-related loss of lean muscle seems to be primarily responsible for the reductions in physical capacities of masters athletes. We specifically recommend that masters team sport athletes place emphasis on training practices that maintain lean mass and type II muscle fibres. Therefore, high-intensity strength training together with sport-specific aerobic training drills such as SSGs that allow athletes to work on the physical, technical and tactical aspects of teams sports are fundamental for masters athletes. Furthermore, older age can lead to impaired recovery and may require modifications to training programs both in the pre- and in-season periods.

Nutritional factors are also important for effective training and performance in competition. Masters team sport athletes need to focus on achieving adequate energy intake from carbohydrates, particularly leading into match day and during the recovery in the days following match play. There may also be a requirement for increased protein intake in team sport athletes during periods of intense training and in the recovery periods following matches. Therefore we recommend that masters team sport athletes consume quality essential amino acids consumption to aid in muscle recovery.

Finally, team sports may provide older sedentary adults with an alternative exercise mode capable of improving factors related to cardiac health, physical functioning and body composition management. Indeed, the social engagement that is provided through team sports provide positive motivation and social factors that facilitate individual compliance and persistence, contributing to maintaining a physically activity and healthy lifestyle for older individuals.

18.8 IMPLICATIONS FOR SPORTS MEDICINE PROFESSIONALS AND CLINICIANS

Activity across the lifespan is a popular term used to describe the continued engagement in structured physical activity despite increasing age [89]. The health benefits purported to be gained by continued engagement in physical activity are often highlighted by the maintenance of functional capacity, glycaemic control, blood lipid profile and body composition [103–105], all of which are noted predictors of the development of preventable chronic diseases. The vast array of research literature reporting the above outcomes often incorporates exercise programs that are complicit with the American College of Sports Medicine recommendations of the volume and intensity of the weekly dose of exercise [89]. Indeed, to comply with such recommendations many studies understandably incorporate controlled, laboratory-based exercise modes such as stationary ergometer cycling or single-joint machine-based resistance exercises. Given the cultural importance, popularity and continued engagement in team sport exercise, it is surprising the lack of research attention devoted to both performance and health outcomes of these exercise modes [15,92].

18.8.1 Medical Issues and Contraindications

Due to the intense nature of team sports, there are a number of medical issues and contraindications that should be considered prior to participating in team sports. Typical exercise-related contraindications typically include cardiovascular complications, orthopaedic injury, sprains and strains [106]. With increasing age these contraindications may be of greater importance to the mature athlete [106]. However, it is important to avoid isolated scrutiny of respective contraindications, as overall health benefits may outweigh localised potential problems. Specifically, the potential health benefits of regular exercise are proposed to represent a dose–response effect, with increased exercise volume resulting in a lower relative risk for cardiovascular disease and all-cause mortality, regardless of potential acute contraindications. For example, elite endurance (aerobic) and mixed sports (aerobic and anaerobic) athletes are reported to exhibit lower mortality rates and higher longevity in comparison to the general population [107].

18.8.2 Cardiovascular Complications

Atherosclerotic coronary artery disease is the most prevalent cardiovascular disease within the older population (>50 years old) and is a major risk factor for angina, myocardial infarction and arrhythmia [106]. Cardiovascular complications during exercise may be triggered acutely by the physiological stress of exercise and thus it is important to distinguish absolute risk from relative risk. Epidemiological research suggests the risks of fatal and nonfatal events during maximal exercise testing in apparently healthy individuals are rare (approximately <1 per 10,000 hours of testing) [108–110]. However, the risk that a non-smoking, non-diabetic, 50-year-old man will have a myocardial infarction is approximately 1 per 1 million hours [108]. Notably, the relative risk increases as both the individuals level of fitness declines and with increases in exercise intensity in that heavy physical exertion would increase 100 times over the baseline value, despite the absolute risk remaining <1 per 10,000 hours [108].

For team sport athletes, the variable intensities resulting in heart rate (HR) responses ranging up to 90% of HR_{max} may elevate the risk of those complications. However, the actual incidence of adverse events in masters athletes is extremely low. For example, a report from the 2005 World Masters Games highlighted that within 20,000 participants, only one (0.05 per 1000 athletes) cardiac arrest and no deaths occurred, with a total of nine cardiac complaints (0.42 per 1000 athletes) [111].

There is little data available on cardiovascular events in masters team sports. However, given the intense nature of team sports, previous research suggests that vigorous exercise 3 days a week increases the risk of a myocardial infarction from 1.3% to 1.6% in 79-year-old women and 3.9% to 4.8% in 90-year-old men [112]. Additionally, this risk is attenuated by 25%–50% in individuals who have prior experience with increased levels of physical activity, particularly vigorous exercise [110]. Collectively, to minimise the risk of cardiovascular complications during exercise each individual masters athlete should take into account and show pre-participation screening of personal history, family history and a physical examination to plan their exercise intensity and thus team sports activities accordingly [113].

18.8.3 Musculoskeletal Implications

Multiple age-related factors have been attributed to the observed functional decline in older athletes which may present as risk factors for the onset of acute, chronic and/or overuse musculoskeletal injuries [114]. These factors include declines in reaction time, flexibility, range of motion, skeletal size, body composition, bone mineral density, recovery time, coordination, aerobic endurance, and muscular strength [89,114]. Furthermore, data from the 2002 World Masters Games indicated cycling as the sport associated with the most serious injuries, while team sports such as hockey, baseball, volleyball and basketball had the highest injury rates (reported as personal communications in Franc-Law [111]). As evidence, data from the 2005 World Masters Games reported an injury rate of 8.0% for basketball and 7.5% for rugby, although most injuries were reported as minor with these injury rates being identified as low risk. However, masters teams sports athletes should still ensure correct training and match preparation to reduce the risk of musculoskeletal contraindications resulting from competitive team sports [111,115]. Having a well periodised training program, allowing gradual progressions of training loads and avoiding consecutive days of intense training early in a program will assist in reducing these risks.

Despite masters athletes representing high levels of functional capabilities in comparison to age-matched non-athletic populations, the most common reported conditions are lower-back pain (25.3%), hypertension (22.9%) and knee osteoarthritis (15.3%) [114]. Additionally, a survey of football (soccer) related injuries showed that of the 128 reported injuries, the most common were lower limb (82%), including lower leg (23%), ankle (18%), hamstring (17%), knee (15%), Achilles tendon (15%) and groin (7%) [115]. Notably, 67.3% of these injuries occurred during matches and 32.7% occurred during training. These injuries resulted in a reported injury-enforced median time off training or competition of 2 days (range 0–365) with physiotherapy (47%) and massage therapy (12%) forming the majority of injury treatment [115].

Additionally, osteoarthritis in the hip and shoulder, lumbar spinal stenosis, rotator cuff tendinopathy/tear and lateral elbow tendinopathy are all common musculoskeletal considerations for masters athletes [106]. Furthermore, factors such as training intensity, body mass index, occupation, previous injury, playing conditions (inadequate equipment, poor field condition and foul play), player positions and sporting type contribute to the specific injury type and location within the older athlete [114,116,117]. Taken as a whole, risk factors and injury mechanisms involve intrinsic (athlete-related risk) and extrinsic (environmental) factors, which can be modifiable and non-modifiable. As non-modifiable risk factors such as age and gender need to be recognised, modifiable factors such as physical training and behavioural approaches specific to the team sporting environment is important and should be the main focus in minimising sporting injuries in masters athletes playing team sports [118,119].

Readers interested in increasing their knowledge in this area are encouraged to look at a number of published reviews [120–126].

18.9 IMPLICATIONS FOR MASTERS ATHLETES AND COACHES

- Success in team sports are influenced by a complex relationship between physical and physiological characteristics, the technical and tactical abilities of a player and their team and the influence of the opponent and the environment. The physical, physiological and technical/tactical abilities of team sport athletes of all ages can be improved by well designed training programs.
- Age-related losses in lean mass and specifically type II muscle fibres appear to be responsible for the loss of physiological capacities such as muscular strength, power, speed and even aerobic fitness that all contribute to team sport performance. These reductions in physical capacity and performance may be minimised through life-long participation in team sports.
- Performance in team sports relies on the complex interactions between physical, technical and tactical abilities. Well-designed, sport specific SSGs can train each of these factors concurrently are recommended as an essential component of training programs for masters team sport athletes.
- Muscular strength, speed and power are important physical characteristics that are markedly affected by ageing. Since strength training helps prevent the age-related losses in muscle mass, training programs should consist of regular strength training (~ twice weekly) for masters team sport athletes.
- Older athletes have higher perceived soreness following intense training and a slower rate of recovery from exercise. To assist with recovery and reduce the risk of injury, training should be modified during periods of intense training and following competition. Moreover, recovery strategies such as cold water/ice therapy, compression garments and so forth need to be encouraged in masters team sport athletes.
- To maintain physical performance, muscle mass and optimise recovery, team sport athletes must consume sufficient energy to meet the demands of competition and training. Insufficient

energy intake reduces the benefits of training and can lead to weight loss, poorer performance and increased injury risk.

- Current evidence suggests that once athletes have healthy and balanced eating habits, then specific supplementation with agents such as creatine, alkalising agents and caffeine and possibly β-alanine can help improve team sport performance. Master team sport athletes may benefit from these supplements, but these should only be used as an adjunct as to a well-balanced diet. Athletes should also verify if supplements comply with the World Anti-Doping Agency (WADA) anti-doping code.

18.10 FUTURE RESEARCH DIRECTIONS

- There have been very few studies that examined the physical and physiological requirements of team sport in older athletes. Additionally, the few studies that attempted this have used a cross-sectional design which limits our ability to establish causality between performance/physiological changes and ageing. To better understand the relationships between ageing on team sport performance and its determinants, there is need for more longitudinal studies.
- Whilst regular endurance training can slow the loss of muscle mass with ageing, high-intensity training may be more protective against this loss, especially in fast type II fibre size. Since team sports have require both endurance and high-intensity efforts, future research should examine the influence of this mode compared to other modes of training as an effective method of preventing the loss of muscle mass in older athletes.
- Older team sport athletes appear to have a reduced tolerance to heavy training and poorer recovery following intense training and competition. The physiological basis of diminishing trainability with age is still unclear. Future studies are required to examine the effects of specific nutritional and recovery interventions on training tolerance and recovery from intense exercise in masters athletes.
- There are no data available on the physical characteristics, training or competition demands or the influence of team sport training on health and performance in older female team sport athletes. Future studies are required to examine these factors so that evidence-based training and nutritional interventions can be developed for this group.
- One important aspect of team sports in masters athlete is the social and motivational factors which might assist long-term exercise adherence. Further studies are required to better understand these factors and investigate how recreational team sports can be used as a panacea for the deleterious combined effects of a sedentary lifestyle and ageing.

REFERENCES

1. Reilly, T. and Gilbourne, D., Science and football: A review of applied research in the football codes, *J. Sports Sci.* 21(9), 693–705, 2003.
2. Bangsbo, J., Team sports, in *Nutrition in Sport*, R. Maughan, eds., Blackwell Science Ltd, Oxford, United Kingdom, 2000, pp. 574–87.
3. Bangsbo, J., The physiology of soccer with special reference to intense intermittent exercise, *Acta Physiol. Scand.* 151(Suppl 619), 1–156, 1994.
4. Bangsbo, J., Physiology of intermittent exercise, in *Exercise and Sport Science*, W.E. Garrett and D.T. Kirkendall, eds., Lippincott, Williams & Wilkins, Philadelphia, 2000, pp. 53–65.
5. Di Salvo, V., Gregson, W., Atkinson, G., Tordoff, P. and Drust, B., Analysis of high intensity activity in Premier League soccer, *Int. J. Sports Med.* 30(3), 205–12, 2009.
6. Rampinini, E., Impellizzeri, F.M., Castagna, C., Coutts, A.J. and Wisløff, U., Technical performance during soccer matches of the Italian Serie A league: Effect of fatigue and competitive level, *J. Sci. Med. Sport* 12(1), 227–33, 2009.

7. Sullivan, C.J., Bilsborough, J.C., Cianciosi, M., Hocking, J., Cordy, J. and Coutts, A.J., Match score affects activity profile and skill performance in professional Australian Football players, *J. Sci. Med. Sport* 17(3), 326–31, 2014.
8. Stølen, T., Chamari, K., Castagna, C. and Wisløff, U., Physiology of soccer: An update, *Sports Med.* 35(6), 501–36, 2005.
9. Reaburn, P. and Dascombe, B., Endurance performance in masters athletes, *Eur. Rev. Aging Phys. Act.* 5, 42–52, 2008.
10. Reaburn, P. and Dascombe, B., Anaerobic performance in masters athletes, *Eur. Rev. Aging Phys. Act.* 6, 39–53, 2009.
11. Maharam, L.G., Bauman, P.A., Kalman, D., Skolnik, H. and Perle, S.M., Masters athletes: Factors affecting performance, *Sports Med.* 28(4), 273–85, 1999.
12. Tessitore, A., Tiberi, M., Cortis, C., Rapisarda, E., Meeusen, R. and Capranica, L., Aerobic-anaerobic profiles, heart rate and match analysis in old basketball players, *Gerontology* 52(4), 214–22, 2006.
13. Tessitore, A., Meeusen, R., Tiberi, M., Cortis, C., Pagano, R. and Capranica, L., Aerobic and anaerobic profiles, heart rate and match analysis in older soccer players, *Ergonomics* 48(11–14), 1365–77, 2005.
14. Izquierdo, M., Ibanez, J., Gorostiaga, E. et al., Maximal strength and power characteristics in isometric and dynamic actions of the upper and lower extremities in middle-aged and older men, *Acta Physiol. Scand.* 167(1), 57–68, 1999.
15. Cortis, C., Tessitore, A., Lupo, C., Perroni, F., Pesce, C. and Capranica, L., Changes in jump, sprint and coordinative performances following a senior soccer match, *J. Strength Cond. Res.*, 2013.
16. Faulkner, J.A., Larkin, L.M., Claflin, D.R. and Brooks, S.V., Age-related changes in the structure and function of skeletal muscles, *Clin. Exp. Pharmacol. Physiol.* 34(11), 1091–6, 2007.
17. Andersen, J.L. and Aagaard, P., Effects of strength training on muscle fiber types and size: Consequences for athletes training for high-intensity sport, *Scand. J. Med. Sci. Sports* 20(Suppl 2), 32–8, 2010.
18. Martin, J.C., Davidson, C.J. and Pardyjak, E.R., Understanding sprint-cycling performance: The integration of muscle power, resistance, and modeling, *Int. J. Sports Physiol. Perform.* 2(1), 5–21, 2007.
19. Perez-Gomez, J., Rodriguez, G.V., Ara, I. et al., Role of muscle mass on sprint performance: Gender differences? *Eur. J. Appl. Physiol.* 102(6), 685–94, 2008.
20. Stewart, A.D., Assessing body composition in athletes, *Nutrition* 17(7–8), 694–5, 2001.
21. Maughan, R.J., Relationship between muscle strength and muscle cross-sectional area. Implications for training, *Sports Med.* 1(4), 263–9, 1984.
22. Häkkinen, K. and Keskinen, K.L., Muscle cross-sectional area and voluntary force production characteristics in elite strength- and endurance-trained athletes and sprinters, *Eur. J. Appl. Physiol. Occup. Physiol.* 59(3), 215–20, 1989.
23. Maughan, R.J., Watson, J.S. and Weir, J., Relationships between muscle strength and muscle cross-sectional area in male sprinters and endurance runners, *Eur. J. Appl. Physiol. Occup. Physiol.* 50(3), 309–18, 1983.
24. Hart, C.L., Ward, T.E. and Mayhew, J.L., Anthropometric correlates of bench press performance following resistance training, *Res. Sports Med.* 2(2), 89–95, 1991.
25. Chelly, S.M. and Denis, C., Leg power and hopping stiffness: Relationship with sprint running performance, *Med. Sci. Sports Exerc.* 33(2), 326–33, 2001.
26. Veale, J.P., Pearce, A.J., Buttifant, D. and Carlson, J.S., Anthropometric profiling of elite junior and senior Australian football players, *Int. J. Sports Physiol. Perform.* 5, 509–20, 2010.
27. Spencer, M., Lawrence, S., Rechichi, C., Bishop, D., Dawson, B. and Goodman, C., Time-motion analysis of elite field hockey, with special reference to repeated-sprint activity, *J. Sports Sci.* 22(9), 843–50, 2004.
28. Mohr, M., Krustrup, P. and Bangsbo, J., Match performance of high-standard soccer players with special reference to development of fatigue, *J. Sports Sci.* 21(7), 519–28, 2003.
29. Bangsbo, J., Nørregaard, L. and Thosøe, F., Activity profile of competition soccer, *Can. J. Sport Sci.* 16, 110–6, 1991.
30. Varley, M.C. and Aughey, R.J., Acceleration profiles in elite Australian soccer, *Int. J. Sports Med.* 34(1), 34–9, 2013.
31. Osgnach, C., Poser, S., Bernardini, R., Rinaldo, R. and di Prampero, P.E., Energy cost and metabolic power in elite soccer: A new match analysis approach, *Med. Sci. Sports Exerc.* 42(1), 170–8, 2010.
32. Spencer, M., Rechichi, C., Lawrence, S., Dawson, B., Bishop, D. and Goodman, C., Time-motion analysis of elite field hockey during several games in succession: A tournament scenario, *J. Sci. Med. Sport* 8(4), 382–91, 2005.
33. Balsom, P.D., Seger, J.Y., Sjodin, B. and Ekblom, B., Physiological responses to maximal intensity intermittent exercise, *Eur. J. Appl. Physiol. Occup. Physiol.* 65(2), 144–9, 1992.

34. Bangsbo, J., Iaia, F.M. and Krustrup, P., Metabolic response and fatigue in soccer, *Int. J. Sports Physiol. Perf.* 2(2), 111–27, 2007.
35. Krustrup, P., Mohr, M., Steensberg, A., Bencke, J., Kjaer, M. and Bangsbo, J., Muscle and blood metabolites during a soccer game: Implications for sprint performance, *Med. Sci. Sports Exerc.* 38(6), 1165–74, 2006.
36. Bangsbo, J., Mohr, M. and Krustrup, P., Physical and metabolic demands of training and match-play in the elite football player, *J. Sports Sci.* 24(7), 665–74, 2006.
37. Korhonen, M.T., Suominen, H. and Mero, A., Age and sex differences in blood lactate response to sprint running in elite master athletes, *Can. J. Appl. Physiol.* 30(6), 647–65, 2005.
38. Reaburn, P., Nutrition issues for the aging athlete, in *Clinical Sports Nutrition*, L. Burke and V. Deakin, eds., McGraw-Hill, Sydney, Australia, 2010, pp. 547–77.
39. American College of Sports, M., Sawka, M.N., Burke, L.M. et al., American College of Sports Medicine position stand. Exercise and fluid replacement, *Med. Sci. Sports Exerc.* 39(2), 377–90, 2007.
40. Al-Jaser, T.A. and Hasan, A.A., Fluid loss and body composition of elite Kuwaiti soccer players during a soccer match, *J. Sports Med. Phys. Fit.* 46(2), 281–5, 2006.
41. Duffield, R., Coutts, A.J. and Quinn, J., Core temperature responses and match running performance during intermittent-sprint exercise competition in warm conditions, *J. Strength Cond. Res.* 23(4), 1238–44, 2009.
42. Duffield, R., McCall, A., Coutts, A.J. and Peiffer, J.J., Hydration, sweat and thermoregulatory responses to professional football training in the heat, *J. Sports Sci.* 30(10), 957–65, 2012.
43. Shirreffs, S.M., Aragon-Vargas, L.F., Chamorro, M., Maughan, R.J., Serratosa, L. and Zachwieja, J.J., The sweating response of elite professional soccer players to training in the heat, *Int. J. Sports Med.* 26(2), 90–5, 2005.
44. Best, S., Caillaud, C. and Thompson, M., The effect of ageing and fitness on thermoregulatory response to high-intensity exercise, *Scand. J. Med. Sci. Sports* 22(4), e29–37, 2012.
45. Rolls, B.J. and Phillips, P.A., Aging and disturbances of thirst and fluid balance, *Nutr. Rev.* 48(3), 137–44, 1990.
46. Kenney, W.L. and Fowler, S.R., Methylcholine-activated eccrine sweat gland density and output as a function of age, *J. Appl. Physiol.* 65(3), 1082–6, 1988.
47. Cormack, S.J., Newton, R.U. and McGuigan, M.R., Neuromuscular and endocrine responses of elite players to an Australian rules football match, *Int. J. Sports Physiol. Perf.* 3(3), 359–74, 2008.
48. Mohr, M., Krustrup, P., Nybo, L., Nielsen, J.J. and Bangsbo, J., Muscle temperature and sprint performance during soccer matches—Beneficial effect of re-warm-up at half time, *Scand. J. Med. Sci. Sports* 14(3), 152–62, 2004.
49. Duffield, R., Murphy, A., Snape, A., Minett, G.M. and Skein, M., Post-match changes in neuromuscular function and the relationship to match demands in amateur rugby league matches, *J. Sci. Med. Sport* 15(3), 238–43, 2012.
50. Girard, O., Lattier, G., Maffiuletti, N.A., Micallef, J.P. and Millet, G.P., Neuromuscular fatigue during a prolonged intermittent exercise: Application to tennis, *J. Electromyogr. Kinesiol.* 18(6), 1038–46, 2008.
51. Rampinini, E., Bosio, A., Ferraresi, I., Petruolo, A., Morelli, A. and Sassi, A., Match-related fatigue in soccer players, *Med. Sci. Sports Exerc.* 43(11), 2161–70, 2011.
52. Fell, J., Reaburn, P. and Harrison, G.J., Altered perception and report of fatigue and recovery in veteran athletes, *J. Sports Med. Phys. Fit.* 48(2), 272–7, 2008.
53. Coutts, A.J., Charmari, K., Rampinini, E. and Impellizzeri, F.M., Contrôle et suivi de l'entraînement: Périodisationet charges d'entraînement, in *De L'entraînement à la Performance en Football,* A. Dellal, ed., De Boeck Universite, Paris, France, 2009, pp. 242–63.
54. Slattery, K.M., Wallace, L.K., Bentley, D.J. and Coutts, A.J., Effect of training load on simulated team sport match performance, *Appl. Physiol. Nutr. Metab.* 37(2), 315–22, 2012.
55. Andersson, H., Bohn, S.K., Raastad, T., Paulsen, G., Blomhoff, R. and Kadi, F., Differences in the inflammatory plasma cytokine response following two elite female soccer games separated by a 72-h recovery, *Scand. J. Med. Sci. Sports* 20(5), 740–7, 2010.
56. Andersson, H., Raastad, T., Nilsson, J., Paulsen, G., Garthe, I. and Kadi, F., Neuromuscular fatigue and recovery in elite female soccer: Effects of active recovery, *Med. Sci. Sports Exerc.* 40(2), 372–80, 2008.
57. Rowsell, G.J., Coutts, A.J., Reaburn, P. and Hill-Haas, S., Effects of cold-water immersion on physical performance between successive matches in high-performance junior male soccer players, *J. Sports Sci.* 27(6), 565–73, 2009.
58. Rowsell, G.J., Coutts, A.J., Reaburn, P. and Hill-Haas, S., Effect of post-match cold-water immersion on subsequent match running performance in junior soccer players during tournament play, *J. Sports Sci.* 29(1), 1–6, 2011.

59. Dupont, G., Nedelec, M., McCall, A., McCormack, D., Berthoin, S. and Wisloff, U., Effect of 2 soccer matches in a week on physical performance and injury rate, *Am. J. Sports Med.* 38(9), 1752–8, 2010.
60. Dellal, A., Lago-Penas, C., Rey, E., Chamari, K. and Orhant, E., The effects of a congested fixture period on physical performance, technical activity and injury rate during matches in a professional soccer team, *Br. J. Sports Med.*, 2013.
61. Fell, J. and Williams, D., The effect of aging on skeletal-muscle recovery from exercise: Possible implications for aging athletes, *J. Aging Phys. Act.* 16(1), 97–115, 2008.
62. Manfredi, T.G., Fielding, R.A., O'Reilly, K.P., Meredith, C.N., Lee, H.Y. and Evans, W.J., Plasma creatine kinase activity and exercise-induced muscle damage in older men, *Med. Sci. Sports Exerc.* 23(9), 1028–34, 1991.
63. Clarkson, P.M. and Dedrick, M.E., Exercise-induced muscle damage, repair, and adaptation in old and young subjects, *J. Gerontol.* 43(4), M91–6, 1988.
64. Fell, J., Haseler, L., Gaffney, P., Reaburn, P. and Harrison, G., Performance during consecutive days of laboratory time-trials in young and veteran cyclists, *J. Sports Med. Phys. Fit.* 46(3), 395–402, 2006.
65. Asp, S., Kristiansen, S. and Richter, E.A., Eccentric muscle damage transiently decreases rat skeletal muscle GLUT-4 protein, *J. Appl. Physiol.* 79(4), 1338–45, 1995.
66. Costill, D.L., Pascoe, D.D., Fink, W.J., Robergs, R.A., Barr, S.I. and Pearson, D., Impaired muscle glycogen resynthesis after eccentric exercise, *J. Appl. Physiol.* 69(1), 46–50, 1990.
67. Kumar, V., Atherton, P., Smith, K. and Rennie, M.J., Human muscle protein synthesis and breakdown during and after exercise, *J. Appl. Physiol.* 106(6), 2026–39, 2009.
68. Norris, S.R. and Smith, D.J., Planning, periodization, and sequencing of training and competition: The rationale for a competently planned, optimally executed training and competition program, supported by a multidisciplinary team, in *Enhancing Recovery: Preventing Underperformance in Athletes*, M. Kellmann, ed., Human Kinetics, Champaign, IL, 2002, pp. 121–41.
69. Impellizzeri, F.M., Rampinini, E., Coutts, A.J., Sassi, A. and Marcora, S.M., Use of RPE-based training load in soccer, *Med. Sci. Sports Exerc.* 36(6), 1042–7, 2004.
70. Wrigley, R., Drust, B., Stratton, G., Scott, M. and Gregson, W., Quantification of the typical weekly in-season training load in elite junior soccer players, *J. Sports Sci.* 30(15), 1573–80, 2012.
71. Coutts, A.J., Sirotic, A.C., Knowles, H. and Catterick, C., Monitoring training loads in professional rugby league, in *Science and Football VI*, T. Reilly and F. Korkusuz, eds., Routledge, London, 2009, pp. 272–7.
72. Stone, N.M. and Kilding, A.E., Aerobic conditioning for team sport athletes, *Sports Med.* 39(8), 615–42, 2009.
73. Hill-Haas, S.V., Coutts, A.J., Dawson, B. and Impellizzeri, F.M., Small-sided games training in football: A systematic review, *Sports Med.* 41(3), 199–220, 2011.
74. Cortis, C., Tessitore, A., Perroni, F. et al., Interlimb coordination, strength, and power in soccer players across the lifespan, *J. Strength Cond. Res.* 23(9), 2458–66, 2009.
75. Nedelec, M., McCall, A., Carling, C., Legall, F., Berthoin, S. and Dupont, G., Recovery in soccer: Part I—Post-match fatigue and time course of recovery, *Sports Med.*, 2012.
76. McLean, B.D., Coutts, A.J., Kelly, V., McGuigan, M.R. and Cormack, S.J., Neuromuscular, endocrine, and perceptual fatigue responses during different length between-match microcycles in professional rugby league players, *Int. J. Sports Physiol. Perform.* 5(3), 367–83, 2010.
77. Andersson, H., Karlsen, A., Blomhoff, R., Raastad, T. and Kadi, F., Active recovery training does not affect the antioxidant response to soccer games in elite female players, *Br. J. Nutr.* 104(10), 1492–9, 2010.
78. Nedelec, M., McCall, A., Carling, C., Legall, F., Berthoin, S. and Dupont, G., Recovery in soccer: Part II—Recovery strategies, *Sports Med.* 43(1), 9–22, 2013.
79. Akermark, C., Jacobs, I., Rasmusson, M. and Karlsson, J., Diet and muscle glycogen concentration in relation to physical performance in Swedish elite ice hockey players, *Int. J. Sport Nutr.* 6(3), 272–84, 1996.
80. Mujika, I. and Burke, L.M., Nutrition in team sports, *Ann. Nutr. Metab.* 57(Suppl 2), 26–35, 2010.
81. Halson, S.L., Nutrition, sleep and recovery, *Eur. J. Sports Sci.* 8(2), 119–26, 2008.
82. Plews, D.J., Laursen, P.B., Kilding, A.E. and Buchheit, M., Evaluating training adaptation with heart rate measures: A methodological comparison, *Int. J. Sports Physiol. Perform.* 8(6), 688–91, 2013.
83. Nutrition for football: The FIFA/F-MARC Consensus Conference, *J. Sports Sci.* 24(7), 663–4, 2006.
84. Balsom, P.D., Wood, K., Olsson, P. and Ekblom, B., Carbohydrate intake and multiple sprint sports: With special reference to football (soccer), *Int. J. Sports Med.* 20(1), 48–52, 1999.
85. Zimmet, P., Alberti, K.G. and Shaw, J., Global and societal implications of the diabetes epidemic, *Nature* 414(6865), 782–7, 2001.

86. Conn, V.S., Hafdahl, A.R. and Mehr, D.R., Interventions to increase physical activity among healthy adults: Meta-analysis of outcomes, *Am. J. Public Health* 101(4), 751–8, 2011.
87. Cameron, A.J., Dunstan, D.W., Owen, N. et al., Health and mortality consequences of abdominal obesity: Evidence from the AusDiab study, *Med. J. Aust.* 191(4), 202–8, 2009.
88. Blatter, J.S. and Dvorak, J., Football for health—Prevention is better than cure, *Scand. J. Med. Sci. Sports* 20(Suppl 1), v, 2010.
89. American College of Sports Medicine, Chodzko-Zajko, W.J., Proctor, D.N. et al., American College of Sports Medicine position stand. Exercise and physical activity for older adults, *Med. Sci. Sports Exerc.* 41(7), 1510–30, 2009.
90. Andersen, L.J., Hansen, P.R., Sogaard, P., Madsen, J.K., Bech, J. and Krustrup, P., Improvement of systolic and diastolic heart function after physical training in sedentary women, *Scand. J. Med. Sci. Sports* 20(Suppl 1), 50–7, 2010.
91. Andersen, L.J., Randers, M.B., Westh, K. et al., Football as a treatment for hypertension in untrained 30–55-year-old men: A prospective randomized study, *Scand. J. Med. Sci. Sports* 20(Suppl 1), 98–102, 2010.
92. Krustrup, P., Aagaard, P., Nybo, L., Petersen, J., Mohr, M. and Bangsbo, J., Recreational football as a health promoting activity: A topical review, *Scand. J. Med. Sci. Sports* 20(Suppl 1), 1–13, 2010.
93. Mendham, A.E., Coutts, A.J., and Duffield R., The acute effects of aerobic exercise and modified rugby on inflammation and glucose homeostasis within Indigenous Australians, *Eur. J. Appl. Physiol.* 112(11), 3787–95, 2012.
94. Krustrup, P., Nielsen, J.J., Krustrup, B.R. et al., Recreational soccer is an effective health-promoting activity for untrained men, *Br. J. Sports Med.* 43(11), 825–31, 2009.
95. Knoepfli-Lenzin, C., Sennhauser, C., Toigo, M. et al., Effects of a 12-week intervention period with football and running for habitually active men with mild hypertension, *Scand. J. Med. Sci. Sports* 20(Suppl 1), 72–9, 2010.
96. Krustrup, P., Christensen, J.F., Randers, M.B. et al., Muscle adaptations and performance enhancements of soccer training for untrained men, *Eur. J. Appl. Physiol.* 108(6), 1247–58, 2010.
97. Rampinini, E., Impellizzeri, F.M., Castagna, C. et al., Factors influencing physiological responses to small-sided soccer games, *J. Sports Sci.* 25(6), 659–66, 2007.
98. Kelly, D.P. and Drust, B., The effect of pitch dimensions on heart rate responses and technical demands of small-sided soccer games in elite players, *J. Sci. Med. Sport* 12, 475–9, 2009.
99. Castagna, C., Romualdo, B., Abt, G.A., Coutts, A.J., Impellizzeri, F.M. and Lacapprice, F., Cardiovascular responses during recreational 5-a-side indoor-soccer, *J. Sci. Med. Sport* 10(2), 89–95, 2007.
100. Krustrup, P., Hansen, P.R., Andersen, L.J. et al., Long-term musculoskeletal and cardiac health effects of recreational football and running for premenopausal women, *Scand. J. Med. Sci. Sports* 20(Suppl 1), 58–71, 2010.
101. Spencer, M., Bishop, D., Dawson, B. and Goodman, C., Physiological and metabolic responses of repeated-sprint activities: Specific to field-based team sports, *Sports Med.* 35(12), 1025–44, 2005.
102. Randers, M.B., Petersen, J., Andersen, L.J. et al., Short-term street soccer improves fitness and cardiovascular health status of homeless men, *Eur. J. Appl. Physiol.* 112(6), 2097–106, 2012.
103. Halbert, J.A., Silagy, C.A., Finucane, P., Withers, R.T., Hamdorf, P.A. and Andrews, G.R., The effectiveness of exercise training in lowering blood pressure: A meta-analysis of randomised controlled trials of 4 weeks or longer, *J. Hum. Hypertens.* 11(10), 641–9, 1997.
104. Jeon, C.Y., Lokken, R.P., Hu, F.B. and van Dam, R.M., Physical activity of moderate intensity and risk of type 2 diabetes: A systematic review, *Diabetes Care* 30(3), 744–52, 2007.
105. Pedersen, B.K. and Saltin, B., Evidence for prescribing exercise as therapy in chronic disease, *Scand. J. Med. Sci. Sports* 16(Suppl 1), 3–63, 2006.
106. American Academy of Family Physicians, American Academy of Orthopaedic Surgeons, American College of Sports Medicine et al., Selected issues for the master athlete and the team physician: A consensus statement, *Med. Sci. Sports Exerc.* 42(4), 820–33, 2010.
107. Teramoto, M. and Bungum, T.J., Mortality and longevity of elite athletes, *J. Sci. Med. Sport* 13(4), 410–6, 2010.
108. Mittleman, M.A., Maclure, M., Tofler, G.H., Sherwood, J.B., Goldberg, R.J. and Muller, J.E., Triggering of acute myocardial infarction by heavy physical exertion. Protection against triggering by regular exertion, *New Engl. J. Med.* 329(23), 1677–83, 1993.
109. Maron, B.J., Thompson, P.D., Ackerman, M.J. et al., Recommendations and considerations related to preparticipation screening for cardiovascular abnormalities in competitive athletes: 2007 update. A scientific statement from the American Heart Association Council on Nutrition, Physical Activity, and Metabolism: Endorsed by the American College of Cardiology Foundation, *Circulation* 115(12), 1643–455, 2007.

110. Goodman, J.M., Thomas, S.G. and Burr, J., Evidence-based risk assessment and recommendations for exercise testing and physical activity clearance in apparently healthy individuals, *Appl. Physiol. Nutr. Metab.* 36(Suppl 1), S14–32, 2011.
111. Franc-Law, J.M., A community-based model for medical management of a large scale sporting event, *Clin. J. Sports Med.* 16(5), 406–11, 2006.
112. Gill, T.M., DiPietro, L. and Krumholz, H.M., Role of exercise stress testing and safety monitoring for older persons starting an exercise program, *JAMA* 284(3), 342–9, 2000.
113. Maron, B.J., Araujo, C.G., Thompson, P.D. et al., Recommendations for preparticipation screening and the assessment of cardiovascular disease in masters athletes: An advisory for healthcare professionals from the working groups of the World Heart Federation, the International Federation of Sports Medicine, and the American Heart Association Committee on Exercise, Cardiac Rehabilitation, and Prevention, *Circulation* 103(2), 327–34, 2001.
114. Wright, V.J. and Perricelli, B.C., Age-related rates of decline in performance among elite senior athletes, *Am. J. Sports Med.* 36(3), 443–50, 2008.
115. Newsham-West, R., Button, C., Milburn, P.D. et al., Training habits and injuries of masters' level football players: A preliminary report, *Phys. Ther. Sport* 10(2), 63–6, 2009.
116. McKean, K.A., Manson, N.A. and Stanish, W.D., Musculoskeletal injury in the masters runners, *Clin. J. Sports Med.* 16(2), 149–54, 2006.
117. Best, T.M. and Hart, L., A growing concern: The older athlete, *Clin. J. Sports Med.* 18(6), 477–8, 2008.
118. Bahr, R. and Holme, I., Risk factors for sports injuries—A methodological approach, *Br. J. Sports Med.* 37(5), 384–92, 2003.
119. McNoe, B.M. and Chalmers, D.J., Injury prevention behaviour in community-level soccer players, *J. Sci. Med. Sport* 14(6), 482–8, 2011.
120. Dziedzic, C.E. and Higham, D.G., Performance nutrition guidelines for international Rugby Sevens tournaments, *Int. J. Sport Nutr. Exerc. Metab.* Jan 17 (Epub ahead of print), 2014.
121. Bishop, D. and Girard, O., Determinants of team-sport performance: Implications for altitude training by team-sport athletes, *Br. J. Sports Med.* 47(Suppl 1), i17–21, 2013.
122. Girard, O., Mendez-Villanueva, A. and Bishop, D., Repeated-sprint ability—Part 1: Factors contributing to fatigue, *Sports Med.* 41(8), 673–94, 2011.
123. Bishop, D., Girard, O. and Mendez-Villanueva, A., Repeated-sprint ability—Part 11: Recommendations for training, *Sports Med.* 41(9), 741–56, 2011.
124. Dawson, B., Repeated-sprint ability: Where are we? *Int. J. Sports Physiol. Perform.* 7(3), 285–9, 2012.
125. McMaster, D.T., Gill, N., Cronin, J. and McGuigan, M., The development, retention and decay rates of strength and power in elite rugby union, rugby league and American football: A systematic review, *Sports Med.* 43(5), 367–84, 2013.
126. Kilduff, L.P., Finn, C.V., Baker, J.S., Cook, C.J. and West, D.J., Preconditioning strategies to enhance physical performance on the day of competition, *Int. J. Sports Physiol. Perform.* 8(6), 677–81, 2013

Index

Page numbers followed by f and t indicate figures and tables, respectively.

F

G

H

I

K

L

M

Q

R

S